THE SCIENCE OF LABORATORY DIAGNOSIS

THE SCIENCE OF LABORATORY DIAGNOSIS

Edited by

David Burnett
Institute of Research and Development, University of Birmingham Research Park,
Vincent Drive, Edgbaston, Birmingham, UK

John Crocker
Department of Histopathology, Birmingham Heartlands Hospital,
Bordesley Green East, Birmingham, UK

I S I S
MEDICAL
M E D I A

Oxford

© 1998 Isis Medical Media Ltd.
59 St Aldates
Oxford OX1 1ST, UK

First published 1998

British Library Cataloguing in Publication Data.
A catalogue record for this title is available from
the British Library

ISBN 1 899066 62 4

Crocker, J. (John)
The Science of Laboratory Diagnosis
John Crocker and David Burnett (eds)

Isis Medical Media staff
Commissioning Editor: John Harrison
Editorial Controller: Maren White
Production Manager: Julia Savory

Typesetting and reproduction by
Expo Holdings Sdn Bhd, Malaysia

Produced by Phoenix Offset, HK
Printed in China

Distributed in USA by
Books International, Inc. 22883 Quicksilver Drive,
Dulles Virginia 20166, USA

Distributed in the rest of the world by
Plymbridge Distributors Ltd, Estover Road,
Plymouth, PL6 7PY, UK

"Faith" is a fine invention
When Gentlemen can *see* —
But *Microscopes* are prudent
In an Emergency

Emily Dickinson

CONTENTS

CONTRIBUTORS LIST

Derek Allen MD MB BCH MRCPath
Consultant Histopathologist and Cytopathologist, Histopathology Laboratory, Belfast City Hospital, Belfast BT9 7AD, UK

Hazel Appleton BSc PhD
Principal Microbiologist, Enteric and Respiratory Virus Laboratory, PHLS Central Public Health Laboratory, 61 Collindale Avenue, Collindale, London NW9 5HT, UK

Dugald R Baird MA MRCP FRCPath Dipl. Bact
Consultant Microbiologist, Hairmyres and Stonehouse Hospitals NHS Trust, Eaglesham Road, East Kilbride G75 8RG, UK

Diana M Barnes BSc PhD
Consultant Biochemist, Hedley Atkins, ICRF Breast Pathology Laboratory, Guy's Hospital, St. Thomas St., London SE1 9RT, UK

Supratik Basu MB BS MD MRCP (UK) MRCPath (UK)
Consultant Haematologist, Pathology Laboratory, Warwick Hospital, Lakin Road, Warwick CV34 5BJ, UK

A Graham Bird PhD FRCP FRCPath
Consultant Immunologist, Oxford Radcliffe Hospital Trust, Churchill Hospital, Headington, Oxford OX3 7LJ, UK

Paul C Boreland BSc PhD CBiol MIBiol FIBMS
Principal Microbiologist, Microbiology Department, Antrim Hospital, 45 Bush Road, Antrim, Northern Ireland BT41 2RL, UK

Brian Boullier BSc DPhil
Co-ordinator, Educational Development Innovation Centre, University of Bradford, Bradford, West Yorkshire BD7 1DP, UK

Eric Y Bridson MPhil FIBiol FIBMS
Technical Consultant, Oxoid Ltd., 3 Bellever Hill, Camberley, Surrey BU15 2HB, UK

David Burnett BSc PhD FRCPath
Micropathology Ltd., Institute of Research and Development, University of Birmingham Research Park, Vincent Drive, Edgbaston, Birmingham B15 2SQ, UK

CH Stuart Cameron PhD
The Queen's University of Belfast, Institute of Pathology, Grosvenor Road, Belfast BT12 6BL, UK

Catherine Caveen FISMS
Haematology Department, Warwick Hospital, Lakin Road, Warwick, CV34 5BJ, UK

Gordon S Challand BSc MA PhD MCB CChem FRSC FRCPath
Consultant Biochemist, Clinical Biochemistry Department, Royal Berkshire Hospital, Reading RG1 5AN, UK

Ian Chant BSc PhD
Department of Haematology, Warwick Hospital, Lakin Road, Warwick CV34 5BJ, UK

Janine Clover MSc FIBMS
Senior BMS Department of Histopathology, Birmingham Heartlands Hospital, Bordesley Green East, Birmingham B9 5SS, UK

John Crocker MA MD FRCPath MRCP
Honorary Professor to Birmingham University and Consultant Histopathologist, Birmingham Heartlands Hospital, Bordesley Green East, Birmingham B9 5SS, UK

Roger P Eglin PhD
Clinical Scientist, Head of Virology, Public Health Laboratory, Bridlepath, York Road, Leeds LS15 7TR, UK

Mohammad S Enayat BSc MSc PhD CBiol MIBiol
Principal Clinical Scientist, Head of Molecular Haemostasis Laboratory, The Birmingham Children's Hospital NHS Trust, Ladywood, Birmingham B16 8ET, UK

Dave I Fish BA MSc FIBAS
Operational Manager Biochemistry/Haematology Department, North Manchester General Hospital, Delaunays Road, Crumpsall, Manchester M8 5RB, UK

Cheryl E Gillett BSc PhD FIBMS
Senior Scientific Officer, Hedley Atkins/ ICRF Breast Pathology Laboratory, Guy's Hospital, St. Thomas St., London SE1 9RT, UK

Robert WA Girdwood MB ChB FRCPath DTM&H
Director, Scottish Parasite Diagnostic Laboratory, Stobhill NHS Trust, Stobhill Hospital, Balornock Road, Glasgow G21 3UW, UK

Ian M Gould BSc MBChB FRCPE MRCPath
Department of Medical Microbiology, Medical School, Foresterhill, Aberdeen, AB9 2ZB, UK

Trevor Gray FIBMS CMLM
Dept. of Histopathology, Queen's Medical Centre, University Hospital, Nottingham NG7 2UH, UK

Peter Hamilton BSc PhD
Department of Pathology, The Queens University of Belfast, Grosvenor Road, Belfast BT12 6BL, UK

Neil Hand MPhil
Department of Histopathology, Queen's Medical Centre, University Hospital, Nottingham NG7 2UH, UK

Mark Hathaway PhD
Liver Research Laboratories, Queen Elizabeth Hospital, Edgbaston, Birmingham B15 2TH, UK

Andrew J Hay MB ChB MSc MRCPath
Consultant Microbiologist, Raigmore Hospital NHS Trust, Perth Road, Inverness IV2 3UJ, UK

Ivor Hickey BSC PhD
School of Biology and Biochemistry, The Queen's University of Belfast, Medical Biology Centre, 97 Lisburn Road, Belfast BT9 7BL,UK

Alan D Hirst BSc MCB FRCPath
Top Grade Biochemist, Biochemistry Department., Bradford Royal Infirmary, Duckworth Lane, Bradford BD9 6RJ,UK

Carl Holland FIBMS
Department of Haematology, South Warwickshire Hospitals NHS Trust, Lakin Road, Warwick CV34 5BJ,UK

Richard E Holliman BSc MSc FRCPath MD
Reader in Clinical Microbiology, Department of Medical Microbiology, St George's Hospital and Medical School, Blackshaw Road, London SW17 0QT,UK

Darrel Ho-Yen BMSc MBChB FRCPath MD
Consultant Microbiologist, Raigmore Hospital NHS Trust, Perth Road, Inverness IV2 3UJ and Honorary Clinical Senior Lecturer, Aberdeen University,UK

Mervyn Humphreys BSc
Senior Clinical Scientist, North Ireland Regional Genetic Centre, Leukaemia Cytogenetic Laboratory, Floor A, Belfast City Hospital, Tower Block, Lisburn Road, Belfast BT9 7AB,UK

William L Irvine MA MB Bchir MRCP PhD MRCPath
Reader in Clinical Virology, University Hospital, Queens Medical Centre, Nottingham, UK

Julie D Johnson CBiol MIBiol FIBMS MSc
Chef Medical Laboratory Scientific Officer, Department of Medical Microbiology, St. George's Hospital, Blackshaw Road, London SW17 0QT, UK

Alex WL Joss BSc PhD
Consultant Clinical Scientist, Microbiology Department, Raigmore Hospital NHS Trust, Perth Road, Inverness IV2 3UJ, UK

Paul E Klapper BSc PhD MRCPath
Principal Clinical Scientist, Clinical Virology, Manchester Central Laboratory Services, 3rd Floor, Clinical Sciences Building, Manchester Royal Infirmary, Oxford Road, Manchester M13 9WL, UK

Goura Kudesia MBBS FRCPath
Consultant Medical Virologist, PHLS Honorary Clinical Lecturer, Public Health Laboratory, Northern General Hospital NHS Trust, Herries Road, Sheffield S5 7BQ, UK

Robert J Landers MB BCh BAO BSc MRCPath
Lecturer, Dept. of Pathology, The University of Sheffield Medical School, Beech Hill Road, Sheffield S10 2RX, UK

William J Marshall MA PhD MSc MB BS FRCP FRCP Edin FRCPath
Senior Lecturer in Chemical Pathology, Dept. of Clinical Biochemistry, King's College School of Medicine & Dentistry, Bessemer Road, London SE5 9PJ and Honorary Consultant Chemical Pathologist, King's Healthcare NHS Trust, London, UK

Siraj A Misbah MBBS MSc MRCP MRCPath
Consultant Clinical Immunologist, Yorkshire Regional Immunology Service, The General Infirmary at Leeds, Old Medical School, Thoresby Place, Leeds, West Yorkshire LS2 9JT and Honorary Senior Clinical Lecturer in Immunology, University of Leeds, UK

Jonathan North MBBS MD MRCPath
Consultant Immunologist, Department of Immunology, City Hospital, Dudley Road, Birmingham B18 7QH, UK

Marie M Ogilvie MD BSc MRCPath
Senior Lecturer/Honorary Consultant Virologist, Department of Medical Microbiology, University of Edinburgh Medical School, Teviot Place, Edinburgh EH8 9AG, UK

John J O'Leary MD DPhil MSc BCs MRCPath
Director of Pathology, The Coombe Women's Hospital, Dublin, Ireland

Jacqueline C. Osypiw BSc MSc PhD
Senior Biochemist, Clinical Biochemistry Department, Royal Berkshire Hospital, Reading, Berks RG1 5AN, UK

David Parratt MBChB MB FRCPath
Senior Lecturer/Honorary Consultant Microbiologist, Department of Medical Microbiology, Ninewells Hospital and Medical School, Dundee DD1 9SY, UK

Steven J Picton BSc PhD
Scientist, Perrin-Elmer, Applied Biosystems, Kelvin Close, Birchwood Science Park North, Warrington WA3 7PB, UK

Paul Revell BSC MRCP MRCPath FRCPCH
Consultant Haematologist, Staffordshire General Hospital, Weston Road, Stafford ST16 3SA, UK

Bernard F Rocks MSc PhD FRSC
Consultant Clinical Scientist, Department of Clinical Pathology, Royal Sussex County Hospital, Brighton BN2 5BE and visiting research fellow Trafford Centre for Medical Research, University of Sussex, UK

Peter Rose FRCP FRCPath
Consultant Haematologist, Pathology Laboratory, Warwick Hospital, Lakin Road, Warwick CV34 5BJ, UK

Anne Sermon FIBMS
Department of Haematology, Nottingham City Hospital, Hucknall Road, Nottingham NG5 1PB, UK

Roy A Sherwood MSc DPhil
Consultant Biochemist, Department of Clinical Biochemistry, King's College School of Medicine and Dentistry, Bessemer Road, London SE5 9PJ, UK

Ivan Silva BA
Research Fellow, Dept. of Pathology, Cornell University Medical College, The New York Hospital, 1300 York Avenue, New York, NY 10021, USA

Barrie Sims JP FIBMS
Department of Histopathology, Staffordshire General Hospital, Weston Road, Stafford ST16 3SA, UK

Paul J Smith FIBMS
Department of Histopathology, Birmingham Heartlands Hospital, Bordesley Green East, Birmingham B9 5SS, UK

Andrew Taylor BSc MSc PhD CChem MRSC MRCPath
Consultant Clinical Biochemist, Trace Element Laboratory, School of Biological Sciences, University of Surrey, Guildford, GU2 5XH and the Clinical Laboratory, Royal Surrey County Hospital, Guildford, GU2 5XX, UK

Peter G Toner DSc MB ChB FRCP FRCPath
Professor, Department of Pathology, Queens University, Royal Hospital, Grosvenor Road, Belfast BT12 6BL, UK

Volker Uhlmann Dip Chem
Visiting Fellow, Dept. of Pathology, Cornell University Medical College, The New York Hospital, 1300 York Avenue, New York, NY 10021, USA

Steven Walton MSc FIMLS
Haematology Department, Pathology Laboratory, Warwick Hospital, Lakin Road, Warwick CV34 5BJ, UK

Adrian T Warfield MB ChB MRCPath
Consultant Histopathologist & Cytopathologist, Department of Histopathology, Birmingham Heartlands Hospital, Bordesley Green East, Birmingham B9 5SS, UK

David W Warnock BSc PhD FRCPath
Consultant Clinical Scientist, PHLS, PHL, Mycology Reference Laboratory, Myrtle Road, Kingsdown, Bristol BS2 8EL, UK

Keith Whaley MBBS MD PhD FRCP FRCPath
Professor, Department of Immunology, Leicester Royal Infirmary, Leicester LE1 5WW, UK

Dedication

"With love to our families"

FOREWORD

It has been the experience of ourselves and our colleagues for some years that people at all levels come to work in our laboratories but have no experience of such environments. We have felt that there was a need for a text, across all disciplines of Pathology, which would explain the 'whys and wherefores' of laboratory medicine. We emphasize that this text is not intended to be a 'recipe book'; its purpose is, however, very much to explain the basic principles of laboratory techniques and the interpretation of results obtained from them. We have tried to ensure that this book is of use to as diverse a range of readers as possible. This should include undergraduate and postgraduate students, trainee pathologists, surgeons and physicians, as well as laboratory scientific staff.

The contents are multidisciplinary and there is overlap between some chapters and sections. This is deliberate as it reflects the true state of modern pathology. We feel that it is important that pathologists in each sub-specialty should be more aware of activity in their colleagues' laboratories. This book intends to represent standard methods and fairly recent advances within them. It is again stressed that compartmentalization of pathology and laboratory medicine is artificial although often convenient. However, it is our hope that workers in one speciality will be stimulated by reading other sections. For example, histopathologists working in the field of lymphoma need to understand large area of haematology and microbiology. The former, of course, impinges on the management of lymphoma patients, as does microbiology when opportunist infections occur after chemotherapy. Furthermore, clinical chemists need to relate their findings in relation to haematology and so on.

Another feature of this book is that there is, in some areas, overlap between chapters and sections; this is wholly intentional and again reflects the present state of laboratory medicine. Also, the applications, contexts and interpretation of shared methods will inevitably differ depending upon the discipline. The reader will notice this particularly in sections covering subjects such as electron microscopy and molecular techniques where methodologies are shared extensively between different disciplines. Indeed, failure to engage in cross-field communication will have an inevitable deleterious effect on advances in routine and research methodologies. To our knowledge this book is unique and we hope it will give insight to many people training and trained in laboratory medicine concerning not only their own field but also those of others. Most chapters include a list of principal articles although in some cases this has been deemed unnecessary; furthermore, the occasional chapter has an extended reading list which may reflect its complexity or wide-ranging content.

We should, of course, like to express our gratitude to all of our section editors and chapter authors. Naturally, we are indebted to our Publisher, John Harrison and his staff. Our thanks are also extended to Mrs Ruth Fry, Mrs Vivien Garland and Mrs Valerie Griffiths for secretarial help and for answering endless telephone calls.

John Crocker
David Burnett

SECTION 1
HISTOPATHOLOGY

1 SPECIMEN HANDLING AND PREPARATION FOR ROUTINE DIAGNOSTIC HISTOPATHOLOGY

Paul J Smith and Janine Clover

Introduction

Diagnostic histopathology is a speciality that, even nowadays, has remained a particularly labour-intensive faculty benefitting over the years from only a modest development in time-saving, automated technology. Tissue processing and section staining machines, an integral part of any routine histology laboratory, have become increasingly more sophisticated in terms of their application and their contribution to the health and safety conscious environment in which we work. The manual inscription of tissue processing cassettes and microscope slides is fast becoming antiquated since the introduction of stand-alone and computer-linked transcription systems. Automatic coverslipping is also commonplace in many laboratories, minimizing personal exposure to organic solvents and allowing staff, otherwise involved in section mounting, to concentrate their efforts in the remaining manual areas of the department.

The modern routine histopathology laboratory, although having benefitted from a degree of automation and continually evolving enhancements to its standard equipment, remains an area that is sensitive to increases in workload activity. Spare capacity relates directly to processing capability and the number of staff available to perform the associated tasks required to produce stained histopathological sections for subsequent microscopical examination and diagnosis by a pathologist. Many modern laboratories have experienced significant increases in workload activity over the past few years as a result of waiting list initiatives, mergers and GP purchasing ability, without a directly proportional rise in staffing levels. It is inevitable that these laboratories have had to streamline their methodologies and repertoires in order to exist in today's highly active, competitive working environment and still continue to provide an efficient and effective quality service.

Specimen Management Systems

Computer-based information systems

Manual data entry

Automatic cassette markers and slide writers

It is the intention of this chapter to provide a simple insight into tissue preparation in the modern histopathology laboratory (previously described) with the emphasis on efficiency, effectiveness and quality of service. It is not the intention of this chapter to explain in any particular depth the philosophy, chemistry or minor details of the processes involved in tissue preparation, but to give an overall picture of these processes and thus enable the reader to put the techniques into perspective as an aid to the standardization of routine histopathology in the diagnostic laboratory.

Specimen Management Systems

Most modern histopathology laboratories have their own departmental information technology system for the storage and retrieval of patient demographic and specimen data. The manual or computerized patient registration system should be situated within the booking-in area of the laboratory. This accommodation should be separate from the 'cut-up' room and, ideally, housed in an office environment, either self-contained or integrated into the clerical area of the laboratory.

Computer-based information systems
One of the fundamental functions of a computer-based specimen management system is to facilitate the allocation of unique hospital and laboratory patient/specimen-specific identifiers – the patient hospital registration number and the laboratory number. The hospital registration number should be present on the histology request form and the accompanying specimen. The laboratory number is usually allocated automatically by the software but may be manually entered. The laboratory number remains with the specimen throughout the histological process and is transferred to the request form, specimen pot(s), tissue cassette(s), microscope slide(s) and the final diagnostic report belonging to the patient.

The pathologists, laboratory manager, secretaries and laboratory areas require terminals to facilitate the input and coding of diagnostic reports, patient/specimen enquiry, work list generation, input of additional technical procedures, specimen/request tracking (audit trail), tissue/condition-specific list generation and the collection of data for workload activity, weighted activity and costing.

Manual data entry
Manual data entry, using a surgical day book, and the manual labelling of tissue cassettes and microscope slides, has more drawbacks than a computerized laboratory system. Manual systems rely on neat, clear handwriting and the accurate allocation of progressive laboratory numbers by an individual. Transcription errors may occur during the transfer of the laboratory number to tissue cassettes and microscope slides if the handwriting in the day book, or on the request form, is of a poor standard. Poor or illegible marking of tissue cassettes may result in the mismatching of tissue blocks with request forms and slides resulting in the worst scenario, in a patient being misdiagnosed if similar tissues are involved or in the wasting of precious laboratory time while the situation is rectified. It is essential in all laboratories, regardless of whether a manual or a computerized system is the order of the day, that stringent control measures are in place to ensure the integrity of the final diagnostic report.

Manual systems require provision of a cross-reference file for report retrieval, a diagnostic index and ample storage facilities for the filing of reports and request forms.

The quality of information processed by the service department is only as good as the quality of information on the request form and/or the information provided by the hospital patient administration, or order communications systems in the case of computer networking.

Automatic cassette markers and slide writers
Cassette markers and slide writers are commercially available and can be utilized by all laboratories. Manual data entry laboratories

would rely on manual input into these machines as would those laboratories with less common generic computer systems. Laboratories with more sophisticated systems can interface specifically with these machines so that cassette marking and slide writing become totally automatic procedures linked to, for example, data entry and worklist generation respectively. The advent of these machines has enabled clear, concise labelling of cassettes and slides and has reduced transcription error to a minimum.

On completion of data entry the request forms are matched with their respective specimen pot(s) and the pots themselves marked indelibly with the laboratory number. Some laboratories may allocate the laboratory number, prior to booking in, using pre-printed rolls of self-adhesive sequential numbers.

Specimen Receipt and Handling

The trimming or cut-up room
A purpose-designed room, the 'cut-up' or 'trimming' room, should be available for the receipt and handling of all tissue specimens requiring histopathological diagnosis. This room should be totally separate from other laboratory accommodation, well illuminated, well ventilated and providing areas for specimen unbagging and matching and specimen dissection. The storage of formalin-fixed ('wet') tissues, following dissection, may also be a function of the cut-up room. Custom-built, ventilated specimen stores are commercially available and can be incorporated into larger cut-up rooms or be conveniently housed in a separate, enclosed area used specifically for specimen storage.

The containment of formaldehyde fumes is of prime concern in this area and is legislated for under the *Health and Safety Act, 1974* in conjunction with the *Containment of Substances Hazardous to Health (COSHH) Regulations*. Formaldehyde is the most commonly used of all fixatives in the modern histology laboratory and will be discussed later.

Hitherto, the specimen cut-up area should be provided with an extraction facility in the form of either an over-bench fume hood or a dissection bench fitted with an extraction system that pulls fumes away from the user. The bench should include an integral sink, with hot and cold running water, for washing specimens and cleansing the area after disinfection with the appropriate chemical agent. The dissection area of the bench should slope towards the sink to facilitate the drainage of formalin away from the fixed specimens and should include a polypropylene, or cut resistant, dissection board for the examination and trimming of the fixed biopsies and whole organs.

A standard cut-up kit should include a stainless steel ruler, scalpel and PM40 handle and blades, steel-handled knives, a brain knife, scissors, bowel scissors, probes, a magnifying illuminator, bowel clamps and forceps (tweezers) for the handling of biopsies and tissue slices. Personal protective equipment (PPE) should include gowns or theatre pyjamas, aprons, surgical and cut-resistant gloves, goggles, visors, surgical masks and respirators (used in conjunction with specimen discard).

The cut-up room may, where space is available, house the tissue processing machines. Processors can be of the totally enclosed variety, and health and safety approved, or of the open variety which should be enclosed in a ventilated cabinet in order to contain solvent fumes. The room may also contain a polythene heat-sealing unit for the containment of specimens requiring transport to another hospital or department.

Fixation

When tissues are removed from the body they undergo a series of degenerative changes known as autolysis and putrefaction. Autolysis is the breakdown of cells and tissue components by the body's own enzymes and putrefaction is the degenerative change brought about in tissue as a consequence of bacterial action.

The aims of fixation

Fixation should arrest autolysis and putre-faction and preserve the cells and tissue components in as lifelike a state as possible. The fixative should not cause excessive shrinkage, swelling or hardening of the tissue and should stabilize the tissue against the rigours of processing. Finally, the fixative should complement and enhance subsequent histological staining and immunohistochemical procedures. This is broadly the remit of an 'ideal' fixative. However, in reality fixation is a compromise of these various requirements.

Types of fixative

Simple fixatives are a single chemical solution e.g. methanol, ethanol, glacial acetic acid and formaldehyde, which have no additives and which, used on their own, may produce some of the artefacts mentioned previously. Compound fixatives are mixtures of simple fixatives which have been formulated to offset and minimize fixation artefacts, e.g. Carnoy's fluid (ethanol–chloroform–acetic acid) which is recommended for the fixation of nucleic acids.

Simple and compound fixatives react with proteins in two ways. Coagulants, as suggested by their name, coagulate tissue protein, e.g. ethanol. Non-coagulant fixatives, e.g. formaldehyde, form cross-links with tissue protein.

Duration of fixation

The length of fixation depends on the density of the tissue and the speed of penetration of the fixative. Softer, less dense tissues are penetrated more quickly than dense fibrous tissues and bone. The penetration rate of fixatives varies, e.g. Carnoy's fluid is more rapid in its action than formaldehyde. It is common practice in histology laboratories to describe and slice large dense specimens (e.g. spleen), prior to tissue sampling, and leave them for an appropriate length of time to facilitate thorough fixation.

Formaldehyde as the routine fixative of choice

The most widely utilized fixative in routine histopathology departments is 10% formalin (4% formaldehyde) and its derivatives. Formaldehyde is soluble in water to a maximum of 40% by weight (100% formalin) and is commercially available as a 40% solution to which 10–14% methanol has been added as a stabilizer. Ten parts of 100% formalin is normally diluted with 90 parts water, physiological saline or phosphate buffer to obtain the 10% working solution. Non-buffered formalin becomes acidic on standing due to the formation of formic acid. Formic acid reacts with blood, in blood-rich tissues such as spleen, to produce a black pigment called acid formalin haematin. This usually occurs after prolonged fixation and the use of buffered formalin solutions will alleviate this fixation artefact.

Formalin has a pungent odour, is a strong eye, skin and mucous membrane irritant and, in some workers, may cause contact dermatitis. Personnel using formalin should undergo an annual respiratory sensitizer screening. Maximum recommended exposure limits are one part per million and exposure levels should be monitored on a regular basis. Formalin solutions should be carefully handled in well-ventilated rooms or fume hoods and protective clothing such as gloves, laboratory coats, goggles and respirators should be worn.

Formalin reacts to form cross-links between proteins. Soluble proteins are fixed to structural proteins giving strength to the tissue and enabling subsequent processing. Formalin does not fix carbohydrates but it does fix glycogen when it is held to a fixed protein. It is a good fixative for complex lipids.

Heat and agitation speed up the process of fixation. The recommended time for fixation of tissues in formalin is 24–48 hours, the optimum time being 7–10 days. Modern enclosed tissue processing machines allow for the heating of reagents at 40–45°C during processing to expedite the process of fixation. Tissues received in the laboratory should be completely submerged in 5 to 10 times their volume of fixative.

No fixative is ideal but 10% formalin has the advantage of preserving a wide range of tissues. It is tolerant and adequate histochemistry can be subsequently performed. Tissue may be stored for long periods without harmful effects on the nucleus, cytoplasm or overall morphology of the tissue. It is not the fixative of choice for immunohistochemistry, but many of the problems may be overcome with appropriate pre-digestion of the tissue prior to staining.

Other commonly used fixatives

Glutaraldehyde is often the fixative of choice for tissue requiring electron microscopy, as it gives good preservation of the ultrastructure of the cell. It is a respiratory sensitizer and is strongly linked to industrial asthma. Appropriate safety measures should be observed when handling glutaraldehyde. Its use as a disinfectant has, in the main, been outlawed in hospital laboratories.

Osmium tetroxide is used as a secondary fixative in electron microscopy, usually after primary fixation in glutaraldehyde. It fixes lipids and also preserves the fine structure of the cell. Osmium tetroxide is toxic and appropriate safety precautions should be taken when handling it.

Potassium dichromate may be used to identify adrenal medullary tumours, both macroscopically and microscopically. It reacts with adrenal medullary catecholamines, producing a black or brown precipitate which is water insoluble. It is not suitable as a general fixative as it penetrates tissue slowly and causes shrinkage.

Alcohol penetrates tissue rapidly and may be used in conjunction with other fixatives to increase the speed of fixation. *Absolute ethanol* preserves glycogen but it causes distortion of nuclear detail and shrinkage of cytoplasm. Carnoy's fixative is a good fixative for nucleic acids but causes shrinkage of the tissue and lysis of red blood cells. It consists of absolute ethanol, chloroform and glacial acetic acid.

Various additives in fixatives may be used. For example, tannic acid, phenol or heavy metal solutions may be added to formalin to increase the rate of penetration, improve preservation or enhance subsequent staining procedures.

Vapour fixation using volatile fixatives enables retention of soluble substances *in situ*, by converting them into insoluble products before they come into contact with solvents. This method is often used in conjunction with freeze drying. Suitable fixatives for this technique include formaldehyde, osmium tetroxide and alcohol.

Microwave ovens can be used in fixation, either to preserve the tissue with the action of the heat itself or to speed up the process of a fixative solution.

Tissue Processing and Embedding

Fixed, stabilized tissue will subsequently undergo microtomy involving the preparation of 1–6 μm thick tissue sections for examination microscopically. To facilitate this process the tissue must be supported internally and externally. Although freezing protocols are available for both fixed and unfixed tissue samples, these methods are normally utilized for the demonstration of fixation-labile components or for rapid diagnostic techniques. For general histopathological diagnosis tissues are commonly subjected to a series of reagents culminating in their infiltration and subsequent envelopment by a rigid support medium. The most widely used fixatives are variations of 10% aqueous formalin and it is the aim of tissue processing to substitute the aqueous fixative within the specimen by non-water miscible paraffin wax. To achieve this the specimen is subjected to the following stages:- (a) **dehydration**, in which alcohol replaces the aqueous fixative within the tissue; (b) **clearing**, in which an ante medium such as xylene replaces the alcohol; (c) **infiltration**, in which paraffin wax replaces the clearing agent and infiltrates the tissue; and (d) **embedding**, in which infiltrated tissue is encapsulated by paraffin wax to provide a rigid support for microtomy.

Tissue Processing and Embedding

Factors affecting tissue processing

Dehydration, clearing, infiltration and embedding

To ensure good tissue processing it is essential that tissue slices are no more than 2–3 mm thick for rapid/urgent processing schedules and 3–5 mm thick for routine overnight and weekend schedules. Poor processing will occur if tissue is crammed into the processing cassette, by prohibiting the reagents to circulate adequately. Tiny biopsies may be placed into commercially available biopsy bags or mesh biopsy cassettes which, in turn, are placed inside the processing cassette (see Fig. 1.1).

Factors affecting tissue processing
Temperature
At low temperatures processing reagents are more viscous and hence their tissue diffusion rates are slower. An elevated processing temperature increases the kinetic energy of reagent molecules, decreases reagent viscosity and increases the rate of diffusion of reagent into the tissue. Gentle heating of the dehydration and clearing reagents, in the range 37–45°C, will substantially reduce processing times but may increase tissue shrinkage due to the effect of heat on collagen.

High temperatures at the infiltration stage may cause undue tissue shrinkage and hardening. This can be resolved by employing temperatures of 2–3°C above the melting point of the infiltration media to minimize these effects. However, blood and muscle may still become brittle during infiltration and the combined effect of the fixation regime, the dehydrating agent and tissue type must also be considered.

Vacuum and pressure
Modern enclosed tissue processing machines incorporate a switchable vacuum and pressure cycle. In practice the application of pressure during dehydration and clearing has little effect on diffusion of reagents, although it may have an increased effect at the infiltration stage. However, the application of a vacuum enhances dehydration, clearing and infiltration.

Agitation
The maximum surface area of tissue should be available for fluid/reagent exchange and circulation during processing. This is not achieved in situations where tissue cassettes lie at the bottom of a container, are static in the reagent or are packed tightly into the processing basket. Maximum surface area for fluid exchange is impaired and circulation of reagent around the tissue is impeded resulting in stagnation, i.e. the reagent surrounding the tissue remains at a lower concentration and a much longer time is required for satisfactory processing.

To achieve consistent processing results the tissue cassettes should be loosely packed, suspended and agitated in the reagent to prevent stagnation and to allow circulation of the medium. Agitation can be facilitated by magnetic stirrers and rotors for manual processing whereas modern processing machines utilize rotational, up and down, side to side and/or tidal flow motion.

Dehydration, clearing, infiltration and embedding
Dehydration
The majority of tissue fixatives are made up in aqueous solution and the function of the dehydrating agent is to remove free and bound water molecules from the tissue specimen. The most commonly employed dehydrating agent, for routine paraffin processing, is 99.85% ethanol which, due to its expense, is purchased by laboratories in the form of the less expensive 99% industrial methylated spirit (IMS)

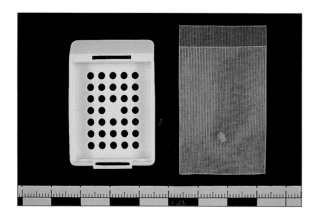

Figure 1.1: Tissue processing cassette and biopsy bag.

containing 2% methanol. Certain lipids and water-soluble proteins are removed from the tissue during this stage.

Tissues are processed through a rising concentration gradient of ethanol to 99% IMS (absolute ethanol). The fixation regime employed and the tissue type will dictate the strength of the first IMS bath. Routine histological processing schedules employ 70% IMS as the first step in tissue dehydration. Delicate tissues may need to be processed slowly from 50% IMS, whereas tissues that have been fixed in an alcoholic reagent such as Carnoy's fixative may be immersed directly into several changes of 99% IMS.

Dehydration time is dependent on the size and type of tissue specimen. In general tissue blocks of 1 mm thickness require 30 minutes in each graded alcohol and tissue blocks of 5 mm thickness require up to 90 minutes in each alcohol.

Clearing

The clearing agent is a reagent that is miscible with paraffin wax and acts as a link between the wax-immiscible dehydrating agent and the paraffin wax itself. The most commonly used clearing agents for routine tissue processing are hydrocarbons such as xylene, toluene, chloroform and petroleum solvents. These reagents are all controlled substances under the COSHH regulations, are flammable, cause skin degreasing and have varying degrees of toxicity. Toluene is a possible carcinogen, chloroform has a narcotic effect and xylene, although not proved to be a carcinogen, may cause headaches as a side-effect from inhalation of the vapour where adequate extraction facilities are not provided (usually in coverslipping and manual staining areas).

For the reasons stated previously, xylene is probably the most widely used clearing agent. It is compatible with all the major enclosed tissue processors and is relatively cheap. Xylene should be purchased as the benzene- (carcinogenic) and sulphur-free reagent. Prolonged exposure to xylene may cause excessive tissue hardening and tissue processing schedules should be formulated to minimize this effect. Tissues of 1–2 mm thickness require two to three changes of xylene over 30 minutes to one hour and specimen blocks of 3–5 mm

thickness require three changes over a two to four-hour period for normal processing. The heat and vacuum facilities on modern tissue processing machines will substantially reduce these times.

Infiltration

Paraffin wax is the infiltration and embedding medium of choice for routine histopathology. It is a mixture of polycrystalline straight-chain hydrocarbons produced from the distillation and cracking of crude mineral oil. Paraffin wax is categorized by its melting point which, in turn, reflects the admix of molecular weights of its constituent hydrocarbons. Melting points, though not wholly accurate, are in the range 39–68°C and, as a general rule, the higher the melting point the harder the wax. Softer tissues benefit from infiltration by lower melting point waxes and harder tissues from infiltration by those with a higher melting point. However, routine histopathological processing is partly a compromise due to the variation in size and hardness of the tissue samples to be processed and the preferred clearing agent. To this end, paraffin wax of melting point 56–58°C is normally employed. Infiltration times are illustrated later in Table 1.1. Infiltration times are greatly reduced by the application of a vacuum. This is essential for specimens of lung where the vacuum forces out trapped air molecules from the tissue.

Additives have been included in some paraffin waxes to improve their crystalline constituency by reducing their hardness and brittleness and, hence, improve their cutting (microtomy) characteristics. These substances include, among others, thermoplastic resins, plastic polymers and dimethyl sulphoxide (DMSO) which aids infiltration and allows thin sectioning.

Embedding

Paraffin wax for tissue embedding should be clean, filtered and held at 2–4°C above its melting point. On completion of processing the tissue basket is transferred to a heated reservoir or free-standing bath of paraffin wax. Tissues are removed from their cassettes, one at a time only, with heated forceps and placed face down

Tissue Processing and Embedding

Dehydration, clearing, infiltration and embedding

Table 1.1: Schedules for automatic tissue processing.

Reagent	Open tissue processor			Enclosed tissue processor		
	Routine Overnight	Rapid	Vacuum	Routine Overnight	Rapid	Vacuum
10% formal saline	1 hour	30 minutes	No	30 minutes*	15 minutes	Yes
70% alcohol	1 hour	Nil	No	30 minutes*	Nil	Yes
95% alcohol	1 hour	Nil	No	30 minutes*	15 minutes	Yes
100% alcohol	1 hour	15 minutes	No	30 minutes*	15 minutes	Yes
100% alcohol	1 hour	15 minutes	No	30 minutes*	15 minutes	Yes
100% alcohol	1 hour	30 minutes	No	1 hour*	15 minutes	Yes
100% alcohol	1 hour	30 minutes	No	1 hour*	15 minutes	Yes
Xylene	30 minutes	15 minutes	No	30 minutes*	10 minutes	Yes
Xylene	1 hour	15 minutes	No	30 minutes*	15 minutes	Yes
Xylene	1 hour	30 minutes	No	30 minutes*	15 minutes	Yes
Paraffin wax	1 hour	30 minutes	No	30 minutes	15 minutes	Yes
Paraffin wax	1 hour	30 minutes	Yes	1 hour	30 minutes	Yes
Paraffin wax	1.5 hours	30 minutes	Yes	1 hour	30 minutes	Yes

*Processing temperature 45°C

in a pre-filled mould of molten paraffin wax. The mould is placed on a refrigerated surface or ice tray to facilitate the clamping of the tissue to its base. A variety of moulds are available and include stainless steel moulds of graded capacities which receive the processing/embedding cassette, the latter acting as the tissue support platform, Leuckhart's L pieces, ice trays, metal boats and peel-away plastic moulds. Moulds are left on the coldplate until the wax solidifies or, where a form of refrigeration is not available, can be immersed in cold water once a thick enough crust has formed on the surface of the wax.

Commercial embedding centres, which combine a heated mould store, a molten wax reservoir/dispenser and a coldplate, are readily available (Fig. 1.2).

Once the wax has solidified the tissue blocks may be gently removed from their moulds and prepared for microtomy.

It is a general rule, for appropriate orientation of tissue specimens, that the surface of the tissue facing downward in the cassette should be placed face down in the mould. Orientation is extremely important for effective diagnosis. A skin biopsy should be embedded at right angles to its surface to give the correct plane for sectioning. Cylindrical or tubular tissue such as Fallopian tube or vas deferens should be embedded on end in order that transverse sections may be cut through their walls and lumina. Dyes or special inks can be utilized to mark resection planes and allow for correct tissue orientation.

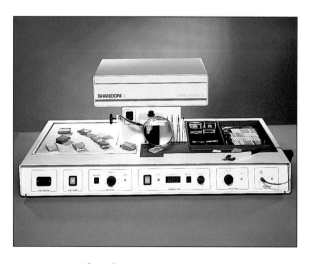

Figure 1.2: Shandon Histocentre 2 tissue embedding centre.

Dehydration, clearing, infiltration and embedding

Automatic tissue processors

Carousel type 'open' tissue processors (Fig. 1.3a) are rapidly being replaced by 'enclosed' (Fig. 1.3b) Health and Safety compliant, processing machines with larger cassette capacities. Open processors release reagent vapours into the atmosphere as the tissue basket moves between stations and, therefore, should be contained within a well-ventilated area or extraction facility. Agitation is effected by a rotational or dunking motion and vacuum is available on the final wax infiltration baths. Tissues are processed through the solvents at room temperature.

Enclosed processors are stand-alone or modular units which fully contain reagent fumes during tissue processing by means of water or vapour traps and charcoal adsorption filters. Reagents are pumped into and out of a processing chamber or retort. Agitation is provided in the form of tidal flow of reagents in and out of the retort or by a side to side rotational motion. Ingress of reagents can be enhanced by alternating, programmable vacuum and pressure cycles, of which vacuum is the most effective, and the dehydrating and clearing steps can be substantially reduced by the ability to heat the reagents (25–45°C). Microprocessor technology enables multiple processing schedules to be stored and retrieved and, on some machines, allows for simultaneous use of add-on units running a variety of schedules under the control of a command module.

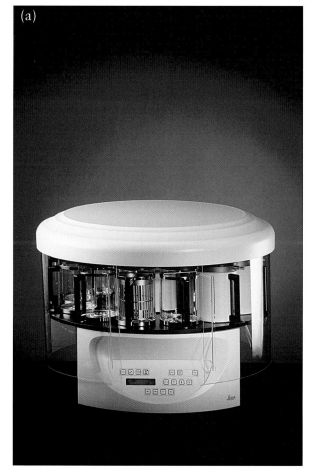

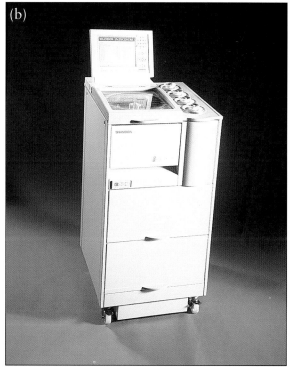

Figure 1.3: *(a) Leica TP1020 tissue processor and (b) Shandon Pathcentre enclosed tissue processor.*

Microtomy

Microtomes

Microtome knives

'Routine overnight' and 'rapid' tissue processing schedules

Table 1.1 shows a comparison of 'routine overnight' and 'rapid' schedules for open and enclosed automatic tissue processing.

The replenishment of processing reagents and infiltration media is dependent on the volume of reagent used per step and the quantities of tissue cassettes being processed. Appropriate safety precautions should be taken and the use of personal protective equipment is essential when decanting these solutions.

Microtomy

Microtomy is the production of thin sections, 1–5 μm in thickness, from paraffin wax embedded tissue blocks. This process utilizes a microtome in conjunction with a microtome knife or disposable microtome blade and blade holder. Microtomes are of the 'rotary' or 'base sledge' variety and are commercially available from a large number of laboratory equipment suppliers. The microtome knife has largely been superseded, in routine histopathology departments, by the disposable microtome blade. Microtome knives need to be specially sharpened, either manually (a highly skilled procedure) or by machine, which can be extremely time-consuming in an age where workload activity demands the streamlining of histopathology services.

Microtomes

The rotary microtome (Fig. 1.4) is a general purpose machine for the production of semi-thin tissue sections for light microscopy. The manual rotation of the laterally mounted wheel causes the advance mechanism to move the block holder towards the rigidly mounted knife at a pre-set thickness of cut (section thickness). The block moves up and down through the knife in a vertical plane with the production of flat sections on the downward stroke, usually 3–5 μm for routine histological purposes. The speed of the block through the knife is controlled by the rate at which the hand wheel is rotated. Heavy duty, motorized, rotary

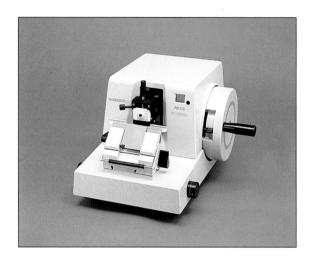

Figure 1.4: Shandon AS325 rotary microtome.

microtomes are also available for use in conjunction with the production of semi-thin (0.5–1 μm) resin embedded sections for light microscopy where the constant speed of the block through the knife can be controlled automatically. The section thickness range of these microtomes is usually 0.5–60 μm.

The sledge microtome, although best suited for the sectioning of hard tissues and some softer resins, is equally suitable for the sectioning and ribboning of soft tissues and biopsies. The heavy construction of these machines means that they do not succumb easily to vibration and the knife clamp can be angled away from the direction of cut which aids in sectioning hard tissues. The block holder is mounted on two parallel runners and the block holder advanced by either a manual specimen advance on the handle itself or by a lever mounted on the side of the block carrier which moves against a static stanchion. The block is passed forwards and backwards through the knife using a push and pull motion. Sections are cut at 3–5 μm for routine histology.

Microtome knives

Conventional steel microtome knives have, in the main, been replaced by disposable blades for routine histopathology.

Steel knives are manufactured from a high grade carbon or tool quality steel that should be free from impurities and rust resistant. Knives are tempered (hardened) from the tip inwards and the degree of hardness measured using the Vickers scale (usually 400–900 on the scale). The degree of hardness can vary between manufacturers and between individual knives from the same manufacturer. A hardness of 700 is desirable, 400 being soft and 900 being considered brittle, for routine use. Steel knives come in a variety of profiles dependent on their intended use (Fig. 1.5).

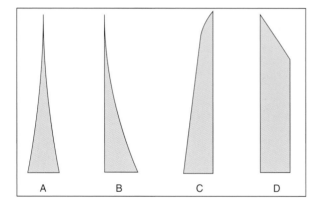

Figure 1.5: Microtome knife profiles.

Profile A: is biconcave and was employed for sectioning celloidin embedded tissues. It is rarely used in routine histopathology.

Profile B: is planoconcave and can be used to section wax-embedded soft tissues, celloidin embedded tissues and botanical specimens. Profiles A and B produce the sharpest edges.

Profile C: is wedge shaped and is the most commonly utilized steel knife for routine histopathology. It is a more rigid knife than profiles A and B and is used for paraffin wax sectioning of all tissues as well as being employed in cryostats for sectioning frozen material (see later). This profile cannot be ground as sharp as profiles A and B.

Profile D: is tool-edged or plane-shaped and is used for sectioning hard materials such as resins and extremely hard paraffin wax tissue blocks. This knife produces the least sharp edge when ground.

Methods for the sharpening and honing of the above knives are to be found in the further reading section.

Disposable blades are modified, thickened razor blades produced from high quality stainless steel and give reproducible, compression free, good quality sections. The thin blade is held rigidly in its own special holder to minimize vibration during microtomy. The blades may be coated with platinum or chromium for a longer cutting life. These blades appear to be the first choice, nowadays, for routine histopathology.

Other knives include tungsten carbide for resin work and production of undecalcified bone sections, glass, diamond and sapphire knives for use with araldite and epoxy resin embedded material for electron microscopy or for small, narrow blocks of acrylic or polyester resin embedded tissues for light microscopy.

Paraffin wax sectioning

A microtome knife or disposable blade with a sharp, blemish-free edge is essential for quality sectioning. All operations concerning the placement or removal of the block into and out of the block holder should be carried out with the safety of the user in mind. Blades are extremely sharp. The hand wheel of rotary microtomes should be clamped and the block carrier on sledge microtomes should be positioned, and clamped where available, at the end of the microtome furthest from the blade during these procedures.

Some laboratories employ a 'rough-cutting' microtome to trim down the tissue block until a representative cross-sectional area of the tissue is obtained. Sections are removed at 10–15 μm intervals until the full face of the tissue is available, followed by several sections at 4–5 μm to ensure a smooth block surface (avoids rough cutting artefact). The block holder of the rough cutter is set in the same plane as the rest of the laboratory microtomes. Rough cutting and sectioning may be performed on the same microtome or even the same blade. Section cutting should be performed on a separate area of the blade or knife to that which was used for rough cutting purposes.

Blocks for diagnostic sectioning are precooled on an ice tray or chiller plate prior to cutting. Chilling causes compression of the block and offers a more rigid block face to the knife for ease of sectioning. Section thickness is commonly set at 3–5 μm. As the block face passes through the knife edge the tissue sections move up (sledge microtome) or down (rotary microtome) the knife face. As the block hits the knife edge the friction produced causes a 'melting front' in the wax and, thus, subsequent sections adhere to each other creating a ribbon. This ribbon of sections is supported, removed from the knife edge and floated on to a water bath (48–50°C) with cutting forceps. The sections are teased apart at their points of adhesion and attached to glass microscope slides by part submersion of the slide in the water. Excess water is drained from the slide and the slide left to dry face up on a 60°C hotplate, not in direct contact, until all traces of water have disappeared. The slide is then placed in contact with the hotplate for 5–10 minutes to facilitate adhesion of the paraffin wax section to the glass. Sections are now ready for staining by haematoxylin and eosin and a whole host of other tinctorial and immunocytochemical methods that the histologist has at his or her disposal. Section mounting, as mentioned earlier, may be automated.

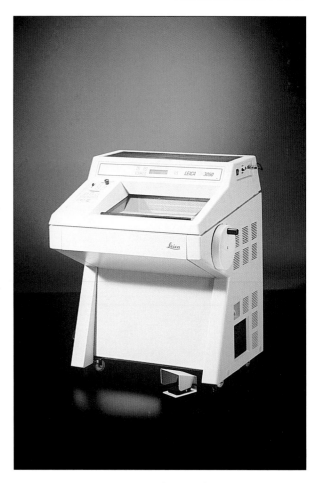

Figure 1.6: Leica CM3050 Cryostat.

Special Techniques

Frozen sectioning of fresh tissues
The majority of routine histopathology laboratories include amongst their repertoires a diagnostic frozen section service for suspected tumour patients. A diagnosis can be phoned to the surgeon within 10–20 minutes of receipt of the tissue sample and, hence, aid the clinical management of the patient. The *cryostat* (Fig. 1.6) a rotary or rocking microtome housed within a refrigerated chamber, is utilized for this procedure. The temperature of the specimen and specimen holder, knife and chamber, can normally be set independently or a single temperature may be pre-selected for the whole. Fresh tissue for rapid diagnosis is received from the operating theatre, frozen on to the specimen holder using carbon dioxide, liquid nitrogen or a commercial freezing spray, and transferred to the cryostat for sectioning. If conditions are optimal for the tissue being sectioned, then it is possible to cut sections as thin as 1 μm. Fresh tissues should be dissected and frozen in the confines of a microbiological safety cabinet. Most modern cryostats incorporate a four-hour formalin decontamination cycle for the disinfection of the chamber after sectioning unsuspected infectious cases (some tuberculous lesions can closely mimic tumour macroscopically).

The *freezing microtome* (Fig. 1.7) may be utilized for the semi-thin sectioning of fresh tissues, where there is a requirement to demonstrate substances that are normally removed

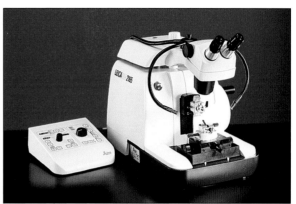

Figure 1.8: *Leica RM2165 motorized heavy duty rotary microtome.*

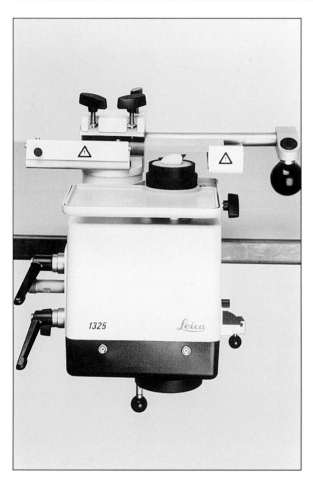

Figure 1.7: *Leica Freezing Microtome.*

during routine processing (e.g. lipids). This type of microtome has a static specimen holder with the knife itself being manually drawn across the surface of the tissue as the specimen holder is advanced by a preset thickness. The tissue is frozen *in situ* by means of an attached carbon dioxide cylinder or a circulating coolant. Consistent thin sections are difficult to obtain.

Undecalcified bone sectioning

This requires the production of 4–5 µm sections of undecalcified bone embedded in an acrylic or polyester resin. Although a base sledge microtome may be used for this purpose, it is more common to employ a *heavy duty*

motorized microtome (Fig. 1.8) D profile (tool edge), tungsten, glass or diamond knives are commonly used for the sectioning of this tissue.

Electron microscopy

Electron microscopy requires the production of ultra-thin resin embedded sections using an *ultramicrotome*. Hard epoxy or araldite resins are usually employed and section thickness is measured in nanometres. Sectioning is facilitated by the use of glass or diamond knives and section thickness monitored by observing the interference colour produced by the section in contact with water i.e. gold (90–120 nm), silver (60–90 nm) and grey (< 60 nm). Sections are picked up and stained on special copper and/or rhodium grids. Stains employ heavy metal salts, such as lead citrate and uranyl acetate, which impregnate certain tissue structures. These heavy metals deflect an electron beam, produced by the electron microscope. This results in shades of black and grey areas within the tissue section where ultra-structural elements have been impregnated by the heavy metals. The electron microscope incorporates a camera system that can photograph areas of interest within the section, the final result being the electron micrograph. This is an extremely simplistic overview of electron microscopy. See Chapter 5 for a full description.

Acknowledgements

Photographs by courtesy of Shandon Lipshaw
(A Life Sciences International company), Leica
UK Ltd and Dr A. Warfield, Histopathology,
Birmingham Heartlands Hospital.

Further Reading

Bancroft John D, Stevens A; *Theory and Practice of Histological Techniques, 4th edn 1996: Churchill Livingstone, Edinburgh.*

Woods Anthony E, Ellis Roy C; *Laboratory Histopathology: A Complete Reference, 1994: Churchill Livingstone, New York.*

2   GENERAL STAINS

Barrie Sims

Why Stain?

The refractive indices of tissue structures in thin sections are so similar that it is necessary to enhance the visibility and improve the contrast by the use of staining procedures.

The majority of diagnostic routine histopathology is performed on paraffin wax sections, with the exception of frozen sections, which are used for rapid diagnosis or the demonstration of substances, such as lipids and enzymes, removed by processing. Wax present in the sections obscures the tissue structure and is poorly permeable to stains. It is therefore necessary to remove the paraffin wax from the sections. The sections are first treated with xylene to dissolve the paraffin wax. Treatment with alcohol will remove the xylene, which is not miscible with water or low-grade alcohols, and will allow the section to be hydrated in water. This process is often referred to in methodology books by various terms, for example, de-wax sections; sections to water; hydrate sections.

Basic Staining Mechanisms

In diagnostic histopathology, staining methods may be grouped into four main processes (vital staining is rarely used, if at all).

Elective solubility

This is the process by which stains that are dissolved in a solvent are more soluble in the tissue structure than they are in the solvent. This method is primarily used for the demonstration of fat droplets. The dyes used are usually of the Sudan type category (Sudan III; Sudan IV). Because paraffin wax processing will remove the majority of fats the technique is usually performed on frozen sections.

Metallic impregnation

The deposition of metallic silver onto tissues may be used for the demonstration of a wide range of structures and substances.

Cells which have the ability to reduce ammoniacal silver to produce a visible deposit are termed 'argentaffin'. Melanin and Kultschitzky cells of the intestinal gland are typical examples. Cells or structures that require the use of an external reducer to produce the deposit are termed 'argyrophil'. Metallic impregnation is used widely for the demonstration of reticular fibres, nerve cells and their processes, micro-organisms and cellular pigments.

Basic Staining Mechanisms

Histochemical reactions

Staining with dyes

Histochemical reactions

These are methods in which there is a clear understanding of the chemical mechanisms involved in the production of the final reaction product. The final reaction products may or may not be dyes. Perl's reaction for ferric iron will produce a deep blue coloured deposit (Prussian blue), whereas the reaction produced by Schiff's reagent in the periodic acid Schiff procedure is a deep magenta dye. Many enzymes may be demonstrated by the incubation of sections (frozen or paraffin) in substrates containing a substance upon which the enzyme reacts, producing a primary reaction product (PRP). A second reagent then couples with the PRP to produce a coloured deposit. Tissue sections known to contain (or not contain) the substance are used to control the specificity of the method. Substances known to inhibit the reaction will also be utilized to improve specificity.

Staining with dyes

The majority of staining procedures in routine histopathology will fall into this group. The nature of the staining mechanism in many cases is not clearly understood and results often depend upon the skill of the histotechnologist.

Dyes may be classified into natural and synthetic. Natural dyes include haematoxylin, whilst synthetic dyes will include the greater majority of dyes used in histotechniques (e.g. eosin, methylene blue and basic fuchsin). Dyes may also be classified as acidic, basic or neutral.

Acidic dyes will be attracted to tissue elements of a basic nature such as the cytoplasm of cells. Basic dyes will be attracted to structures of an acidic nature such as the DNA in nuclei. Thus the basic dye haematoxylin is attracted to the acidic nature of DNA whilst the acid dye eosin will stain the cell cytoplasm. This essentially forms the mechanism of the haematoxylin and eosin stain for general structure. Neutral stains are produced by the combination of acid and basic dyes. The resulting product will stain both acidic and basic structures, forming the basis of Romanowsky stains such as Giemsa.

Dyes which combine with certain tissue structures and produce a colour different to that of the original dye are called metachromatic. Metachromatic staining methods may be used for the demonstration of connective tissue mucins, mast cell granules, amyloid and cartilage.

The vast majority of staining methods are examined by light microscopy at the visible end of the spectrum. Dyes which have the ability to absorb ultraviolet light and then transmit in the visible spectrum are termed fluorescent. Fluorescent staining methods may be used for the demonstration of *Mycobacterium tuberculosis*, amyloid and tissue antigens.

Dyes which have the ability to combine with tissue structures from simple aqueous or alcoholic solutions are termed direct dyes. Eosin and many other aniline dyes exhibit this property. However, dyes which require the use of an intermediary substance to allow adequate staining to take place are termed indirect. The intermediary substance is known as a 'mordant'. The dye and the mordant combine to produce a coloured 'lake' which then combines with the tissue structure to produce a dye–mordant–tissue complex. Haematoxylin without the use of a mordant is a weak histological dye. By the addition of metals such as aluminium potassium sulphate or ferric chloride, haematoxylin can be made into a powerful versatile stain.

Haematoxylin staining

Haematoxylin usually requires oxidation to haematein in order to stain tissues. Oxidation may be induced chemically by the addition of an oxidizing agent such as sodium iodate, or naturally by sunlight (which can take several months). As described above, in order to stain tissues haematoxylin requires the use of a mordant. Depending upon the mordant used, haematoxylin can be made to demonstrate a variety of substances, as follows.

Alum haematoxylins are produced by the combination of haematoxylin with aluminium potassium sulphate or aluminium ammonium sulphate. These combinations are used to stain nuclear material blue. There are various formulae available such as Harris's, Ehrlich's, Mayer's, Delafield's, Cole's and Gill's.

Iron haematoxylins are produced by combination with iron salts such as ferric chloride or ferric ammonium sulphate. This combination produces a dense black stain which may be used to demonstrate nuclei, elastin, myelin and muscle striations. The structure stained will be dependent upon after-treatment. Iron haematoxylins are much more resistant to acid extraction and are used when acid counterstains are required. Alum haematoxylins may be converted into iron haematoxylins by sequential staining, firstly with a weak nuclear stain made up in iron alum, followed by an alum haematoxylin. The celestine blue-haemalum sequence is such a method.

Lead haematoxylin solutions have been used for the demonstration of endocrine cells.

Phosphotungstic acid haematoxylin may be used to demonstrate muscle striations, fibrin, nuclei, myelin, cilia, neuroglial cells and amoebae. The haematoxylin is combined with a solution of phosphotungstic acid. By using haematein instead of haematoxylin the oxidation process is avoided.

Many haematoxylin solutions are now commercially available, avoiding the need for time-consuming preparation in the laboratory and the need to handle toxic substances. In addition new formulae have removed some of the environmentally harmful substances from the preparation, making disposal to the sewers acceptable.

Regressive and progressive staining

Stains which overstain tissue structures and are then subsequently selectively removed are termed 'regressive'. The removal of the excess stain is called differentiation. This may be achieved by the use of solvents (e.g. alcohol), acid solutions (e.g. acid alcohol), or the mordanting solution (e.g. iron alum). 'Progressive' staining does not overstain the tissues and the staining period is stopped after a given period of time. Mayer's haemalum stain for nuclei is a common example.

Common Staining Methods

Routine staining methods may be grouped broadly into the following nine categories: general structure; connective tissue fibres; carbohydrates and mucosubstances; demonstration of pigments; micro-organisms; extracellular substances (fibrin and amyloid); lipids; cytoplasmic granules; neurological tissues.

General structure
Haematoxylin and eosin (H&E)
The haematoxylin and eosin method is the most popular general structure stain in diagnostic histopathology. An alum haematoxylin is most commonly used. Following haematoxylin staining the excess dye is removed (differentiated) using a dilute acid alcohol (commonly 0.5% to 1%) until only the nuclei are stained. At this stage the nuclei are stained red. By washing in tap water or an alkaline solution, the pH of the stain is moved towards alkalinity. This has the effect of changing the haematoxylin stain from red to blue (an action similar to litmus). The process is termed '*blueing*'. The application of eosin will stain the cytoplasm and other structures within the section. The procedure of dehydrating in alcohol (which may be preceded by washing in water), prior to 'clearing' in xylene for coverglassing, will also remove some of the eosin staining. By careful timing of these steps the eosin can be removed selectively

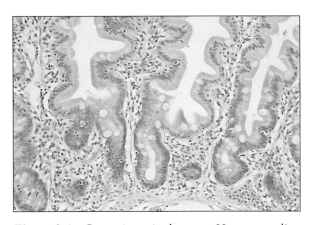

Figure 2.1: Gastrointestinal tract – Haematoxylin and eosin.

Common Staining Methods

Connective tissue fibres and muscle

from the section thereby demonstrating muscle, collagen, red blood cells and acidophilic structures differentially. The choice of solvent and concentration of eosin will depend upon local conditions such as alkalinity of tap water.

Simple staining solutions

A basic dye, such as methylene blue, will stain tissue structure blue. By selective removal of the dye using water and alcohol the various components can be demonstrated in various shades of blue. This type of method is often used as a counterstain to another technique which may be demonstrating specific elements (e.g. *Mycobacterium tuberculosis*) in the tissues. These stains often enable the observer to orientate the position of the elements within the tissues.

Connective tissue fibres and muscle

The connective tissues most commonly demonstrated include collagen, reticular fibres, muscle, basement membranes and elastin.

Collagen and muscle

van Gieson is perhaps one of the most commonly used stains for collagen and muscle. The stain is a combination of picric acid and acid fuchsin. Due to the acidic nature of the van Gieson counterstain an iron haematoxylin (e.g. Weigert's or celestine-blue haemalum) is used to stain nuclear detail. Collagen is stained red whilst muscle and red blood cells are stained yellow, and nuclei are black.

Trichrome staining demonstrates collagen and muscle differentially. Muscle staining is red whilst the collagen stain may be blue or green depending upon preference. Fixation in a mercury-based fixative usually gives superior results to formalin fixation. The stain is more complex to perform than the van Gieson and requires skill in assessing the various staining stages. The theory behind trichrome staining is varied and complex and beyond the reaches of this chapter.

Phosphotungstic acid haematoxylin will stain muscle striations and myofibrils blue.

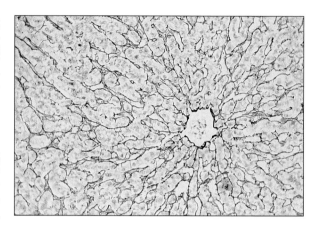

Figure 2.2: Reticular fibres – Gordon and Sweet's silver impregnation method.

Reticulin

Reticular fibres are demonstrated primarily by silver impregnation techniques. There are a wide variety of methods of silver preparation but the methodology is similar. Sections are usually oxidized with potassium permanganate followed by bleaching; sensitized with iron alum; impregnated with ammoniacal silver nitrate; reduced in formalin and fixed in sodium thiosulphate. Toning in gold chloride is optional and dependent upon preference. Reticular fibres are blackened whilst other structures may vary from yellow to brown (grey if toned) to colourless. In some instances nuclei may be impregnated by the silver. Reticulin fibres may also be demonstrated by the PAS technique.

Basement membranes

Glomerular basement membranes are most commonly demonstrated when looking for glomerular disease. The basement membrane is oxidized with periodic acid and then treated with a methenamine silver solution. Basement membranes are progressively blackened and the technique halted at the appropriate degree of impregnation. Thin sections, 1 to 2 μm thick, are preferred to enable fine structures or projections to be visualized. The PAS technique will also demonstrate basement membranes.

Elastin

Popular stains for elastin include Verhoeff's elastin stain and the resorcin fuchsin methods such as Weigert's and its variants (e.g. Miller's). Verhoeff's elastin stain is an iron haematoxylin method in which the fibres are differentiated using the mordant ferric chloride. Muscle and collagen are stained with the van Gieson method. A problem with the Verhoeff method is that it is difficult to demonstrate both coarse and fine fibres in the same section. Methods based upon Weigert's elastin method will stain both coarse and fine fibres. Collagen and muscle may again be demonstrated with van Gieson. Additionally these stains may be purchased commercially removing the need for sometimes messy and lengthy preparation.

Carbohydrates and mucosubstances
The periodic acid Schiff reaction (PAS)
The PAS reaction is widely used throughout histology. Periodic acid will break the carbon bonds of adjacent 1:2 glycol groups, turning them into aldehydes. The aldehydes recolour the colourless Schiff reagent, staining the sites of activity magenta. Since many substances will, on oxidation by periodic acid, reveal aldehyde groups, the specificity of the method is controlled by digestion or blocking of the tissue elements in duplicate sections. Sites of activity are determined by comparing the two sections. The PAS reaction may be combined with other stains to demonstrate composite structures such as acid and neutral mucins using alcian blue.

Glycogen
The routine demonstration of glycogen is frequently by the use of the PAS reaction. However, as described above the PAS reaction will demonstrate many other substances which contain aldehydes. To determine sites of glycogen deposition a duplicate section is pre-treated with diastase before the PAS technique. This will digest glycogen from the diastase-treated section which, upon staining with the PAS technique, will show an absence of staining. Methenamine silver can be substituted for Schiff reagent which will demonstrate glycogen black instead of magenta. Another popular stain for glycogen is Best's carmine.

Mucosubstances
Mucosubstances are often found as mixtures and include mucins. Mucins are found in many sites in tissues (e.g. glandular, connective). The demonstration of the mucins will depend upon their particular nature. Neutral mucins may be stained with the PAS reaction and acid mucins with alcian blue.

Alcian blue prepared at different pHs will differentiate between general acid mucins and sulphated mucins. Alcian blue prepared with differing concentrations of magnesium chloride will differentiate substances such as hyaluronic acid, chondroitin sulphate, keratin sulphate and heparin. Connective tissue mucins may be demonstrated with metachromatic dyes such as toluidine blue whilst Southgate's mucicarmine

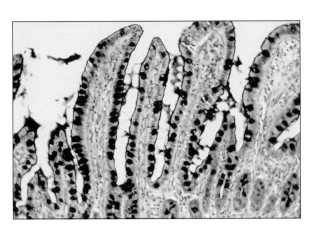

Figure 2.3: *Gastrointestinal tract – Periodic acid Schiff reaction.*

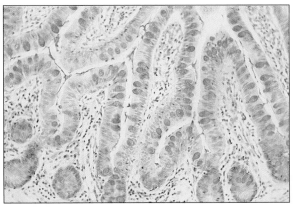

Figure 2.4: *Gastrointestinal tract – alcian blue method for acid mucopolysaccharides.*

Common Staining Methods
Demonstration of pigments

Micro-organisms

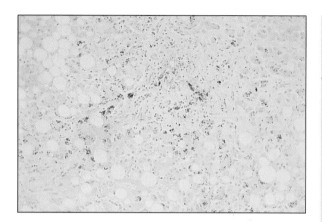

Figure 2.5: *Haemosiderin deposits – Perl's Prussian blue reaction.*

will demonstrate carboxylated or weakly acidic mucins.

Blocking techniques to prevent staining of particular chemical groups (e.g. carboxyl) are used to increase specificity by the absence of staining in treated sections.

Demonstration of pigments
Pigments may be found in normal and pathological tissues and may be formed naturally or as an *artefact* of tissue preparation.

Artefactual
These usually occur during fixation and may be caused by acid solutions of formalin reacting with haematin (formalin pigment) or deposits of mercury salts following mercury-based fixation (e.g. Zenker). These pigments are easily removed prior to staining.

Staining methods for pigments
Table 2.1 gives some common pigments which may be present in tissues, and methods to demonstrate them.

Micro-organisms
Micro-organisms that can be demonstrated histologically include bacteria, viral inclusions, fungi and spirochaetes. Simple stains such as methylene blue will often provide a quick and easy means of identifying the presence of organisms but will only provide information concerning morphology.

Table 2.1: Demonstration of some common pigments.

Pigment	Demonstration
Haemosiderin	Perl's Prussian blue
Bile pigment	Gmelin
Melanin	Masson Fontana
Lipofuscins	Schmorl's ferric ferrocyanide
	PAS
	Masson Fontana
	Sudan black
	Long Ziehl–Neelsen
APUD cell granules	Lead haematoxylin
	Masson Fontana
	Diazo
	Grimelius
	Bodian
Chromaffin cells	Chromaffin reaction
	Giemsa
Copper	Rubeanic acid
	Rhodanine
Asbestos	Perl's Prussian blue
	Birefringence

APUD = Amine Precursor Uptake and Decarboxylation

Bacteria can be divided into Gram-positive and Gram-negative according to their staining reaction with Gram's crystal violet stain. Gram-positive bacteria will retain the stain following differentiation in either alcohol or acetone whilst Gram-negative bacteria are decolorized. Iodine is used in the technique either as a mordant or as a means of precipitating the dye within the cytoplasm of Gram-positive bacteria. Gram-negative bacteria are demonstrated with a contrasting counterstain e.g. neutral red. It is possible to over-differentiate bacteria and careful control of the technique is required.

Acid-fast bacilli are most commonly demonstrated by the Ziehl–Neelsen method (ZN). Basic fuchsin and phenol are combined to produce strong carbol fuchsin. Following application of the dye, the section is differentiated with a mixture of acid and alcohol until the section is decolorized. A counterstain (blue or green) is applied to demonstrate other bacteria, cells and nuclei. A fluorescent method is also available using a mixture of the dyes auramine and rhodanine. Under ultraviolet light the bacilli will fluoresce. This procedure may improve the location of the organisms particularly if present in scanty amounts.

Viral inclusions have no specific staining methods as many of the stains will also stain other structures. Phloxine tartrazine has been used to demonstrate inclusion bodies and orcein is commonly used for the demonstration of hepatitis B.

Fungi may be quite apparent in H&E stained sections but can be more selectively stained by the PAS method, Grocott's methenamine silver technique, Southgate's mucicarmine (*Cryptococcus*), Gram's stain, Ziehl–Neelsen, and Giemsa.

Spirochaetes are most difficult to demonstrate in tissue sections. The classical method of Levaditi is performed on tissue blocks which are subsequently embedded and sectioned. There are many silver impregnation methods described, all of which require a degree of expertise to perform successfully. Some of these methods have been adapted for the demonstration of *Helicobacter*.

Extracellular substances (fibrin and amyloid)

Fibrin stains strongly with eosin and is moderately PAS positive. Fibrin threads stain strongly with phosphotungstic acid haematoxylin. 'Fibrinoid' is a term given to a hyaline substance found to give similar staining reactions to those of fibrin. A popular stain in routine use is Lendrum's martius scarlet blue (MSB) method. This will demonstrate younger fibrin and fibrinoid red, red blood cells yellow and collagen and older fibrin blue. The method requires skilful differentiation. Although formal mercury fixation was originally recommended, acceptable results are achieved with non mercury-containing formaldehyde mixtures.

Amyloid stains pink in haematoxylin and eosin preparations, is moderately PAS positive and stains yellow to brown with van Gieson. Amyloid may be demonstrated with congo red, metachromatic methods and thioflavine T fluorescence. There are several congo red formulations in routine use producing pink to red amyloid staining. Congo red stained amyloid is dichroic with polarized light producing a yellow green birefringence. Methyl violet or toluidine blue will exhibit purplish-red to red metachromasia. Thioflavine T is a fluorescent dye which exhibits a bright yellow fluorescence with ultraviolet light. The method is not specific but is highly sensitive.

Lipids

Lipids are found in both normal and pathological tissues. Simple lipids are normally lost during paraffin wax processing and, therefore, frozen sections are required. Compound lipids, in which other products are present (e.g. phospholipids), may resist processing and be demonstrable in paraffin sections. Simple lipids are demonstrated using fat soluble dyes (e.g. Sudan dyes). The principle of staining relies on the fact that the dye is more soluble in the fat than it is in the solvent it is made up in (elective solubility). Compound lipids are demonstrated by a variety of methods depending upon the nature of the lipid, for instance phospholipids (e.g. myelin) can be demonstrated with luxol fast blue whilst sudan black B will demonstrate compound lipids in paraffin sections.

Cytoplasmic granules

Mast cell granules are metachromatic and can be demonstrated using toluidine blue, thionin or azure A. The granules exhibit purple to red metachromasia with nuclei and other structures stained blue. Other connective tissue and some epithelial mucins may also be demonstrated. The granules are also demonstrated using a variety of alcian blue staining methods. Bancroft recommends chloroacetate esterase as the method of choice.

Paneth cell granules are acidophilic and easily seen in well-differentiated H&E stained sections. The phloxine tartrazine method of Lendrum demonstrates the granules red against a yellow background.

Pancreatic cell granules are now largely demonstrated by immunocytochemical methods. Zymogen granules are acidophilic and PAS positive. The cells of the islets of Langerhans have traditionally been demonstrated by chrome alum haematoxylin (B cells); aldehyde fuchsin (B cells); Grimelius (A cells); Hellerström & Hellman (D cells).

Pituitary cell granules are again now primarily demonstrated using immunocytochemical methods. Traditional staining methods include PAS–orange G (basophil cells PAS positive, acidophil cells orange and chromophobes unstained). Further subdivisions are available using performic acid and alcian blue. Other methods include Mallory's trichrome and its variants and pontamine sky blue.

Eosinophils are acidophilic, seen clearly in well-differentiated H&E stained sections and demonstrated using chromotrope and Romanowsky stains.

Neurological tissues
In routine diagnostic histopathology the demonstration of neurological elements by conventional staining methods is largely confined to those of nerve cells, their processes and myelin sheaths. Immunocytochemical methods have largely replaced some of the more capricious silver impregnation techniques for neuroglial elements. Myelin in routine paraffin sections is commonly demonstrated using luxol fast blue or solochrome cyanin. Degenerate myelin is demonstrated by its absence of staining with these methods. Nerve fibres may be demonstrated using a variety of silver impregnation techniques. Nissl substance is often demonstrated using cresyl fast violet, as part of the luxol fast blue technique.

Conclusions
Conventional staining methods still have a significant role to play in the diagnosis of tissue pathology. Routine laboratories use a combination of staining methods and immunocytochemistry to provide the necessary information. The morphology presented by haematoxylin and eosin staining is the precursor to subsequent investigations. Although immunocytochemistry is superseding a number of historical staining methods there are still a large number of investigations which rely solely on conventional staining with dyes.

Further Reading

Bancroft J D, Stevens A. *Theory and Practice of Histological Techniques*, 4th. edn. 1996: Churchill-Livingstone, Edinburgh, London.

Culling C F A, Allison R T, and Barr W T. *Cellular Pathology Technique*, 4th. edn. 1985: Butterworth, London.

Drury R A B, Wallington E A. *Carleton's Histological Technique*, 4th edn. 1980: Oxford University Press.

3 ENZYME HISTOCHEMISTRY

Trevor Gray and Neil Hand

Introduction

Enzymes are large tertiary proteins that act as catalysts for most biological reactions that are vital in cellular metabolism and maintaining homeostasis in man. There are over 700 known enzymes, each catalyzing a specific reaction by acting on specific molecules (substrates). The resulting reaction product may act as a new substrate for a different enzyme, as illustrated by the Krebs cycle which gives a 'cascade' of reactions. After each metabolic reaction, the enzyme in each case is left unaltered for further interactions.

Biochemists study enzyme levels routinely in solutions derived from body fluids, tissue cultures, and resected tissue for diagnostic and research investigations. These give valuable evidence in detecting and monitoring disease processes and assessing drug-induced physiological changes. Biochemical analysis however, does not give specific cellular values as most tissues are heterogeneous. A more accurate assessment of intracellular enzyme location and biological activity can be undertaken using enzyme histochemistry. This relies on applying an enzyme detection system to tissue sections or smears. These techniques produce a final coloured reaction product that is localized to the cells and has an intensity proportional to enzyme activity, although unlike biochemical methods, accurate quantitative results are difficult to generate. Nonetheless, the qualitative microscopic appearances as seen by an experienced pathologist are important in the detection and assessment of several disease processes.

The main problem with enzyme histochemistry is the retention of enzyme function during tissue preparation and histochemical staining. Numerous histological methods have been developed for specific enzymes, and though these methods are not difficult, the non-standard tissue handling procedures required have resulted in the techniques being performed in specialist laboratories. Other non-enzyme histochemical methods for enzyme detection on standard paraffin sections include immunohistochemistry and m-RNA *in situ* hybridization. These methods can identify the presence or production of cellular enzymes, but neither can show the biological activity of the molecule.

Structure and Classification

Structure
Enzymes are high molecular weight globular proteins that may be found free within the cytoplasm (*lysoenzymes*) or bound to cellular membranes (*desmoenzymes*). Nonproteinous components (*prosthetic groups*) may be attached to the enzyme, which may help form an active quaternary structure. The functional property of the enzyme depends on maintaining the shape and charge of its 'active site' at the site of enzyme–substrate interaction.

Various *co-factors* are necessary for most enzyme reactions. *Activators* such as ions of calcium, magnesium, manganese, sodium, potassium and others help with electron transfer during the enzymatic reaction. *Co-enzymes* are molecules that combine with a non-active *apoenzyme* producing a sterically active site by altering the apoenzyme's quaternary structure. The co-enzyme can also combine with the substrate and may play an active part in the metabolic reaction. Most of the B-vitamins are co-enzymes.

Classification
There are several ways of classifying enzymes, the most accurate being the enzyme code number based on the systematic name of the enzyme. This contains the name of the specific substrate reacted upon, followed by a word with the suffix -*ase* specifying the type of reaction involved. In diagnostic enzyme histochemistry a shorter trivial name is more commonly used due to the small number of enzymes investigated.

Six major enzyme groups are classified according to their effect on the substrate and are named oxidoreductases, transferases, hydrolases, lyases, isomerases and ligases. Probably the most important groups to the diagnostic enzyme histochemist are oxidoreductases (previously known as oxidases and dehydrogenases) and hydrolases. These are often called oxidative and hydrolytic enzymes respectively.

Preservation and Preparation

Enzyme preservation
The cumulative effects of the processing stages required in the production of a conventional paraffin wax-embedded tissue block, such as fixation, dehydration and embedding are not conducive to preserving functional enzymes. This process usually results in complete loss of enzyme activity, although chloroacetate esterase and peroxidase are sufficiently resistant to damage by paraffin processing. Consequently, the demonstration of most enzymes is usually performed on frozen sections, but other preparations, such as smears, may also be employed.

It is important to remember that various enzymes react differently to external influences but most are rapidly lost if fresh tissue is left at room temperature. Many oxidative enzymes which are diagnostically important when investigating muscle diseases are located in mitochondria. When fresh tissue is deprived of oxygen, the mitochondrial membranes are soon damaged and reduction in enzyme activity occurs. It is therefore important to quickly freeze the tissue, which is usually fresh, as most oxidative enzymes cannot withstand conventional fixation. Hydrolytic enzymes are contained in lysosomes, but are damaged by freezing and subsequent thawing of blocks or sections, with a release of enzymes. Diffusion of hydrolytic enzymes can be minimized and localization improved if the tissue is treated with a fixative before cryotomy, although some enzyme loss will occur.

In practice, enzyme histochemical staining is often carried out on unfixed cryostat sections, especially in clinical circumstances where a delay in diagnosis is undesirable or different enzymes are required to be demonstrated in the same sample. However, localization of some enzymes may be improved by briefly fixing the tissue section after cryotomy.

If fixation is employed, the fixative should be at 4°C and used for the shortest time possible. Formol calcium is often recommended for tissue blocks as this helps maintain cell membrane integrity. Cryotomy and enzyme activity may be improved further by washing the fixed tissue in a sucrose buffer solution before freezing. For optimal results, it is important to keep these solutions close to physiological pH. A variety of fixatives, in addition to formol calcium, have been used on smears and cryostat sections, including acetone, formalin vapour, and formalin–alcohol mixtures. The choice of fixative depends on the particular enzyme investigated, and is a compromize between enzyme activity and morphological appearance. Even after short fixation times most oxidative enzymes are rendered inactive.

Tissue preparation

Several different methods are available for the examination of enzymes, but in this chapter only frozen sections, smears and paraffin wax-embedded sections are considered. As outlined previously the type of preparation employed is mainly determined by the enzymes required to be demonstrated.

Frozen sections

The most common specimen preparation in enzyme histochemistry is the use of frozen sections, usually cut with a cryostat. Tissue is required to be rapidly 'snap frozen' as slow freezing will causes ice crystal artefacts: faster freezing produces smaller ice crystals. Muscle biopsies which usually require diagnostic enzyme histochemistry samples, yet are very prone to ice crystal artefact. The most suitable method for freezing tissue is the use of isopentane that has been frozen with liquid nitrogen and allowed to partly thaw. The solid fraction acts as a thermal buffer keeping the temperature of the liquid fraction stable (–150°C) during freezing of the tissue. The tissue (fixed or unfixed) is orientated on a cork disc in OCT gel and immersed in the thawing isopentane until the gel and specimen freezes. The cork is attached similarly to the block holder using OCT and then placed inside the cryostat ready for sectioning at –23°C. Liquid nitrogen alone should not be used, as it has a low rate of thermal conductivity producing a gaseous thermal barrier around the tissue.

Smears

Smears may be prepared by various means from blood, bone marrow and tissue cell sus-

pensions. Imprint smears of tissue, e.g. lymph nodes, are also useful where fresh tissue is cut and the new surface touched gently against a clean glass slide. Smears are air-dried and usually lightly fixed (depending on the enzymes required) for a few seconds before cytochemical staining of the cells.

Paraffin wax sections

Most enzymes will not withstand the effects of standard paraffin wax-processing and therefore this mode of preparation is not often useful. Peroxidase and chloroacetate esterase are however sufficiently hardy to survive routine paraffin wax-embedding and may easily be shown. Some other enzymes may partly be preserved using a specialized schedule with waxes of a low melting point but this is seldom used.

Histochemical Techniques

These histological methods are unique in that the enzymes are never stained, only the reaction products are demonstrated. For meaningful results careful optimization of the enzyme reaction and colouring of the reaction product is essential.

The process involves cleavage of a substrate by the tissue-bound enzyme to form a primary reaction product (PRP). This PRP can then react with a chemical known as a 'capture agent', to form a final reaction product (FRP), which should be insoluble at the site of the enzyme.

Numerous factors influence the reactions and all must be carefully controlled. The pH of the incubating solutions is critical for most enzyme reactions and is maintained using suitable buffers. Temperature can be used to alter the enzyme reaction rate, with some methods requiring incubation at 37°C, while others are performed at room temperature. This lower temperature gives time for completion of FRP formation with the PRP and capture agent, by decreasing the enzyme reaction rate. Substrates and capture agents should be chosen to prevent interactions and both should be readily diffusible across cell membranes. Both substrate and capture agent should be used at a concentration that would prevent local depletion

27

<u>Histochemical Techniques</u>
Enzyme reaction methods
Demonstration methods

during rapid enzyme activity, but not at a concentration that would inhibit the enzyme reaction. The selection of a capture agent is dependent upon the enzyme method used and the type of tissue in which the enzyme is found. For example, when using the metal precipitation method on muscle, the calcium salt is preferred to the lead salt as the latter can bind non-specifically with the muscle. Often there is also a choice of substrates, but many naturally-occurring substrates, although cheap, may be non-specific or produce PRPs that are not totally insoluble. Specially synthesized substrates usually produce superior results.

It is important to include positive control tissue during histochemical staining so that the quality of the reagents and the accuracy of the protocol employed can be assessed. Omission of the substrate from the incubating medium or the inclusion of specific inhibitors will act as a negative control.

Enzyme reaction methods
In histopathology, most enzymes are demonstrated using either simultaneous coupling or post-incubation coupling.

Simultaneous coupling
Simultaneous coupling requires only one solution containing both the substrate and a capturing agent, with the required co-factors. The tissue-bound enzyme reacts with the substrate in solution to produce a PRP. Here the PRP may be either insoluble or soluble as the capture agent, also in solution, binds with the PRP instantaneously to form an FRP. This insoluble FRP is bound to the enzyme site and may be coloured or colourless, although the latter would require an additional colouring step for visualization.

Post-incubation coupling
Occasionally it is not possible to have the substrate and capturing agent in one solution, as the conditions required for PRP production may be different from those required for FRP production. Sometimes the capturing agent may also interfere with or inhibit the enzyme function. In post-incubation coupling methods, the initial solution only contains the substrate

and any co-factors required. The PRP produced must be insoluble as false negatives or gross diffusion of the FRP will occur. A secondary solution which contains the capture agent is then applied to produce the FRP as above. In practice it is difficult to find suitable substrates for post-incubation coupling methods, with a result that simultaneous coupling is more popular.

Demonstration methods
The coloured FRPs are normally produced by one of the following methods: metal precipitation; azo-dye; tetrazolium salt; indigogenic method.

Other methods include: the oxidation of 3,3′-diaminobenzidine (DAB) by cytochrome oxidase or the peroxidases to form a brown pigment; the metabolism of glycogen by phosphorylase to produce a polysaccharide that is coloured blue-black with iodine.

Metal precipitation methods
Metal precipitation methods are used routinely to identify phosphatases, e.g. acid phosphatase, alkaline phosphatase, and adenosine triphosphatase (ATPase). The PRP in these cases is phosphate ions released from the substrate which that reacts with lead or calcium salts in solution (capture agent), to form the insoluble FRP of lead or calcium phosphate.

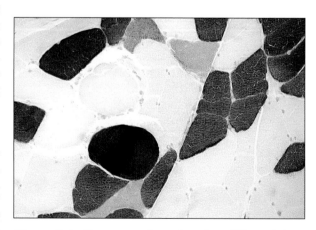

Figure 3.1: *Frozen sections showing differential staining of muscle fibres stained for ATPase at pH 4.2 with a metal precipitation technique.*

Lead phosphate is colourless, but is blackened with ammonium sulphide solution to form lead sulphide. Calcium phosphate is soluble at alkaline pH and needs to be converted to cobalt phosphate with cobalt chloride solution (which is insoluble at alkaline pH), before treating with ammonium sulphide to form the black pigment of cobalt sulphide. Both of these methods are liable to fade with time but may be recoloured with ammonium sulphide.

The acetylcholinesterase method, using the substrate acetylthiocholine, can be regarded as a metal precipitate method that produces a PRP of thiocholine, which reacts with copper sulphate and potassium ferricyanide respectively to form the brown pigment of copper ferrocyanide.

Azo-dye methods

The azo-dye methods are used to identify acid and alkaline phosphatases, non-specific esterase and chloroacetate esterase. The different substrates contain a naphthol group that can be cleaved by one of the above enzymes. Various diazonium salts or freshly hexazotized pararosaniline are used, which react with the naphthol group to form a coloured insoluble azodye. Typically the diazonium salts used include Fast Red TR, Fast Blue RR, Fast Blue B and Fast Garnet GBC, which have to be aqueously mounted. The azo-dye formed from the hexazotized pararosaniline is the method of choice, as it can be mounted in a synthetic resin which improves localization at light microscopy. Diazonium salts may be used with either simultaneous or post-incubation coupling methods.

Tetrazolium salt methods

Tetrazolium salts are colourless, water-soluble salts that accept enzymatically released hydrogen from the substrate to form highly coloured, water-insoluble microcrystalline deposits known as formazans. Many oxidative enzymes such as succinic dehydrogenase are demonstrated using tetrazolium salts, such as methylthiazolyldiphenyl tetrazolium (MTT) and nitro blue tetrazolium (NBT). As with diazonium salts, several factors influence their selection,

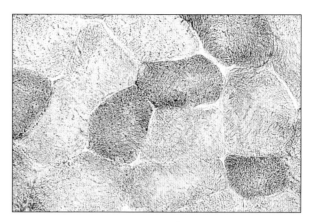

Figure 3.2: *Frozen section of muscle stained for NADH diaphorase using the tetrazolium salt MTT.*

but NBT is often used in preference to MTT as it can be mounted in a synthetic resin.

Indigogenic method

The various substrates contain an indoxyl group which is released as a PRP, which in turn is oxidized by the capture agent potassium ferricyanide to form a turquoise FRP. The incubation solution also includes potassium ferrocyanide which prevents over-oxidation of the FRP.

Main Diagnostic Applications

The use of enzyme histochemistry in diagnostic pathology has several important applications, which may be summarized as follows: pathology of skeletal muscle; gastrointestinal tissue to assess malabsorption; nerves and ganglia in suspected Hirschsprung's disease; lymphoid and myeloid cell identification.

Skeletal muscle

The use of enzyme histochemistry in the diagnosis of neuromuscular diseases and congenital myopathies has become firmly established, with many histopathological appearances only recognized and described after the introduction of enzyme histochemistry.

<u>Main Diagnostic Applications</u>

Gastrointestinal tissue to assess malabsorption

Nerves and ganglia in suspected Hirschsprung's disease

Traditional tinctorial staining of striated muscle is sufficient to show inflammatory responses and variation in fibre size, but is unable to differentiate between the various muscle fibre types. This is important as many disease processes are confined to, or show alteration of, specific muscle fibre types. This can be in the form of atrophy, hypo or hyperplasia, and in certain diseases alteration of the internal cellular structure. The application of enzyme histochemical methods on transversely cut skeletal muscle enables several different fibre types to be distinguished, which in conjunction with examining their distribution and size, can assist in diagnosis.

Striated muscle fibres may broadly be divided into Type 1 and Type 2 depending on the level of myofibrillar ATPase activity shown at pH 9.4. If the ATPase staining is applied after pre-incubating in a buffer at pH 3.2 or 3.6, further differentiation of Type 2 fibres into subtypes 2A, 2B and 2C may be achieved. Another useful enzyme to demonstrate is phosphorylase which in McArdle's disease is deficient, but its presence in smooth muscle of blood vessels is unaffected and serves as a useful inherent control. NADH diaphorase is used to study the internal structure of muscle cells as it demonstrates mitochondria and the sarcoplasmic reticulum network. When this is compared with the myofibrillar distribution shown by ATPase, various pathological conditions may become apparent. Abnormal enzyme distribution patterns are often described in terms of their appearances that are specific to a particular disease entity, such as 'target fibres', 'ring fibres', and 'central cores'. Cytochrome oxidase, succinic dehydrogenase, and lactate dehydrogenase are more specific for mitochondria and may prove helpful in identifying mitochondrial myopathies. A summary of the differential enzyme staining of skeletal muscle is shown in Table 3.1.

Gastrointestinal tissue to assess malabsorption
To achieve a definitive diagnosis on gastrointestinal biopsies where malabsorption is suspected, morphological information alone is insufficient. Various enzymes on the brush border of villi are useful, but the disacchari-

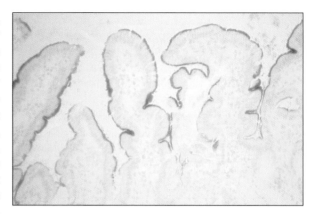

Figure 3.3: Frozen section of jejunum showing lactase activity on the micro villi stained turquoise using the indigogenic method.

dases lactase and sucrase are particularly important. These enzymes reflect changes to enterocyte injury; lactase is the most sensitive whereas sucrase is the most resistant and therefore histochemical staining for these two diasaccharidases is helpful. These methods can also be used to detect primary lactase or sucrase deficiencies.

Acid phosphatase, found in the lysosomes of enterocytes and in macrophages in the lamina propria, may also be a useful enzyme to demonstrate when considering malabsorption. To assess and monitor malabsorption properly, jejunum is required to be orientated so that the villi are sectioned longitudinally.

Nerves and ganglia in suspected Hirschsprung's disease
In normal colon and rectum, ganglion cells and associated nerves are present which are responsible for colonic motility. In Hirschsprung's disease in children there is an absence of ganglia from between the circular and longitudinal smooth muscle junction (myenteric plexus) and in the submucosa. There is also a marked increase in the number and thickening of non-argyrophilic nerve fibres in the submucosa and the lamina propria. These ganglion cells and nerve fibres contain cholinesterase and may be demonstrated using the acetylcholinesterase method. Identification is normally required to confirm the initial diagnosis

Table 3.1: Diagnostic enzyme histochemistry.

Tissue	Enzyme	Method	Substrate	pH	Colour	Demonstrates

Striated muscle	Myofibrillar ATPase	• Metal precipitation (calcium chloride)
		• Metal precipitation (calcium chloride) preincubation @ pH 4.6
		• Metal precipitation (calcium chloride) preincubation @ pH 4.2
			Adenosine triphosphate (ATP)	9.4	Black/brown	• Type 1 fibres – pale
						  Type 2a & 2b & 2c fibres – dark
						• Type 1 – dark
						  Type 2b & 2c fibres – intermediate
						  Type 2a fibres – pale
						• Type 1 fibres – dark
						  Type 2c fibres – intermediate
						  Type 2a & 2b fibres – pale

	NADH diaporase	Tetrazolium salt (MTT)	NADH	7.0	Black	Mitochondria (Type 1 fibres – darker) Sarcoplasmic reticulum
	Succinic dehydrogenase	Tetrazolium salt (MTT)	Sodium succinate	7.0	Black	Mitochondria (Type 1 fibres – darker) for mitochondrial abnormalities
	Cytochrome oxidase	Oxidation of DAB	Cytochrome C	7.4	Brown	
	Myophosphorylase	Metabolism of glycogen (iodine)	Glucose-1-phosphate	5.9	Purple/black	Negative staining muscle fibres in McArdle's disease
	Myoadenylate deaminase	Tetrazolium salt (NBT)	Adenosine 5-monophosphate (AMP)	6.1	Blue	Absent in some metabolic disorders
	Aldolase		Disodium fructose 1,6-diphosphate	8.6		
	Phosphofructokinase		Fructose 6-phosphate	7.0		
Nerves	Acetylcholinesterase	Potassium ferricyanide – copper sulphate reaction (metal precipitation)	Acetylthiocholine iodide	6.0	Red/brown	Nerve fibres & cells in colon (Hirschsprung's) and muscle diseases
Jejunum	Lactase	Indigogenic method (potassium ferricyanide)	5-Bromo-4-chloro-3-indoxyl-β-D-fucoside	6.0	Turquoise	Reduced or negative with malabsorption
	Sucrase	Azo dye (pararosaniline)	6-Bromo-2-naphthyl-α-D-glucoside	6.0	Red	

Main Diagnostic Applications
Lymphoid and myeloid cells

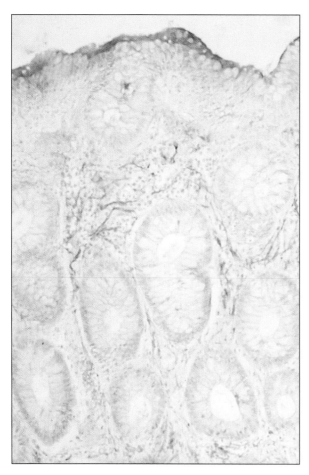

Figure 3.4: Frozen section of rectal tissue with Hirschsprung's disease, stained for acetylcholinesterase demonstrating the thickened nerve fibres.

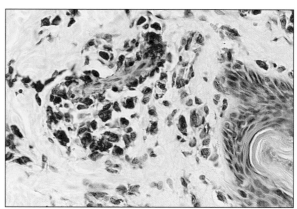

Figure 3.5: Paraffin wax section of skin showing mast cells in the dermis stained red for chloroacetate esterase using naphthol AS-D chloroacetate and hexazonium pararosaniline.

and at a later stage the resection boundaries during removal of the abnormal bowel. As this is performed during surgery using small rectal suction biopsies, speed is important. Cryostat H&E stained sections are usually sufficient to detect the absence or presence of the large ganglion cells. Inadequate biopsies do not have to be discarded, as the acetylcholinesterase method is able to show the abnormal nerve fibres in the lamina propria.

Lymphoid and myeloid cells
Several enzymes including non-specific esterase, acid phosphatase, and chloroacetate esterase

Table 3.2: Enzyme histochemical staining for white blood cells.

Enzyme	Method	Substrate	pH	Colour	Comments
Chloroacetate esterase	Azo dye (pararosaniline)	Naphthol AS-D chloroacetate	6.3	Red	Mast cells stain first followed by eosinophils and neutrophils
Acid phosphatase	Azo dye (pararosaniline)	Naphthol AS-B1 phosphate	5.0	Red	Monocytes stain diffusely; T-cells have a single focal spot
Alkaline phosphatase	Azo dye (Fast Red TR)		8.0	Red	Neutrophils
Non-specific esterase	Azo dye (pararosaniline)	α-Naphthyl acetate	7.6	Red	Monocytes

are used for the cytochemical identification and evaluation of cells in smear preparations, as shown in Table 3.2. In addition to enzyme activity, specific cells may be differentiated by their staining pattern, i.e. focal or diffuse. Immunohistochemistry is now the method of choice for identifying these cells in histopathology, but many haematology departments still use the enzyme histochemical methods. Chloroacetate esterase, which as mentioned previously survives paraffin wax-embedding, can distinguish between lymphoid and myeloid cells as the former are not demonstrated. Mast cells are recognized easily by their strong staining, morphology and granularity.

Conclusion

Enzyme histochemistry still plays a vital role in histopathology, especially in the detection and diagnosis of muscle disease. It is also used routinely as a detection system in immuno-cytochemistry and molecular biology. The formazan method for succinic dehydrogenase has been used successfully on fresh macro heart slices to identify infarction on post-mortem tissue. In research, a much wider range of enzymes is studied, using diverse techniques such as electron microscopy and flow cytometry, in addition to light microscopy.

Further Reading

Bancroft J D. Enzyme histochemistry. In: *Theory and Practice of Histological Techniques*, 4th edn 1996: Eds Bancroft J D, Stevens A. Churchill-Livingstone, London, pp. 391–410.

Bancroft J D, Hand N M. *Enzyme Histochemistry*. RMS microscopy handbook No. 14, 1987: Oxford University Press.

Filipe M I, Lake B D. *Histochemistry in Pathology*, 2nd edn 1990: Churchill-Livingstone, Edinburgh.

Hayhoe F G J, Quaglino D. *Haematological Cytochemistry*, 2nd edn 1988: Churchill-Livingstone, Edinburgh.

Stevens A, Palmer J B. Enzyme histochemistry: diagnostic applications. In: *Theory and Practice of Histological Techniques*, 4th edn 1996: Eds Bancroft J D, Stevens A. Churchill-Livingstone, London, pp. 411–420.

4 IMMUNOHISTOCHEMISTRY

John Crocker

Introduction

In terms of normal function and of disease states, study of the simple morphology of sections or cells is generally sufficient for analysis. As described in Chapters 3, 5 and 8, ancillary techniques, such as histochemistry, enzyme histochemistry and electron microscopy may be most helpful in understanding further the nature and functional state of a cell or tissue type. However, in the 1970s it became apparent that more detailed assessment of the products of cell function was both necessary and possible. In histopathology, the advent of immunohistochemistry (IHC) was exciting and opened large new vistas in the investigation of biopsy and surgical excision specimens. The principle which underlies all IHC is that of demonstrating antigen by means of its binding to an antibody which, in turn, is linked to a molecule which can be visualized histologically. Thus, the site of the antigen in question is highlighted.

IHC methods can conveniently be classified into three main groups, namely: direct, indirect and complex, and range from those visualized in ultraviolet light to those which are chromogenic. In addition, particulate material, such as heavy metal, may be used at both the light and electron microscope levels.

Direct methods

In these, antibody directed against a certain molecule or part of a molecule (epitope) is bound to a section. The antibody has its 'reporter agent' bound to it and the antigen is thus visualized directly. The method is relatively insensitive in that there is no 'amplification' of the antigenic signal involved. The direct technique has largely been abandoned, although it is still used where chimaeric 'humanized' genetically engineered antibodies are used against human tissue sites.

Indirect methods

The indirect methods involve a further layer of antibody to demonstrate the antigen con-

Introduction

Multi-stage methods

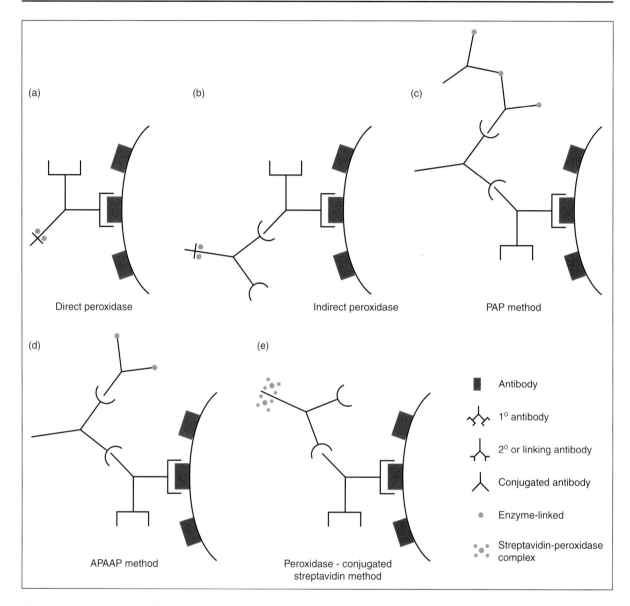

(a)
Direct peroxidase

(b)
Indirect peroxidase

(c)
PAP method

(d)
APAAP method

(e)
Peroxidase - conjugated
streptavidin method

- ▪ Antibody
- ⋎ 1° antibody
- ⋏ 2° or linking antibody
- ⋏ Conjugated antibody
- ● Enzyme-linked
- ∴ Streptavidin-peroxidase complex

Figure 4.1: *Schematic diagram to show some of the more commonly used IHC sequences. These are of varying complexities and sensitivities.*

cerned. This is illustrated classically by the build-up of layers of antibodies directed against antigens of differing species specificity, giving an 'inverted cone' of molecules, thus amplifying the original signal greatly. Thus, for example, rabbit anti-human antigen as the first step is further reacted with, say, swine anti-rabbit antibody. This gives greater sensitivity than direct methods but, again, has been overtaken to a large extent by more complex sequences.

Multi-stage methods

Examples of this range of methods are illustrated by the peroxidase–antiperoxidase (PAP) and alkaline phosphatase–anti-alkaline phosphatase (APAAP) techniques. Variants are also encountered in sequences using complexing of other molecules bound to the antibodies concerned. In all of these reactions the signal sensitivity is much greater than in direct and indirect techniques, the 'inverted cone' of amplification being much greater with multilayering of molecules. Figure 4.1 summarizes the main sequence types used in IHC.

Reporter and Linkage Molecules

To be able to visualize the antigen, albeit indirectly, it is necessary to give a visual signal to localize the binding site in the cells or tissues. Accordingly, a range of 'reporter' systems has been developed over the years. These are described, more or less chronologically, below.

Fluorescent molecules

The original reporter was the fluorescent dye, fluorescein, tagged to the appropriate antibody. The antigen could then be visualized by means of a microscope using ultraviolet light (see Chapter 6). One of the main problems with this method is that the fluorescence is quenched by various molecules; furthermore, it gradually fades on exposure to daylight. (However, it should be noted that the antigenic rather than fluorescent properties of fluorescein have recently been used to good effect in IHC.) Other fluorescent molecules, such as rhodamine (which gives a red colour in contrast to the green fluorescence of fluorescein) have been utilized, especially in double-labelling reactions (see below) to demonstrate two different antigens in the same sample. Immunofluorescence has relatively limited use in the diagnostic laboratory today but is still seen in the assessment of renal and skin biopsies, perhaps because the material lends itself to the demonstration of linear or membranous antigen (Fig. 4.2).

Fluorescent labelling is said, perhaps anecdotally, to be more sensitive than other methods but this may not be true with the advent of techniques such as the avidin–biotin complex sequence (or tyramide signal amplification).

Peroxidase

Horseradish peroxidase (HRP) is an extraordinarily well-suited molecule for the investigation of human disease. Firstly it is not of mammalian origin, being derived, of course, from a plant! This means that the chances of antigenic

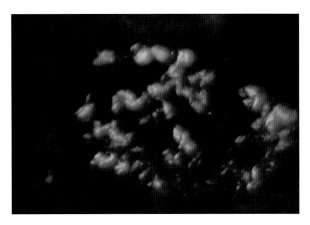

Figure 4.2: A photomicrograph of a glomerulus from a renal biopsy. The patient had IgA glomerulopathy and delicate immunostaining can be seen in this frozen section, reacted for IgA (fluorescent green).

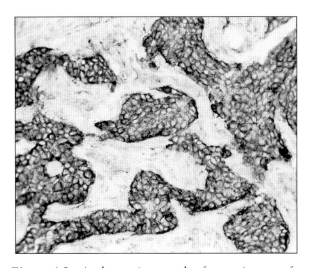

Figure 4.3: A photomicrograph of a carcinoma of the lung, showing a positive reaction with a monoclonal antibody to cytokeratins 8/18, by means of the ABC method.

cross-reaction are lessened; however, it must be noted that the enzymatic activity of HRP is similar to that in mammals and this can cause problems when the enzyme is demonstrated in tissues or cells (see below). Secondly, it can be demonstrated readily by virtue of its chemically stable brown product when reacted with the substrate 3,3′-diaminobenzidine (DAB) in the presence of hydrogen peroxide. Finally, it is a

Reporter and Linkage Molecules

Alkaline phosphatase

Gold–silver

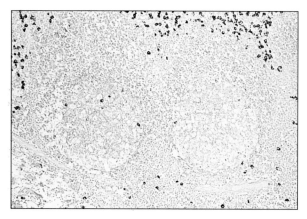

Figure 4.4: A photomicrograph of a paraffin section palatine tonsil, reacted with a monoclonal antibody to κ Ig light chain. The careful application of the sensitive ABC method has enabled the demonstration of both surface and cytoplasmic Ig.

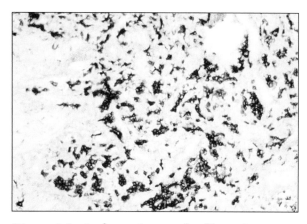

Figure 4.5: A photomicrograph of lung tissue stained with a monoclonal antibody to CD68, showing intense red positivity of alveolar macrophages by means of the APAAP method.

molecule which can be used at the ultrastructural level.

HRP-labelling has been used in direct, indirect and multi-stage techniques. For some years, the mainstay of histopathology laboratories was the indirect, peroxidase–antiperoxidase (PAP) method. However, this has probably been overtaken generally by the more 'amplifying' avidin–biotin complex (ABC) technique (Figs 4.3 and 4.4).

A problem with the use of HRP lies in the presence of peroxidatic activity endogenous to human and other tissues, which will lead to a positive reaction with, for example, DAB. Fortunately, this activity can largely be blocked by pre-treatment of sections with certain reagents, notably hydrogen peroxide or hydrochloric acid in methanol. Even when this is done, certain cells, notably neutrophil polymorphs and mast cells, which are very rich in peroxidase, may still give false-positive results.

Alkaline phosphatase

Alkaline phosphatase (AP) is another enzyme which has widespread use in IHC, especially in cell preparations. This latter is largely because of the high sensitivity of the resulting alkaline phosphatase–anti-alkaline phosphatase (APAAP) interaction. AP can give vivid colour reaction products (Fig. 4.5) with certain substrates but in general these suffer from the problem that, unlike (say) the DAB reaction product, they are not stable in ethanol (and such reagents as xylene and ethanol, etc.). This means that sections must be mounted in aqueous media, which are are non-permanent. Again, there may be problems with endogenous tissue alkaline phosphatase but this may be blocked with certain agents, such as levamisole.

Gold–silver

Antibodies can be bound to fine, uniform aggregates of the element gold and this will in turn react with silver from argentous compounds, by virtue of differing electropositivity. This gives a very sensitive reaction sequence which found extensive use at the light microscope level in the mid 1980s, when it was used in some studies as a labelling method for certain low-expression epitopes, such as those on cell surfaces (Fig. 4.6). It must be stated, however, that the method never found widespread diagnostic application and generally remained as a research tool. Furthermore, it has largely been replaced by the avidin–biotin complex (ABC) series of methods. However, a major use of immunogold technique lies in the field of immuno-electron microscopy, where metallic particles can be seen to localize on antigenic sites (Fig. 4.7); indeed, it is possible to demonstrate more than one antigen in the same preparation by using antibodies linked to gold particles of different sizes.

IMMUNOHISTOCHEMISTRY

Avidin–biotin

Newer methods

Non-specific Antibody Binding

Antigen Retrieval Methods

Enzyme pre-treatment

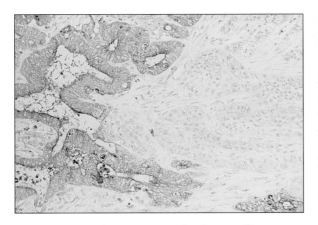

Figure 4.6: A photomicrograph of a paraffin section of colonic carcinoma, reacted with a monoclonal antibody to carcinoembryonic antigen (CEA), demonstrated by means of the immunogold–silver (IGSS) technique. The surface CEA is seen as a thin black line on the cancer cell surfaces.

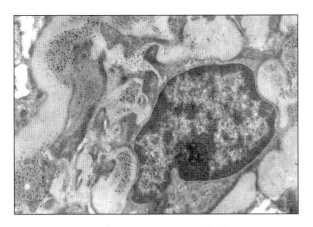

Figure 4.7: An electron micrograph showing tiny black dots of gold lying over the glomerular mesangium and basement membrane. This is, as in Fig. 5.2, a case of IgA nephropathy and the primary antibody was directed against IgA. The photograph was given kindly by Dr G R Newman, Medical Microscopy Sciences, University of Wales College of Medicine, Heath Park, Cardiff.

Avidin–biotin

Although neither biotin nor avidin is used as a chromogen proper, they have found much application as an intermediate stage in high-amplification and sensitivity methods, such as ABC. Avidin (or streptavidin) and biotin have an exquisitely high level of mutual binding and can be used to bridge between different layers in IHC. The secondary antibody is generally biotinylated and avidin (or streptavidin) is conjugated to, say, HRP or AP in the third layer, forming the complex. The ABC method has found widespread use in research and diagnostic laboratories and is probably the standard in most at present (Figs 4.3 and 4.4).

Newer methods

As described above, fluorescein has found favour recently as a coupling reagent, not by virtue of its fluorescence but as antigen: this molecule has the obvious advantage that it clearly does not have a human analogue!

Another novel method involves the use of tyramine and gives very striking signal amplification, up to 10^3 times greater than other methods. In this system, HRP acts as a catalyst in the deposition of tyramide, bound to fluorochrome or biotin in direct or indirect sequences respectively.

Non-specific Antibody Binding

Readers should note that primary antibodies may bind non-specifically to tissue sections, largely by means of their Fc fractions. The problem is much more likely to occur with polyclonal than monoclonal reagents. This can generally be overcome by means of blocking with the appropriate non-immune serum.

Antigen Retrieval Methods

Enzyme pre-treatment

In the late 1970s it was found that immunostaining could often be enhanced by pre-treatment of sections with certain proteolytic enzymes, such as pronase or trypsin. The precise basis for such processes is uncertain but it is assumed that certain antigenic groups are 'unmasked' biochemically by removal of obscuring side-chains resulting from fixation, enabling access of the primary antibody. The enzymes are highly lytic and 'titration' prior to regular use is essential to avoid tissue disruption.

Microwave pre-treatment

In the 1990s it became apparent that certain epitopes could conveniently be unmasked by the use of controlled microwave irradiation of tissue sections in aqueous media. As with enzyme pre-treatment, the mechanism behind the success of microwaves is far from clear; nonetheless, this technique has found very wide application in the last few years. Like enzyme methods, microwave treatment not only in some cases improves visualization of certain antigens but may also enable detection when *none* was possible before. As with enzyme treatment, titration of microwave timing is necessary.

Another recent development has been the use of pressure-cooking of sections to improve immunostaining. This is presumably rather more hazardous than the careful use of microwave ovens! (Note, however, that it is now possible to obtain plastic pressure cookers to use in microwave ovens.)

Controls

It is most important to set up certain essential controls before testing any new antibody and, ideally, at least some of these constraints should be applied on a day-to-day diagnostic basis. *Positive controls* involve the inclusion of sections known to have elements reactive with the antibody in question. This is the most important and regularly used control in everyday diagnostic IHC. It is useful sometimes to prepare a composite paraffin wax-embedded tissue block containing an assortment of small pieces of known positive controls and mounted on the same slide as the test section. This enables the pathologist to see both positively and negatively stained structures at the same time.

When a new antibody or antiserum is being evaluated prior to diagnostic or research use, a range of more rigorous controls is required. The stringency of this field is potentially substantial but the important constraints here include: blocking with the pure antigen/epitope (affinity purification); omission of the 1° anti-body or further antibodies in the sequence and application of the chromogenic reaction alone. Such controls check for the specificity of 1° antibody binding and the need for its presence in a positive reaction result.

Dual Labelling Methods

It is often important to be able to demonstrate more than one antigen or epitope in a particular cell or tissue. An example lies in the demonstration of κ and λ light chains in an individual lymphocytoid cell. The question asked is, of course, 'Is it a section of benign or malignant lymphoid tissue?' The exhibition of monoclonality in or on cells from a section must in everyday terms indicate malignancy, and the ability to demonstrate or fail to demonstrate this will influence patient management. To demonstrate more than one antigen or epitope, chromogenic substrates of different hues are used and the preparation assessed accordingly (Fig. 4.8). IHC can also be combined with other techniques, such as the AgNOR method (see Chapter 8), conventional histochemistry and *in situ* molecular reactions (Fig. 4.9).

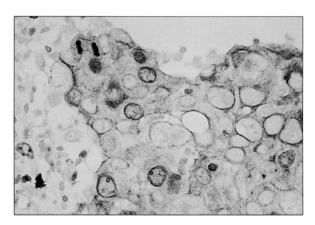

Figure 4.8: A photomicrograph double-stained to show both cytokeratin (blue, cell membrane) and Ki67 epitope (brown, nuclear) expression in a lymphoepithelioma. The photograph was given kindly by Miss Jane Oates, Department of Histopathology, Birmingham Heartlands Hospital.

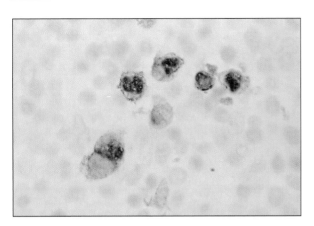

Figure 4.9: *A photomicrograph of a section of Hodgkin's disease tissue, double-stained by means of an immunohistochemical reaction for Epstein–Barr viral latent membrane protein (mauve, cytoplasmic) and by means of* in situ *hybridization for EBERs (brown, nuclear). The photograph was kindly given by Jane Oates, Department of Histopathology, Birmingham Heartlands Hospital.*

Polyclonal Versus Monoclonal Antibodies

The early work on IHC was performed using ployclonal antisera, raised in mammals against antigenic preparations. These antisera were polytypic and thus tended to give staining patterns which were often not 'clean' on sections, with binding of different constituent antibodies to rather variable microscopic sites. With the advent of monoclonal antibodies, far 'cleaner' and more specific localization of epitopes was possible and thus better delineation of cell and tissue species. The method of affinity purification, where the polyclonal antibody was run through a column containing the target antigen, bound to matrix, improved the specificity of the reagents.

A major early problem, however, was that unlike many polyclonal antibodies, most monoclonal antibodies could not successfully be applied to routine, archival paraffin wax-embedded sections. Accordingly, most early studies depended upon the availability of frozen section material, with its relatively poor morphological preservation. Nowadays, however, with the advent of higher affinity monoclonal antibodies, many can successfully be applied to paraffin sections, especially following the use of antigen retrieval methods. Nonetheless, frozen sections may still offer an advantage over paraffin sections in that the former can offer better visualization of *surface* antigens.

Applications of Immunohistochemistry

It would be far beyond the scope and intent of this book to give a comprehensive account of the myriad applications of IHC in the diagnostic laboratory. In brief, this technology has enabled us to distinguish between lymphomas and small cell carcinomas, melanomas and seminomas, mesotheliomas and adenocarcinomas, and B- and T-cell lymphomas. Furthermore, we can identify microorganisms as far-ranging as cytomegalovirus to toxoplasma and, as discussed in Chapter 8, we can assess cell proliferation state. In addition, hormones, hormone receptors, growth factors, adhesion molecules and oncogene products can be demonstrated by IHC, as can ligands for certain molecules. Some examples of the applications of the use of IHC are given in Table 4.1. As a caveat, however, it must be stressed that shared epitopes do not necessarily indicate shared lineages. For example, the Reed–Sternberg cells of Hodgkin's disease and adenocarcinoma cells both express CD15, yet it is not suggested that these cell types are of common lineage!

Quality Control

In today's world of tightening laboratory standards, external quality control as well as routine internal surveillance are highly desirable. In general, the external system depends on the assessment of staining of selected antigens by the target laboratory. The specimens are a combina-

Quality Control

Automation

Table 4.1: Some examples of diagnostic uses of monoclonal and polyclonal antibodies in histopathology.

CD designation	Example clone or name of target antigen	Target cell
CD3		T-cells
CD20	L26	B-cells
CD79a		B-cells
CD30	BerH2	Reed–Sternberg/Hodgkin cells
CD68		Histiocytes
CD45RA	Leukocyte common antigen (LCA)	White cells in general
—	Cytokeratins	Epithelial cells
—	Epithelial membrane (EMA)	Epithelial cells; some histiocytes; some Reed–Sternberg/Hodgkin cells
—	S-100 protein	Melanocytes; neural and neuroendocrine cells; some histiocytes
—	Ig light chains	Clonality of B-cells
—	Chromogranin A	Neuroendocrine cells
—	Oestrogen receptors	Status of breast carcinoma for therapy
—	Ki67	Cell proliferation state

tion of straightforward cases and of sections where more difficulty may be expected (for example, the staining of surface Ig light chains on antigen-presenting cells). This sort of quality control is related to pathological cases but an equally important type of control, probably in wider use at present, lies in the specific testing of the ability to detect antigens. This should enable workers to improve and standardize their technique in the light of peer review.

their predecessors but are microprocessor-controlled, programmable to the user's requirements and enable the processing, in some instances, of sections simultaneously with others undergoing different types of staining. Figure 4.10 shows a typical modern automated immunostaining device.

Automation

Immunohistochemistry came into the arena of automation relatively late. This was probably because initially relatively few antibodies were available that were suitable for routine use. Recently, however, any busy laboratory will have a large panel of reagents being applied to numerous sections in any diagnostic run and the call for automation has risen. The earlier devices were semi-automated and largely served to save time, manipulation and reagent volumes by reducing, for example, the tedium of multiple buffer washes and so forth. Later, more automated machines have come onto the market. These are much more expensive than

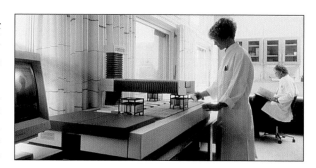

Figure 4.10: An illustration of an automated immunostainer, capable of staining many slides, in many procedures, at any one time. The photograph was given kindly by Sharon Law, on behalf of DAKO Ltd, High Wycombe, Bucks.

Acknowledgement

I am most grateful to Miss Janine Clover for reading this chapter and for her creative comments.

Further Reading

Jasani B, Schmid K. *Immunohistochemistry in Diagnostic Histochemistry*. 1993: Churchill-Livingstone, Edinburgh, London.

Leong S-Y. *Applied Immunohistochemistry for the Surgical Pathologist*. 1993: Edward Arnold, London, Boston, Melbourne, Auckland.

Newman G R, Hobot J A. *Resin Microscopy and On-Section Immunocytochemistry*. 1993: Springer-Verlag, Berlin, Heidelberg, New York.

Polak JM, Van Noorden S. Introduction to Immunocyto-chemistry. 1997; Bios Scientific Publishers Ltd, Oxford.

Most of the major pathology journals publish numerous papers, either wholly or partly involving IHC in each issue. Such journals include: *The Journal of Pathology, Histopathology, The Journal of Clinical Pathology, Molecular Pathology, Human Pathology, Modern Pathology, The American Pathology* and *The American Journal of Pathology*.

5 ELECTRON MICROSCOPY IN PATHOLOGY

C H Stuart Cameron and Peter G Toner

Introduction

Morphological examination is at the centre of tissue diagnosis, the pathologist traditionally combining gross description with an interpretation of the microscopic appearances, to reach a definitive diagnosis. Cancer therapy relies upon a precise microscopically verified diagnosis, which is fundamental to rational medical and surgical care. While light microscopy remains the foundation of histological diagnosis, newer technologies such as immunohistochemistry, electron microscopy (EM) and molecular and cytogenetic studies can now provide additional information and further refinement of disease classifications. Electron microscopy bridges the gap between light microscopy and the domain of molecular organization.

The importance of diagnostic electron microscopy, or ultrastructural pathology, is widely recognized by pathologists and clinicians in most major medical centres. Most modern specialist texts on pathology record the ultrastructural features of key conditions. Specialist handbooks on the diagnostic applications of electron microscopy are also widely available, along with monographs and other material produced by groups such as the Ultrapath Society, Eurocell Path, the Clinical Electron Microscopy Society of Japan and the Australian Society for Electron Microscopy. The continuing activities of these specialist groups leave one in no doubt that ultrastructural pathology is alive and well.

The extent to which EM is used in a routine diagnostic department is partly determined by the expertise and facilities available. There are those who argue that electron microscopy is now of little practical relevance in tissue diagnosis, particularly in relation to soft tissue tumours, where immunohistochemistry and molecular genetics are claimed to be more efficient and cost effective. Others, however, have suggested that EM can be more helpful and cost effective than immunohistochemistry in diagnostically challenging tumours. Our own experience and that of others is that EM can contribute to diagnosis to a greater or lesser extent in up to 5% of cases, depending upon the range of tissues received and the particular interests and commitments within the pathology department.

Both electron microscopy and immunohistochemistry must be selectively applied to areas where they can be most rewarding; these two techniques for phenotypic analysis should be seen as complementary rather than competitive. The areas where electron microscopy can most often and most effectively be deployed by pathologists are summarized in Table 5.1.

Table 5.1:	The place of electron microscopy in pathology.
Diagnosis	• establishing or redefining diagnostic criteria
	• identifying poorly differentiated neoplasms
	• refining tumour classification
	• correlating tumour ultrastructure with biological behaviour
	• identifying specific subcellular changes in non-neoplastic disease
	• delineating new variants of neoplastic and non-neoplastic disease
Quality assurance	• monitoring of certain light-microscopic diagnoses
Research	• clinical research and trials
	• laboratory research on organs, tissues and cells
	• epidemiological studies
Education	• undergraduate education and basic vocational training
	• postgraduate medical education in histopathology and cytopathology
	• postgraduate research training

Technical Considerations

Ultrastructural pathology uses transmission electron microscopy (TEM) and to a lesser extent scanning electron microscopy (SEM) to determine specific subcellular features, or alterations to those features, which may be related to disease or subsequent treatment. Allied to basic morphology are the 'functional' techniques of X-ray microprobe analysis, immunocytochemistry, electron histochemistry and morphometric analysis. These additional techniques expand the scope of subcellular imaging by contributing additional data on cell differentiation at the molecular level.

The primary justification for electron microscopy is the barrier produced by the limitation of light microscopic resolution, which had been largely reached in routine practice by the end of the nineteenth century. The much smaller effective wavelength of electrons makes EM resolution of less than 0.3 nm attainable, compared to around 200 nm for the light microscope, thus in effect providing the pathologist with a new 'objective lens' for the study of tissue sections, up to a thousand times more powerful than the best light microscope.

With the transmission electron microscope, the electrons of the illuminating beam either pass directly through the specimen unhindered, or are deflected from their path by areas of varying electron density within the tissue section. The result is therefore a shadow image reflecting the various densities that exist within the specimen. In the scanning electron microscope, the beam of electrons is scanned in a square grid pattern, or raster, across the surface of the specimen and the emerging electrons are collected by a detector and converted to a topographical image which is viewed on a cathode ray tube. Surface scanning images have a three-dimensional quality due to the great depth of focus obtainable with this form of microscopy. Unlike the light microscope, electron images are not viewed directly, but are displayed on a fluorescent screen or cathode ray tube and then recorded on photographic film, or digitized and stored electronically.

Glutaraldehyde, a protein cross-linking dialdehyde, has remained the primary ultrastructural fixative of choice since 1963, but the practical pathologist cannot afford to be too perfectionist, particularly when examining soft tissue tumours. Many cases come retrospectively to electron microscopy and the pathologist can often supplement the histological appearances by selecting for EM the most suitable area within the retained formalin-fixed tissue. It is practicable to retrieve tissue from stored necropsy specimens and even paraffin blocks, although the quality of the results may be too poor for any but the most straightforward analysis. Techniques are also available which enable stained tissue sections and smear preparations to be retrieved from glass slides, though these are rather unrewarding

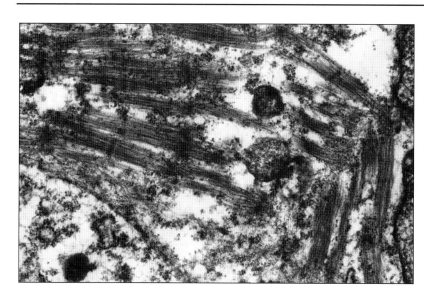

Figure 5.1: Aggregates of thick myosin filaments displaying sarcomeric organization with z-band formation are easily recognized within the cytoplasm of a tumour cell despite the tissue being retrieved from paraffin wax. A diagnosis of rhabdomyosarcoma was made on the basis of the EM findings in this oral biopsy from a 10-year-old boy. ×31 500.

generally. The pathologist must adapt to the technical imperfections of the available material and interpret the cellular appearances accordingly. Specific cellular features such as premelanosomes, neurosecretory granules, cytoplasmic filaments, microvilli and cell attachments usually survive reprocessing from paraffin wax in recognizable form, even though their preservation is poor (Fig. 5.1). If available, stored frozen tissue, which can then be fixed specifically for EM, is much superior to paraffin wax-retrieved tissue.

Such a pragmatic approach is less acceptable in cases where the diagnosis rests solely upon the identification of specific and often rather subtle fine structural alterations. Such examples would include disorders of cilia and cell metabolism or genetic disorders of skin involving keratinization or mechanobullous conditions. Biopsies from the central and peripheral nervous systems and from cardiac and skeletal muscle, as well as peripheral blood samples, usually require their fine structure to be optimally preserved by prompt primary glutaraldehyde fixation, if electron microscopy is to make a meaningful contribution to diagnosis.

Not all specimens come as solid tissue blocks. The electron microscopy laboratory must be familiar with a wide range of preparative methods to ensure that samples as diverse as cell aspirates, peripheral blood and other body fluids, nasal and bronchial brushings, as well as hair, nails and even faecal samples, are optimally prepared to answer the diagnostic question being posed.

The goal of a universal fixative suitable for both morphological and functional studies has been only partially met by the use of buffered formaldehyde; it is unlikely that the divergent needs of immunohistochemistry and electron microscopy can ever be fulfilled by a single fixative. Thus the method of study which is initially thought likely to be the most rewarding for a particular specimen will continue to dictate the primary method of fixation. All pathologists should at least be aware of the potential uses of electron microscopy in tissue diagnosis and of the competing technical requirements of this and other techniques. The special interests and different requirements within individual pathology departments will also influence protocols for tissue sampling and specimen fixation.

Tissue preparation for electron microscopy must not only be reproducible and cause minimal artefact, but must also impart electron density to ultrathin tissue sections. This is routinely achieved through the use of osmium tetroxide as a secondary fixative and uranium and lead salts as electron dense stains. Heavy metals bind differentially to subcellular structures, providing more effective scattering of the electron beam and thus enhancing image contrast. The primary role of osmium is not as a fixative but to impart general contrast to the tissue components; it has an affinity for lipopro-

Technical Considerations

teins, enhancing particularly the contrast of cell membranes. Uranyl salts show a preference for nucleic acids over proteins, while following post-fixation in osmium, lead salts bind to a wide range of cellular structures, enhancing the overall contrast of the tissue section.

The sections for electron microscopy must be thin enough to permit the passage of electrons. This is achieved by first dehydrating the fixed

blocks and then embedding in epoxy resin, which allows thin sections (typically 60 nm) to be cut from the surface of the polymerized tissue block using glass or diamond knives. Sections are subsequently mounted and dried on copper mesh support grids prior to staining.

Processing schedules for EM are now comparable in time-scale to routine paraffin procedures. Tissues can be processed overnight using

Table 5.2: Ultrastructural markers of differentiation which assist in the identification and classification of certain tumours.

Cell Type	Ultrastructural Features
Squamous epithelium	Desmosomes, tonofibrils
Glandular epithelium	Apical junctional complex, microvilli, mucin granules
Neuroendocrine	Dense-cored granules
Schwann cell	Complex interleaving processes, external lamina closely applied
Mesothelium	Long sinuous microvilli
Smooth muscle	Fine myofilaments, focal densities, external lamina
Striated muscle	Sarcomeres, actin and myosin filament arrays
Fibroblast	Rough ER, Golgi
Endothelium	Weibel–Palade bodies
Langerhans cells	Birbeck granules
Melanocyte	Pre-melanosomes
Pancreatic α-cell	Double-density granules
Pancreatic β-cell	Crystalline granules
Type II pneumocyte	Myelinosomes
Juxtaglomerular cell	Rhomboidal granules
Lymphocyte	The ultimate 'undifferentiated' cell
Plasma cell	Prominent concentric cisternae of rough ER with perinuclear Golgi

Figure 5.2: (a) The premelanosome, a marker for melanocytic differentiation, is identified by its characteristic internal cross-striations or ribbed appearance. The transverse striations have a periodicity of 8–10 nm. In amelanotic melanomas, premelanosomes may be extremely infrequent, or may lose their internal architectural arrangement. The cross-striations provide the framework for melanin storage and become obliterated by melanin pigment in the mature granule. ×97 000. (b) Weibel–Palade bodies are a characteristic feature of normal endothelial cells and are used as a marker for endothelial cell differentiation within neoplasms. However, they can often be absent or poorly represented in less well differentiated vascular tumours. Weibel–Palade bodies are usually rod-shaped and display an internal linear arrangement of fine tubules, giving them a periodicity sometimes mistakenly confused with that of the premelanosome. In suspected cases, care must be taken to ensure that the Weibel–Palade bodies are present in the neoplastic cell population, rather than in the accompanying stromal microvasculature. ×55 500. (c) Langerhans cell granules, occasionally referred to as Birbeck granules, are unique organelles which provide useful markers for normal and neoplastic Langerhans cells. They are involved in endocytic transport to the golgi apparatus and are formed through invagination of the cell membrane. They are known to be discoid in shape, but are usually seen in section as thin rod-like structures having short cross-striations giving them a zipper-like appearance. They occasionally resemble a tennis racket, when one end of the granule becomes dilated. ×178 500. (d) Sezary cells. The gross nuclear irregularities displayed by these circulating lymphocytes are said to be characteristic of those associated with mycosis fungoides and Sezary's syndrome. The nuclei are often described as having a cerebriform pattern (C). ×4000.

automated systems and the embedded blocks polymerized in one hour at 90°C. Furthermore, the capacity of microwave technology allows for the rapid fixation and same day EM reporting of really urgent biopsy specimens. Staining of ultrathin sections can also be achieved to good effect in a matter of seconds in the microwave. Readers should consult Bozzola & Russell (1992) and Hayat (1989) for more detailed information on specimen preparation.

Morphological Examination of Pathological Specimens

Electron microscopy is rarely undertaken in isolation. The pathologist must have all relevant clinical information and should be acquainted with the initial histological appearances. Having ensured that the areas selected for ultrastructural examination are representative of the condition, the pathologist uses the

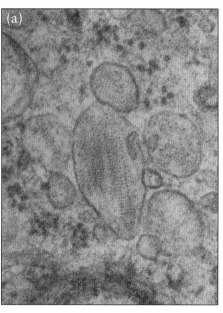

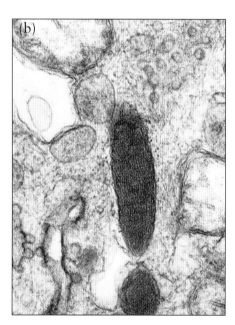

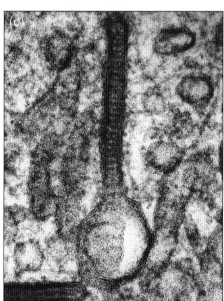

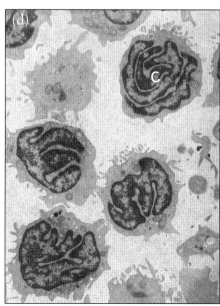

Morphological Examination of Pathological Specimens

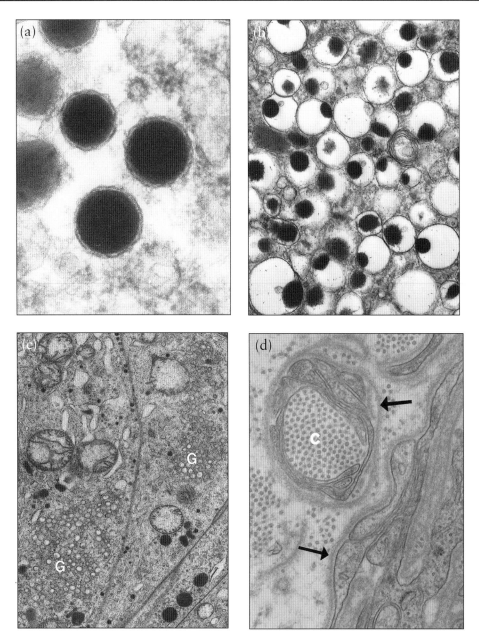

Figure 5.3: (a) The identification of neuroendocrine granules assists the ultrastructural diagnosis of neuroendocrine tumours. Although they may be round or ovoid and vary in size, they typically contain a dense matrix which is separated from the limiting membrane by a narrow halo or electron lucent rim. In poorly differentiated neoplasms the granules are often depleted and are sometimes difficult to identify with confidence. ×86 000. (b) The noradrenaline-containing neuroendocrine granules in a phaeochromocytoma are characterized by a dense eccentric core within an enlarged electron lucent matrix, giving them a typical 'bull's-eye' appearance. ×24 000. (c) The cells in a pituitary adenoma from a 75-year-old female are seen to contain a prominent honeycomb golgi apparatus (G). This unique feature is only associated with the 'feminizing' gonadotroph cell adenoma and is not seen in any other pituitary adenoma. ×9500. (d) Acoustic Schwannoma or neurinoma occurring in a 32-year-old male. Long branching processes emanating from the cell bodies in an Antoni A area are seen to be enveloped by a continuous external lamina (arrows), while in one area the cell processes are seen to wrap around a bundle of collagen fibrils (C). ×33 000.

Morphological Examination of Pathological Specimens

high resolution of the EM to determine structural abnormalities or patterns of cell differentiation at the subcellular level.

The detection and recognition of specific cytoplasmic organelles and matrix components relies on a detailed knowledge of ultrastructural anatomy, which forms the essential basis of diagnostic electron microscopy. Most differentiated cells have specific architectural and cytoplasmic features (see Table 5.2) and it is the recognition of these features, however poorly represented they may be, which allows a more precise identification of various poorly differentiated or undifferentiated tumours than is possible by light microscopy. In practice, as well as allowing the identification of some anaplastic tumours previously regarded as unclassifiable by light microscopy, electron microscopy is also useful in supporting a difficult or unexpected light microscopic diagnosis, or in refining a differential diagnosis, such as those which occur with small round cell, or spindle-cell malignancies. Electron microscopy can also assist in determining the primary site of metastatic neoplasms. In central nervous system tumours, the identification of meningeal, Schwannian, neuronal, glial or ependymal features provides important assistance to the neuropathologist, since immunohistochemistry has only limited value in such cases. Some examples of the role and specificity of organelle identification in tumour diagnosis are shown in Figs 5.2, 5.3.

With the increasing use of fine-needle aspiration biopsies, electron microscopy is well placed to handle the small solid 'floaters', or 'microbiopsies' that are drawn off into the syringe. EM is said to provide a major diagnostic contribution in about 20% of such cases. As the practice of obtaining smaller biopsy specimens becomes more widespread, so the overlapping technologies of plastic histology and EM may take on greater diagnostic significance. Many laboratories already use such a dual approach for the examination of bone marrow trephines in addition to liver and kidney biopsies. The role of electron microscopy as a means of internal audit should also not be overlooked.

Electron microscopy can have a substantial and occasionally solitary role to play in the identification and classification of a wide range of non-neoplastic conditions (see Table 5.3). Here the pathologist looks for specific alterations or defects in cell or tissue fine structure as an indication of a particular pathological condition. In many instances, the changes are beyond the resolution of light microscopy, while in others the characteristic nature of the defect becomes more clearly defined by electron microscopy. Some examples of the application of EM to non-neoplastic conditions are shown in Fig. 5.4.

Most specialists agree that electron microscopy has an essential diagnostic role in the majority of renal biopsies, through the detailed analysis of changes occurring within the walls of the glomerular capillaries and in the mesangium. Similarly, EM is invaluable in the identification of certain myopathies, while it has expanded our knowledge and understanding of many skin disorders, more accurately reflecting the varied clinical presentations than was possible by light microscopy. For example, EM has revealed much greater morphological heterogeneity within such conditions as ichthyoses and mechanobullous disorders than was previously suspected. In both of these conditions it is the recognition at ultrastructural level of specific fine structural defects either in keratinization, or which occur with blister formation following mechanical stress, that enables the diagnosis to be made.

The diagnostic application of EM to inborn errors of metabolism is based upon the recognition of metabolites in abnormal quantities or at an abnormal location, or the excessive accumulation of cell byproducts, usually as the result of a metabolic block in normal catabolism, or the accumulation of abnormal metabolites which are not produced by healthy cells. The consequent morphological manifestations are often characteristic of a particular condition or group of conditions (see Fig. 5.5). EM is therefore particularly helpful in the identification of various metabolic disorders, particularly where the exact biochemical defect remains undetermined. A skin biopsy provides an easily accessible source of material rich in epithelial, neural and mesenchymal elements, while providing fibroblasts for culture, storage and future analysis. Conjunctival, liver and rectal biopsies offer suitable alternatives.

Morphological Examination of Pathological Specimens

Table 5.3: Application of electron microscopy to non-neoplastic conditions.	
Renal disease	• intrinsic changes in glomerular basement membrane • electron dense deposits in immune complex disease • essential for diagnosis of Alport's syndrome and thin basement membrane disease • useful for staging disease progress
Neuromuscular disorders	• particularly mitochondrial, congenital and metabolic myopathies
Skin disorders	• disorders of keratinization • mechanobullous dermatoses • hair and nail defects
Connective tissue disorders	• stromal disorders involving alterations of collagen, proteoglycans and elastin • amyloidosis
Haematopoietic disorders	• platelet disorders • granulocytic anomalies
Inborn errors of metabolism	• accumulation of metabolites • potential for prenatal detection
Paediatric liver biopsies	• metabolic liver disease • Reye's syndrome
Endomyocardial biopsies	• cardiomyopathies • amyloidosis
Respiratory diseases	• ciliary abnormalities • identification of lung particulates
Disorders of the central and peripheral nervous system	• dementias, neuropathies
Infective agents	• parasites • fungi • bacteria • viruses

Figure 5.4: *(a) Epidermolysis bullosa simplex in a 24-year-old male. Early blister formation (B) has occurred within the basal cell layer. Some cell remnants (C) remain attached to the underlying basal lamina (arrow heads). ×5250. (b) Mitochondrial myopathy in a 27-year-old female. Accumulation of abnormal mitochondria is seen at the periphery of a skeletal muscle fibre. The mitochondria are increased in size and number as well as being structurally abnormal. Many contain paracrystalline inclusions or have concentrically arranged cristae, giving the mitochondria a 'Catherine-wheel' appearance. ×11 500. (c) Defective cilia in a six-year-old boy with Kartagener's syndrome. The cilia display an absence of dynein arms, which are normally located on the outer and inner aspects of the microtubular doublets and which are necessary for ciliary movement. ×166 000. (d) Amyloidosis. Accumulation of amyloid fibrils in a myocardial biopsy from a 22-year-old female with a history of familial Mediterranean fever. The deposits (A) are seen at higher power (inset) to consist of randomly arranged non-branching rigid filaments approximately 9 nm in diameter. Other studies have shown the fibrils to have a hollow core. Electron microscopy is particularly useful in cases such as this, where the amyloid deposits are small and cannot be identified by conventional microscopical techniques. ×5750. Inset ×53 000.*

Morphological Examination of Pathological Specimens

Antenatal diagnosis can be achieved from cells harvested from amniotic fluid, while blood leukocytes can provide an early means of detecting some metabolic storage disorders.

In some instances the identification of a defective organelle can be central to the recognition of certain diseases. Two such examples are the detection of abundant and abnormal mitochondria in mitochondrial myopathies and ciliary defects in immotile cilia syndrome (Fig. 5.4(b), (c)). Working at magnifications of around 100 000 and using a goniometer stage, the defective macromolecular organization of dynein arms and radial spokes can be identified.

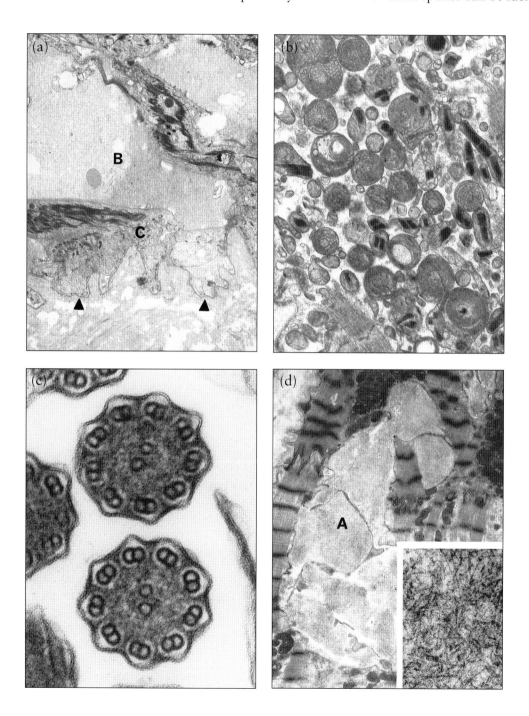

53

Morphological Examination of Pathological Specimens

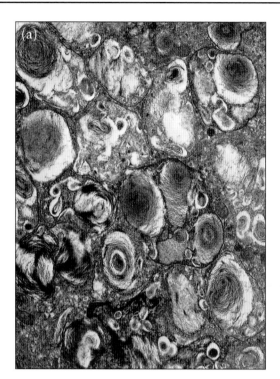 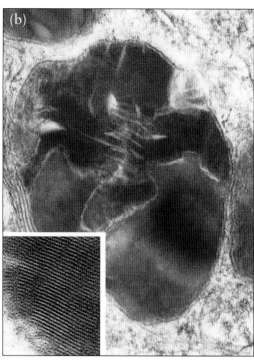

Figure 5.5: *Inborn errors of metabolism. (a) An hepatocyte in a liver biopsy from a 10-month-old girl is loaded with lysosomes displaying the characteristic lamellar appearance associated with Niemann–Pick's disease. ×8000. (b) One of many dense lysosomal inclusions found in endothelial cells in a skin biopsy from a 14-year-old boy. The inclusion is highly osmiophilic and at higher magnification (inset) displays the closely packed myelinated appearance typical of that seen in Fabry's disease. ×66 500. Inset ×188 000.*

Electron microscopy can be a useful adjuvant in the identification of microorganisms, often providing a useful 'screening' approach, in contrast to the more focused testing using microbiological antigens. Due to the small size and distinctive ultrastructural features of viruses, EM has an important role in their identification and, where it is not possible to grow an organism, EM may be the only method available. Clinically relevant viruses can often be recognized in ultrathin sections of fixed and stained tissue (Fig. 5.6(a)). Many display a dense nucleic acid core surrounded by a protein shell or capsid, which in turn may be enveloped by the cell membrane as the virus particle leaves the cell. Although morphology plays an important part in viral recognition, it has its limitations in subclassification, while virus identification in sections becomes more difficult where viral assembly is incomplete. The literature contains various unsubstantiated claims of 'viral-like particles', due to the difficulties of interpretation of subcellular images of this sort. In these and other instances, immunoelectron microscopy may provide useful support.

The identification of 'live' virions in negatively stained preparations from body fluids and faecal samples has provided a useful screening method, which is both rapid and simple, since it does not involve tissue processing, embedding and sectioning. Unlike the positive staining used in tissue sections, negative staining does not require protein–stain interaction. Instead, the heavy metal stain such as phosphotungstic acid or uranyl acetate is simply mixed for a few moments with a small drop of the particulate viral suspension on a formvar-coated grid and rinsed before drying. The contrast medium penetrates the hydrophilic regions of the viral surface and when dried imparts electron density to these areas, thereby providing a unique map of the macromolecular arrangement of surface proteins [Fig. 5.6(a), (b)].

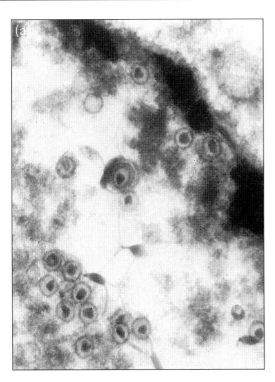 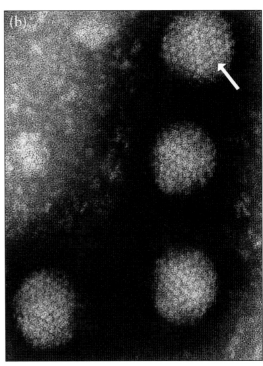

Figure 5.6: (a) Herpes viral particles within a portion of a hepatocyte nucleus. The dense protein core is often polygonal or bar-shaped and the outer capsid, which is icosahedral, appears round, hexagonal or pentagonal in tissue sections. ×55 000. (b) Negative stained preparation of 'live' adenoviruses showing the typical geometric organization of closely packed 7–9 nm diameter capsomers. Note the triangular pattern formed by the capsomeres (arrow). The size of the virus (80 nm) together with its capsomere arrangement allows for identification, despite the difficulty often encountered in recognizing the hexagonal outline characteristic of an icosahedral virus. ×250 000.

Other Imaging Modalities

The diverse interactions which occur when primary electrons interact with the specimen provide additional information on specimen composition. Through the use of various types of electron detectors to collect the emerging signals, or by adjusting the operational mode of the microscope, it is possible to view the specimen in a variety of ways. Modalities such as secondary and backscattered electron imaging, electron diffraction and X-ray microanalysis are among the most useful and will be discussed in greater detail below. Other operating modes such as specimen tilt and scanning transmission electron microscopy have only limited practical value in pathological diagnosis, while dark field electron microscopy is rarely used.

The detection of ciliary abnormalities requires the use of a goniometer stage in which the ultrathin sections can be tilted ±30° in order to determine the presence or absence of dynein arms. Specimen tilt can also aid the identification of paracrystalline inclusions or resolve interpretative difficulties due to plane of section. In general, tilting has a greater role in electron diffraction studies, which are relatively little used in diagnosis.

With scanning transmission electron microscopy (STEM), the image is formed not by the projector lenses but by an electronic system similar to that of the SEM. A fine diameter beam (2 nm) is scanned in a raster pattern across a small area of the ultrathin section. The electrons which pass through the specimen are collected by a detector placed at the bottom of

<u>Other Imaging Modalities</u>

Electron diffraction

Scanning electron microscopy

---

the microscope column. The signal from this detector is then amplified and displayed on a cathode ray tube, synchronized with the scanning electron beam. Because there are no final image-forming and magnifying lenses, chromatic and spherical aberration are virtually eliminated. This factor, together with the increased penetration of the beam, allows much thicker sections (< 0.5 μm) to be examined and specimen contrast can be generated in part by electronic means, reducing reliance on heavy metal stains. Most modern TEMs have a STEM facility as an optional accessory; because of the degree of control such systems attain over the beam spot size, it is used in conjunction with X-ray microprobe analysis, using relatively thick sections of unosmicated tissues in order to obtain the maximum analysable mass of the target substance while minimizing spectral interference from the heavy elements used in routine fixation and staining.

Electron diffraction
When a specimen is bombarded with electrons, the incident electrons may be deflected or diffracted from their normal path. If the specimen is crystalline, the constituent atoms, molecules, or clusters of molecules will have a distinct repeating array in at least two dimensions; the diffracted electrons will then produce a characteristic diffraction pattern of bright spots or rings located at varying distances from the beam centre, which can be visualized in the back focal plane of the objective lens. Because the atoms or molecules within amorphous material are randomly arranged with no distinct repeat, the diffraction pattern in this case will contain no distinct maxima (bright spots) and will show only diffuse scattering. Electron diffraction is therefore able to provide information regarding the structure of the specimen from the arrangement and spacing between the atomic sites represented by the pattern of bright spots or rings in the recorded image. A knowledge of crystallography is required for the interpretation of the structural information obtained in this way. For that reason, most pathologists prefer to rely upon X-ray microanalysis for particle identification, although X-ray diffraction has a useful contribution to

make to the identification of xenobiotics, where it can distinguish between some non-fibrous particulates, such as silicates, which may have similar chemical compositions. On the other hand, while chrysotile fibres apparently have a particularly distinctive diffraction pattern, it is not possible to distinguish between the various amphibole asbestos fibres. The structural features of many cellular and matrix components such as cytoplasmic filaments, enzymes, nucleic acids, collagens and polysaccharides, as well as viruses, have been studied by electron diffraction, yet apart from the identification of xenobiotics, this technique is currently little used in pathological diagnosis.

Scanning electron microscopy
When a high energy incident electron enters a specimen and collides with an orbiting electron of an atom, the orbital electron will probably be knocked out of the atom to become a free electron. If this inelastic scattering event occurs within a few nanometers of the specimen surface, the free electron will leave the specimen. Such electrons have low energy (< 50 eV) and are known as secondary electrons. There is no means of distinguishing precisely between secondary and backscattered electrons, but electrons leaving the specimen surface with energies greater than 50 eV are generally classed as backscattered.

The production of backscattered electrons is dependent upon the energy of the incident electrons and the elemental composition of the specimen. High energy incident electrons will penetrate deeper into the specimen and are more likely to be released as backscattered electrons. Also, should the incident electrons collide with high atomic number elements within the specimen, they will be deflected upwards and leave the specimen with energies approaching that of the primary beam. In general the production of backscattered electrons is related to the atomic number of the elements present within the specimen and therefore provides what is known as atomic number or Z contrast. Because of their high energy, backscattered electrons are difficult to deflect and the detector must therefore be positioned close to the specimen surface. Generally,

Other Imaging Modalities
Electron diffraction
Scanning electron microscopy

backscattered electron detectors are either solid angle or annular type scintillation detectors which function in a similar manner to secondary electron detectors.

Due to their low energy only those secondary electrons produced within approximately 10 nm of the surface actually escape. Since they provide important topographical information, secondary electron emission is therefore regarded as the normal imaging mode for most purposes in the SEM. The low energy negatively charged secondary electrons are easily attracted towards the detector located within the side of the specimen chamber, by applying a variable positive voltage across the front of the detector. The electrons strike the glass scintillator forming the detector tip and a light pulse is produced which is proportional to the energy of the free electron. The pulse is then reflected down a light pipe to a photomultiplier, where it is amplified and converted back into an electrical signal, which is then fed to a cathode ray tube.

During the operation of the SEM, the electron beam is scanned in a square grid or raster pattern across the surface of the specimen by means of a series of deflection coils, in synchrony with the raster of the receiving cathode ray tube. Each location on the specimen surface is represented by an image point on the screen. As the image magnification is determined by the relative dimensions of the scanned surface and the cathode ray display tube, the magnification (10 × to 200 000 ×) is increased by reducing the area scanned by the beam on the specimen surface. Images are traditionally recorded from the CRT on roll film using slow scan speeds, but increasingly many modern SEMs are linked to high resolution printers to good effect, or to optical disc image archiving systems.

The majority of biological specimens require to be fixed and their water content removed before they can be examined in the high vacuum environment of the SEM. Preparative methods such as critical point drying, or drying from organic solvents at low temperature, have been employed in the past. More recently, simple air drying methods using either hexamethyldisilazane (HMDS) or tetramethylsilane

(TMS) have generally proved adequate and have become more popular.

To date, other more specialized means of examining biological specimens such as the use of cryogenic stages, or variable pressure SEMs, have not been widely applied to the study of surgical material. In contrast, specimens which contain little water, such as hair, nails, teeth and occasionally bone, can be examined directly with minimal preparation. However, all biological specimens are poor conductors of electrical charge; to prevent image distortion due to uneven surface charging, the specimens are routinely fixed to the metal specimen stub with conductive glue and vacuum-coated with a thin evaporated conducting layer, using metals such as gold, palladium or platinum.

Although the SEM is ideally suited to the examination of natural biological surfaces, it has so far failed to meet its potential in the clinical context and as a result has had a limited diagnostic role. Its main contribution has been in the characterization of hair shaft abnormalities, many of which have specific genetic or systemic implications (Fig. 5.7). When combined with X-ray microanalysis, the SEM has provided an extremely rapid and simple method for identifying unexplained xenobiotics and endogenous deposits in body fluid residues, or in paraffin or frozen sections. In such situations, backscattered imaging (BSI) facilitates the identification of high atomic number elements, including those which lie just beneath the specimen surface and which would not otherwise be easily recognized. Similarly, because of the high signal emitted from colloidal gold particles, BSI offers improved resolution and three-dimensional localization of surface antigens on specimens prepared for immuno EM.

The role of SEM in the identification of neoplastic cells is less clear-cut and is often controversial. The diagnostic basis for SEM relies heavily upon the identification of cell-specific surface features and thus requires a uniform and reproducible method of preparation which will minimize surface artefact. In practice, the diagnostic application of SEM is rather restricted, as only a small number of normal cells can be reliably identified on the basis of their topographical features. With their neo-

Other Imaging Modalities

Electron microprobe analysis

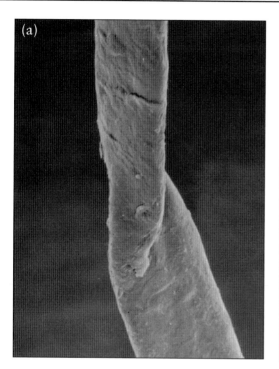
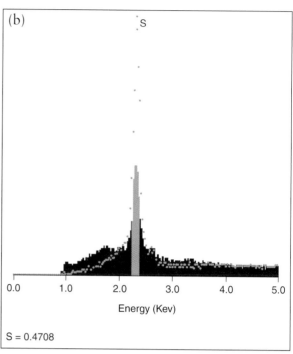

S = 0.4708

Figure 5.7: *Trichothiodystrophy associated with lamellar ichthyosis (Colloidin baby) in a two-week-old infant. (a) The hair shaft is severely flattened, having a ribbon-like appearance with loss of the normal cuticle pattern. In addition to trichoschisis and partial fractures, the hair shafts show pronounced axial twisting. ×550. (b) This rare autosomal condition is associated with a marked reduction in the sulphur content of the hair. X-ray microanalysis showed that the sulphur content of the affected hair was 47% of that found in an age-matched control (dotted line).*

plastic counterparts, such distinguishing features are extremely variable and often poorly represented or absent, making identification difficult if not impossible. There have been some claims for SEM as a means of screening for malignant cells in body fluids, especially where routine cytology has failed to identify any malignancy, or where ambiguous cells have been noted. Reports have shown a distinction between reactive mesothelial cells and those from metastatic adenocarcinoma and between lymphoid cells and cells from small cell carcinoma of lung in body fluid preparations.

While SEM may advance the scientific basis of our understanding of some pathological processes by providing a useful adjunct to other imaging modalities, it would appear to have a limited diagnostic role, with little to offer either in the identification of neoplasms, or in non-neoplastic diagnosis, beyond that which light microscopy and TEM already provides.

Electron microprobe analysis

While conventional electron microscopy is used to study the morphology of cells and tissues, the ancillary technique of microprobe analysis can determine the spatial distribution of chemical elements within a specimen. In other words, it provides specific information regarding elemental composition in relation to fine structure.

X-ray microanalysis relies upon the interaction of high velocity incident electrons with inner shell orbiting electrons within the specimen. This results in the removal of the bound electron from the atom, or from its normal energy level. The atom becomes energetically unstable and, in order to restore stability, an electron from a higher energy shell moves to fill the inner shell vacancy. As a result, the excess energy is emitted as an X-ray photon. The principal vacancies occur within the three inner K, L and M shells and several 'electron jumps' can

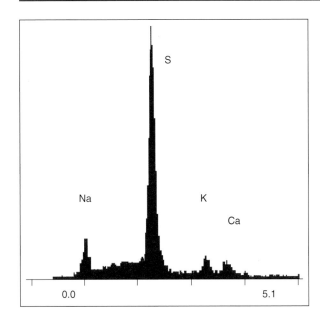

Figure 5.8: An energy spectrum obtained by X-ray microprobe analysis. Distinct peaks are identified at differing energy levels along the horizontal scale for Na (1.041 keV), S (2.307 keV), K (3.313 keV) and Ca (3.691 keV), corresponding to K-shell spectral emissions.

take place at any one time, producing a variety of X-ray photons of differing energies. Thus not only will an inner K shell photon of, say, sulphur (N16) have a higher energy than one emerging from the L or M shells, it will have an energy level which is also characteristic of that element and which is higher than that of a corresponding K shell photon from sodium (N11), but lower than those emerging from potassium (N19), or calcium (N20) (Fig. 5.8). However, with high atomic number elements such as uranium (N92) it is not always possible to produce spectral K lines, particularly when the energy of the primary electrons does not exceed the excitation potential of the orbiting K shell electrons. In such instances the lower energy L and M lines are generated and can be used effectively.

There are two distinct methods for the collection and counting of the emerging X-ray photons, wavelength dispersive (WDX) systems and energy dispersive (EDX) systems. EDX systems are currently the more popular because of their ease of use and greater collection efficiency.

The WDX system relies upon the principle that X-rays leaving the specimen have a waveform which is proportional to their energy. X-rays within a narrow range of wavelengths are deflected by a diffracting crystal into a gas-flow proportional counter. A major disadvantage of this system is that usually only one particular wavelength is strongly reflected at a given angle, to the exclusion of all others (Bragg's law). A variety of crystals are therefore used in succession and the diffracted X-ray photons are focused into the detector by varying the angle of the curved diffracting crystal until maximum intensity is obtained and the element is identified.

In contrast, the EDX system allows X-rays of all energies to be detected and displayed simultaneously. The tip of the detector, which is placed within a few millimetres of the specimen, usually contains a lithium-drifted silicon or germanium crystal which the X-rays strike, producing charge pulses within the detector that are proportional to their energy. The pulses are amplified, then digitized, separated and stored according to their amplitude in the memory channels of a computer. The resultant spectrum accumulated during a single analytical run is displayed on a monitor with the energy value of the X-ray photons expressed as electronvolts (eV) on the horizontal scale and the number of photons per energy channel counted on the vertical axis (Fig. 5.8).

With many Si (Li) detectors a thin beryllium window is used to maintain the integrity of the vacuum system. This limits detection to elements with an atomic number above that of sodium (N11). This limitation can be overcome using windowless detectors, but these must be protected during specimen changing in the microscope. More recently, the introduction of thin polymeric windows has allowed for the detection of elements down to beryllium (N4).

Electron energy loss spectroscopy (EELS) provides an additional means of elemental analysis which is particularly sensitive to the detection of biologically relevant low atomic number elements. The system measures the energy losses which occur when electrons have been transmitted through a thin specimen. Electrons interacting with high atomic number elements will lose

Other Imaging Modalities

Electron microprobe analysis

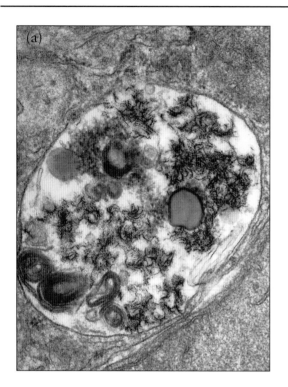

more of their energy and be deflected to a greater degree than those which interact with lighter elements and which produce a high signal. The EEL spectrometer, which is placed beneath the specimen, filters out electrons within a selected energy band. Although, in theory, EELS is ideally suited to the detection of low atomic number elements, it is currently less popular than WDX or EDX systems, but further improvements related to specimen thickness and minimizing radiation damage should see its expansion as a unique investigative tool with potential applications in pathology.

Conventional microanalysis systems combined with either scanning or transmission electron microscopy have shown a mass sensitivity approaching 10^{-19} g. The results may be either qualitative or quantitative and microanalysis systems also have the facility to produce digitized X-ray maps, which display the spatial distribution of elements within the specimen by way of computer-aided imaging. The limita-

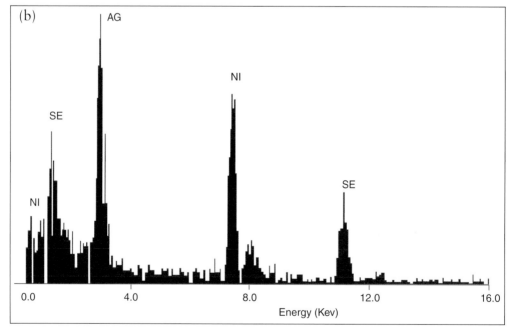

Figure 5.9: (a) A lysosomal inclusion within the cytoplasm of a tubular epithelial cell in a kidney removed from a 72-year-old male with renal carcinoma. The dense particles display a fine curvilinear or leaf-like arrangement within the lysosomal inclusions. ×40 500. (b) X-ray microanalysis undertaken on a similar inclusion in unosmicated and unstained sections identified the presence of gold (Au) and selenium (Se). The nickel peak (Ni) is from the specimen grid. Selenium is often an accompaniment of heavy metal deposits. On follow-up, it was found that the patient had previously received gold therapy for rheumatoid arthritis.

Table 5.4:   Applications for microprobe analysis in pathology.

Identification of xenobiotics

- Particulates
  - mineral pneumoconioses; asbestosis, silicosis
  - hard metal disease
  - unexplained particulates
  - unexplained granulomas

- Drugs, metals and unexplained pigments
  - skin and dental amalgam tattoos
  - toxic elements: lead, silver, arsenic
  - chrysotherapy: gold
  - contrast medium: thorium, barium

- Failure of prosthetic devices
- Adverse reaction to surgical implants including teflon, silicon

Identification of endogenous substances
- Urinary stones
- Metabolic disturbances; haemochromatosis, Wilson's disease
- Crystalline inclusions; cystinosis
- Cell injury, ion shifts

Forensic pathology
- Gunshot residues
- Particulate identification

Enzyme histochemistry
- Reaction products

tions of the technique include the inherent physical constraints affecting resolution, as well as the preservation and detection of biologically relevant low atomic number elements, which are inevitably lost or redistributed during conventional fixation and embedding.

Although cryogenic techniques offer the best means of preserving diffusible ions, such technical perfection is seldom required for the investigative pathologist, whose tissue is often already fixed or embedded. Nevertheless, before undertaking microprobe analysis, some thought must be given to avoid artefactually introducing elements during specimen preparation which may distort the analysis, or mask the identification of those elements of interest. For this reason, the choice of buffer and fixative should be considered, as well as the method of preparation and embedding.

Ultrathin sections are usually examined unstained, while the tissue blocks of bulk specimens are mounted on carbon rather than alu-

minium stubs and the conducting metal film is replaced by a layer of carbon.

The pathologist uses microprobe analysis to identify xenobiotics or endogenous substances which may give rise to, or which occur as a result of, disease and which can have a diagnostic, medico-legal, therapeutic or even environmental or social significance (Fig. 5.9). Among the most common applications are the identification of unexplained pigments and inclusions, the study of certain metabolic disorders, and the analysis of urinary stones and lung particulates (see Table 5.4).

Often the analysis is made retrospectively for the purposes of particle identification. In such cases, high resolution elemental localization is usually unnecessary and the analysis is undertaken on contiguous unstained paraffin or cryostat sections, which are mounted on carbon planchets and examined in the SEM (Fig. 5.10). As a general rule, successful identification and analysis can be achieved with paraffin or cryo-

Other Imaging Modalities
Electron microprobe analysis

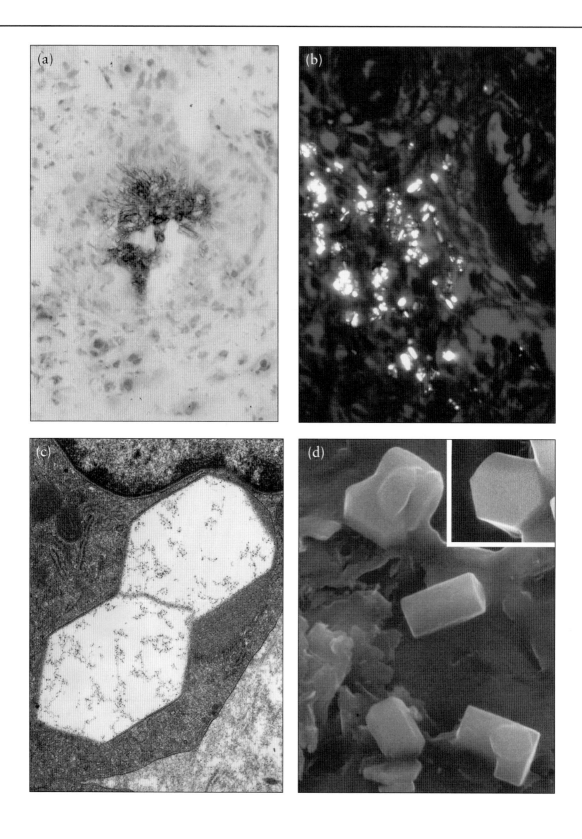

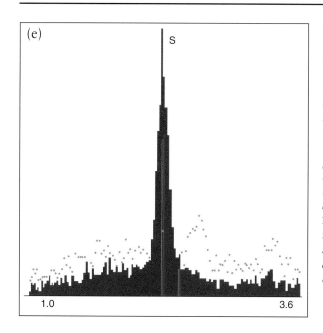

Figure 5.10 (a) to (e): Birefringent rectangular or needle-shaped crystals in a cryostat section from a transplanted kidney removed from a 15-year-old boy homozygous for cystinosis. (a) H&E. (b) Polarized light microscopy. (c) Hexagonal-shaped profiles of dissolved cystine crystals are seen within an interstitial macrophage in a portion of the kidney routinely prepared for TEM. ×17 500. (d) A cryostat section mounted on a carbon planchet and examined immediately in the SEM. Although the tissue architecture is lost, hexagonal-shaped crystals characteristic of cystine are clearly identified within the amorphous mass. ×3750. Inset ×7000. (e) X-ray microanalysis undertaken on individual crystals showed a solitary peak representing sulphur. An analysis of an adjacent control area is represented by the dotted line.

stat sections where the particles or deposits can be visualized by LM. In all other instances, a suitable area from the paraffin block can be reprocessed, or stored frozen, or formalin-fixed material can be prepared and viewed by TEM, although sectioning may occasionally prove difficult.

In pulmonary pathology, EDX has proved to be indispensable in the detection and identification of inhaled inorganic particles, such as those found in asbestos exposure and in hard metal lung disease. In such cases, the residues from digested lung samples are deposited onto a membrane filter and examined in the SEM, or in the TEM after the filter has been dissolved onto a plastic-film-coated grid.

Modern EDX systems also have the capacity to incorporate image analysis. Computer-driven SEM–image analysis–microanalysis systems have evolved, in which the computer software drives the motorized stage of the SEM, successive images are captured and digitized and particles are detected and classified according to their size, shape and elemental composition. The results can then be calculated as the number of particles per gram dry or wet weight of tissue.

Specialized Staining Procedures

Occasionally the pathologist finds it necessary to revert to specialized or selective staining procedures, such as immunoelectron microscopy or electron histochemistry, in order to enhance or identify particular subcellular structures or functions within cells. Both techniques have expanded the scope of cellular identification and have become well-established routine procedures in many diagnostic EM laboratories.

Immunoelectron microscopy

The elegance of immunohistochemistry is aptly demonstrated by combining it with electron microscopy. Together, they provide the investigative pathologist with an Aladdin's cave of applications and techniques, not all of which will be technically demanding or have a direct diagnostic significance. While its practical diagnostic value may currently be limited, the scientific value of immuno EM cannot be in doubt. Problems do exist, principally the apparently conflicting demands of preserving immunoreactivity and tissue ultrastructure; these are further complicated by the unavoid-

Specialized Staining Procedures

Electron histochemistry

able fact that diagnostically important studies must often be undertaken retrospectively on imperfectly preserved human material. However, in reality, simple post-embedding procedures undertaken on less optimally preserved tissues can often successfully provide a diagnostic solution. Alternatively, in situations such as with endocrine tumours, where the need for immuno EM can be anticipated, a portion of the fresh specimen can be finely diced into small (< 1 mm^3) blocks and given a brief fixation in dilute paraformaldehyde or acrolein/glutaraldehyde solutions before being embedded in LR White resin from 70% ethanol. In some instances, it is even possible to achieve satisfactory labelling from routinely embedded material by removing the osmium and etching the epoxy resin sections with hydrogen peroxide.

The techniques of immuno EM are many and varied. The use of colloidal gold as an electron dense particulate marker has greatly enhanced immuno EM, particularly as it facilitates high resolution labelling without masking the tissue fine structure, while through the use of different sized gold particles ranging from 1 to 40 nm in diameter, two or more antigens can be localized within the same preparation (Fig. 5.11).

The principal diagnostic value of immuno EM currently lies in the identification of the secretory nature of neoplastic cells. In poorly differentiated tumours, where light microscopic immunohistochemistry proves equivocal, the secretory granules are often sparse or atypical. The granules may also lack clear distinguishing features and it can often be impossible to determine on morphological grounds alone whether the dense vesicles represent lysosomes, or neurosecretory granules, or whether they contain mucin, or a glycoprotein such as milk fat protein, or a variety of peptides. In such instances, cell identification can rest solely upon the results of immuno EM. Electron immunocytochemistry is much more sensitive than its LM counterpart and is able to correlate more fully with the clinical and biochemical behaviour of an endocrine tumour, as often more than one secretory protein can be packaged within the same cell or secretory granule.

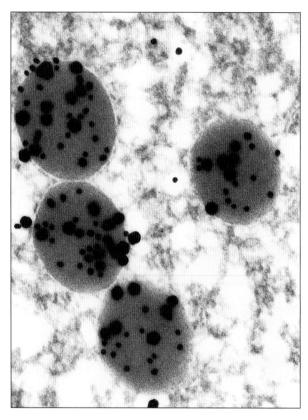

Figure 5.11: Double immunogold labelling in a pituitary adenoma from a 42-year-old male with acromegaly showing colocalization of growth hormone (10 nm gold) and prolactin (20 nm gold) within the same secretory granules. ×66 500.

Other practical applications of immuno EM include the localization of immunoglobulins in certain bullous skin disorders and in some renal biopsies where the immunofluorescence results are unclear. Furthermore, it is possible to undertake LM, TEM and immuno-labelling at light and at ultrastructural level on a single renal biopsy embedded in LR White, with the same glomerulus being studied in each of the three modalities. The pathologist should be ready to adapt to such an approach where the amount of tissue is limited.

Electron histochemistry

Without the use of electron microprobe analysis, the range of histochemical methods available to the electron microscopist is limited to those in which the final reaction product is

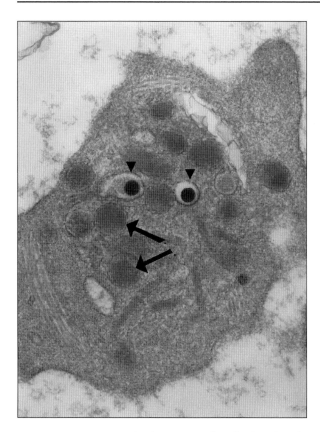

Figure 5.12: Dense bodies (arrowheads) localized within a platelet in a suspected case of Hermansky–Pudlak syndrome following fixation in Weiss's calcium-rich fixative. Differences between dense bodies and alpha granules (arrows) are clearly demonstrated. ×4600.

aldehyde can be tolerated. Aldehyde purity is important and for that reason usually paraformaldehyde or distilled glutaraldehyde is used. No single fixative is universally suitable, though hydroxyaldehyde has been found to have more widespread use in retaining enzymatic activity. In other instances, principally in the demonstration of carbohydrates by silver impregnation techniques, formaldehyde is less likely than glutaraldehyde to cause non-specific staining through the introduction of free aldehydes. It must be borne in mind that post-fixation in osmium tetroxide is not always desirable. It is sometimes omitted, as it can introduce non-specific staining, while in other instances its use is essential in order to stabilize the final reaction product. Whatever histochemical method is being contemplated, it is important first to consider the consequences of fixation, even in situations where there is no choice of fixation method.

Limitations are imposed not only by fixation, but also by many of the histochemical procedures. The reaction product must not diffuse out or translocate and, while many staining techniques can be applied directly to ultrathin sections of either expoxy or water-miscible embedded material, a good many, particularly enzymatic reactions, must be undertaken *en bloc* prior to embedding. Although 20–30 μm thick tissue slices are used to facilitate rapid access for the reagents, there is still the problem of uneven penetration. Adequate controls are thus essential to validate the staining reaction, although it must be remembered that not all histochemical methods are equally specific.

Because of their high affinity for specific carbohydrate moieties, lectins have been seen as an important adjuvant to electron histochemistry, particularly as they can be attached to colloidal gold probes and applied directly to tissues or tissue sections. Unfortunately, their large size hinders diffusion through tissues and thus limits their appeal. More recently, the localization of enzymes and other cell metabolites by immuno EM offers an exciting alternative, with the potential of high specificity coupled to high resolution.

Despite the sophistication and wealth of available histochemical techniques, only a few

sufficiently dense to be localized at the ultrastructural level. Despite this restriction, many techniques are available from the very simple, such as the addition of calcium ions to the primary fixative to enhance dense bodies in platelets in suspected cases of Hermansky–Pudlak syndrome (Fig. 5.12), to the more complex and demanding enzyme localization methods. In truth, however, it is likely that the simpler histochemical methods will have more of a direct diagnostic contribution than those involving the ultrastructural localization of enzymatic sites, where once again a compromise is sought, this time between preserving chemical integrity and cell fine structure.

Fixation has a detrimental effect on all enzymes and only the slightest exposure to any

---

seem likely to contribute diagnostically at the ultrastructural level.

Conclusion

This chapter has attempted to outline the techniques and rationale involved in diagnostic electron microscopy. It is fair to say that the development of immunocytochemical markers of phenotype and the emergence of genotypic markers in tumour pathology have recently reduced the demand for electron microscopy in routine diagnosis. Despite this, however, EM remains essential for targeted studies in many important areas.

Both in diagnosis and in biomedical and pathological research, the increasing sophistication of EM and its related techniques continues to offer unique insights into the structure and function of tissues and cells. The range of available techniques now goes far beyond conventional TEM and extends from the very simple to the highly sophisticated, involving new operational modes of the EM, or the use of additional instrumentation and procedures. The investigative pathologist should be acquainted with the many modalities available within the field of electron microscopy, as well as with their possible application, in order to realize to the full the continuing diagnostic potential of electron microscopy.

Acknowledgements

We wish to thank Rhona Cooley, Roy Creighton and Brendan Kelly for technical support and Dawn Wylie for secretarial assistance.

We would also like to thank Dr E Dermott for Fig. 5.6b and Dr C Hill for Figs 5.10a and b.

Further Reading

Bozzola J J, Russell L D. *Electron microscopy. Principles and techniques for biologists.* 1992: Jones & Bartlett, Boston.

Erlandson R A. *Diagnostic transmission electron microscopy of human tumours.* 1994: Raven Press, New York.

Ghadially F N. *Ultrastructural pathology of the cell and matrix.* 4th ed. 1997: Vol 1. Butterworth-Heinemann, Boston.

Hayat M A. *Principles and techniques of electron microscopy: Biological applications,* 3rd Ed. 1989: Macmillan Press, London.

Henderson D W, Papadimitriou J M, Coleman M. *Diagnosis and classification of human neoplasia by electron microscopy.* 2nd Ed. 1986: Churchill Livingstone, London.

Ingram P, Shelburne J D, Roggli V I. *Microprobe analysis in medicine.* 1989: An Ultrastructural Pathology Publication Series, Hemisphere, New York.

Lewis P R, Knight D P. Cytochemical staining methods for electron microscopy. In: *Practical methods in electron microscopy.* 1992: A M Glauert (Ed) Vol 14. Elsevier Science, Netherlands.

Papadimitriou J M, Henderson D W, Spagnolo D V. *Diagnostic ultrastructure of non-neoplastic diseases.* 1992: Churchill Livingstone, London.

Polak J M, Priestley J V. *Electron microscopic immunocytochemistry. Principles and practice.* 1992: Oxford University Press, Oxford.

6 LABORATORY MICROSCOPY

Brian Boullier

Introduction

The light microscope has come a long way since Hans and Zacharias Janssen created the first compound microscope in 1590. Unlike a simple magnifying glass, it consisted of a tube with a separate lens at each end. Clinical scientists have subsequently benefited from radical improvements in microscope design, construction and technique, particularly during the past 100 years.

The compound light microscope is the standard workhorse of every modern clinical laboratory, with specimens most commonly observed using brightfield illumination. However, the rapidly increasing availability of diagnostic tools, such as fluorescently-labelled monoclonal antibodies (see Chapter 4), has required the clinical scientist to become routinely proficient in a broader range of microscope techniques in recent years.

This chapter shall introduce the basic concepts of microscope design, briefly explain the rationale behind the most common procedures currently encountered in the clinical laboratory, and discuss various areas of application. The reader may wish to consult additional references for a more extensive description and fuller explanation of each technique.

Basic Microscope Design

At its simplest, the compound microscope consists of two lens systems: the objective lens which forms a real image of the specimen and the eyepiece which forms an image at infinity that can be viewed by the operator. The overall magnification is the product of the magnification of these two groups of lenses. In practice the typical laboratory microscope contains additional lens groups which may or may not affect overall magnification, but which invariably improve the optical performance of the instrument and/or convenience of operation

(by slanting the eyepieces towards the operator, for example).

Microscope performance is more correctly described in terms of resolving power – the capability of the microscope to discriminate between two points separated by a minute distance. At best, the unaided human eye can resolve two points as close as 150 μm apart. The wavelength range of visible light and the numerical aperture of microscope lenses together combine to constrain the maximum theoretical resolution of the light microscope to 0.22 μm, irrespective of maximum magnification.

Modern microscopes are modular in construction. This offers several benefits to the user, including the facility to expand the capa-

Basic Microscope Design

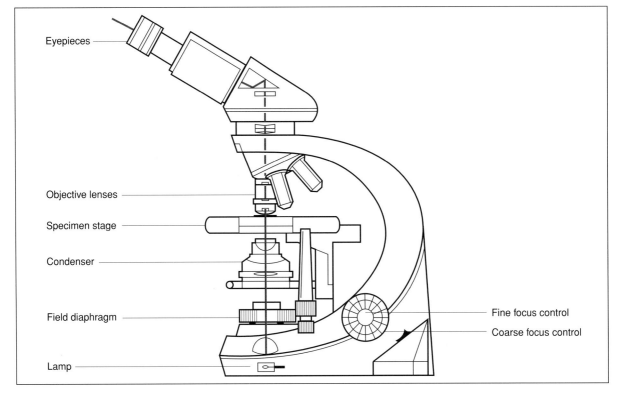

Figure 6.1: *Cross-sectional diagram of a typical laboratory microscope (Courtesy of Leica UK Ltd.).*

bilities of the microscope to meet future demands. Perhaps more importantly, this allows the initial purchase budget to be biased towards obtaining the highest quality optics possible – after all, a fully-featured microscope is only as good as the quality of its lens systems.

Figure 6.1 illustrates the major parts of the typical laboratory microscope. Several parts deserve explanation, namely the objective lenses, eyepieces, condenser, field diaphragm, and light source(s).

The *objective lenses* are the most important part of the microscope, determining the various magnifications possible and defining the optical quality achievable from the rest of the instrument. Typically 10×, 40× and 100×, objective lenses are attached to a rotating turret. This gives overall magnifications of 100×, 400× and 1000× respectively when 10× eyepieces are used.

The properties of each objective lens are usually inscribed on the lens barrel. Markings can include:

- the manufacturers' name;
- 'Fluotar', 'Fluor', 'Neofluar' or 'UV' which mean that the lens will transmit ultraviolet light and is therefore suitable for fluorescence microscopy;
- 'Phaco', 'Phase' or 'Ph' which indicates the presence of a phase ring and that the lens is suitable for phase contrast microscopy (an accompanying number, e.g. Ph 2, specifies the phase contrast condenser aperture to use);
- 'Plan' which means that the lens produces a 'flat field' image in which everything is in focus across the whole field of view;
- 'Apo' which means that the lens is highly corrected for chromatic aberration, which otherwise produces visible colour fringing around fine points in the image;
- lens magnification and numerical aperture (essentially the light gathering power of the lens) e.g. 40×/0.85;
- tube length (which is the effective distance between the eyepiece and the objective, and

is usually 160 mm) and required cover-slip thickness (in mm) e.g. 160/0.17;

- 'oel', 'Imm' or 'Oil' which means that the lens is designed for use with immersion oil between the final lens element and the cover-slip;
- 'DIC' which means that the lens is specifically designed for Nomarski 'differential interference contrast'.

The *eyepieces* further magnify the image produced by the objective lenses, usually by a factor of 10×. The image they produce is focused at infinity which allows the operator to comfortably view the image as if in the distance. 'High eyepoint' eyepieces are useful for spectacle wearers because they are designed to allow the full image to be viewed from several centimetres above the eyepiece.

The *condenser* is an important part of the illumination system. When adjusted correctly, it focuses a uniform cone of light onto the specimen (at low magnifications a 'swing out' lens above the condenser may have to be removed from the light path to ensure that the whole field of view is illuminated). Correct adjustment of the condenser diaphragm ensures an optimal balance of image resolution, contrast and depth of field.

The *field diaphragm* is centred and its aperture adjusted so that only the observed region of the specimen is illuminated. This minimizes unnecessary light scatter otherwise produced within the unobserved outer regions of the specimen.

The most commonly used *light source* in modern laboratory microscopes is a low voltage tungsten/halogen bulb. This provides stable and intense illumination in the visible spectrum. The bulb may be housed within the body of the microscope or within an external lamp housing. Fluorescence microscopy usually exploits the more suitable spectral characteristics of the high pressure mercury arc lamp which emits strongly in the ultraviolet (UV) region of the spectrum.

Types of Microscopy

Brightfield illumination

Brightfield illumination remains the most commonly used form of microscopy in the clinical laboratory. Other methods including fluorescent, phase contrast and increasingly darkfield, polarized light and Nomarski microscopy are finding varied application in laboratory diagnosis. The cost and relative complexity of the confocal microscope, however, has largely restricted its application to research applications. Each of these types of microscopy will now be discussed in turn.

As its name suggests, brightfield illumination presents the observer with an image of the specimen set against a bright background. To work effectively the specimen must absorb sufficient light to produce an acceptable degree of contrast. Stains are commonly employed to increase specimen contrast and reveal further structural detail.

Köhler illumination

Köhler illumination, introduced early this century by August Köhler, has become the universally used form of brightfield illumination because of the quality of image produced. However, optimum image quality requires regular adjustment of the microscope. Unfortunately, many instruments are not used to their full potential because of a disregard for the need to readjust the microscope when changing objective lenses and general ignorance of the required technique. In Köhler illumination two sets of light rays contribute to the final image, one set called the illuminating rays and the other called the image-forming rays. Both are derived from the incandescent lamp filament. (In practice a ground glass filter is usually fixed in front of the lamp filament to provide a more even source of illuminating rays.)

Figure 6.2 illustrates the separate paths followed by illuminating rays and image-forming rays in a microscope correctly set up for Köhler illumination. Most notably: (1) the illuminating rays are parallel at the specimen plane to provide the desired wide area of illumination; (2) the illuminating rays are finally focused on the eye lens before diverging to

Types of Microscopy

Fluorescence microscopy

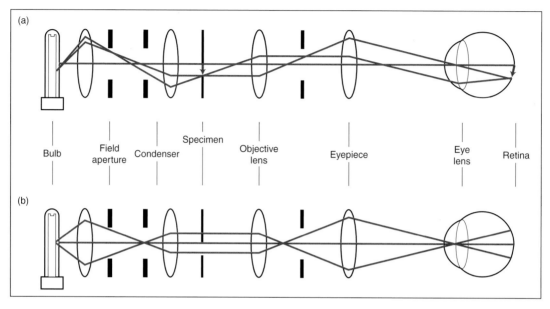

Figure 6.2: The compound microscope set up for Köhler illumination: (a) paths of image forming rays; (b) paths of illuminating rays.

provide a wide area of illumination on the retina; (3) the image-forming rays converge on the specimen plane, resulting in a magnified but inverted image of the specimen at the primary image plane below the eyepiece; (4) the eyepiece lenses invert the specimen image-forming rays again before they enter the eye and are focused on the retina to produce an image of the specimen.

In this way Köhler illumination provides a large, evenly illuminated field of view on the observer's retina together with a focused and magnified image of the specimen.

Fluorescence microscopy

Fluorescence microscopy takes advantage of the property of molecules called fluorochromes to emit light of a particular wavelength when excited by incident light of shorter wavelength. These fluorochromes may be native to the specimen under study, but more commonly the specimen is treated either directly or indirectly with fluorescing dyes. For example, the DNA-specific 4′,6-diamidino-2-phenylindole (DAPI) may be used directly to reveal the extracellular presence of DNA-containing mycoplasma which frequently contaminates cell cultures. Cellular components, e.g. the cytoskeleton,

may be stained indirectly using highly specific probes created by conjugating fluorochromes such as fluorescein isocyanate with monoclonal antibodies.

Fluorescence microscopy requires relatively simple upgrading of the conventional light microscope. High pressure mercury arc lamps are commonly used to provide intense illumination in the ultraviolet (UV) region of the spectrum which excites fluorescence in many important fluorochromes. The use of UV also requires the use of special objective lenses capable of UV transmission. This is because in the typical fluorescence microscope configuration the objective lenses also serve to focus the illuminating rays onto the specimen. Because the illuminating rays pass through the objective and are incident on the specimen (rather than being transmitted through it from below) this technique is known as epi-illumination.

An appropriate combination of excitation filter, chromatic beam splitter and barrier filter must be used for each fluorochrome(s) in use (Fig. 6.3). The excitation filter is located in front of the mercury lamp and is chosen to allow transmission of a narrow range of wavelengths of light which includes the wavelength required to excite fluorescence.

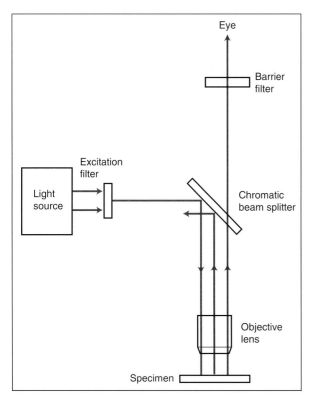

Figure 6.3: *Light path in an epi-fluorescent microscope.*

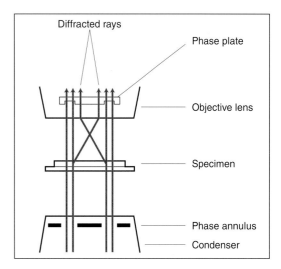

Figure 6.4: *Light path in phase contrast microscopy.*

The chromatic beam splitter must reflect excitatory wavelengths of light onto the specimen and stop reflected incident light reaching the eyepieces. As its name suggests, the barrier filter ensures that only light emitted by the fluorochrome reaches the eyepieces (UV light can damage the eyes and unprotected skin).

Phase contrast microscopy

Phase contrast microscopy allows unstained biological specimens with little inherent contrast – which includes living specimens – to be studied. The technique exploits the phase differences which arise between light passing through a biological specimen and light which passes uninterrupted through the surrounding medium. In biological materials this difference is about $1/4\lambda$. The phase contrast microscope requires a special condenser with a series of annular apertures at their front focal plane and matched objective lenses with phase rings at their rear focal plane (Fig. 6.4). This arrange-

ment introduces a further relative phase shift of $1/4\lambda$ to the light already diffracted through the specimen, resulting in a total $1/2\lambda$ phase retardation relative to the background light. The destructive interference that is produced results in refractive specimen details appearing darker than the background, an effect known as 'positive phase contrast'. Conversely 'negative phase contrast', in which specimen details appear brighter than the background, results when constructive interference is produced by retarding the background light by $1/4\lambda$.

Phase contrast microscopes are excellent for observing living specimens with minimal disturbance, including cultured animal cells in closed, sterile containers and motile spermatozoa in Petri dishes.

Darkfield microscopy

Darkfield microscopy reveals structural details as bright objects on a dark background. A special condenser is used to provide oblique illumination which, if unaltered by the specimen, fails to enter the objective lens. Only those parts of the specimen which deflect light into the objective lens present an image at the eyepieces. Two types of condenser facilitate darkfield illumination. A simple 'patch stop' may be used to obscure the central portion of the illumination provided by a conventional condenser, leaving only oblique rays incident

Types of Microscopy

Polarized light microscopy

Nomarski differential interference contrast microscopy

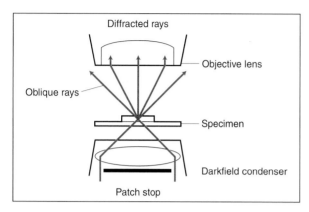

Figure 6.5: *Light path in darkfield microscopy.*

on the specimen (Fig. 6.5). Special 'mirror condensers' provide the best image quality, but are only suitable for darkfield illumination.

Darkfield microscopy does not provide a fully representative image of the specimen – many intracellular structures may not be evident. However the method is useful for revealing further details of fine line structures which are difficult to observe using brightfield illumination because of their lack of contrast. Furthermore, since staining is unnecessary (as with phase contrast and Nomarski microscopy), this method of illumination is useful for observing live specimens – spermatozoa and flagellated protozoa offer fascinating images when observed in this way.

Polarized light microscopy

Polarized light microscopy represents another modification of the conventional light microscope. The light emanating from a light source may be thought of as many sine waves oscillating in any one of an infinite number of planes around a central axis – in other words it is not polarized. The polarization microscope includes two polarizing filters. The 'polarizer', which can usually be rotated, is located between the lamp and the condenser and hence provides illuminating rays to the specimen which oscillate in only one plane. Secondly, the 'analyzer', which is usually fixed, is located between the objective lens and the eyepiece. Assuming no specimen is in the light path, then there will be a single position of the polarizer where the transmitted planes coincide and the image will appear

brightest. Conversely, at 90° to this orientation the two transmitted planes are crossed, resulting in the extinction of light reaching the eyepieces.

The polarizing microscope exploits the property of 'birefringent' specimens to split the polarized incident light into two components which oscillate in planes parallel to the two directions of refractive index. The two components are retarded differently within the specimen which introduces a phase difference. Since these components do not share the same plane this does not lead to interference. However on reaching the analyzer only the components that are parallel to the analyzer are transmitted and since they now share the same plane they can interfere. Rotating the specimen stage allows the amount of constructive interference to be varied, resulting in a consequent change in the brightness of birefringent structures under observation.

Objects of known birefringence called compensators, which include quartz and the 'first-order red plate' filter, can be inserted into the light path and used to calculate the birefringent properties of unknown structures, so assisting in their identification. The polarization microscope also benefits from the use of specialized 'strain-free' objective lenses which minimize the amount of birefringence introduced by the optical system itself. Polarizing microscopy has found application in differentiating between sodium acid urate and calcium pyrophosphate dihydrate in synovial fluid, for example. Generally, however, the applications for polarizing microscopy in laboratory diagnosis are limited and infrequent.

Nomarski differential interference contrast microscopy

Nomarski (DIC) microscopy represents a combination of polarization and phase contrast microscopy. Successful application requires a specially designed instrument which includes crossed polarizer and analyzer filters, and two Wollaston prism beam splitters. In combination with the phase differences introduced by the beam splitters, the additional light retardation imposed by the specimen produces an image in which the background is grey, left-hand edges are bright, central areas are grey and right-hand edges are dark. This gives objects in the light path an almost three-dimensional appearance with organelles such as mitochondria and nucleus being clearly defined. DIC microscopy is ideally suited to the study of living organisms. It has also found favour in the routine study of wet specimens such as urinary sediment.

Confocal microscopy

No discussion of modern microscopical technique would be complete without at least brief reference to confocal microscopy. Confocal microscopy represents an important modification of epi-fluorescent microscopy. The major difference between confocal microscopy and previously discussed methods is that it relies on point illumination rather than field illumination. This is provided by a finely focused laser beam, which is scanned through the specimen at a specific depth (Fig. 6.6). The image produced is a computer-generated composite built up from the differing intensities of light emitted by different regions of the specimen. Thus image quality is finally dependent on the light sensitivity and resolution of the electronic camera as well as the quality of the microscope optical elements and instrument set-up. Confocal microscopy can provide very sharp images devoid of the out-of-focus blur associated with conventional fluorescence observation and from within relatively thick (<100 μm) specimens.

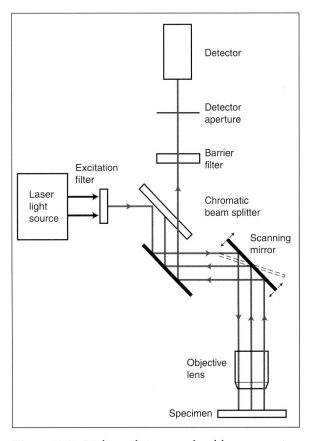

Figure 6.6: *Light path in a confocal laser scanning microscope*

ing. Photomicrography is particularly useful for recording fluorescently-stained specimens which tend to fade with time. Electronic cameras, which have become generally both more light-sensitive and affordable in recent years, are increasingly popular for this purpose.

The quality of conventional photomicrographs is dependent upon several factors. The recorded resolution is obviously affected by the quality of the optical components of the microscope, but also depends on the size of the film 'grain' which determines the sharpness of the photographic image. Unfortunately the light sensitivity or speed of photographic film is inversely related to grain size, making the correct choice of suitable film a compromise between these two parameters. The accurate rendition of specimen colour requires careful consideration, primarily because the spectral sensitivity of photographic emulsions differs

Photomicrography

Good photomicrography remains something of an art in scientific laboratories, and is dealt with in more appropriate detail in several texts. The ability to create a permanent and convenient record of microscope-derived images is important in most fields of diagnostic pathology and consequently most laboratories possess one or more photomicroscopes. These range from laboratory microscopes with a conventional 35 mm camera body attached by means of a simple adapter, to instruments with sophisticated light metering systems and several integral cameras designed to allow the simultaneous use of different types of film as well as video-record-from that of the human eye. Hence careful selection of colour compensating filters regarding the 'colour temperature' of the illuminating light (which varies as the lamp voltage is adjusted) is also necessary to record a faithful representation of the original specimen's appearance.

Further Reading

Determan H, Lerpusch F. *The Microscope and Its Application*. 1988: Wild Leitz, Wexlar, Germany.

Lacey A J. *Light Microscopy in Biology*. 1989: IRL Press, Oxford, UK.

Rawlins D J. *Light Microscopy*. 1992: Bios Scientific Publishers, Oxford, UK.

Smith R F. *Microscopy and Photomicrography*. 1990: CRC Press Boca Raton, USA.

7 MORPHOMETRY IN PATHOLOGY

Peter W Hamilton and Derek C Allen

Introduction

The practice of measurement is central to nearly all aspects of scientific investigation as it provides a means to compare observations in an objective, reproducible and reliable fashion. Diagnostic pathology from its outset has been largely based on the visual assessment of tissue morphology by microscopy, the use of visual diagnostic clues to classify a given case and the use of descriptive, linguistic criteria to convey how this process can be achieved. This is a subjective process which often results in poor reproducibility in diagnostic classification, both between pathologists and by the same pathologist on different occasions.

It has long been recognized that the measurement of histological and cytological features can provide objective data which can significantly improve our ability to make diagnostic decisions in pathology. Measurement in pathology has a number of distinct advantages. It allows us to describe in numerical terms the morphological changes we see with the naked eye. This provides us with quantitative data which are objective, reproducible and can be used to test statistically certain hypotheses about changes in tissue morphology. In addition, measurement allows the detection of subtle, 'subvisual' features, not readily apparent to the naked eye. In both instances, measurement can be an invaluable tool for the objective interpretation of morphological abnormalities and for the quantitative classification of human disease.

Methods

There are a variety of methods available that allow us to extract quantitative information from microscopic scenes. These range from very simple linear measurements that can be made with an eye-piece graticule to the very complex which require computerized image analysis.

Graticules

Eye-piece graticules are small pieces of engraved glass which can be fitted into the ocular tube of any microscope. A variety of different engravings can be used (Fig. 7.1) and when inserted into a microscope are visualized as overlaying the specimen. This is an extremely useful tool for obtaining quantita-

Methods

Graticules

Stereology

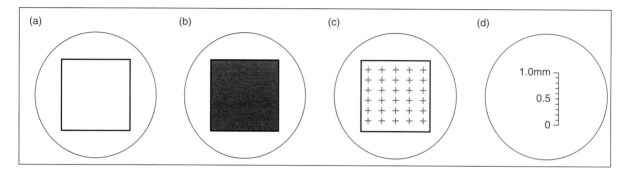

Figure 7.1: Examples of graticules.

tive information about the specimen. For example, an engraved linear rule [Fig. 7.1(d)] can be used to measure lengths or distances within the specimen such as nuclear diameter, muscle fibre diameter (see Fig. 7.12) or depth of tumour invasion (see Fig. 7.10). It must be remembered that the graticule is in the eyepiece and so must be scaled to the objective magnification. This can be done by comparison with a slide graticule which is viewed at the given objective magnification. Other types of graticule can be used to facilitate the counting of objects and stereological estimates of area and volume.

Stereology

Stereology is a technique that allows the quantitative evaluation of three-dimensional components from two-dimensional sections taken through those components. The techniques were originally described in the field of geology for estimating mineral composition in polished rock slices but are particularly appropriate for the analysis of tissues from two-dimensional tissue sections. Stereology is based on the principle of statistical geometry which states that in a random two-dimensional section through a three-dimensional structure, measures of area, profile length and number have a mathematical relationship to the volumes, surfaces and number of structures in three-dimensional space, respectively.

Acquisition of stereological data can be achieved easily through the use of geometric probes, a typical example being the point probe. By overlaying a tissue section with a

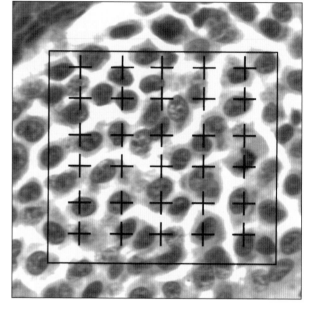

Figure 7.2: The use of a point grid to determine the percentage of area occupied by nuclei. The grid consists of 30 points, 14 of which fall within nuclei, giving a value of 47%.

series of points and counting the number of points that fall within a given structure as a fraction of the total number of points, the percentage of the field occupied by that structure can be precisely estimated. In the example shown in Fig. 7.2, 47% of the field is occupied by nuclei. If this is measured over several fields, the percentage can be reliably extrapolated to the third dimension by stating that 47% of the biopsy is occupied by nuclei.

Advocates for stereology state that such measurements are more precise and provide an unbiased estimate of the dimensions we are trying to assess.

A variety of techniques are currently available for the unbiased measurement of volume, surface area, length and number in three dimensions. The probes and grids used can now be purchased in the form of eye-piece graticules for direct microscopic evaluation or can be photocopied onto acetate sheets and overlaid onto photomicrographs. In addition, computer systems can be used to facilitate the use of stereology through the generation of digital grids for overlay onto on-line or digitally recorded images.

Computers

Computers have had a major impact in many aspects of medical practice and research. This is also true in pathology and specifically when we consider their role in tissue and cellular measurement. When presented with information on the profile of an object, e.g. a nucleus, a computer program can very rapidly calculate a variety of measurements relating to that profile such as area, perimeter, maximum diameter, minimum diameter, shape factor, etc. (Fig. 7.3). This information can be readily stored in a database and information on a series of nuclear

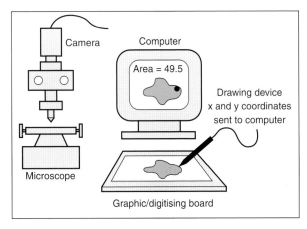

Figure 7.4: Interactive image analysis system. Profiles traced on the digitizing board or from the computer monitor are stored and used to compute geometric characteristics.

profiles collected. Two types of approach can be broadly identified which determine how the profile of an object is defined.

Interactive computer systems

Interactive systems are relatively simple technology which completely rely on the human user to trace or mark the regions that need to be measured. They consist of a computer with an attached drawing device which could be the mouse or a more specialized digital pen and drawing tablet (Fig. 7.4). By tracing the boundary of a given object, the x,y coordinates are registered by the system and the morphometric characteristics of the object computed. Images can be in the form of photomicrographs or alternatively can be relayed to a TV monitor by a video camera, where an on-screen cursor can be manoeuvred and used to trace structures viewed on the screen (Fig. 7.4). Digitally recorded images (see next section) can also be viewed on-screen and objects interactively traced. Interactive systems are relatively cheap and reliable and have been used in a wide variety of applications.

Digital image analysis

The ability to record images digitally has had a great impact on our ability to retrieve quantitative histological data. This requires the

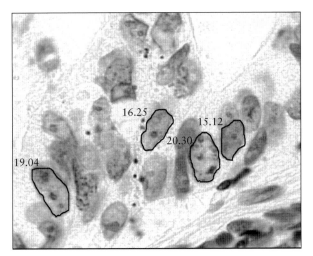

Figure 7.3: Identifying the profile of nuclei allows their area to be computed.

Methods

Computers

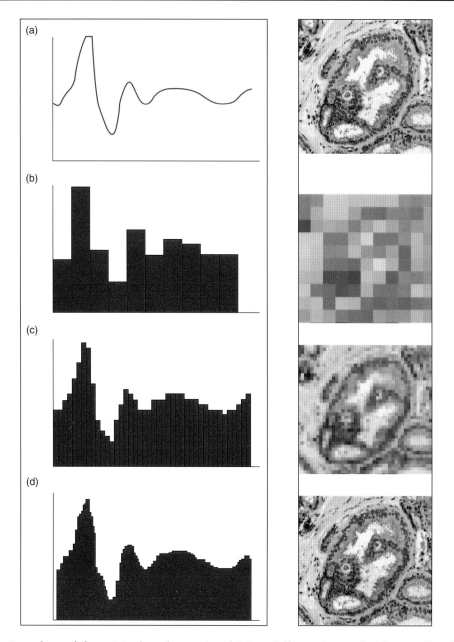

Figure 7.5: *Sampling of the original analogue signal (a) at different intervals. The smaller the interval the more precise the digital representation (b, c and d). The resulting image is shown on the right.*

conversion of the analogue video signal to a digital signal which can be stored and processed within a computer. The analogue video image is essentially a series of horizontal scan lines each represented by a continuous electronic charge pattern which is determined by the variation in the density of the image across that line. This analogue signal must be sampled at regular intervals in order to generate a digital representation. The number of samples taken over the signal determines how precise the digital representation will be (Fig. 7.5).

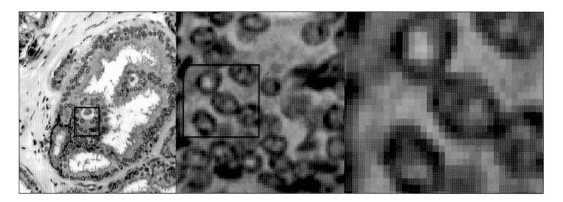

Figure 7.6: Illustrates the pixel composition of a digital image with each pixel comprising a single grey value.

Most analogue to digital converters (ADC) sample the video line 512 times. Each sampling unit is called a pixel and if we take a digitally recorded image and enlarge a given area we can see how it is made up of pixels (Fig. 7.6).

While the number of pixels in an image determines its spatial resolution, we also need to determine how many values we allow for density representation. In Fig. 7.6, we see that each pixel is represented by a single grey value. In most systems, each pixel can be allocated any one of 256 possible grey values depending on the density of that point in the original image, where 0 = black and 255 = white. As the human eye can only reliably distinguish about 64 grey values the use of 512×512 pixels and 256 grey values usually gives a precise representation of the original image. A digital image is therefore simply represented as a matrix of numbers which can be stored and retrieved for display on a computer monitor.

Having a digital representation of a histological image allows us to carry out numerous procedures not possible with an analogue image. By drawing a grey level frequency histogram of the image we obtain a summary of density information within the image. By setting a threshold on this histogram we can get the computer to select out all those pixels which fall above or below the threshold. This is called grey level thresholding and allows us to specifically identify objects within the image that have certain density characteristics, e.g.

nuclei (Fig. 7.7). The identification of objects in this way is often called segmentation. The computer can automatically derive the profile boundary of the objects it segments and from these morphometric features can be derived.

The setting of a single grey level threshold does not always result in the accurate segmentation of all nuclei. In Fig. 7.7, we can see that some nuclei which have been lying close together have been identified as a single object. If the area of these objects were to be automatically measured by the computer, the results would be inaccurate. However, since we have the information stored in a digital format, there are a variety of procedures that can be used to resolve this problem. Each suspected nuclear profile can be examined independently for its morphometric (size, shape, etc.) characteristics. If these fall within defined limits, then the object can be accepted as a nucleus. If, however, the object features fall outside the defined range, it can be processed further to determine whether a better segmentation result can be obtained. For example, we can search the profile of the object for sharp transitions in direction (termed 'cusps'). If two are found to occur on opposite sites of the object, a splitting function can be called and the object divided (Fig. 7.8). An extensive library of image processing algorithms is available which allow us in most circumstances to reliably segment objects within a histological or cytological image. This identification of important image

Methods

Computers

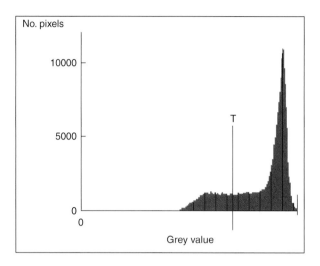

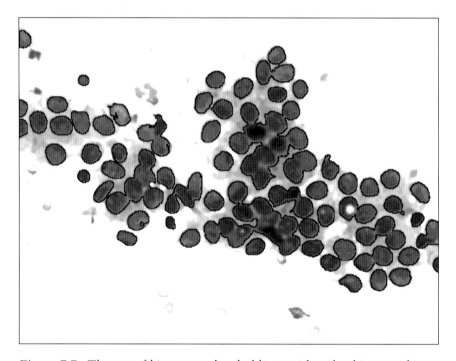

Figure 7.7: *The use of histogram thresholding to identify objects within the image.*

components and their measurement can be carried out in an automated fashion limiting the need for human intervention. This has a number of distinct advantages as discussed under Automation.

Densitometry and texture

As we have seen, when images are digitally recorded, quantitative information is stored on the density of each pixel within the image. In pathology, this information can be used

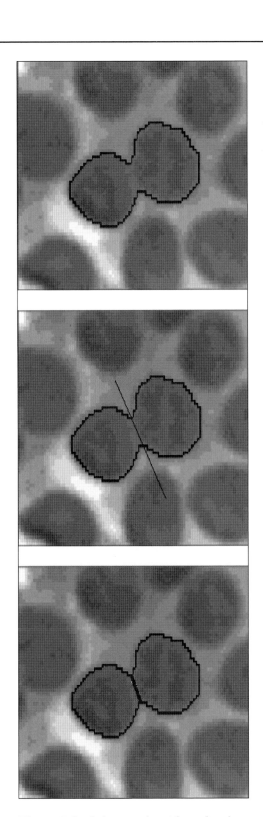

Figure 7.8: Splitting algorithms for the accurate segmentation of nuclei.

effectively to quantify the optical density (OD) of a given staining reaction. This is achieved by measuring the grey value of a series of OD filters and drawing a calibration curve to convert grey value to OD. Measurement of OD is only really valuable when the staining reaction is stoichiometric, i.e. when the density of the stain is proportional to the substrate being assessed. This is found when using the Feulgen reaction to label DNA, where the measurement of integrated nuclear optical density by image densitometry provides a quantitative measure of DNA content. As DNA content is disturbed, particularly in malignant disease, this measurement has been extensively explored as a useful quantitative clue in diagnosis and prognosis.

In conventional diagnosis, the distribution of nuclear chromatin is a visual clue that provides information on the biological behaviour of a cell. Using the numerical information provided to us through digital imagery, we can quantify chromatin organization by assessing the spatial distribution of grey values within a nucleus (Fig. 7.9). This is commonly called textural analysis which entails the measurement of a series of quantitative features including the co-occurrence and the run length pattern of grey values within a nucleus. As well as providing quantitative support for visually apparent changes in chromatin organization, these measures have been shown to illustrate chromatin characteristics that are not apparent to the naked eye. These features have been used extensively in the identification of malignancy associated changes (MACs) which are discussed later.

Automation
The ability to measure tissue and cellular characteristics and to use these to classify a given case, begs the question whether this can be done in an automated fashion. Automation has developed rapidly in other laboratory disciplines such as haematology and clinical biochemistry but has been slow in pathology. The lack of automation in diagnostic pathology to date is not altogether unjustified. Diagnostic pathology requires direct visualization of

Applications

Breslow's measure of melanoma thickness

Bone biopsy

Muscle biopsy

Breast cancer

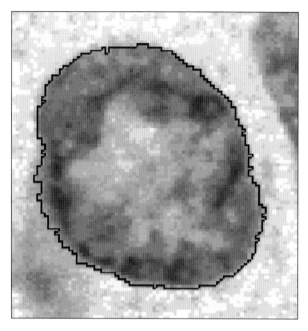

Figure 7.9: The analysis of nuclear chromatin texture involves the examination of the spatial relationships of grey values within a stained nucleus.

complex tissue and cellular structures using the standard light microscope, making the process of automation extremely difficult in comparison to the use of biochemical tests or cell counts. However, with developments in computerized image analysis and machine vision, automating the task of morphological interpretation and diagnostic classification is theoretically possible. The major effort in this field has been in the development of automated cervical screening devices (discussed later) but is now being extensively explored in tissue histology.

Applications

Breslow's measure of melanoma thickness
This represents one of the most commonly used measurements in diagnostic histopathology and is the measure of the depth of melanoma invasion below the granular cell layer of the skin (Fig. 7.10). This method and its prognostic value was defined by Breslow. Measurements

can be made with an eye-piece graticule and it has now become accepted practice to define malignant melanoma as being thin (<0.76 mm), of intermediate thickness (0.76–1.5 mm) or thick (>1.5 mm) with the percentage disease-free survival being 100%, 70% and 40% respectively.

Bone biopsy
Morphometric analysis can provide extremely valuable data for the diagnosis of metabolic bone disease. Bone biopsies are taken from the iliac crest and analysis carried out using undecalcified sections and microscopy with transmitted, cross-polarized and ultraviolet light. Measurements of trabecular and osteoid volume, osteoid, and mineralized surfaces, and osteoid thickness can be easily made and have been found to be useful in the diagnosis of osteoporosis and osteomalacia (Fig. 7.11). These can be made using point/line grids and stereological procedures. The use of computerized image analysis is now becoming a more attractive means of measuring these features. It has been argued that every health-care region should have the facilities to perform bone morphometry.

Muscle biopsy
The assessment of muscle fibre characteristics in longitudinal and transverse sections is central to the diagnosis of neuromuscular disorders including congenital, metabolic and destructive myopathies and muscular dystrophy. The morphometric measurement of muscle fibre size and number on transverse sections, stained differentially for fibre type using the myosin ATPase reaction, can enhance the objective classification of these disorders (Fig. 7.12). Fibre atrophy and hypertrophy is determined by the measurement of fibre size which is conventionally taken as the muscle fibre diameter across the lesser aspect of the profile.

Breast cancer
The Bloom & Richardson method of grading breast cancer was an attempt to introduce simple 'semi-quantitative' criteria into histopathological diagnosis. This requires the subjective grading of nuclear pleomorphism, an estimation of the percentage of tubule forma-

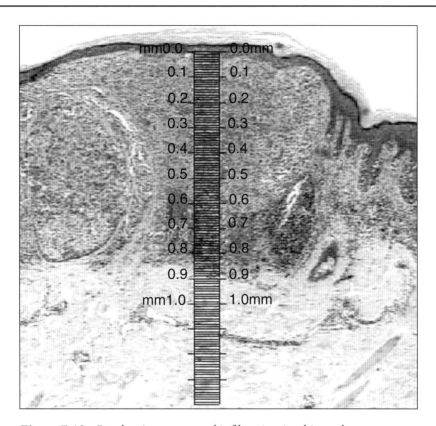

Figure 7.10: *Breslow's measure of infiltration in skin melanoma.*

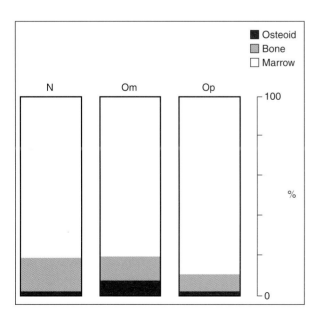

Figure 7.11: *Quantitative estimation of bone, osteoid and marrow in bone biopsies allows the identification of osteomalacia (Om) and osteoporosis (Op).*

tion and counting the number of mitoses per ten high-powered fields. The number of mitoses appears to be particularly relevant in predicting prognosis in patients with breast cancer. It has been shown in large-scale clinical trials that the calculation of a mulivariate prognostic index based on mitotic counts, tumour size and lymph node status can provide a valuable measure of prognosis in breast cancer, particularly in premenopausal women. The analysis of architectural characteristics of duct architecture and epithelial pattern assessment can provide useful data on the discrimination of intraductal hyperplasia and ductal carcinoma *in situ*.

Endometrium

The measurement of nuclear size and shape is of value in the discrimination of normal endometrium, atypical hyperplasia and endometrial carcinoma. These benefits can be supplemented by the quantitative analysis of

83

Applications

Endometrium

Automated cervical cytology

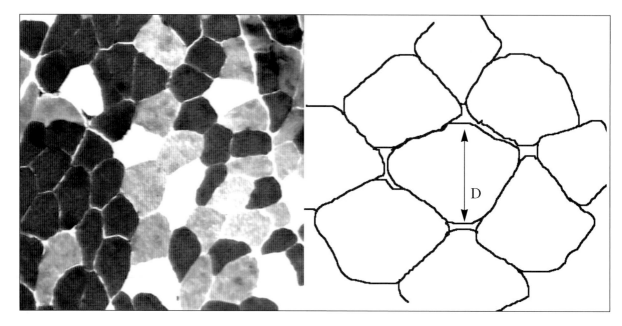

Figure 7.12: *Muscle biopsy morphometry in the assessment of neuromuscular disorders. D is the lesser aspect of the muscle fibre diameter.*

architectural features which in combination allow the identification of cases of atypical hyperplasia that progress to cancer. A multivariate morphometric scoring system has been shown to correlate strongly with depth of myometrial invasion and to be more specific than subjective classification schemes such as the Kurman classification. In the Netherlands, morphometric analysis of endometrial curettings or hysterectomy specimens is carried out routinely in an attempt to reduce overtreatment of these lesions. It has been estimated that in 1996, this could save approximately 15 million US dollars per year. The combination of the mean shortest nuclear axis, DNA ploidy and depth of myometrial invasion has also been shown to have significant prognostic value, particularly in FIGO I endometrial cancers.

Automated cervical cytology

Automated cervical cytology represents one of the major efforts over the past thirty years to introduce automation into a visually demanding diagnostic process. The motivation for this came from the significantly reduced mortality from cervical cancer after the introduction of cervical cancer screening programmes and the demanding workload that this initiated. It was clear that overworked cytotechnicians and clinical cytologists could misdiagnose difficult cases. Work on the development of computer-based scanning devices began in the late 1950s but only recently have we seen the commercial release of systems with automated capabilities in this area.

These systems mostly work on the same principle where slides are mechanically fed into an imaging microscope, mechanically scanned, sequential images of the smear are digitally recorded, cells are identified and segmented and are then subjected to quantitative analysis (Fig. 7.13). A variety of features are recorded including nuclear size, shape, density, texture, etc. Each nucleus is then classified as normal or potentially abnormal. This information can then be handled in a number of ways. Some systems are designed to store all images of the abnormal events which must then be reviewed by the cytologist at a later date to confirm a diagnosis

MORPHOMETRY IN PATHOLOGY

Applications
Automated cervical cytology
Malignancy associated changes (MACs)

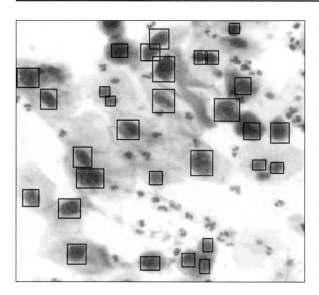

Figure 7.13: *Automatic identification of cervical cell nuclei from a smear preparation. Quantitative characterization allows classification of cell type and identification of malignant cells.*

of malignancy. This retains human expertise in the final decision-making process but significantly reduces the workload as suspicious fields are automatically selected by the machine.

Alternatively, the system can arrive at a diagnostic classification independently from human intervention. This totally automated classification of cervical smears can be used for a number of purposes.

Quality control

Cervical cytology screening demands an assessment of quality by the systematic rescreening of at least 10% of slides or rapid rescreening of all slides. This is conventionally carried out by experienced individuals within the cytology team and is a time-consuming process. An automated cervical screening system can be used to re-examine a proportion of slides, relieving the cytologist from this task. Discrepancies between human and machine classification of the same case will be highlighted and an explanation requested. Given that the machine will have a defined

classification accuracy this will ensure that the quality of diagnostic procedures will be maintained above this level.

Prescreening

Up to 95% of cervical smears are normal. Automated systems could potentially select out a large proportion of perfectly normal smears leaving the more visually complex samples to be assessed by the human cytologist. This again could represent a significant reduction in the workload of a given laboratory while at the same time enriching the job of screening by providing the cytologist with the more challenging cases.

Full automation

Completely automated devices which provide a definitive diagnosis on all presented smears have been advocated for many years and are now a possibility. There are medico-legal issues to be overcome but full automation could have a part to play in providing cervical screening services in countries where no screening programme currently exists.

The use of automation imaging systems in diagnostic cytology of the cervix and other sites is likely to develop rapidly over future years. Such systems have already been introduced in some laboratories as quality control devices and are currently being promoted as prescreening systems. With advances in computer technology, machine vision and classification procedures, it is likely that fully automated systems will perform at levels which exceed the best human screeners.

Malignancy associated changes (MACs)

Subtle alterations in nuclear chromatin organization have not only been demonstrated in malignant cells but in apparently 'normal' cells from patients with a malignant tumour. These changes have been termed malignancy associated changes or MACs. They can be reliably measured using computerized texture analysis of nuclei (Fig. 7.9) and often highlight nuclear

Applications

Malignancy associated changes (MACs)

Automation in tissue histology

characteristics which are not apparent to the naked eye. For example, in cervical cytology, it has been shown that in an analysis of only 30 normal appearing cells per sample, 70% of samples with moderate or severe dysplasia could be identified. This advocates their role in automated cervical screening devices and many of the current systems employ nuclear texture as a diagnostic feature. MACs have also been demonstrated in the colon, bladder, breast and lung. It is unclear, whether these changes in apparently normal cells indicate a primary pre-malignant change in the cell or are secondary changes due to exposure of surrounding cells to tumour-related proteins. The fact that MACs can disappear after the removal of a tumour suggests the latter, at least in some tissues. Recent work has suggested that MACs can be used as a potential method for the screening of lung cancer. Analysis of MACs in histologically normal lung biopsies allowed the correct identification of over 80% of cancer patients. In addition, the identification of textural disturbances in normal appearing cells from sputum samples has been advocated in the screening of patients for lung cancer. Textural characteristics may also allow the identification of chemosensitive tumours which have the propensity to apoptose in the presence of chemo- or radiotherapeutic insult.

Automation in tissue histology
The automated analysis of cytological preparations is a demanding task. Even more difficult is the automated interpretation and analysis of histological scenes due to the complexity of the imagery. Until recently, automated analysis of histological imagery was considered an insurmountable task, except in the most simple applications. However, with development in computer processing power and the use of expert system methodology, the development of machine vision systems for complex imaging tasks is now possible. This requires the definition of knowledge concerning the components which comprise the image and their relationships to each other. These are defined in a knowledge file and are used to drive the actions of a scene segmentation expert system. Objects are accepted or rejected as histological compo-

Table 7.1: List of potential sources of variation in a morphometric/photometric study.	
Microscope	Light source
	Field aperture settings
	Condenser settings
	Kohler illumination
	Objective quality
Video Camera	CCD array characteristics
	Automatic gain control
Specimen	Fixation
	Paraffin wax embedding
	Tissue section thickness
	Staining
	Mounting and coverslip thickness

nents on the basis of defined quantitative criteria. Rejected objects can be selected for further image processing to facilitate their identification. Once all objects are identified, the histological scene is reconstructed allowing the measurement of relevant histometric features. This methodology has now been applied successfully in colon, prostate and breast (Fig. 7.14).

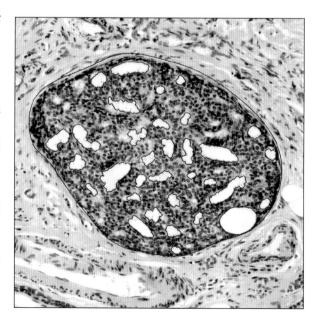

Figure 7.14: *Automated identification of intraductal breast lesion using knowledge guided segmentation.*

Standardization and control

There are a number of factors which can significantly influence the reliability of measurement data. These range from the fixation of the tissue specimen to the settings of the microscope and are listed in Table 7.1. These factors can introduce variation (or noise) into a study, so reducing our ability to detect the changes (signal) we are looking for. It is the aim of most scientific studies therefore to reduce the variation from external factors, so improving our ability to resolve the effect of the specific factor we are interested in testing. We therefore aim to increase the signal to noise ratio. While the list of potential sources of error may seem daunting, quality of results can be ensured by using standardized and properly calibrated equipment, control samples with known results and by ensuring consistency in the processing of tissue.

Conclusion

Measurement in pathology clearly enhances conventional visual interpretation. However, the incorporation of techniques into routine practice has been, and continues to be, slow. A number of factors are responsible, not least of which are the lack of large-scale clinical trials to test the efficacy of measurement in given diagnostic problems, the expense associated with computerized equipment, and the lack of familiarity of diagnosticians with computer systems. The latter two are becoming less of a problem, with the rapid development of computer technology, the associated reduction in cost and the fact that all but the most stubborn of professionals has had some hands-on experience with computers. It is likely that within the next few years most pathologists will have access to a computer workstation which is more than capable of performing simple measurement tasks, digitally recording microscopic images and perhaps have automated capabilities for the interpretation and analysis of complex histological scenes. This could significantly influence how pathology is practised and, while not immediately replacing his/her diagnostic ability, will provide valuable objective support in diagnostic decision-making.

Further Reading

Anderson N H, Hamilton P W, Bartels P H, Thompson D, Montironi R, Sloan J M. Computerised scene segmentation for the discrimination of architectural features in ductal proliferative lesions of the breast. *J Pathol* 1997; **181**:374–380.

Baak J P A. Diagnostic, prognostic and therapeutic impact of quantitative pathology in endometrial hyperplasia and carcinoma. (Abstract) *10th International Conference on Diagnostic Quantitative Pathology*, 1996; 145.

Baak J P A, van Diest P J, Ariens Ath, *et al*. The Multicentre Morphometric Mammary Carcinoma Project (MMMCP). A nationwide prospective study on reproducibility and prognostic power of routine quantitative assessments in The Netherlands. *Pathol Res Pract* 1989; **185**:664–670.

Bartels P H, Thompson D. Scene segmentation. Marchevsky A M, Bartels P H (eds). *Image Analysis: A Primer for Pathologists*. Raven Press Ltd: New York, 1994;57–77.

Bartels P H, Thompson D. The video photometer. Marchevsky A M, Bartels P H (eds). *Image Analysis: A Primer for Pathologists*. Raven Press Ltd: New York, 1994;29–56.

Bocking A, Striepecke E, Auer H, Fuzesi L. Static DNA cytometry. Biological background, technique and diagnostic interpretation. *Compendium on the Computerized Cytology and Histology Laboratory*. Edited by Wied G L, Bartels P H, Rosenthal D L, Schenk U (ed.). Chicago: Tutorials of Cytology 1994, pp. 107–128.

Breslow A. Prognosis in cutaneous melanoma: tumour thickness as a guide to treatment. *Pathol Ann* 1980; **15**:1–22.

Dubowitz V. *Muscle Biopsy. A Practical Approach*. 1985: London, Bailliere Tindall.

Grohs H K, Husain O A N (eds). Automated Cervical Cancer Screening. 1994: New York, Igaku-Shoin.

Further Reading

Gundersen H J, Bendtsen T F, Korbo L, Marcussen N, Müller A, Nielsen K, Nyengaard J R, Pakkenberg B, Sørensen F B, Vesterby A, *et al*. Some new, simple and efficient stereological methods and their use in pathological research and diagnosis. *APMIS*, 1988; 5:379–94.

Hamilton P W. Designing a morphometric study. Hamilton P W, Allen D C (eds). *Quantitative Clinical Pathology*. 1995: Blackwell Science: Oxford, 311–315.

Palcic B, MacAulay C. Malignancy associated changes. Can they be employed clinically? *Compendium on the Computerized Cytology and Histology Laboratory*. Wied G L, Bartels P H, Rosenthal D L, Schenk U (ed.). Chicago: Tutorials of Cytology 1994, pp. 157–172.

8 PROLIFERATION MARKERS IN HISTOPATHOLOGY

Cheryl E Gillett and Diana M Barnes

Introduction

It is well recognized that in human tumours the rate at which cells are proliferating has a profound effect on prognosis. Since proliferative activity was first crudely estimated by measuring the change in size of a mass over a period of time, the whole subject of proliferation and how to measure it has exploded and there are now hundreds of publications on the subject. There is a continuous stream of papers introducing new markers, combining established markers, varying the demonstration techniques and advocating novel approaches to evaluation. Such a mass of information is a daunting prospect to the inexperienced who wants to measure proliferation and usually prompts the question 'what's the best way of doing it?'

Before describing some of the different ways of measuring proliferation it is important to have a basic understanding of the cell cycle, as all markers demonstrate a particular aspect. The cycling or 'growth fraction' stage has four phases, Gap 1 (G_1), DNA synthesis (S), Gap 2 (G_2) and mitosis followed by cytokinesis (M). During the cycling stage the cell produces sequentially the necessary proteins to allow replication of its DNA and subsequent nuclear and cell division. 'Checkpoints' exist at all phases of the cycle to assess the condition of the cell before entering the next phase. Only cells in which the DNA is in perfect condition are allowed to progress to the next stage. Those cells not in good shape are arrested until the DNA has been repaired or are directed towards programmed cell death (apoptosis). All cells can enter a stage of non-proliferation or non-cycling; this is known as Gap 0 or (G_0). Here, the cells retain their viability and can move back into the cycle as required.

The term 'proliferation rate' is frequently used to describe the 'amount' of a proliferation marker in clinical material. These measurements are usually made on a piece of tissue at one given point in time, thus the term 'rate' is inappropriate. Proliferative 'activity' should be used as a more accurate expression of this kind of evaluation and the term 'rate' reserved for methods which provide more kinetic information.

Proliferation Markers

The number of so-called proliferation markers continues to grow. Outlined below are those which are reasonably well established and have been shown to provide prognostic information.

Mitotic count (MC) or mitotic activity index (MAI)

Mitoses are the only proliferative marker which can be identified and quantified in a conventional haematoxylin and eosin (H & E) stained section (Fig. 8.1). However, they are not always easy to recognize and can be confused with either hyperchromatic nuclei or nuclei in the early stages of apoptosis. Inadequate fixation, poor section cutting and overstaining can all lead to difficulties in the recognition of mitoses. These factors as well as the concern that mitotic activity may continue prior to fixation, could give an inaccurate score.

Estimating the proliferative activity of a piece of tissue according to the numbers of mitoses present may, at first, appear to be a very straightforward task. However, several different methods of evaluation have developed over the years and, despite the well-recognized value of mitoses as markers of proliferation, there remains as much debate as ever over the 'correct' method of evaluation. A mitotic 'count' was the first formal method of evaluation used, a step up from an overall estimate or the 0,+, ++ system used by so many pathologists. An MC literally counts the numbers of mitoses present in a number of high power fields (HPFs) and presents the results as the mean number of mitoses per HPF. In order to make the method more reproducible refinements have been made, including evaluating the cells at the periphery of the lesion, making the count in consecutive fields and defining the area of the HPF. The mitotic count is an integral part of grading infiltrating mammary carcinomas, using the modified Bloom and Richardson criteria, and is also used to determine the diagnosis and prognosis of soft tissue sarcomas.

To overcome some of the inconsistencies associated with a mitotic count, the idea of mitotic activity index was introduced. With this method of evaluation the numbers of mitoses are expressed as a proportion of the number of interphase cells. The total numbers of interphase cells and mitotic figures are counted in consecutive HPFs until the section has been sampled sufficiently well. As the MAI measures the proportion of mitoses in the lesion it is not related to or affected by the area of the HPF. It also takes into account variations in both the cellularity of the lesion and the cell size. Thus, it is a more accurate way of comparing the proportion of mitoses present between tumours.

Antibodies have been developed, such as MPM2, which recognize mitotic figures. These are aimed at not only reducing the chances of including apoptotic bodies in a mitotic count but also lend themselves to automated analysis.

Nucleolar organizer regions (NORs)

NORs are the sites of rDNA genes and are present in groups on a number of specific chromosomes. By having several sites of transcription the cell can keep up with demand for ribosomes whenever necessary. The NOR-associated proteins, as the name implies, lie in very close proximity to the NORs and it is these proteins which are demonstrated as markers of proliferation. The NOR-associated proteins are argyrophilic and are demonstrable using a silver-binding technique and are thus referred to as AgNORs. They can be seen as small black dots within the nucleus (Fig. 8.2).

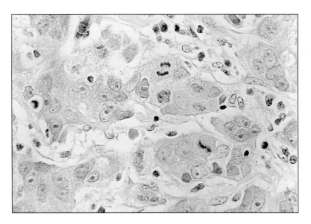

Figure 8.1: Mitotic figures in a conventional haematoxylin and eosin (H & E) stained section (×400).

Proliferation Markers

Immunohistochemical demonstration of cell proliferation

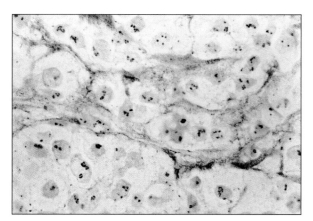

Figure 8.2: Nucleolar organizer region associated proteins – AgNORs, demonstrated using a silver technique (×1000).

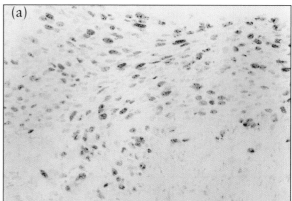

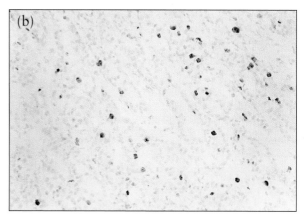

Figure 8.3: Ki67 Antigen detected using monoclonal Ki67 antibody in frozen tissue from (a) a rapidly proliferating and (b) a slowly proliferating tumour (×200).

The numbers of AgNORs present are considered to reflect ribosome production and hence protein synthesis within the cell. The resultant AgNOR assessment has been portrayed as not only a marker of proliferative activity but also a method of distinguishing between benign and malignant lesions, a measure of tumour ploidy and grade of malignancy.

AgNORs are laborious to count and some earlier papers also endeavoured to describe their pattern within the nucleolus, referring to 'clusters' and 'satellite AgNORs'. Evaluation was not reproducible, which accounted for much of the variation reported in their prognostic value. There have been many publications which have used image analyzers to quantify the presence of AgNORs, many of which have shown that the mean area occupied by AgNORs within the nucleus provides prognostic information.

Immunohistochemical demonstration of cell proliferation

The first antibody to be recognized widely as a marker of proliferating cells was monoclonal Ki67 (mKi67). The function of the Ki67 protein has remained elusive and for many years was known to have only a structural role within the nucleus. Despite this, it has been shown that the protein is expressed during all phases of the cycling cell but not during the non-cycling stage. mKi67 has been used in many studies and the resultant measure of proliferative activity compares well with other established markers of proliferation, including mitotic counts and thymidine labelling index [Fig. 8.3(a) and (b)]. Some studies have shown that it also relates to AgNOR scores. However, the drawback with mKi67 antibody is that the area of the antigen which it recognizes is very fixation-sensitive and antigenicity is lost following standard formalin fixation, paraffin wax-embedding procedures. Prognostic studies using mKi67, therefore, had to be undertaken prospectively using fresh frozen tissue.

The potential of mKi67 as a proliferation marker provided the impetus to produce

Proliferation Markers

Immunohistochemical demonstration of cell proliferation

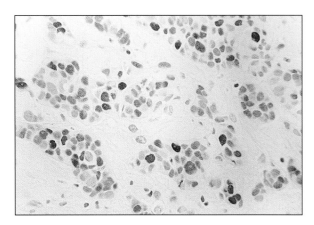

Figure 8.4: Proliferating cell nuclear antigen detected by PC10 antibody in formalin fixed, paraffin wax-embedded tissue (×400).

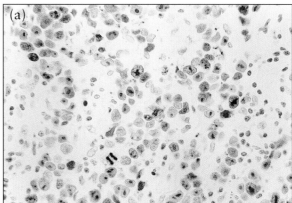

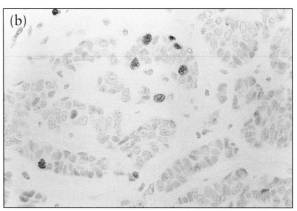

Figure 8.5: Ki67 Antigen detected using KiS1 antibody in formalin fixed, paraffin embedded tissue from (a) a rapidly proliferating and (b) a slowly proliferating tumour (×400).

similar antibodies to proteins which played a part during the cell cycle but were robust enough to survive formalin fixation and paraffin wax processing, thus giving the marker a far wider application. Antibodies to proliferating cell nuclear antigen (PCNA) and another against the Ki67 antigen (KiS1) were developed at about the same time and both were hailed as the fixative-resistant equivalents of mKi67 [Figs 8.4, 8.5(a) and (b)]. However, after the initial excitement both were found to have their own drawbacks. PCNA (also confusingly known as cyclin in some papers) has a role in both DNA replication and DNA repair. This duality has led to considerable variation in claims as to its value as a proliferation marker. Its expression appears to be related to proliferation in tissues which have active stem cells but the relationship is less clear-cut in epithelial lesions. The protein also has a long half-life and therefore it continues to be detected long after its functional time slot within the cell cycle. KiS1, like other antibodies against the Ki67 antigen, detects those cells which are cycling. However, this antibody also detects part of the protein which is still present after the cell has completed the cycle and is in a non-cycling state. More recently KiS5 antibody has been raised, which has similar binding properties to KiS1 but with improved specificity. There continues to be a steady flow of publications using

these antibodies with modifications to both the method and the evaluation procedure which are claimed to provide more accurate and reproducible proliferative information.

More recently the polyclonal Ki67 (pKi67) and monoclonal MIB1 have been heralded as the 'best' antibodies for detecting proliferating cells. Both recognize part of the Ki67 structural protein and can continue to bind to the antigen following fixation and paraffin wax-embedding (Fig. 8.6). Both MIB1 and pKi67 expression have proved to be associated closely with mKi67 antibody and their proliferative activity information correlates well with other established proliferation markers. Coupled with the development of these antibodies has been the recent improvement in antigen retrieval

<u>Proliferation Markers</u>

Thymidine (TLI) and bromodeoxyuridine labelling index (BrdULI)

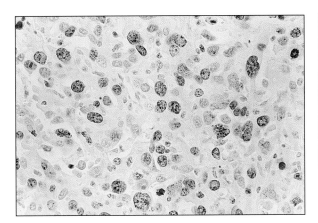

Figure 8.6: Ki67 Antigen detected using MIB1 antibody in formalin fixed, paraffin wax-embedded tissue from a rapidly proliferating tumour (×400).

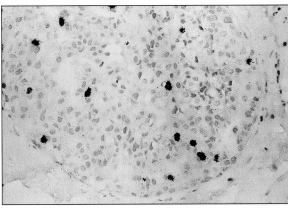

Figure 8.7: Autoradiographic detection of thymidine incorporated into the nuclei of proliferating cells (×200).

methods beyond that of proteolytic digestion. Heat-mediated antigen retrieval is essential for the use of both antibodies in formalin-fixed paraffin wax-embedded material. Even the mKi67 can be used in paraffin wax-embedded material following antigen retrieval, although the results are not as good as with either pKi67 or MIB1.

Thymidine (TLI) and bromodeoxyuridine labelling index (BrdULI)

Both of these techniques involve the incorporation of a nucleotide during S-phase, which can then be demonstrated. In the case of TLI, the thymidine is tritiated and its uptake is demonstrated using autoradiography (Fig. 8.7). For BrdU, uptake is demonstrated using immunocytochemistry with an anti-BrdU antibody (Fig. 8.8). A disadvantage is that both methods need viable material in order to incorporate the nucleotides into the DNA. Furthermore, detection of radiolabelled thymidine brings with it the problems of balancing accuracy with speed of development of autoradiographs and with safety aspects of the technique. However, results are good when carried out by experienced practitioners and provide an accurate evaluation of the proportion of cells in S-phase. These are specialized techniques and are not introduced easily into histopathology laboratories with any degree of reliability.

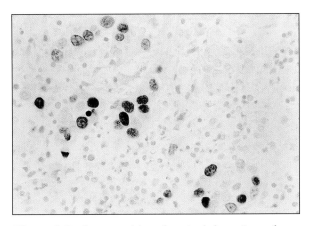

Figure 8.8: Immunohistochemical detection of bromodeoxyuridine incorporated into the nuclei of proliferating cells (×400).

BrdU labelling in combination with flow cytometry has more recently been used to measure proliferation *in vivo*, providing a true measure of proliferation rate. Patients are injected with BrdU, which becomes incorporated into cells during DNA synthesis. The lesion is biopsied several hours after injection and from this tissue both the presence of BrdU incorporation and DNA content can be measured for individual cells. The relationship between the time between injection and sampling, BrdU uptake and DNA content allows the rate at which the cells in the lesion are proliferating to be determined.

Flow cytometry

Flow cytometry is one of the most reliable and reproducible methods of measuring proliferative activity and can be used on cytological, fresh or fixed, paraffin wax-embedded material. By measuring the amount of DNA in individual nuclei which have been disaggregated from a piece of tissue, a histogram can be generated showing the numbers of cells with similar amounts of DNA. Computerized analysis of these histograms allows the proportion of cells in each phase of the cell cycle to be calculated. As far as proliferative activity information is concerned, it is the proportion of cells in S-phase or the S-phase fraction which is of most interest.

Flow cytometry is one of the most objective methods of assessing proliferative activity but as the tissue has to be disaggregated before analysis the results cannot be related to morphology and the sample may include normal, benign and non-specific elements of the tissue under study. Furthermore, when using paraffin wax-embedded material a substantial piece of tissue is needed and even then the numbers of incomplete or poorly preserved nuclei in the sample means that about a quarter of the histograms cannot be interpreted with any degree of accuracy. The capabilities of the flow cytometer have developed considerably since the early days of measuring a single parameter, DNA content. It now has facilities for multiple measurements and its use has become even more specialized (see Chapter 32). The measurement of DNA content is more likely to be carried out in conjunction with the measurement of one or more proteins detected by immunofluorescence, providing information about the relationship between phase of the cell cycle and protein expression. The technique of flow cytometry and computerized analysis of the results appears to give a more accurate approach to assessing proliferation; however, a number of studies have shown that similar information can be obtained by careful counting of mitoses, Ki67- and MIB1-cell positivity, all of which can be carried out in histopathology laboratories without special equipment.

Other markers

There continues to be a steady flow of potential markers of proliferation; many of these are antigens labelled by antibodies which have been raised against proteins expressed during the cell cycle. In a similar fashion to Ki67 and PCNA, it is assumed that if an antigen is present during a specific phase or phases of the cell cycle, then its detection means that it can be used to identify cells which are proliferating. Amongst these putative markers have been the cyclins and their associated cyclin-dependent kinases (CDKs), retinoblastoma protein (pRb), transferrin receptor and the proliferation-associated nuclear antigens p105 and p120.

However, many of these cell cycle-associated markers have an altered expression in malignant cells because of changes in the regulatory pathway of proteins controlling the cell cycle and are not suitable markers of proliferative activity. As a result of the high level of interest in control of the cell cycle, novel antibodies are being developed and marketed at a far greater pace than they can be evaluated. Care must be taken when using any new antibody to ensure that it has been validated adequately before being accepted as a proliferation marker.

In situ hybridization has also been used to demonstrate proliferative activity. Expression of histone 3 (H3) mRNA has been recognized as such a marker for a number of years and compares well with other markers which provide prognostic information. Histones are the major protein component of chromatin and have a role in packaging strands of DNA into a compact form, the nucleosome. As histones are so closely associated with DNA, they also have to be manufactured during DNA synthesis. Hence, detection of increased levels of H3 mRNA in S-phase reflects the proliferative activity of the tissues. Levels of H3 mRNA are known to decrease rapidly during G_2 and no synthesis occurs once the cell enters G_0, which makes it one of the most specific markers of proliferative activity. However, this method is not widely used, primarily because the *in situ* hybridization technique needed to detect mRNA is not readily available to most laboratories, but also because the results are not significantly better than other markers which do not require a specialized method. *In situ* hybridization techniques (in particular those

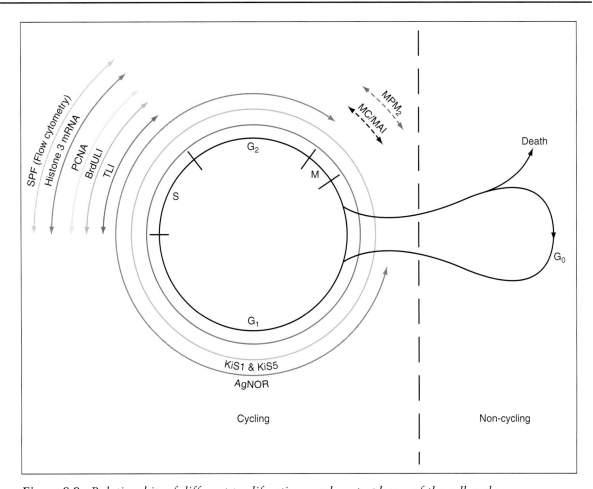

Figure 8.9: Relationship of different proliferation markers to phases of the cell cycle.

using non-isotopic methods) are being introduced gradually into more laboratories, so it may be that in the future information relating to proliferation will be more frequently obtained using H3 mRNA.

Figure 8.9 shows how the different markers of proliferative activity relate both to each other and to the different phases of the cell cycle.

Practical use of markers

The choice of method for measuring proliferative activity is very much dependent upon the type of material being assessed. If a retrospective study is being undertaken using paraffin wax-embedded material, methods such as TLI, BrdULI and mKi67 cannot be used.

Points to consider regarding tissue preparation should include the type of fixative used, since all markers are influenced by this, and the effect that a delay in fixation may have. Mitotic figures are very difficult to distinguish from apoptotic bodies following the use of alcohol-based fixatives; likewise, AgNORs can be difficult to identify. Antigen expression is reduced and even lost in some fixative solutions despite the use of heat-mediated antigen retrieval. Even in flow cytometry, the nuclear dyes are unable to bind to chromatin when a metal-containing fixative has been used. Some studies have shown that a delay in fixation reduces the numbers of mitoses in the tissue and would, therefore, underestimate proliferative activity. Finally, section thickness is usually not considered to have a significant effect on the demonstration and evaluation of markers. Nevertheless, as well as altering the quality of staining, both mitotic and AgNOR counts will vary according to the thickness of the section and in immunohistochemistry the resultant staining will vary in intensity. This latter is an important factor if it is included as part of the evaluation. All sections which are to undergo a heat-mediated antigen-retrieval step must be put onto adhesive coated slides and baked on, otherwise the sections will lift and some will become totally detached.

Method of Evaluation

Once the most suitable proliferation marker has been selected and the method carried out, the next question is 'how do I count it?' This is often considered to be the final and easiest stage of the whole technique but it requires a methodical approach to obtain consistent and reproducible results. It is at this stage that flow cytometry has a distinct advantage over the other markers, as thousands of cells can quickly be assessed with a satisfactory degree of consistency between samples. All other methods in which a proliferation marker is demonstrated in a histological section have a number of similar criteria which must be met.

Firstly, the time taken to carry out the evaluation must be balanced against the value of the information being obtained. It would be pointless to spend 20 minutes carrying out a formal count on a section, when similar prognostic information could be obtained using a semi-quantitative method which takes a fraction of that time. Secondly, whatever method of evaluation is used, it must be both reliable and consistent.

Most methods of evaluation used with the markers discussed here are conventional counts or estimates. A number of criteria have to be met in order to reduce any subjectivity associated with the evaluation, thereby allowing comparisons to be made between both samples and evaluators. The following points should always be considered before undertaking any assessment and must not be deviated from during the course of the study.

Which area of the section should be evaluated?

Traditionally the 'growing edge' of a tumour is considered to be the most appropriate area for evaluation. This tends to be the most proliferative and is often the area in which the mitotic count for a histological grade is calculated. An alternative is to use the 'worst' or most poorly differentiated area, which provides potentially the poorest prognostic characteristics. Selecting the growing edge is virtually impossible in some forms of tissue preparations, such as needle core biopsies or trans-urethral resections of prostate. Moreover, both TLI and BrdULI methods require that fresh tissue is cut into very small pieces to allow access of the nucleotides to the nucleus. Again, it is almost impossible to be certain that the growing edge is being evaluated.

If a *formal count* is being made then a sufficient number of cells must be evaluated to be representative of the section as a whole, thus reducing the effect of area selection, whereas if an *estimate* of the frequency of the marker is being made then the entire section is assessed.

Which method of assessment should be used?

It is no longer appropriate to carry out an assessment of proliferation without defining the criteria used to reach the end result. It is important to decide whether intensity of staining is an important feature. Obviously, this will not be a consideration for evaluating either mitoses or AgNORs but with immunohistochemical based markers it may represent an increase in protein expression above its usual base level, such as in the case of PCNA. If intensity of staining is relevant then it should be combined with either a count or an estimate of the proportion of stained cells.

Accurate quantification of any marker requires a formal count to be made both of the cells which are demonstrated and those which are not, thus providing a 'proliferative index'. A quick look at the publications where a count has been undertaken reveals a considerable variation in the total numbers of cells evaluated. To be correct statistically, sufficient numbers of cells must be evaluated in order to reduce the counting error to an acceptable level. This is usually considered to be less than 5%. If only a few cells are evaluated the result could considerably either overestimate or underestimate the true proliferative activity. As more cells are included in the evaluation, then this error is gradually reduced. A universal figure for the number of cells to count cannot be applied to all of the different markers and different types of tissue. In general, counts need to be increased both in heterogeneous tissues and when the incidence of demonstration of the marker is low. For example, MIB1 detects cells in all phases of the cell cycle, except G_0, whereas a mitotic index 'detects' events only in a limited part of the cell cycle. Hence, in any given piece of tissue, the proportion of cells expressing MIB1 will be much higher than those undergoing mitosis. Therefore, in order to achieve the same acceptable level of error for both markers, the total numbers of cells evaluated for the mitotic activity index would need to be much more than for the MIB1 count.

There has been little published work directed at comparing counting methods but in general counts in excess of 1000 cells appear to reduce the counting error to an acceptable level. Sometimes counting as many cells as this can be a problem in very small samples, such as needle core biopsies or when the lesion of interest forms only a small part of the tissue being examined such as mammary ductal carcinoma *in situ* or other intra-epithelial neoplasms. In such cases it may be necessary to evaluate multiple levels of the tissue in order to get an accurate record of the proliferative activity.

As mentioned previously it is important to balance the time spent evaluating a proliferative marker with the amount of information it provides. Thus, although assessing more cells increases accuracy, it is often not practical and it will certainly not endear the technique to a busy histopathologist. Semi-quantitative assessments which have defined criteria are proving popular because of their relative speed of assessment and because they have been shown to correlate well with markers assessed more quantitatively. For many years mitoses have been counted and expressed per high power field, which is in itself a semi-quantitative assessment and has potential problems.

Prognostic information for both breast and smooth muscle tumours has improved with a more stringent approach to counting mitoses, whilst retaining the use of high power fields. There are now guidelines on how many HPFs to examine and which area of the section to assess. The considerable variation in size of HPFs between different microscopes has also been noted, so it is important to quote the area of the HPF which was used to make the mitotic count. By following these general guidelines a considerable reduction in inter-observer variability has been achieved.

If a semi-quantitative assessment is used it is important to remember that it is only an estimation and that the results should not be too precise. Indeed, the use of quartiles is usually sufficient. The advantage with this type of evaluation is that it can be done quickly enough for the whole of the section to be assessed, thus removing the need to define which area of the section has been examined. If appropriate, a measure of intensity of staining can be combined with the proportion of cells staining to give a total score. A direct comparison of the different methods of evaluation and how long both the technique and the evaluation take for the established markers is shown in Table 8.1.

Controls

As with any technique, it is important to have controls throughout the procedure. Not only are methodological control sections required but also checks should be done to ensure consistency both in demonstration and evaluation of markers between samples.

Control material must always be included when demonstrating a proliferation marker. The same control sections should be used throughout a study in order to monitor inter-assay consistency. Internal controls, when the staining patterns of specific tissue elements are known, are also very useful to check the quality of demonstration. They can also be used to make adjustments to the 'score' when the sections are thicker (and hence the staining is more intense) or when the method of fixation is not standardized.

Reproducibility of the evaluation procedure should also be included as part of the quality

Method of Evaluation

Table 8.1: Comparison of time taken to demonstrate and evaluate different markers of proliferative activity.

Marker	Method of evaluation	Time for technique	Time for evaluation (min)
Counting methods			
Mitosis	Mitoses per 10 HPF	5 min	5
	Mitoses per 2000 cells	5 min	15
pKi67	Positive nuclei per 1000 cells	3 hrs	5–10
mKi67			
MIB1			
KiS1			
KiS5			
PCNA	Stronger positive nuclei per 2000 cells	3 hrs	15–20
TLI	Labelled nuclei per 2000 cells	10–14 days (plus 2 hrs incubation prior to fixation)	15–20
BrdULI	Positive nuclei per 2000 cells	3 hrs	15–20
Histone 3 mRNA	Positive nuclei per 2000 cells	24 hrs	15–20
AgNOR	Mean number per 100 cells	15–45 min	20–35
Automated method			
S-Phase fraction (Flow cytometry)	Quantity of nuclear staining per cell in > 10 000 cells	2–3 hrs	>5
Image analysis method			
AgNORs	Mean area of AgNORs occupying nucleus in 150 cells	15–45 min	15–20

control aspect of any study or individual case. If either a new marker or a new evaluation method is being introduced, or someone has not assessed proliferative activity before, then the assessment should also be carried out by an experienced evaluator. A comparison of the data from both assessors provides a guide to the inter-observer variability. Any discordant values can be re-examined with joint consultation. Evaluator skills tend to improve with practice, therefore cases which have been assessed early on in a study should be repeated at the end to ensure that the result is the same and the method of evaluation has remained consistent.

Computer-aided image analysis systems are evolving rapidly and will come to have a particularly important role in the assessment of proliferative markers in the future. There is a steady increase in the numbers of publications which have used image analysis. In particular, the evaluation of AgNORs has benefited from semi-automated analysis. AgNORs are extremely difficult to count with any degree of reliability and their proliferative value has been disputed. Measuring the mean total area of silver deposition per nucleus by image analysis has shown a consistent association with proliferative activity and has considerably improved the credibility of AgNORs.

The recognition of individual cells in a histological section remains a difficult task for an image analyzer and discerning a weakly positive immunostained cell from a negative cell, whilst appearing easy to the human eye, proves difficult for an analysis system. If a slice is taken through a sphere, as when a nucleus is sectioned, then the internal edges of the sphere will be less dense than more central areas. If this is considered in the context of an immunohistochemically stained nucleus, then the nucleus will have a reduced colour intensity at the periphery, which can be difficult to distinguish from the non-staining cytoplasm. Nevertheless, automated analysis continues to make progress. Programmes are being developed which can recognize the various characteristics associated with nuclei undergoing mitosis, and the use of stains with a greater degree of contrast can also make analysis more accurate.

One of the main problems to overcome is that of breaking away from the idea that image analysis should provide information in an identical format to that of a visual assessment. In a number of studies, where immunohistochemical markers have been shown to be prognostically useful, the image analysis systems have compared areas of colour. For example, in each HPF, an analyser compares the total area of brown, which denotes DAB demonstration of a bound proliferation-associated antibody, with the total area of blue, which denotes the haematoxylin-stained nuclei. These parameters are measured over much of the section and the resultant proliferative activity is shown by the ratio of total area of the proliferation marker to total area of nuclei.

Conclusion

The initial confusion which greets most novices in the measurement of proliferative activity can be remedied easily by looking at one aspect of the procedure at a time. First of all some of the markers such as TLI or mKi67 may be discounted if the tissues of interest are fixed and paraffin wax-embedded. The choice of marker is also dependent upon the facilities available in the laboratory. Specific projects, with a limited number of cases, can often be undertaken in conjunction with a laboratory with specialized facilities. This would enable methods like flow cytometric analysis or autoradiography for thymidine labelling to be carried out. However, if measuring proliferation is important, then the type of method used for detecting proliferating cells should be suited to the individuals' own laboratory. For this reason there is a tendency for the more conventional 'morphometric' methods, such as mitoses and AgNORs or immunohistochemical methods to be used in histopathology laboratories.

Currently, the best methods of measuring proliferative activity in histological sections are by the proportion of either mitoses or Ki67 antigen-expressing cells. Both have been well documented in a variety of disorders, are technically easy to demonstrate and, provided that the sections are well prepared, are relatively easy to assess. There remains great discussion on how valid both mitoses and Ki67 positive cells are as markers of proliferative activity. Mitoses obviously only demonstrate a relatively short part of the cell cycle and from the resultant mitotic count or activity index no inferences can be made about the rest of the cell cycle. However, there are certainly no problems with lack of specificity with this marker. MIB1 identifies part of the Ki67 protein which is present virtually throughout the cell cycle, although some cells do not express the antigen early in G_1 and would falsely under represent the proliferative activity in tissues. MIB1 can also be detected if the cell has recently left the cell cycle. New markers, in particular antibodies, are continuing to be developed to overcome some of the problems with specificity. These novel markers will have to provide proliferative and prognostic information beyond that provided by mitoses or MIB1 if they are to be considered as viable alternatives.

The evaluation debate looks set to continue for some time to come. For example, mitoses have been recognized as proliferative markers for decades and yet new 'improved' methods of evaluation are still being promoted. However, once some of the evaluation criteria have been applied, and regardless of which method of assessment is chosen, the 'golden rule' is to be consistent from one case to the next. When automated analysis has proved itself it will no doubt be used to evaluate all proliferation markers in histological sections but, until that time comes, sufficiently accurate results can be obtained using either a formal count or a semi-quantitative evaluation, provided that a consistent approach is taken and adequate controls are used.

Further Reading

Baak J P A. Mitosis counting in tumors. *Hum. Pathol.* 1990; **21**:683–685.

Cattoretti G, Becker M H G, Key G, Duchrow M, Schulter C, Galle J, Gerdes J. Monoclonal antibodies against recombinant parts of the Ki67 antigen (MIB-1 and MIB-3) detect proliferating cells in microwave-processed formalin fixed paraffin sections. *J. Pathol.* 1992; **168**:357–363.

Quirke P. Flow cytometry in the quantitation of DNA aneuploidy and cell proliferation in human disease. In: J C E Underwood (ed) *Current Topics in Pathology – Pathology of the Nucleus.* 1990: Springer-Verlag, Berlin, 215–256.

Rüschoff J, Plate K H, Contractor H, Kern S, Zimmerman R, Thomas C. Evaluation of nucleolus organizer regions (NORs) by automatic image analysis: A contribution to standardization. *J. Pathol.* 1990; **161**:113–118.

SECTION 2
CYTOLOGY

9 CYTOPATHOLOGY

Adrian T Warfield

This chapter is intended to provide a synoptic overview of the general principles of diagnostic cytopathology. This is largely a visual subject and therefore plentiful examples and illustrations are included as appropriate. It is by no means a technical or diagnostic treatise on the subject. For systematic, detailed coverage the interested reader is encouraged to consult one of the many works of reference, some of which are listed at the conclusion of this chapter.

Introduction

Cytology is the scientific study of the structure and function of cells. Cytopathology is a branch of laboratory medicine concerned with the examination of cells in health and disease for screening, diagnostic and research purposes. Screening involves the examination of samples from asymptomatic individuals to detect premalignant or early malignant changes. Diagnostic work involves the assessment of material from patients with established signs or symptoms of disease.

It is a basic premise that the content of a cytology specimen should accurately and reproducibly represent the cell population of the target tissue or lesion. In reality a number of confounding variables sometimes militate against this assumption to a greater or lesser degree.

A careful cytomorphological assessment by light microscopy is fundamental to the practice of diagnostic cytopathology and much information has traditionally been derived from the direct comparison of cell samples with corresponding histological sections. Certain limitations, however, are inherent in such extrapolation studies even in adequately sampled, optimally preserved and well-stained material.

Cell culture utilizes immortalized cell lines to detect viral cytopathic and other toxic effects. This and novel, specialized microscopy, microsuction and microdissection techniques enable insight into the dynamic physiology of living protoplasm. At present, however, these are

103

considered peripheral to mainstream diagnostic cytopathology and are encountered more commonly in viral diagnostic or research work.

Types of Cytology Specimen

Most clinical cytology specimens are obtained by one of the following processes:

Exfoliation

Cells sampled are shed (exfoliated) naturally from an epithelial surface. Examples include cells present in sputum (expectorated), urine (voided or via catheter or cystoscope) and nipple discharge (expressed) (Fig. 9.1, 9.2). Spontaneously exfoliated cells differ in appearance from those forcibly denuded by mechanical means, tending to be disaggregated and individually disposed or in small clusters. Such cells often assume a spherical form dependent upon such factors as the rigidity of the cell membrane, inherent cytoskeletal forces, surface tension, the nature of the local microenvironment and the time since shedding. They are susceptible to a series of degenerative changes involving both the cytoplasm and the nucleus as outlined later.

Abrasion

Cells sampled result from denudation by physical force (abrasion). Examples include brushings (e.g. bronchus, cervix), scrapings (e.g. nipple, skin, cervix) or lavage (e.g. bronchus) where isotonic saline is insufflated and the fluid re-aspirated is submitted for examination. In contrast to naturally exfoliated cells, these cells tend to be better preserved, often in larger groups or cohesive aggregates.

Aspiration

There are few organs or sites in the body which are not readily accessible by needle to yield some sort of cellular material for examination. Radiological imaging techniques may assist in localizing small, deep, mobile lesions that are otherwise difficult to palpate. Cells are obtained through a needle, with or without suction, from a fluid-filled cavity or solid tissue. Examples include tumours, pericardial, pleural

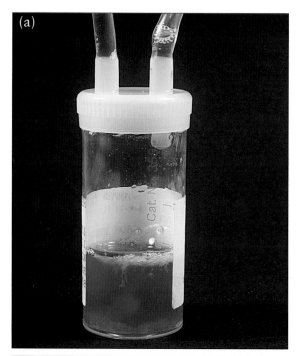

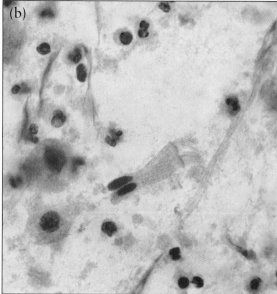

Figure 9.1: Sputum sample. (a) Mucoid, blood-stained sputum obtained by direct suction aspiration ('sputum trap'). This give less contamination by oropharyngeal secretions than an expectorated sample. (b) Bronchial epithelial cells and pulmonary alveolar macrophages here indicate lower respiratory tract sampling. Terminal bars and surface microvilli can be seen at the apices of the bronchial cells amidst a sparse mucoinflammatory background. (Pap × 250).

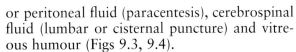

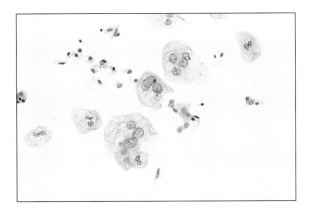

Figure 9.2: Normal superficial transitional cells in urine. These exfoliated uroepithelial cells show variable multinucleation corresponding to 'umbrella cells' in histological sections. Note the uncluttered ('clean') background. (Pap × 100).

or peritoneal fluid (paracentesis), cerebrospinal fluid (lumbar or cisternal puncture) and vitreous humour (Figs 9.3, 9.4).

Fine needle aspiration utilizes a fine bore needle (19 to 25 gauge) firmly attached to a syringe, which is introduced into a lesion. The syringe plunger is partially withdrawn thereby creating a vacuum and aspirating lesional cells. Several passes through a lesion in different directions whilst maintaining suction may be attempted to increase the cellular harvest. Once completed, the plunger is released to equalize the pressure prior to withdrawal of the needle from the lesion. Various 'pistol grip' attachments designed to facilitate single-handed manipulation of the syringe are commercially available, freeing the opposite hand for palpa-

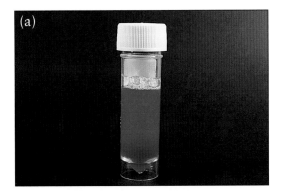

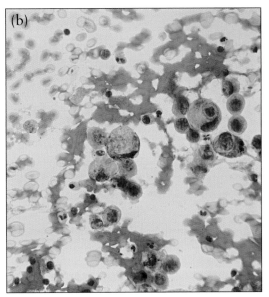

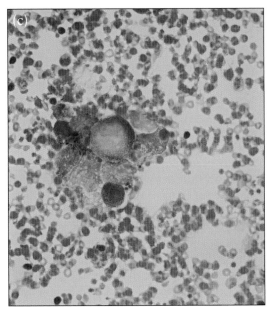

Figure 9.3: Malignant pleural aspirate. (a) Bloodstained sample from a unilateral pleural effusion in a patient who had undergone mastectomy for breast carcinoma. Microscopy (b) and (c) shows dyscohesive pleomorphic adenocarcinoma cells, many possessing a 'signet ring' morphology with abundant intracytoplasmic mucin indenting the peripheral nucleus. (b) Pap × 100 (c) MGG × 100.

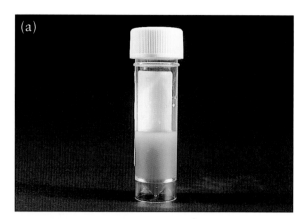

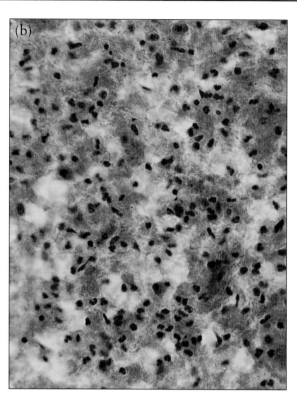

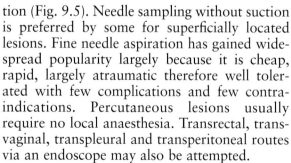

Figure 9.4: *Ascitic fluid. (a) An aliquot of turbid, malodorous ascitic fluid aspirated from a patient with faecal peritonitis shortly prior to death. Microscopy (b) and (c) shows innumerable variform bacteria with pus cells. The debris and pigment are of stercoral origin. (b) Pap × 100 (c) MGG × 100.*

tion (Fig. 9.5). Needle sampling without suction is preferred by some for superficially located lesions. Fine needle aspiration has gained widespread popularity largely because it is cheap, rapid, largely atraumatic therefore well tolerated with few complications and few contra-indications. Percutaneous lesions usually require no local anaesthesia. Transrectal, transvaginal, transpleural and transperitoneal routes via an endoscope may also be attempted.

Bone marrow aspirates are normally the province of the diagnostic haematopathologist.

Failure to obtain a satisfactory aspirate may not necessarily be attributable to poor technique. Desmoplastic, hyalinized or vascular lesions, extensive necrosis, cystic change or haemorrhage may all preclude adequate cell sampling (Fig. 9.6).

Smearing Techniques

The ideal smear should be evenly spread, uniformly thin and flat to enable rapid drying and fixation and to permit optimal penetration of stain. *Direct smear* techniques involve spreading fresh material across a slide utilizing another slide, pick or spatula (Fig. 9.7). *Indirect smear* techniques employ material suspended in fluid e.g. saline or transport medium. A cell concentration procedure may be performed as an intermediary step to increase the yield from a hypocellular specimen.

Clot formation may sequester much of the cellular component of a specimen, preventing adequate transfer of material to a slide. If a clot cannot be dispersed by mechanical means it should therefore be processed as a cell block or

CYTOPATHOLOGY

Specimen Fixation
Wet fixation
Air drying
Cell Concentration Techniques
Centrifugation

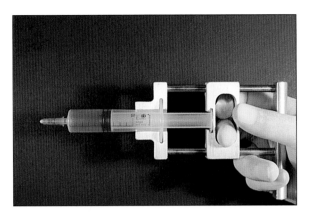

Figure 9.5: *Pistol attachment for fine needle aspiration. Ready with loaded disposable syringe and 23 gauge needle, this allows single-handed manipulation of the syringe, freeing the other hand for palpation.*

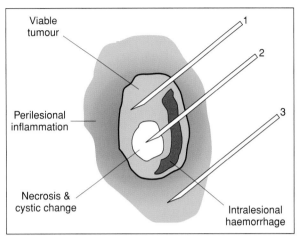

Figure 9.6: *Schematic diagram of a tumour during fine needle aspiration. The viable solid portion of the tumour is pierced by needle 1 to yield potentially diagnostic material; needle 2 piercing areas of necrosis, haemorrhage or cystic change and needle 3 sampling perilesional tissue are unlikely to do so.*

submitted for conventional histology and examined thoroughly (Fig. 9.8).

Cell deposits from transudates, salinated washings and urine may not adhere well to glass slides. Adhesives commonly of proteinaceous (e.g. bovine serum albumin) or ionic (e.g. poly-L-lysine) type may enhance adherence, maximizing the cellular material for examination.

Other techniques less commonly employed include touch imprints, scrapings and squash preparations, the latter popular in peroperative neurosurgical diagnosis in preference to conventional histology on frozen sections.

Specimen Fixation

Wet fixation

Wet fixation dehydrates protoplasm and coagulates protein, usually employing an alcohol-based fluid, either by immersion or coating. Such fixation induces a degree of cell shrinkage in the final preparation. Carnoy's fluid selectively lyses erythrocytes and may be helpful in heavily blood-stained specimens. Other fixatives, e.g. glutaraldehyde or formalin, may be preferred under certain circumstances. Polyethylene glycol in alcohol provides a protective waxy coating for postal despatch which should be thoroughly removed before subsequent staining.

Air drying

Air drying relies upon evaporation which should be rapid and is best facilitated by forced air movement over the slide rather than passively. This method tends to flatten cells with apparent enlargement compared to wet fixation (Figs 9.9, 9.10). Air dried preparations are almost invariably post-fixed in methanol after drying to prevent cross-infection hazards.

Material such as cyst fluid or needle washings following fine needle aspiration may be received in transport medium. It should be remembered that any fresh biological specimen constitutes a potential biohazard to laboratory personnel and recommended health and safety precautions should always be observed.

Cell Concentration Techniques

Centrifugation

This method is suitable for voluminous specimens such as serous effusions, urine or salinated lavage samples.

Cell Concentration Techniques

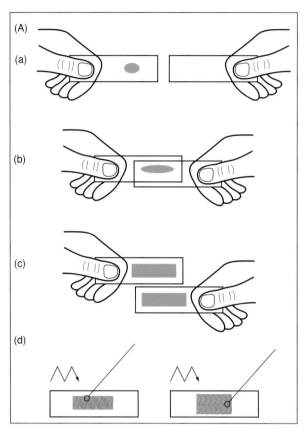

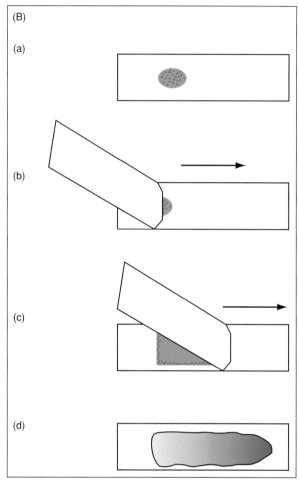

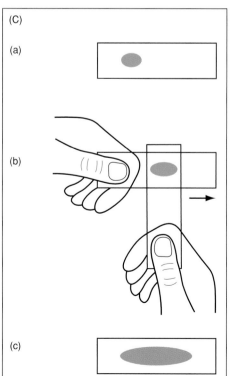

Figure 9.7: *(A) Direct smearing technique for mucoid specimens. (a) A drop of the sample is applied on a slide. (b) A second slide is placed on top with gentle pressure to spread the fluid evenly. (c) The slides are pulled apart and fixed immediately. (d) An alternative method is to spread the specimen as evenly as possible using a pick or spatula. (B) Blood film method for non-mucoid specimens. (a) A drop of the specimen is applied to a slide. (b) A separate spreader slide is drawn towards the sample. (c) The smear is gently made. (d) Cell aggregates tend to be distributed towards the periphery and tail of the smear. (C) Squash method for non-mucoid specimens. (a) A drop of sample is applied to a slide. (b) A separate spreader slide is placed on top of this and with even pressure to the smear drawn out. (c) Cell aggregates tend to be evenly distributed throughout the preparation.*

CYTOPATHOLOGY

Cell Concentration Techniques
Cytocentrifugation
Membrane filtration
Cell block preparation
Staining Methods

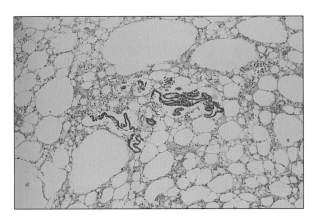

Figure 9.8: *Benign mucinous tumour of ovary. This fibrin clot has sequestered virtually all of the aspirated epithelium from the fluid from this cystic ovary. The corresponding cytopreparations consisted almost exclusively of blood and, in isolation, were deemed unsatisfactory for diagnostic purposes. This illustrates the importance of examining any clot present in fluid aspirates (H & E × 25).*

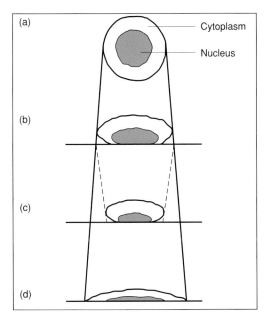

Figure 9.9: *Effect of wet fixation and air drying on cells. (a) An unfixed cell in solution often assumes a spherical shape. (b) This settles onto a slide and partially flattens. (c) Wet fixation ultimately shrinks the cell somewhat. (d) Air drying causes flattening and spreading of the cell with apparent enlargement in its final state. A spherical cell may present a diameter twice its original size whereas a mature squamoid cell will show little apparent increase in size.*

Cytocentrifugation

This utilizes small aliquots of fluid spun directly onto microscope slides to form a localized monolayer of cells (Figs 9.11, 9.12, 9.13). It is suitable for low-volume samples of modest cellularity. Some material is, however, inevitably lost into the filter card. Viscid or cellular specimens are unsuitable.

Membrane filtration

Positive pressure or vacuum filtration is employed by using various types of filter of predetermined pore size, e.g. cellulose acetate or polycarbonate. It is suitable for a wide range of large volume or hypocellular fluid specimens and may yield a greater cell capture than centrifugation methods.

Cell block preparation

Cells are aggregated into a tissue-like state enabling sections to be cut comparable to conventional histology. Methods include plasma thrombin clot utilizing plasma and agar cell block with hot agar. They are suitable for most cell suspensions and allow special staining including immunocytochemistry.

Staining Methods

Many techniques applied to tissue sections may also be performed on cytopreparations. In general the Papanicolaou (Pap) stain is employed for wet-fixed material. The differential staining pattern is useful both for gynaecological and non-gynaecological specimens and permits prolonged periods of microscopy with minimal eye strain.

Romanowsky stains (May–Grünwald–Giemsa (MGG), Diff Quik, etc) are usually performed on air dried preparations and are amenable both to automatic and rapid manual techniques. This method is employed predominantly for non-gynaecological material.

Haematoxylin and eosin staining is favoured by some more familiar with conventional histological sections.

A wide variety of ancillary histochemical stains may be performed as indicated. Examples include periodic acid–Schiff with or without dias-

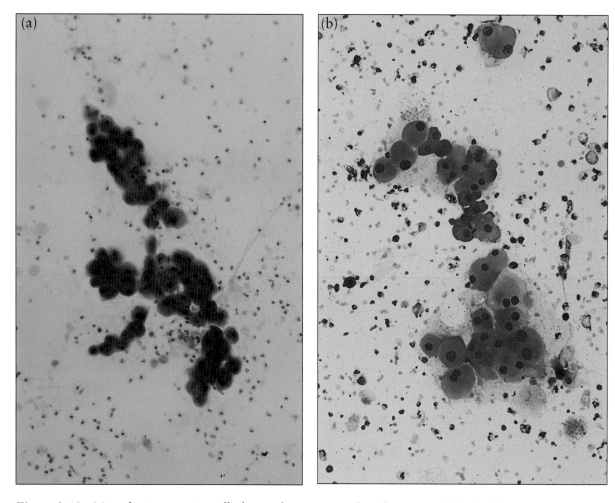

Figure 9.10: Metaplastic apocrine cells from a breast cyst. These benign epithelial cells were present in fluid from a breast cyst and illustrate the complementary nature of the Papanicolaou and May–Grünwald–Giemsa staining. The apparent disparity in the size of the cells at identical magnification is due to wet fixation and dry fixation respectively. [(a) Pap × 50 (b) MGG × 50].

tase predigestion for neutral mucosubstances and glycogen, trichrome stains, Ziehl–Neelsen, Gram and Grocott methenamine silver stains, amongst others.

The repertoire of immunocytological techniques is comparable to that on tissue sections. Immunocytochemistry may be invaluable in ascertaining the presence of microorganisms or in demonstrating tumour cell differentiation (Fig. 9.14).

Cytodiagnosis

The cytodiagnostic procedure is a complex process. It cannot be overemphasized that reaching a final conclusion depends on many factors including detailed site-specific knowledge coupled with experience of normality, familiarity with the manifold appearances of many disease processes, awareness of mimics and artefacts and cognizance of the limitations of the technique, in conjunction with patient-specific details and the clinical context (see Table 9.1). Abundant, well-preserved material

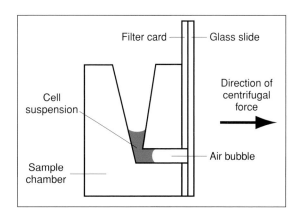

Figure 9.13: *Schematic diagram of cytocentrifuge assembly. Centrifugal force drives the cell suspension through the filter card and onto the glass slide. This is unsuitable for mucoid specimens.*

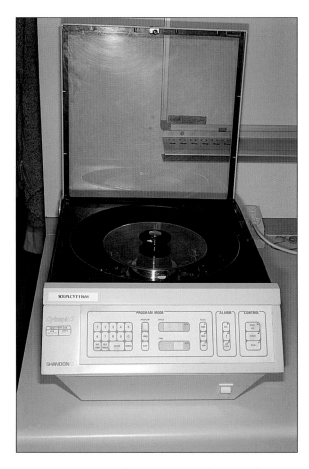

Figure 9.11: *A modern cytocentrifuge machine.*

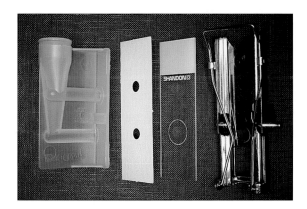

Figure 9.12: *Cytocentrifuge chamber components. Suction chamber, filter card, glass slide and spring clip prior to assembly.*

as ever affords the best opportunity of reaching a definitive diagnosis. Without this background information the cytopreparation is in danger of becoming a two-dimensional, brightly-stained artefact which may be as misleading as it can be potentially helpful. In some instances it may be better to reach an initial 'blind' morphological diagnosis from first principles to avoid preconceived bias. This may then be modified, taking into account such variables as appropriate, before a diagnosis is proffered and any advice on patient management forthcoming.

A cytopreparation is usually a complex admixture of components in varying proportions depending upon the tissue or lesion sampled. Normal and abnormal cells may be present and the cell content, disposition and distribution within a sample should be systematically assessed. Not all features will be relevant to any particular specimen.

Cytomorphology

Much of the diagnostic workload in most laboratories is concerned with discriminating between non-neoplastic, pre-neoplastic and neoplastic lesions. Normal cells are characterized by their morphological uniformity. The nuclear morphology reflects the state of proliferation of a cell and its reproductive capacity. The cytoplasm of a cell generally gives an

Cytomorphology

Specimen cellularity

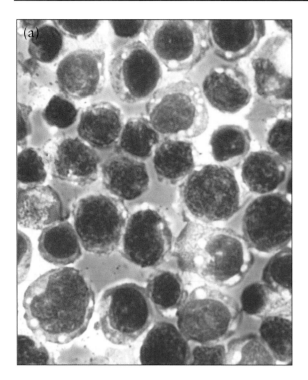

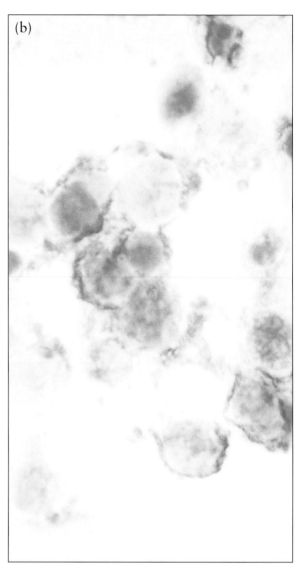

Figure 9.14: *Low-grade non-Hodgkin's lymphoma.*
(a) This aspirate of vitreous humour from the eye
contains innumerable, modestly pleomorphic,
immature-looking lymphocytes with varying
amounts of cytoplasm (MGG × high power)
(b) Immunocytochemistry confirms widespread
CD45 (leukocyte common antigen) reactivity.
(Immunoperoxidase × high power).

indication of its origin, functional state and degree of differentiation.

Increased cell activity may be physiological, such as *hyperplasia*, due to hormonal modulation, or reparative and regenerative in response to damage. An abnormal, uncontrolled proliferative state implies neoplasia.

Decreased cell activity may also be physiological due to atrophy, involutional changes secondary to hormonal influence, senescence or degenerative as in apoptosis.

There is no single cytomorphological criterion or limited set of criteria which in isolation allow a reliable distinction between biologically benign and malignant conditions under all circumstances. The cytonuclear differences between regenerative or hyperplastic cells and low grade neoplastic cells may be subtle and on occasion indistinguishable. Post-radiotherapy, post-chemotherapy, viral and other changes may induce appearances which mimic closely those seen in neoplasia (Fig. 9.15).

Specimen cellularity
The number and type of cells present give important information about the target tissue. Both are subject to lesional and non-lesional factors, particularly the sampling method employed. In general, hypercellularity raises the index of suspicion for a proliferative process,

Table 9.1: Variables which might influence the final interpretation of a cytopreparation.

Patient specific details	Age and sex
	Hormonal status e.g. pregnancy
	Clinical impression
	Previous treatment e.g. radiotherapy, surgery
	Previous material e.g. histology, cytology
	Other laboratory tests
Site specific details	Knowledge of local anatomy
	Radiological features
	Awareness of pitfalls and mimics
	Limitations of technique
Cell population	Degree of cellularity
	Type of cells present e.g. biphasic or single population
	Alien or native populations
	Normal or abnormal morphology
Cytomorphology	Background milieu
	Cell distribution and cohesion
	Individual cell morphology
Ancillary information	Electron microscopy
	Histochemical stains
	Immunocytochemistry
	Image analysis
	Flow cytometry
	Cytogenetics

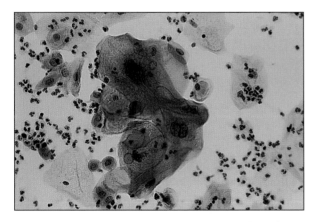

Figure 9.15: Radiation atypia in a vaginal vault smear. Abnormal giant squamous cells ('macrocytes') following radiotherapy. Similar bizarre changes may follow chemotherapy, accompany vitamin B12 or folate deficiency and may occur in viral condylomata. Note the multinucleation and increase in both nuclear and cytoplasmic area. Background inflammatory cells and superficial squamae are useful reference features. (Pap × 100).

either hyperplasia or neoplasia. Conversely however, paucicellularity is not necessarily a reassuring feature, as an absence of abnormal cells by no means excludes serious pathology. Low-grade neoplasms may exfoliate sparsely and yield cells showing minimal deviation from normality. A poverty of adequate material may be a crucial limiting factor in the degree of confidence in interpretation of a sample.

Cytoarchitectural pattern

Many of the architectural clues present in conventional histological sections are often absent in cytopreparations. Larger collections of cells (microbiopsies) if present, often recapitulate the histological pattern of the target tissue (Fig. 9.16). Normal epithelium from many sites is characterized by retained cell polarity and intercellular cohesion. Glandular epithelium yields regularly arranged, monolayered sheets which when viewed *en face* give a 'honeycomb' appear-

Cytomorphology

Nuclear features

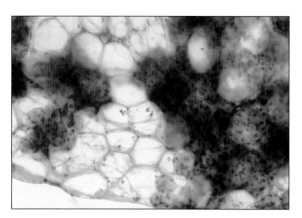

Figure 9.16: *Normal parotid gland. This fine needle aspirate contains a 'microbiopsy' comprising adipose connective tissue intimately admixed with normal acinar secretory tissue from a middle-aged patient. (Pap × 80).*

dyscohesion and disaggregation. Normal lymphoid cells display poor intercellular cohesion as do their neoplastic counterparts (lymphoma) and the dispersed cell pattern of poorly differentiated carcinoma and high grade lymphoma may on occasion be indistinguishable without resort to ancillary techniques. Normal, reactive or neoplastic stromal cells (mesenchyme) may be apparent and adipocytes, capillaries or other connective tissue fragments often emanate from a perilesion site. Benign stromal elements usually manifest as ovoid or fusiform, loosely cohesive cells or bare nuclei (sentinel or bipolar cells) depending on the precise circumstances. Malignant stromal cells (sarcoma) show a similar pattern but with superimposed abnormal nuclear and cytoplasmic features.

Nuclear features

Abnormalities of nuclear morphology are termed *dyskaryosis* and may be graded as mild, moderate and severe or as high-grade and low-grade with increasing deviation from normality. In the normal end-differentiated (mature) cell the nucleus is relatively small compared to the overall volume of the cell, usually of round or ovoid shape with a smooth nuclear contour, evenly distributed, finely granular chromatin and little variation between cells of similar type (isomorphic or monomorphic).

ance and in profile a palisaded 'picket-fence' pattern [Fig. 9.17(a) & (b).] Hyperplastic and benign neoplastic epithelia generally also retain cohesion but may exhibit an unusual outline such as a papilliform, rosette or morular configuration. Syncytium formation with ill-defined cell boundaries and some malorientation is suspect of neoplasia. Malignant epithelial cells (carcinoma) usually present as poorly polarized, overlapping cells, sometimes in three-dimensional clumps (proliferation spheres) with a tendency towards

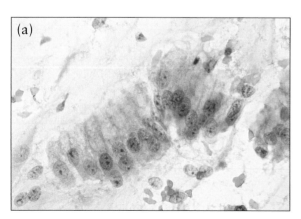

(a)

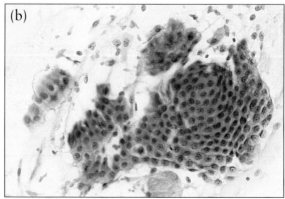

(b)

Figure 9.17: *Normal gastric glandular epithelium. (a) Tall columnar glandular epithelial cells give a regular palisaded or 'picket-fence' appearance when viewed in profile. Note the preserved polarity and round, evenly-spaced nuclei with one or two small nucleoli. (Pap × 80) (b) A monolayer of cohesive, well-orientated, isomorphic glandular epithelium displays a 'honeycomb' pattern when viewed en face. Again, the regularly spaced nuclei with occasional small nucleoli and rounded nuclear contour are well demonstrated. (Pap × 40).*

In a two-dimensional cytopreparation the nuclear size is proportional to the relative nuclear area and may be expressed as the cytonuclear index, nuclear : cytoplasmic ratio or quantified as a percentage. Poorly differentiated cells usually possess enlarged nuclei (karyomegaly or nucleomegaly) and for the same absolute cytoplasmic volume therefore exhibit elevated nuclear : cytoplasmic ratio.

Most normal cells show reasonably homogeneous nuclear chromatin with a finely granular distribution and modest affinity for nuclear dyes. Increased nuclear DNA content results in greater density of nuclear staining (hyperchromasia). Irregularly distributed chromatin with a coarse, clumped texture and thickened nuclear envelope is termed *karyotheca*. Variation in size and shape of nuclei between cells is termed *anisokaryosis* or *anisonucleosis* and with increasing abnormality the nuclear membrane may become irregular in contour with grooving, indentation or crenation. The constellation of abnormal variation in size, shape and intensity of nuclear staining is termed *nuclear pleomorphism* (Fig. 9.18).

Normal nuclei may contain small, discrete nucleoli composed of RNA and associated proteins. Multinucleolation and macronucleoli are observed in proliferation states, both neoplastic and non-neoplastic. Degenerative chromatin

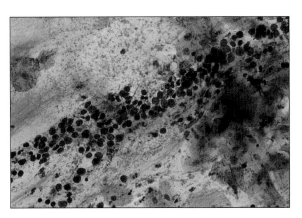

Figure 9.19: *Anaplastic small cell carcinoma in sputum. Loosely cohesive, largely degenerate 'oat cell' carcinoma cells lie within a streak of mucus. In some the finely dispersed ('salt and pepper') chromatin is just discernible as is focal nuclear moulding. They possess minimal cytoplasm with hyperchromatic, karyopyknotic nuclei for the most part. Superficial squamae, erythrocytes and lymphocytes give an indication of relative size. (Pap × 100).*

may appear as a dense, contracted mass (*karyopyknosis*), as dense fragments (*karyorrhexis*) or may undergo dissolution (*karyolysis* or *chromatolysis*). Cytolysis may yield naked or bare, often hypochromatic nuclear remnants and inherent nuclear membrane fragility of some cells results in nuclear streaming or smearing artefact. This often affects lymphoid cells or may be a feature of small cell, anaplastic carcinoma (Fig. 9.19). This may be closely mimicked by *vorticose* damage when cells are forcibly ejected through a fine bore needle onto a slide.

Most cells possess a single nucleus although some, undergoing regenerative or reparative activity, e.g., hepatocytes and chondrocytes, may be *binucleated*. Osteoclasts and syncytiotrophoblast are normally polynucleated. Multinucleation may be a feature both of inflammatory and neoplastic conditions. (Figs 9.20, 9.21).

It is unusual to encounter mitoses in cytopreparations. An increased number of mitoses implies cell proliferation and abnormal spindle forms (tripolar, tetrapolar, etc) are not usually seen in benign conditions.

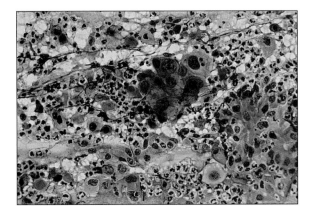

Figure 9.18: *Poorly differentiated squamous cell carcinoma. These malignant cells from bronchial brushings are highly pleomorphic, poorly polarized and demonstrate karyotheca with macronucleolation. Keratinization was more conspicuous in the accompanying bronchial biopsies. (Pap × 100).*

Cytomorphology

Cytoplasmic features

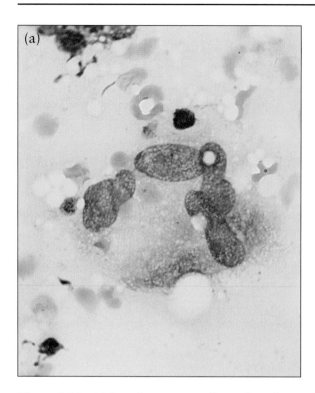

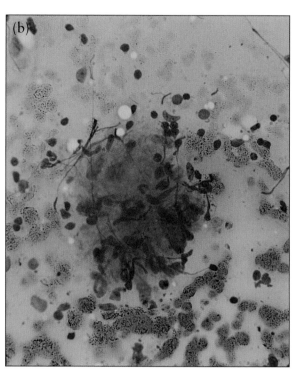

Figure 9.20: *(a) Langhan's giant cell in tuberculosis. This multinucleated giant cell in a fine needle aspirate is of histiocytic origin. The peripheral 'horseshoe' orientation of the nuclei is typical. Other types of giant cell may be observed in a multitude of inflammatory and neoplastic conditions. (MGG × 250) (b) Epithelioid cell granuloma in tuberculosis. This tightly clustered group of ill-defined epithelioid histiocytes from the same fine needle aspirate is evidence of a granulomatous response. Fibrillogranular necrosis was apparent elsewhere and acid/alcohol-fast bacilli were cultured from a similar specimen. (MGG × 100).*

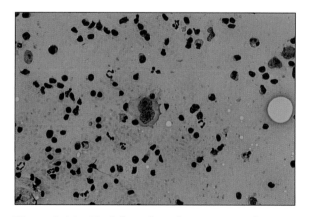

Figure 9.21: *Hodgkin's lymphoma. Central Reed–Sternberg cell showing 'mirror image' binucleation with conspicuous 'owl's eye' macronucleoli. The variform background of eosinophil and neutrophil polymorphs, lymphocytes, plasma cells and histiocytes is characteristic of this condition. (MGG × 100).*

Cytoplasmic features

Variation in the size and shape of similar cells is termed *anisocytosis*. The cytoplasmic volume of an abnormal cell may be larger or smaller than its normal counterpart, thereby influencing the nuclear : cytoplasmic ratio, irrespective of any accompanying nuclear changes. The ultrastructural composition of the cytoplasm, namely the concentration of Golgi apparatus, ribosomes, endoplasmic reticulum, mitochondria and any products of metabolism, exert a major influence on the affinity of various tinctorial staining reactions. Storage products, e.g. mucin, lipid, carbohydrate, hormones or crystalloids, may be highlighted by special stains as appropriate. Mucin globules, foamy microvacuolation, microvillus brush borders and cilia may be discernible in normal or well-differentiated cells. Keratinization indicates squamous differentia-

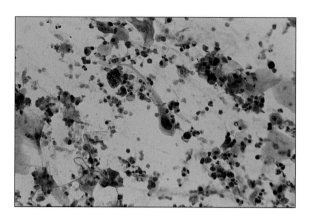

Figure 9.22: Squamous cell carcinoma. This elongated, bizarre squamous cell (caudate, 'tadpole' or 'comet' cell) possesses an enlarged, hyperchromatic nucleus and lies amidst tumour diathesis and degenerate, dyskeratotic squamous cell remnants. Strap-like ('fibre' or 'snake' cell) and brightly orangeophilic ('carrot' cell) forms may sometimes be seen. (Pap × 100).

tion and bizarre elongate or caudate (*non-isodiametric*) cells may be apparent rather than the more usual round or polygonal (*isodiametric*) shapes (Fig. 9.22).

Adjacent cells may demonstrate cytoplasmic moulding or in extreme cases apparent cell engulfment (*embracement* or '*cannibalism*') (Fig. 9.23 (a) & (b)). This is seen both in benign and malignant conditions, but is more common in the latter.

Degenerative cytoplasmic changes include swelling or hydropic change, vacuolation and loss of integrity of the plasma membrane with spillage of cell contents (*cytolysis*).

Background milieu and artefacts
The background content of a cytopreparation may include material both of cellular and non-cellular derivation. This may be either helpful in reaching a diagnosis or a nuisance. Intensely blood-stained material or a vigorous inflammatory response, for example, often obscure the cytonuclear details of any epithelial cell population, limiting the amount of information available.

In addition to the connective tissue stromal components noted earlier, basement membrane material, ground substance, mucus, crystals, fibrinopurulent exudate, colloid, protein-rich

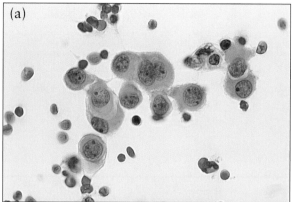
(a)

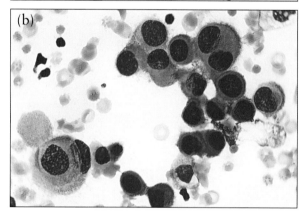
(b)

Figure 9.23: Reactive mesothelial cells arranged both individually and as small groups. Microvillous brush borders are just appreciable around some cells. Empty intercellular spaces ('windows') are a typical feature. Nuclear moulding and apparent cell engulfment (embracement or 'cannibalism') can be seen. [(a) Pap × 250 (b) MGG × 250].

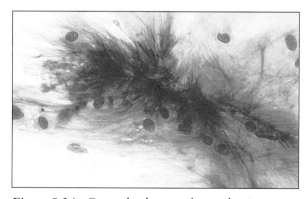

Figure 9.24: Ground substance from a benign salivary pleomorphic adenoma. The epithelial cells are almost obscured by fibrillary ('feathery') Giemsaphilic mucomyxoid ground substance which was much less inconspicuous on Papanicolaou staining. (MGG × 125).

117

Cytomorphology

Background milieu and artefacts

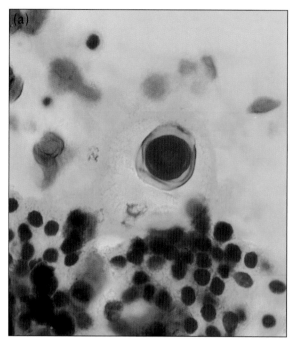

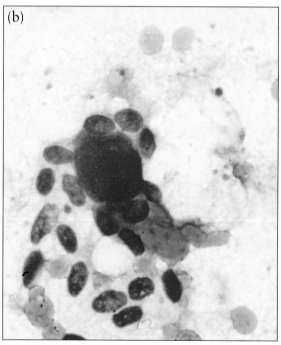

Figure 9.25: Psammoma body. (a) Central psammocalcification exhibiting a typical concentrically laminated, slightly refractile appearance amidst a background of lymphocytes and red blood cells. (Pap × 250) (b) Epithelial-myoepithelial carcinoma of parotid gland. Loosely cohesive, modestly pleomorphic epithelial cells surround densely stained globules of basement membrane material, recapitulating the histological appearances. Similar patterns may be seen in a variety of tumours of salivary and non-salivary gland origin, both benign and malignant. (MGG × 250).

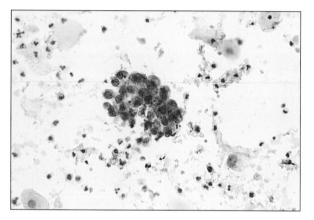

Figure 9.26: Transitional cell carcinoma of bladder. A loosely cohesive, poorly polarized clump of pleomorphic uroepithelial cells. There is nuclear hyperchromasia, an irregular nuclear contour and macronucleolation. Biopsy confirmed high grade transitional cell carcinoma. Note the cytolytic and inflammatory ('dirty') background. (Pap × medium power).

Invasive tumour may be associated with blood, necroinflammatory and degenerate debris (*tumour diathesis*) (Fig. 9.26).

A search for microorganisms or parasites is sometimes indicated. Commensals include *Lactobacillus* in cervicovaginal smears and *Candida* in oropharyngeal specimens. Pathogens include viruses, bacteria, fungi and protozoa amongst others. Some may be directly visible by light microscopy whereas most viral infections are implied by their cytopathic effects. Koilocytosis in human papilloma virus, multinucleation with 'ground glass' nucleoplasm in herpes simplex and 'owl's eye' nuclear inclusions in cytomegalovirus infections are characteristic examples (Fig. 9.27).

fluid or even chondroid tissue microbiopsies may be discernible (Fig. 9.24). Mineralization may manifest as amorphous calcium deposits or sometimes as *psammoma bodies* (Fig. 9.25).

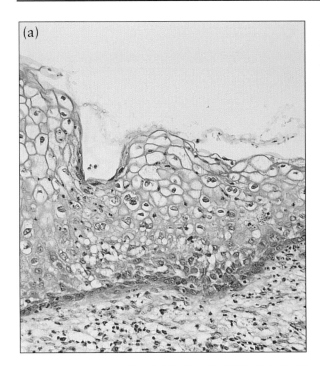

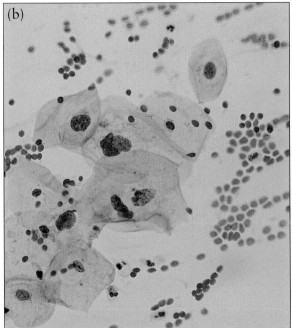

An artefact is an artificial product or morphological change in a cytopreparation arising from physical degradation of a specimen or during sampling, transportation or smear preparation. Contaminants are 'foreign bodies' introduced during these processes. Their importance is due mainly to the fact that they may cause difficulties in accurate interpretation of microscopical appearances. These may be classified as *intrinsic*, arising from an endogenous source, e.g. vegetable or meat fibres and cholesterol crystals, or *extrinsic*, e.g. stain deposits and talc or starch granules from surgical gloves. Poor fixation, particularly initial air drying of subsequent alcohol-fixed, Papanicolaou stained preparations, xylene artefact and air bubbles all give typical appearances (Fig. 9.28). Non-organic elements, e.g. asbestos fibres, are occasionally encountered (Fig. 9.29).

Transfer of cellular material (*cross-contamination*, 'carry over' or 'floaters') from one specimen to another during transport, fixation or staining procedures constitutes a potentially important source of false-positive diagnosis of malignancy and should be avoided at all costs. It is usually preventable by rigorous technique and good laboratory hygiene.

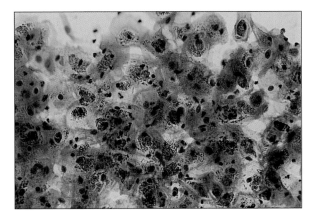

Figure 9.27: Human papilloma virus cytopathic effect. (a) Histology shows multinucleation with clear halos surrounding hyperchromatic, irregular nuclei (koilocytosis). (H & E × medium power) (b) Similar koilocytes present in a cervical smear. Note again the multinucleation, perinuclear clearing of cytoplasm and faint peripheral cytoplasmic condensation. (Pap × 100).

Figure 9.28: 'Cornflake' cells in a cervical smear. A brown, faintly refractile deposit overlies the nuclei and cytoplasm of these squamous cells. This is most commonly seen in cervical smears and is believed to result from air trapping on the surface of cells during mounting. It is rarely so extensive as to render a smear completely uninterpretable. (Pap × 100).

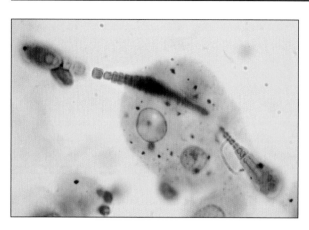

Figure 9.29: Ferruginous body in sputum. A mult-inucleated pulmonary alveolar macrophage partly engulfs a refractile ferruginous body. The brown beaded appearance is due to encrustation of iron pigment upon a colourless fibre, most likely asbestos. The dark intracytoplasmic granules comprise a mixture of anthracotic and haemosiderotic pigment. (Pap × 100).

Spurious environmental contamination is usually of waterborne or airborne origin and may be of biological or non-biological nature (Fig. 9.30).

Accuracy and Limitations of Cytology

Some measure of the reliability and accuracy of diagnostic cytology in various circumstances is useful for comparison and is often expressed statistically (see Table 9.2). Sensitivity (*true positive rate*) is a measure of how successfully a test detects patients with the disease process under consideration. Specificity (*true negative rate*) indicates how well a test excludes those individuals without the disease. *Positive predictive value* and *negative predictive value* give an indication of how accurately the test ascertains the presence or absence of the disease respectively. *A false-negative result* is where the test

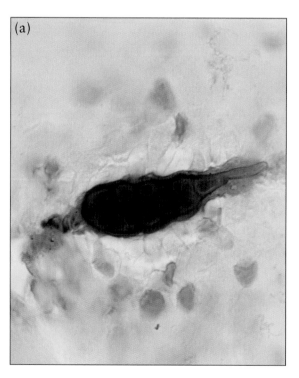

(a)

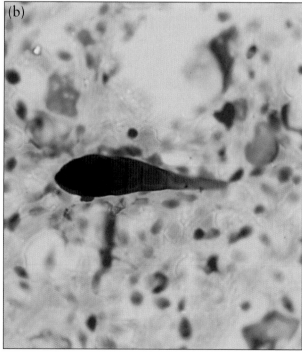

(b)

Figure 9.30: Aerial contaminants. These internally segmented fungal conidia were present at the edge of a smear. They are consistent with Alternaria *spp and are presumed aerial contaminants.*
(a) Pap × 250 (b) MGG × 250.

Table 9.2: Some of the more useful parameters measuring the accuracy of cytology and how they are calculated.

		Disease positive (a + c)	Disease negative (b + d)
Test positive (a + b)		True positive (a)	False positive (b)
Test negative (c + d)		False negative (c)	True negative (d)
Sensitivity	=	$\dfrac{a}{a + c}$	
Specificity	=	$\dfrac{d}{b + d}$	
Positive predictive value	=	$\dfrac{a}{a + b}$	
Negative predictive value	=	$\dfrac{d}{c + d}$	
Accuracy	=	$\dfrac{a + d}{a + b + c + d}$	
Likelihood ratio of a positive test	=	$\dfrac{\text{Sensitivity}}{1 - \text{Specificity}}$	
Likelihood ratio of a negative test	=	$\dfrac{1 - \text{Sensitivity}}{\text{Specificity}}$	

fails to detect subsequently proven disease. This may be due to errors of screening or difficulties in interpretation. A true false-negative is when retrospective review of the material confirms adequacy of the specimen and a genuine negative result. Possible explanations for this include perilesional rather than lesional sampling or the onset of disease following performance of the test procedure (*interval disease*). A *false-positive result* is where the test is reported as positive but the disease cannot subsequently be demonstrated. This may result from difficulties in interpretation or where the appearances of certain conditions may closely resemble each other. The *efficiency* of a test is a measure of how well it correctly classifies those patients who should receive treatment and those for whom treatment is unnecessary.

The absolute statistical values for a particular test may be modulated by the inclusion or exclusion of inadequate or unsatisfactory specimens. Inclusion of these gives an overall indication of clinical effectiveness of the test, whereas excluding these more accurately reflects the laboratory performance.

Gynaecological Cytopathology and Cervical Screening

Cytology specimens from the female genital tract form a major proportion of the routine throughput of most diagnostic laboratories, largely as a result of cervical screening. The prime objective of the cervical smear ('Pap') test is the detection of squamous cell carcinoma and its precursors in asymptomatic women. It is also used in the investigation of women suffering gynaecological symptoms and as part of the monitoring process following treatment. Of secondary importance are the detection of glandular lesions of the cervix or other gynaecological sites, the recognition of a variety of inflammatory and infective conditions and the assessment of hormonal status.

Cervical screening has been demonstrated to be effective in reducing the mortality and morbidity of cervical carcinoma in several countries, albeit not by means of randomized controlled trials. A cervical screening programme has been

Gynaecological Cytopathology and Cervical Screening

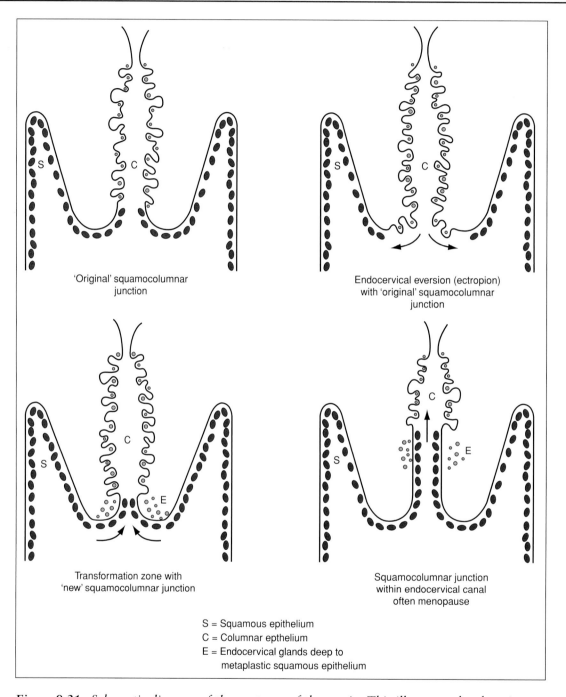

'Original' squamocolumnar
junction

Endocervical eversion (ectropion)
with 'original' squamocolumnar
junction

Transformation zone with
'new' squamocolumnar junction

Squamocolumnar junction
within endocervical canal
often menopause

S = Squamous epithelium
C = Columnar epthelium
E = Endocervical glands deep to
    metaplastic squamous epithelium

Figure 9.31: *Schematic diagram of the anatomy of the cervix. This illustrates the changing morphology of the cervical transformation zone and squamo-columnar junction with advancing years.*

in operation in the UK since 1964. Systematic call and recall of the population was introduced in 1988 under the auspices of the NHS Cervical Screening Programme with establishment of a

national coordinating network. This encourages the uniform classification of abnormalities, standardization of terminology, follow-up of abnormal smears, implementation of quality control mechanisms, evaluates the effectiveness of the Programme via multidisciplinary audit and monitors training of health care professionals.

When all aspects of the screening process are performed optimally the test is a very sensitive method for the detection of precursors of squamous cell carcinoma, less so for invasive carcinoma. It should be remembered, however, that as a screening test it has a low but significant diagnostic error rate. The ultimate goal of eradication of cervical carcinoma has yet to be realized by this route.

The aim of a cervical smear is to representatively sample the cervical transformation zone bordering the squamo-columnar junction, which is the site at greatest risk of neoplastic change (Fig. 9.31). It is ultimately the responsibility of the smear taker to visualize the cervix and ensure that its entire circumference has been sampled whatever the cellularity or cell content of the smear (Fig. 9.32). Indicators of probable transformation zone sampling include immature metaplastic squamous cells and/or endocervical glandular epithelium with mucus. There are no reliable indicators of transformation zone sampling in atrophic smears.

The normal cervical smear

The cytomorphology of superficial, intermediate and parabasal squamous cells largely recapitulates the histological structure of mature stratified squamous epithelium (Fig. 9.33). Mucosal thickness and glycogen content depend upon hormonal activity. Superficial cells usually exfoliate naturally and there is normally no keratinization. They tend to be dyscohesive and individually disposed. Endocervical glandular cells show a wide variation in appearance depending upon their preservation and orientation. They tend to retain cohesion and may show cytoarchitectural patterns comparable to other glandular sites. Subcolumnar reserve cells generally present as bare, isomorphic nuclei. Metaplastic squamous cells are a normal constituent of a smear during the reproductive years. Whilst immature they do not exfoliate spontaneously and when removed by abrasion they often exhibit cytoplasmic projections ('*spider cells*'). Once fully mature they are indistinguishable from the squamous cells of the orig-

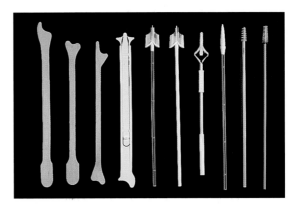

Figure 9.32: Cervical sampling devices. The spatulae, particularly the extended tip type (Aylesbury), give a better cell yield and are recommended for screening. Brush devices for endocervical sampling may be of benefit in addition following an abnormal smear. Sampling technique and visualization of the cervix are of paramount importance irrespective of the design employed.

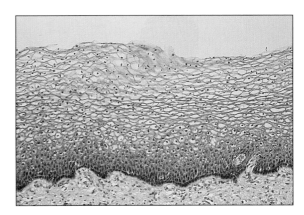

Figure 9.33: Normal mature ectocervical squamous epithelial maturation. Note the ordered polarity from stratum basalis to superficial squamae and the absence of surface keratinization. (H & E × medium power).

inal ectocervix. Endometrial stromal cells, glandular cells and histiocytes ('*exodus*') may be observed from the beginning of menstrual flow until day 12 of the menstrual cycle. Outside this interval they are considered abnormal and such hyperexfoliation may be caused by menstrual irregularities and intra-uterine contraceptive devices in addition to polypi, hyperplasia and neoplasia. Polymorphonuclear leukocytes are

Gynaecological Cytopathology and Cervical Screening

Hormonal cytology

Inflammation and regeneratives changes

Dyskaryosis, CIN, and cervical carcinoma

---

invariably present, most conspicuously around menstruation. Lymphocytes, eosinophils, mast cells and plasma cells are usually scanty. The mere presence of inflammatory cells does not necessarily imply infection. Spermatozoa may persist for several days after sexual intercourse. Trophoblast and deciduoid stroma may be shed during pregnancy or abortion and pseudodeciduoid cells may be the result of hormonal therapy.

Abnormal keratinization (*hyperkeratosis*) yields anucleate, deeply orangeophilic squamae in Papanicolaou preparations. *Parakeratosis* shows spikes ('*sprigs*') or '*pearls*' of similar squamae possessing pyknotic nuclei. Both patterns may be seen in inflammatory and neoplastic conditions. A variety of contaminants including helminths, lice, fungi, pollen and lubricant jelly may be encountered.

Hormonal cytology

Cytohormonal evaluation is based upon the maturation of vaginal squamous epithelium in response to circulating gonadotrophic hormones in combination. The epithelium is thin and immature when deprived of oestrogen and progesterone. Unopposed oestrogen promotes growth and maturation. Progesterone causes desquamation and exfoliation with cytolysis and '*navicular cells*'. Androgens stimulate partial maturation to intermediate cell level in atrophic epithelium with a reciprocal effect in mature epithelium.

Characteristic patterns are recognizable in the postnatal period, during puberty, sexual maturity, pregnancy, post-parturition, lactational, pre-menopausal and established postmenopausal states, modulated by exogenous hormonal influences or abnormal endogenous hormonal sources e.g. ovarian tumours.

Various indices may be used to report hormonal changes including the maturation index, maturation value, karyopyknotic index, eosinophilic index and the folded cell index.

Inflammation and regenerative changes

Inflammation in the female genital tract sometimes has an infective origin and may be of acute, chronic or granulomatous pattern. It is a dynamic process wherein degenerative and regenerative changes are observed synchronously.

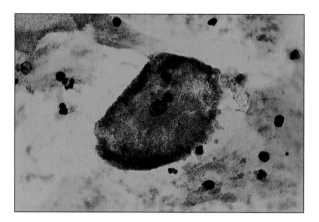

Figure 9.34: '*Clue cell*' *in bacterial vaginosis. Coccoid overgrowth imparts a granular appearance to a superficial squamous cell ('clue cell') in a cervical smear. It is usually due to mixed bacterial flora including* Gardnerella vaginalis. *Their presence is not necessarily an indication of clinical symptoms (bacterial vaginosis). (Pap × 250).*

Commoner infections include follicular cervicitis strongly associated with *Chlamydia* spp, *Lepthothrix* spp often accompanying *Trichomonas vaginalis*, bacterial vaginosis associated with *Gardnerella vaginalis*, *Actinomyces* spp, *Neisseria gonorrhoea*, *Mycobacterium tuberculosis*, *Treponema pallidum*, *Candida albicans*, herpes simplex virus and human papilloma virus, many of which are sexually transmissible (Figs 9.34, 9.35).

Iatrogenic influences include laser ablation, surgery, radiotherapy, hormonal replacement or manipulation and intrauterine contraceptive devices. These may result in various hyperplasias and metaplasias further complicating accurate interpretation of a cervical smear.

Dyskaryosis, CIN, and cervical carcinoma

Invasive squamous cell carcinoma of the cervix is preceded by a prodrome of precancerous changes (*dysplasia*) of the epithelium of the cervical transformation zone, termed cervical intraepithelial neoplasia (CIN). This is a continuous biological spectrum which is arbitrarily subdivided or graded in histological sections into CIN 1, CIN 2 and CIN 3 with increasing severity of dysplasia (Fig. 9.36). These categories correspond to mild, moderate and severe squamous cell dyskaryosis in cervical smear

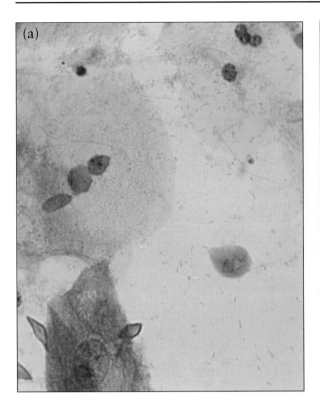
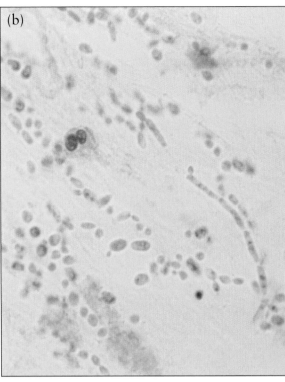

Figure 9.35: Trichomonas *and* Candida *in a cervical smear. (a) Binucleate, flagellate* Trichomonas *protozoon. (Pap × 250) (b) Candidal blastospores and pseudohyphae. (Pap × 250).*

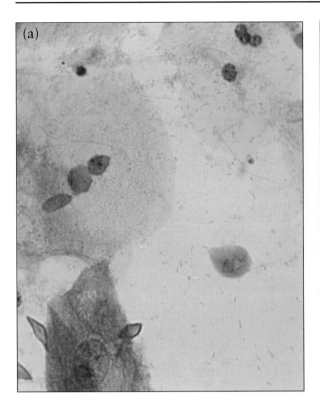

Figure 9.36.: Precursors of invasive squamous cell carcinoma of the cervix. Schematic representation of potential progression of cervical intraepithelial neoplasia to invasive cervical carcinoma.

preparations (Fig. 9.37). The Northern American Bethesda system uses slightly different nomenclature for the same cytomorphological appearances (see Table 9.3). The more severe the degree of abnormality, the greater the statistical risk of progression to invasive carcinoma.

Early stromal invasion, microinvasion and invasive squamous cell carcinoma proper indicate transgression of basement membrane to varying degrees, the latter with tumefaction. This is best assessed by histological examination as the severe dyskaryosis of CIN 3 may be cytomorphologically indistinguishable from the severe dyskaryosis seen in invasive carcinoma. Bizarre dyskeratotic cells and tumour diathesis may be helpful distinguishing features but are neither pathognomonic nor universally present.

Screening programmes to detect breast carcinoma in asymptomatic women have been established in several countries and initial results appear encouraging.

125

Table 9.3: Comparison of current terminologies applied to abnormal squamous cells in cervical cytology.

CIN Grade	WHO	BSCC	Bethesda
		Borderline	Atypia
I	Mild dysplasia	Mild dyskaryosis;	Low grade SIL
II	Moderate dysplasia	Moderate dyskaryosis	High grade SIL
III	Severe dysplasia; Carcinoma *in situ*	Severe dyskaryosis	High grade SIL
	Epidermoid carcinoma	Severe dyskaryosis; ? Invasive carcinoma	Squamous carcinoma

W.H.O.   World Health Organisation
B.S.C.C.   British Society of Clinical Cytology
S.I.L.   Squamous intraepithelial lesion

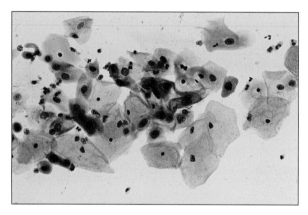

Figure 9.37: Moderate squamous cell dyskaryosis. Note disproportionate nucleomegaly, the nucleus occupying up to two-thirds of the cytoplastic area, nuclear hyperchromasia, irregular nuclear contour and angulated cell borders. (Pap × 100).

Quality Assurance in Diagnostic Cytology

The purpose of a quality assurance programme is to evaluate the diagnostic process as it is practised. Internal quality control indicates a series of procedures within a particular laboratory. This encompasses continuing education, training, review of laboratory procedures and their implementation, rescreening, double screening and audit. External quality assurance indicates performance evaluation against an external peer group, either regionally or nationally, and this may be as part of an accreditation scheme, either voluntary or compulsory.

Ancillary Techniques and Automated Cytology

Cytomorphological assessment is at times a highly subjective process and therefore susceptible to differences in intraobserver and interobserver reproducibility. Attempts to refine and quantify this more rigorously have been undertaken with varying degrees of success.

Flow cytometry involves the automated assessment of cells in suspension, usually for DNA analysis or immunophenotyping purposes. Microfluorimetry enables focus on individual cells in a field to assess the amount of fluorescent activity within nuclei.

Cytogenetic analysis detects chromosomal abnormalities, some of which are characteristic of certain tumours, e.g. t(x:18) in synovial sarcoma, t(11:22) in Ewing's tumour. The majority of neoplasms, however, do not show such typical constant translocations.

Silver stained nucleolar organizer regions (AgNORs) are increased in most malignant nuclei. Unfortunately the overlap between benign and malignant conditions is often considerable.

Scanning and transmission electron microscopy may yield helpful ultrastructural details not discernible by light microscopy which enables more precise classification of cell differentiation, e.g. dense core neurosecretory granules, tight junctions, tonofilaments, etc.

In-situ hybridization techniques may identify viral nuclear material and detect oncogene activation in tumours.

High resolution image analysis systems may be semi- or fully automated. Their main advantage is their potential to obviate the subjectivity of human assessment and reduce error during screening. They may be linked to powerful neural network computer systems and are under continued development.

Confocal laser scanning microscopy gives digital images which may be manipulated further to reconstruct a three-dimensional image of cells within preparations or for quantification purposes.

Acknowledgement

Mrs. V. Garland for her patience and word processing skills.

Further Reading

Clinical Cytotechnology. Coleman D V, Chapman P A (Eds) 1989: Butterworth, London.

Cytopathology. In *Laboratory Histopathology – a complete reference*. Woods A E, Ellis R C (Eds) 1994: Churchill Livingstone, New York, 1994.

Diagnostic Cytopathology. Gray W (Ed) 1995: Churchill Livingstone, Edinburgh.

Fine Needle Aspiration Cytopathology. Young J A (Ed) 1993: Blackwell Scientific Publications, London.

SECTION 3
MICROBIOLOGY: BACTERIOLOGY

10 MICROSCOPY IN BACTERIOLOGY: APPLICATION AND SAMPLE PREPARATION

Dugald R Baird

Introduction

In the late seventeenth century the Dutch draper and amateur scientist Antonie van Leeuwenhoek ground small lenses of extraordinary quality and visualized microorganisms for the first time. Since then microscopy has continued to play a fundamental role in clinical bacteriology. Microscopical examination of clinical specimens is often important in judging the adequacy of a clinical specimen, and may by itself quickly reveal the likely nature of the bacterial pathogen in some critical specimens such as cerebrospinal fluid (CSF) or blood cultures. Methods in a diagnostic clinical laboratory include both light and fluorescence microscopy; specimens may be unstained or stained, depending on the application.

Light Microscopy

Light microscopy may be employed in three ways – ordinary transmitted light (brightfield), darkfield and phase contrast microscopy, of which the first is by far the most commonly used. A modern microscope is capable of achieving a magnification of 1000 times, and a resolving power of approximately 0.2 μm. Most microscopes are designed so that the observer looks through the eyepieces, which are slanted at a convenient angle, down onto the stage containing the object to be viewed. An alternative arrangement (the inverted plate microscope), is designed to examine the subject from below. *Darkfield illumination* effectively increases the resolving power of the light microscope to below 0.2 μm. Specimens are illuminated indirectly, scatter the light and appear bright against a dark background. Using this technique one can visualize bacteria such as spirochaetes, which have a diameter of approximately 0.1 μm. *Phase contrast microscopy* allows examination of the fine internal structure of living unstained bacteria and tissues, the different structures appearing in various shades of grey.

Fluorescence Microscopy

Fluorescence occurs when a molecule is struck by light of a particular wavelength and emits light of a longer wavelength. Fluorochromes (fluorescent dyes) absorb non-visible UV light and emit visible light. A fluorescence microscope uses a mercury vapour lamp which emits high intensity ultraviolet light (*excitation light*) and a mirror directs this onto the specimen from above. Bacteria stained with a fluorochrome absorb this short wavelength light, emit longer wavelength light, and appear as glowing yellow or green objects against a dark background. Fluorescence microscopy allows the use of lower power objectives and hence a much larger area of specimen can be scanned rapidly.

This is important, for example, when searching for mycobacteria in a specimen in which they may be very scanty.

Specimens for Microscopy

These are of two main types: (1) dried smears of fluid specimens or swabs, or of bacterial cultures, spread over an area 1 cm to 2 cm in diameter onto standard 3 in. by 1 in. glass slides and fixed by heat ('films'), and (2) 'wet preparations' of fluids, examined under a coverslip or in special chambers. Swabs contained in transport medium are moist and can be rubbed directly onto the surface of a slide, while films of fluid specimens such as pus, aspirates, cerebrospinal fluid, etc., are made by taking up a loopful and spreading this thinly. Tissue samples are either pressed on to the surface of slides to form imprints, or may be ground up in a small volume of peptone water. Colonies of bacteria growing on solid media are examined by touching the colony with a loop and emulsifying this in a drop of saline on the slide, aiming for a very light suspension so that individual cells can be distinguished clearly.

Examination of Unstained Specimens by Transmitted Light

Examination of fluid specimens in a *counting chamber* or on a slide with a coverslip is routinely used to assess the presence of clues to infection or inflammation in normally sterile body fluids such as urine, cerebrospinal fluid, peritoneal dialysis effluent and joint aspirates. Transmitted light is used, with or without phase contrast, and the sample examined using the ×25 objective for white and red blood cells, organisms, casts or crystals as appropriate to the specimen. Cell counts may be expressed quantitatively if a counting chamber is employed, or semi-quantitatively (e.g. 'per high power field').

Bacteria growing in liquid culture media may be examined for *motility* using a ×50 objective.

Lowering the condenser increases the contrast and makes the organisms easier to see; alternatively, phase contrast microscopy may be used.

Examination of tissue culture cell monolayers for cytopathic effects is mainly the province of virology, but has an application in bacteriology in the detection of *Clostridium difficile* cytotoxin in faecal extracts or culture supernatants.

Cerebrospinal fluid (CSF)

CSF is normally sterile and contains not more than five white cells per mm^3, predominately lymphocytes. The first step in its examination consists of microscopy of uncentrifuged fluid to quantitate the number of cells present and their type. A counting chamber is used, commonly the modified Fuchs–Rosenthal. This is a glass slide containing a well, the floor of which is etched with a grid of nine large squares, each 1 mm^2 in area. Each of these squares is subdivided in turn into 16 small squares. When a coverslip is applied over the counting chamber and fluid run in using a Pasteur pipette, the depth of fluid is 0.2 mm. The volume of fluid overlying five large squares is thus 1 mm^3.

A coverslip is applied to the slide to make a firm uniform seal over the counting chamber, by pressing gently at its edges until the colours of the rainbow are seen uniformly around the sides of the coverslip (Newton's rings), confirming that close and even contact has been made between the coverslip and chamber. CSF is introduced into the chamber using a fine Pasteur pipette applied carefully to the edge, so that fluid runs in to completely fill the chamber, without air bubbles.

After allowing a few minutes to settle, cells are counted using a ×40 objective, the number of squares being examined depending on the number of cells present. CSF containing very large numbers of white cells, or that is heavily bloodstained either as a result of intracerebral haemorrhage, or due to accidental puncture of small blood vessels during lumbar puncture, may have to be diluted before an accurate cell count can be performed. A fluid containing dilute acetic acid and crystal violet is used for this purpose: this lyses erythrocytes and stains the nuclei of the white cells, making them easier to see. Identification of cell types is facilitated by centrifuging an aliquot of the CSF and making a film which is stained using a differential stain such as Leishman's or an equivalent.

Urine

Not all laboratories perform microscopy as a routine on specimens of urine. In specimens taken from patients with catheters (catheter specimens of urine, CSU) this is justifiable, since the absence of pus cells in such samples does not exclude infection. In samples collected cleanly from patients without catheters (midstream urine, MSU), however, the absence of pyuria suggests that the significance of an isolate is at best uncertain; it may be a contaminant and repeat sampling is advised. Microscopy is also useful to detect red cells, casts and crystals, all of which may be of diagnostic significance. The information that can be obtained from urine microscopy is thus valuable, and it should be done whenever possible.

Microscopy is performed on fresh uncentrifuged urine. The visualisation of organisms in such preparations is of secondary importance, since it is quantitation of bacterial growth that is important in assessing the significance of isolates from a urine specimen. Neutrophils are excreted in variable numbers in healthy urine, and only numbers above 10^4 per ml can be considered abnormal in MSUs. Red cells are found as contaminants in the urine of healthy younger females, associated with menstruation, but may also indicate serious renal tract pathology such as calculi, neoplasm or glomerular disease. In the latter case the morphology of the red cells may be abnormal – dysmorphism – the cells exhibiting fragmentation, crenation, or other bizarre shapes.

Laboratories handling small numbers of urine specimens may examine them in counting chambers as described for CSF, but most use a semi-quantitative method. These include simply using an ordinary glass slide and a coverslip, commercially produced disposable counting chambers, or an inverted plate microscope. A ×40 objective is used, and if the area of the field ('high power field') and the depth of the urine is known, the number of cells visible can be translated into counts per ml, although in practice many laboratories express the findings as scanty, moderate or numerous.

The techniques described above may be applied to other normally sterile fluids, such as aspirates from joints (where examination for crystals such as uric acid is also important), serous fluids and peritoneal dialysis effluent.

Microscopy of faeces is employed for the diagnosis of parasitic infections, but has no place in the diagnosis of bacterial gastroenteritis.

Examination of Unstained Specimens using Dark Ground Illumination

This has one application in clinical bacteriology, namely in the examination of material taken from a suspected primary chancre for the presence of the causal organism of syphilis, *Treponema pallidum*. Material is taken from the suspect lesion, a wet film made under a coverslip, and examined immediately for motile treponemes.

Staining of Specimens

Since the refractive index of bacteria is similar to that of their background, it is necessary, when using transmitted light, to increase the contrast by the use of stains. The most widely used method of staining bacteria remains that introduced by Gram in 1884. Although not a stain, but a staining *method*, the term 'Gram stain' is used universally; it exploits the differences in cell wall structure that exist between various classes of bacteria. The material to be stained may be a clinical specimen, broth culture, or a light suspension in saline of an organism taken from an agar plate. In all cases a thin smear is made on a glass slide and allowed to dry naturally or with very modest heat, after which the smear is fixed to the slide either by passing the slide quickly three times through a Bunsen flame, or by the use of a heated plate. Gram's staining method, which has several modifications, involves treating the

Staining of Specimens

Table 10.1: Some examples of bacterial genera classified according to morphology and gram staining.

Shape	Gram-positive	Gram-negative
Cocci (spheres)	Staphylococcus Streptococcus Peptococcus*	Neisseria Moraxella Veillonella*
Bacilli (rods)	Bacillus Listeria Corynebacterium Clostridium*	Enterobacteriaceae Pseudomonas Haemophilus Bacteroides*

* Anaerobic genera

smear successively by (1) a basic positively charged dye, usually crystal violet, (2) mordanting with aqueous iodine, (3) decolorizing with acetone and (4) counterstaining with carbol fuchsin or safranin.

All bacteria are initially stained by the crystal violet and iodine which form insoluble complexes within the bacterial cell. Those bacteria which possess thick layers of peptidoglycan in their cell walls, and hence retain the stain after treatment with acetone and appear purple, are defined as Gram-positive; those with thinner peptidoglycan layers which readily lose the complex with acetone and hence stain with the pink counterstain, are called Gram-negative. Examples of Gram-positive and Gram-negative bacteria are given in Table 10.1. Some bacteria stain only poorly with the Gram stain (e.g. legionella species), some are inconsistent in their staining behaviour (Gram-variable, e.g. *Gardnerella vaginalis*), and others do not stain at all (e.g. mycobacteria).

Special staining methods are required for mycobacteria due to the peculiar composition of their cell walls, which contain high concentrations of mycolic (fatty) acids. The Ziehl–Neelsen stain involves treatment of the film with hot carbol fuchsin, followed by successive decolourization steps with concentrated sulphuric acid and with alcohol, finally counterstaining with methylene blue. Mycobacteria appear red against a blue background (Fig. 10.1).

The other staining method employed for mycobacteria is phenol-auramine. This involves

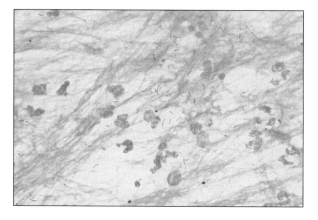

Figure 10.1: Sputum stained by Ziehl–Neelsen's method showing mycobacteria (red) against a blue background. ×1000. [Courtesy of Mr J Winning.]

treating dried and heat-fixed smears of the specimen (usually sputum, pleural and ascitic fluids, early-morning urine, CSF, pus, etc.) with phenol-auramine, decolorizing with 1% hydrochloric acid in industrial methylated spirit, followed by a dilute solution of potassium permanganate. Films are viewed under ultraviolet light using the ×40 objective, and mycobacteria glow green-yellow against a dark background (Fig. 10.2).

Two other staining methods are employed in fluorescence microscopy work – acridine orange, and fluorescein–antibody conjugates. Staining with acridine orange is a useful method for demonstrating bacteria that may not show up

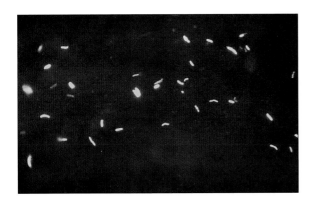

Figure 10.2: The same specimen of sputum as in Fig. 13.1 stained with phenol-auramine and viewed under ultraviolet light. The mycobacteria glow with a green-yellow fluorescence. ×400. [Courtesy of Dr B Watt.]

clearly in a Gram stain (as in blood cultures, below). Under UV light, bacteria appear orange.

Immunofluorescent techniques using fluorescein–antibody conjugates can be used to detect bacteria. Two methods are available, direct and indirect fluorescent antibody tests (DFAT and IFAT respectively). The DFAT utilizes a fluorochrome, commonly fluorescein isothiocyanate, conjugated to a specific antibody which binds directly to the antigen. The IFAT is a two-stage procedure: the specific antibody (e.g. prepared in a rabbit) binds to the antigen and is itself detected by a conjugated antibody (e.g. anti-rabbit). The advantage of the IFAT is that a single conjugated antibody can be used to detect a whole range of specific antibodies.

In bacteriology the major uses of these immunofluorescence techniques are in the detection of (1) Legionella species, which are difficult to grow in the laboratory but can be readily detected in sputum, broncho-alveolar lavages and lung tissue (fresh or formalin-fixed), using either DFAT or IFAT, and (2) for the direct demonstration of chlamydial antigen in genital or respiratory specimens.

Some further examples of the use of microscopy of stained preparations in clinical microbiology are given below.

Specimens from normally sterile sites

It is with these specimens that microscopy can be a powerful tool in predicting the likely causal pathogen. The finding of organisms in cerebrospinal fluid, joint aspirate, or peritoneal dialysis effluent, for example, especially when accompanied by an infiltrate of pus cells, is a virtually certain indicator of infection and the appearance of the bacteria alone may be diagnostic. A very thorough search for bacteria may have to be made, as they are sometimes very scanty in such specimens, which are examined by centrifuging (e.g. at 3000 rpm for ten minutes), discarding the supernatant, and making a film of the deposit which is then stained by Gram's method, and also by auramine or Ziehl–Neelsen if the clinical situation suggests possible mycobacterial infection.

Most laboratories now use some form of semi-automated *blood culture* system, and examination of a Gram-stained drop of broth from a bottle registering positive growth is the first step in the identification of the organism. Microscopy may immediately suggest the diagnosis (e.g. streptococci in the blood of a patient with fever and a heart murmur, see Fig. 10.3). Gram-positive cocci in clusters are staphylococci, but *Staphylococcus aureus* cannot be distinguished by microscopy from the many coagulase-negative species, and

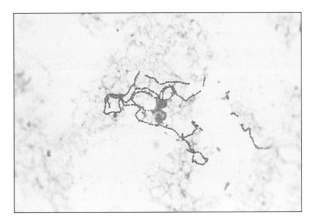

Figure 10.3: Gram stain of a blood culture showing Gram-positive cocci in long chains. The organism turned out to be Streptococcus sanguis, and the patient had infective endocarditis. ×1000. [Courtesy of Dr A McLay.]

Staining of Specimens

Specimens from sites with a normal resident flora

since the latter are the commonest contaminants of blood cultures, the significance of staphylococci in a particular blood culture usually has to await further identification. Gram-negative organisms in blood cultures are sometimes difficult to see against the general background pink staining, and when no organisms are visible it is often useful to perform an acridine stain. When no organisms are seen using this method, it may be that the semi-automated system has registered a *false-positive* result, often because of the metabolic activity of the leucocytes in the broth, especially when the patient has a high peripheral white cell count.

Specimens from sites with a normal resident flora

Oral swabs
Microscopy is the only method of diagnosing Vincent's angina (anaerobic stomatogingivitis), since the causal organisms (which act in synergy to produce the infection) cannot be cultured artificially. Films of oral swabs show many pus cells and large numbers of spirochaetes and fusiform (spindle-shaped) Gram-negative bacilli.

Sputum
All sputum specimens are regarded as potentially hazardous to the operator since they may contain tubercle bacilli, and preparation of films is performed in a safety cabinet housed in a Category 3 containment laboratory. Although sputum originates from the normally sterile lower respiratory tract, it is inevitably contaminated before collection by flora from the upper respiratory tract. Care is needed in interpreting Gram films of sputum, and only rarely can one confidently predict the causal organism of pneumonia on the basis of microscopy alone. Gram films are nevertheless useful in that specimens of 'sputum' which show fewer than 10 neutrophils per squamous epithelial cell are probably saliva rather than sputum, and indicate that culture may be misleading. When mycobacterial infection is suspected, auramine-stained films are examined, and positives confirmed by making fresh films and staining by the Ziehl–Neelsen method.

The disadvantages of sputum are largely overcome by performing broncho-alveolar lavage, a procedure increasingly employed in the diagnosis of pneumonia in patients who are very ill, or who are immunosuppressed. Specimens obtained are free of contaminating upper respiratory tract flora, and can be examined by Gram, auramine and Ziehl–Neelsen stains, and by immunofluorescence techniques for legionella species and a wide range of protozoal, fungal and viral pathogens.

Skin lesions
Microscopy of swabs of skin lesions are rarely of diagnostic value, due to the presence of a normal skin flora, with one important exception. This is the microscopical examination of the purpuric vesicular lesions associated with meningococcal infection, in which the presence of Gram-negative cocci in pairs with their characteristic morphology is diagnostic.

Pus and wound swabs
The value of microscopy of these specimens is variable, depending on a number of factors beyond the control of the laboratory. Pus or pus swabs from such sites as skin or soft tissue infections may suggest infection with staphylococci, streptococci, or anaerobes, whereas similar specimens from intra-abdominal sites may show a highly mixed picture, not always

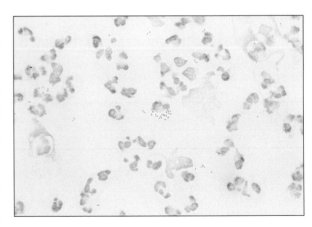

Figure 10.4: *Film of urethral discharge showing numerous intracellular Gram-negative cocci –* Neisseria gonorrhoea ×1000. *[Courtesy of Mr J Winning.]*

easy to correlate with what is subsequently obtained on culture. In many of these cases, prior antibiotic administration may account for the discrepancies. It is, however, often useful to be able to give a provisional report that a pus sample or swab is likely to be, for example, staphylococcal in origin, or alternatively, that it is composed of mixed organisms of probable faecal origin.

High vaginal swabs

Gram films are used to ascertain whether pus cells are present, and also the presence of epithelial cells covered with small Gram-variable bacilli (clue cells). The finding of the latter is a pointer to the condition known as bacterial vaginosis. In genito-urinary medicine, urethral and endocervical swabs are examined for the presence of pus cells containing intracellular Gram-negative cocci in pairs, Neisseria gonorrhoea (see Figure 10.4).

Further Reading

Bishop BJ, Neumann G. The history of the Ziehl-Neelsen stain. *Tubercle* 1970; **51**: 196–206.

Larson HE, Price AB. Pseudomembranous colitis: presence of Clostridial toxin. *Lancet* 1977; **2**: 1312–1314.

Preston NW, Morrell A. Reproducible results with the Gram Stain. *Journal of Pathology and Bacteriology* 1962; **84**: 241–243.

11 CULTURE MEDIA IN BACTERIOLOGY

Eric Y Bridson

Culture Media in Microbiology

The history of plagues and pestilences from the first records of mankind to the early twentieth century has been written by Bulloch. Although the terms 'contagion' and 'infection' were used in mediaeval times, the role of minute infectious agents could not be proved until the work of Louis Pasteur (1822–95). Much of Pasteur's work involved demolishing Galen's theories of infectious disease and that of spontaneous generation of microscopic life.

The father of culture media, however, was Robert Koch (1843–1910; Fig. 11.1) who created methods for the cultivation, isolation and identification of bacteria. Pasteur first showed that bacteria caused infection of humans, animals and food but it took Koch's work to confirm that specific organisms caused specific diseases. The basis of Koch's work was to move away from liquid cultures, with their painstaking dilutions and frequent contamination, to a simple but powerful technique using 'solid' media. By adding gelatin, later agar, to his meat extract broth he created the streak plate with its isolated colonies. He later demonstrated how thorough mixing of suspected material into the molten medium and pouring the plate yielded a quantitative assessment of bacterial numbers, a technique now widely used as the pour plate. Richard Petri, one of Koch's assistants, replaced Koch's glass plate under a bell jar with the Petri dish. This elegant design has remained unchanged for over 100 years.

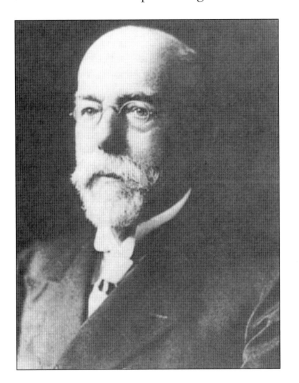

Figure 11.1: Robert Koch (1843–1910). The father of culture media.

Koch was aware that a universal medium for pathogenic bacteria was unlikely. He showed that *Mycobacterium tuberculosis* would not grow on his meat-infusion agar medium. For this organism he used coagulated serum, egg or sliced potato. By the end of the nineteenth century a textbook of medical bacteriology would list about seven media. The most important addition to Koch's meat infusion broth was peptone, a peptic digest of protein which was suggested by Loeffler. He also incorporated 0.5% w/v sodium chloride and his nutrient medium has remained the bedrock of undefined complex culture media for chemo-heterotrophic organisms (i.e. requiring organic carbon compounds for utilization, as opposed to autotrophic bacteria which can synthesize carbon compounds from carbon dioxide).

Many more formulations of culture media arose in the first decades of the twentieth century when enrichment, selection and indicator media were designed for organisms isolated from areas outside medicine, for example agriculture, food and drink manufacture, pharmaceuticals, etc. By 1930 a survey of published media described 2540 formulations, many of them small variations of previously published media. The number has grown enormously since but no similar survey has been repeated.

Formulation of Culture Media

The formulations used for different media may contain as little as three ingredients (Loeffler nutrient broth) to ten times as many in media for fastidious organisms. The number of ingredients has little relationship to its growth performance. 'Simple' culture may be highly complex and totally undefined.

A common structure of culture media for chemo-heterotrophic organisms is as follows.

Amino-nitrogen base (peptone, protein hydrolysate, infusion or extract of protein)
Few organisms can utilize coagulated proteins, and pre-digested or acid-hydrolyzed derivatives are provided. The peptides and amino acids can be transferred into the cell and used as carbon sources for energy or polymerized into functional proteins.

Supplemental growth factors (blood, serum, yeast extract, nucleotides, vitamins)
Microorganisms described as nutritionally fastidious, e.g. *Neisseria*, *Bordetella*, *Legionella*, demand extra growth factors. The considerable benefit of whole blood to these organisms was once attributed solely to the extra growth factors supplied. It is now considered that the major role of whole blood is to protect vulnerable organisms from toxic oxidation processes.

Energy sources, other than peptides (sugars, alcohols and complex carbohydrates)
These substances are usually added to indicator media to enhance pH changes by those organisms that can ferment the energy source. Many other organic molecules can be metabolized by chemo-heterotrophic organisms to provide energy.

Buffer salts (phosphates, acetates, citrates)
Buffers are commonly added to high carbohydrate formulations (e.g. containing soya peptone) to prevent excessive changes in pH levels. Unfortunately, many buffers have a tendency to chelate essential metals and they must be used carefully. Peptides and amino acids can act as buffering agents through the zwitterion effect of the NH_2/COOH groupings.

Mineral salts and metals (phosphates, sulphates, Ca^{++}, Mg^{++}, Fe^{++}, Mn^{++}, trace metals)
These substances may be added separately in macro- or micro-quantities, where particular demands are evident. It is important that the metals are in soluble form and are not complexed into insoluble forms during heat processing. It is usually assumed that hydrolyzed animal or plant tissues contain sufficient minerals and metals for optimal growth.

Selective agents (chemicals, antimicrobials and some aniline dyes)
As the name implies these agents are added at sufficient concentration to inhibit unwanted organisms but allow the selected organisms to

multiply. Extreme care is required to determine the optimum concentration in the medium. All selective agents exhibit some toxicity towards the selected species and can often fail to suppress all unwanted organisms. A general rule is that any increase in nutrients to the medium requires an increase in selective agent and *vice versa*. Selective agents may interact with each other to enhance or diminish their selectivity, e.g., bile salts diminish the toxicity of dyes. Selective agents can also be affected by substances (e.g. most buffers) which chelate cations. For example, certain dyes and bile salts can become more toxic. This effect can be reversed by the addition of cations (Mg/Ca).

Indicator dyes (phenol red, neutral red, bromocresol purple)
These dyes indicate changes in pH value following fermentation, deamination or decarboxylation. Chromogenic culture media developed to indicate colonies producing specific enzyme activities are commonly mixtures of indicator dyes. All dyes require careful titration to avoid selective inhibition.

Gelling agents (agar, gelatin, alginate, silica gel)
Agar, extracted from *Gelidium* species of seaweeds, is the most common gelling agent for chemo-heterotrophic organism growth. Although the quality of agar has improved a great deal from its early beginnings, it cannot be considered to be an inert polymer gel. It contributes metals, minerals and pyruvates which can influence the growth of organisms. Not all agars are similar: differences in agarophyte source and the industrial processes of extraction may cause significantly different growth performance and antibiotic diffusion.

The above eight categories of materials cover almost all the variations in published culture media formulations. Further details on these materials and manufacture can be found elsewhere.

Enrichment and Selection in Fluid Media

The procedures of enrichment and selection in fluid media are not mutually exclusive. Enrichment is generally described as a process of increasing the numbers of an organism from less than 10 cells to detectable levels. Enrichment broths may have supplemental growth factors added to reduce the lag phase of distressed or low numbers of organisms. Blood culturing is the most common example of such an enrichment procedure.

The term 'enrichment' is also used, in a mixed microbial population, when one species is selected for preferential growth. This is arranged by use of preferential formulations including selective or elective chemicals, pH adjustment or favourable temperature of incubation. It is seldom possible in fluid media to specifically enhance the desired organism and to suppress all other organisms present. The dynamics of growth of mixed cultures of organisms in broth are usually complex. Undesired organisms may be retarded for an initial period but they may later overgrow the desired organisms.

Although fixed periods of incubation and subculture are usually set by the working hours of the laboratory, they may not be ideal for the successful recovery of particular organisms. The most important function of enrichment broth is to raise the number of the desired organisms to a level that is sufficient for one loopful of subcultured broth to produce a detectable number of recognizable colonies on selective agar plates. Probably 10^4 organisms per ml in the broth is the minimal figure for detection by this method.

It must be remembered that the function of enrichment broths is usually judged by the results of subculture to a solid selective medium. The interaction of selective chemicals in the broth and those present in the agar plate could be inhibitory to small numbers of organisms. Tetrathionate broth subcultured to MacConkey agar can yield greater numbers of salmonellae or shigellae than when subcultured to deoxycholate-citrate agar.

In summary, the following factors significantly affect the successful enrichment of particular organisms from liquid media: (a) the formulation of the medium and its selective agents; (b) the inoculum size of the desired organism; (c) the competitor-organism numbers and the variety of competitors; (d) the presence–absence of organic material in the broth; (e) the temperature of incubation; (f) the period of time before subculture; (g) the interaction of enrichment broth components with the selective agar plate used for subculture.

It is not surprising that much conflicting opinion has been published on this subject when the complexity of variation possible in the end results is taken into consideration.

Chemically Defined Culture Media Versus Complex Undefined Media

Until the middle of the twentieth century, medical microbiologists accepted the fact that culture media were prepared more as culinary works of art than as scientific formulations. Practically all the ingredients used were undefined, variable natural materials. Growth performance varied widely and this generated a desire for synthetic or chemically defined media, which should yield standard performance. From 1950 to 1975, microbiologists attempted to put together selected amino acids, nucleotides, vitamins, minerals and metals which would grow chemo-heterotrophic organisms at the same speed and with the same characteristics as on undefined media. Microbiological journals of this period contained hundreds of published culture media formulae but they all showed growth performances that were inferior to undefined media or were restricted to a few species only. Not one could be recommended as a general purpose enrichment medium for medical microbes. The sheer difficulty of designing and testing defined media, together with the disappointing results obtained, eventually caused a loss of interest in this ambition. One factor was the replacement of laboratory-prepared raw material media with commercially prepared dehydrated equivalent products. The benefits of better raw material specifications, large-scale controlled manufacture and stringent quality control testing overcame the major problems of media performance variation. More recently, commer-

cially prepared ready-to-use media has replaced much of the culture media preparation that previously took place in microbiological laboratories.

Paradoxically, in 1966, a new undefined blood agar medium was published under the name of Columbia agar. It contained a deliberate mixture of peptones from different protein sources, hydrolyzed by different enzymes, thus creating a broad spectrum of peptides from the largest possible (5000 mol. wt.) to single amino acids (100 mol. wt.). One gram of starch, five grams of sodium chloride and 12 grams of agar made up the formula. Columbia agar, a complex undefined medium, has become the most widely used enrichment medium, in broth and agar forms, for recovering a wide variety of fastidious pathogenic organisms. This appeared to be a triumph of reality over hope for those who wished to replace such media with synthetic or defined formulations.

The dilemma of defined versus undefined media still remains unanswered. It appears that protein hydrolysates and growth factors are the two most likely groups of materials to cause difficulty. It would seem that mixtures of amino acids cannot replace a complex mixture of peptides. It is possible that a wide selection of various growth factors may be required to ensure recovery of stressed or naturally exigenous organisms. It is unlikely that a defined medium comparable to Columbia agar can be developed or justified on a cost-benefit basis.

Growth Environmental Factors

The presence of essential growth nutrients does not by itself guarantee optimal growth of desired organisms. All culture media are susceptible to oxidation if exposed to light, heat and air. This is called photo-, thermo- and chemo-oxidation. It was once considered that chemo-heterotrophic aerobic and facultative anaerobic organisms were little affected by oxidation processes and only obligate anaerobes suffered. It is now evident that all, except a few well-protected species, are vulnerable to oxidation effects. Toxic oxygen radicals (superoxide, singlets, hydroxyls) formed from captured extra electrons can damage nucleic acids and enzymes. Organisms attempt to protect themselves by producing protective enzymes that can neutralize these toxic radicals. Catalase, superoxide dismutase and peroxidases are examples. Some amino acids are effective scavengers of toxic oxidants. Protective agents can be added to culture media for the same purpose, e.g. whole blood, charcoal, pyruvate, reduced iron salts. It may be essential to include these agents for organisms which are particularly vulnerable, e.g. *Neisseria, Bordetella, Campylobacter, Legionella*. Sulphydryl compounds such as thioglycollate and cysteine are added to anaerobic media to reduce the oxidation-reduction potential (Eh) with –SH groups which will neutralize toxic oxidising agents. Some media auto-oxidize on autoclaving, particularly media containing cysteine, glucose, phosphates and some metals.

Water Activity (a_w)

Microorganisms must have 'free' water in which to grow and this especially applies to agar plates. The transfer of nutrients to the colony and the efflux of toxic waste from it depend on free water present in the agar. Water can be 'bound' or complexed so tightly with proteins or polymers that organisms cannot utilize it. Ice is one form of bound water and other forms are often described as quasi-ice.

The biological range of water activity is from 0.97 (1.00 is pure water) to 0.61 (the surface of dried salted fish). Only xerophilic moulds can grow (slowly) at the lowest figure. Fluid media are generally suitable for the growth of all organisms, unless solutes have been added to the medium (sodium chloride or glycerin) to lower the water activity and make it selective for staphylococci or moulds.

Freshly prepared agar plates have satisfactory levels of free water but on storage evaporation reduces the water activity of the agar surface. Overdried or overlong stored agar plates become inhibitory, demonstrate small colonies and fail to recover 'stressed' inocula (Fig. 11.2).

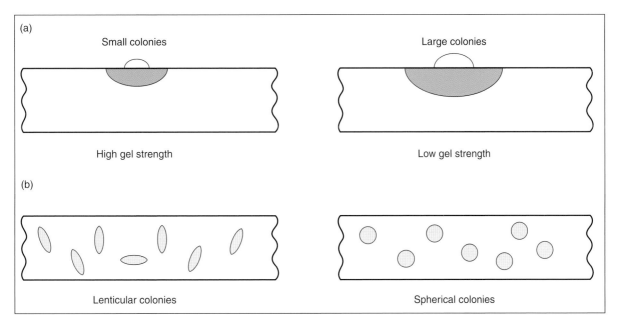

Figure 11.2: *The effect of water loss from agar plates: (a) reduction of size of surface colonies, (b) changes in shape of immersed colonies from spherical to lenticular.*

143

Storage of Culture Media

A good basic rule is that freshly prepared media are better than stored media. However, it is seldom possible to prepare media just prior to to use and some form of storage is inevitable. Stored media should be used strictly in rotation to avoid overlong storage. All containers of media should be dated and batch numbered.

Culture media should be stored away from light to prevent photo-oxidation. All liquid media should be stored in closed tubes or bottles, preferably using screw-capped closures. Store at 2–8°C, except thioglycollate broth which is better kept at 15–22°C. Liquid media, without antibiotics or other labile ingredients, can be stored for many weeks in the cool and away from light.

Poured plates should be stored at 2–8°C wrapped in shrinkfilm. This is preferable to polythene bags which trap all the moisture in the form of pools of liquid in each bag. The shelf life of prepared plates depends on the formulation and on the conditions of storage and transport to the laboratory. With plates wrapped in semipermeable film and stored in expanded polystyrene boxes at the correct temperature, claims have been made of shelf lives of many months. No-one should keep or attempt to use plates of this age. A useful check is to measure the loss of water during storage. A 5% weight loss suggests that the plates have reached a terminal state.

Quality Tests

Most laboratories purchase culture media in dehydrated or prepared form. The product will have been tested by the manufacturer and the user laboratory should undertake a few essential tests only. For autoclaved media, pH value and colour are useful checks. Falling pH values and darkening in colour indicates overheating. Microbiological testing with two or three selected strains of appropriate organisms should be sufficient. Ideally, a strongly and a weakly growing organism should be chosen and some quantitative assessment of growth made. Selective media should be tested for inhibition of unwanted organisms as well as enrichment of selected strains.

If a new supplier is being chosen, or a considerable media contract is being placed, then more extensive testing is called for, preferably using control media alongside. Use small inocula for the tests and include some stressed organisms. Further information on this important subject can be obtained from the PHLS.

The Future of Culture Media

The Koch agar plate, which is cheap, simple and highly versatile, is a very powerful amplifier of small inocula. Properly prepared, it will grow all expected and many unsuspected organisms from samples. Modern diagnostic devices which are forecast to replace conventional microbiology are expensive, complicated and very specific. It is likely that conventional microbiology will continue well into the next century.

Undoubtedly, there will be improvements to the methodology, e.g. semi-automatic labelling, inoculation and signalling, using film technology with confocal laser microscopy for early detection of growth and built-in ID markers for specific enzyme activity. There will be better recovery of damaged organisms at the lag phase of growth. These improved recovery procedures will throw doubt on some existing sterilization kinetics and will solve some of the mysteries surrounding 'viable but non-culturable organisms'. The old bacteriological axiom of 'What does not grow, does not exist' will vanish. It is unlikely that microbiology will be taken over by automation in similar fashion to biochemistry or haematology. Much of the activity in microbiology consists of matching images of colonies or microscope fields with the data bank held in the microbiologist's head. The human brain is incredibly better at this than any computer and it is likely to remain so for a long time. Thanks to the fact that microorganisms are very clever at adaptation and mutation, having been on this planet some 3.5 billion years longer than mankind, there is little fear that microbiologists will become machine minders.

Further Reading

Bridson E Y. *The Development, Manufacture and Control of Microbiological Culture Media*. 1994: Unipath Ltd, Basingstoke, UK.

Brock T D. *Robert Koch – A Life in Medicine and Bacteriology*. 1988; Science Tech. Publishers. Madison WI US.

Bulloch W. *The History of Bacteriology* 1938: Oxford University Press. 1984: Reprinted in New York, Dover Publications.

Ellner P D, Stossel C I, Drakeford E, Vasi F. A new culture medium for medical bacteriology. *Amer. J. Clin. Pathol.* 1966: **45**, 502–505.

Snell J J S, Farrell I D, Roberts C (Eds). *Quality Control – Principles and Practice in the Microbiological Laboratory*. 1991: PHLS, London.

12 IDENTIFICATION OF BACTERIA

Andrew J Hay

Introduction

The ability to identify bacteria quickly and accurately is a skill requiring many years of experience at the laboratory bench to acquire. The purpose of this chapter is to demystify the approaches adopted by clinical laboratories in the identification of common bacteria of medical importance. It is hoped that the reader will gain greater insight into the working of a laboratory and will be able to consult the excellent detailed texts with confidence.

Pure Culture

The first step in identifying a bacterium is to establish a pure culture. Failure to do this is a common error, leading to delayed or misleading laboratory reports.

Clinical material should be plated on primary isolation media in such a way that much of the growth consists of well-isolated colonies (Fig. 12.1). The colonies thus obtained should be examined carefully with a magnifying hand lens under good lighting, and single colonies for investigation picked and transferred to a non-selective medium using a straight wire and a steady hand! If this process fails to yield adequate growth of a pure culture, it should be repeated. Short-cuts taken at this stage will delay identification, waste reagents and possibly produce misleading results, to the frustration and aggravation of bacteriologist and clinician, and wrong treatment for the patient.

A non-selective medium must be used at this stage as selective or inhibitory primary isolation media often interfere with subsequent biochemical and other identification techniques.

The Art of Identification

When faced with a primary isolation plate that may contain up to a dozen or so different species of commensal bacteria, and the knowledge that almost any bacterium can cause disease, the novice bacteriologist must despair

The Art of Identification

Preliminary identification

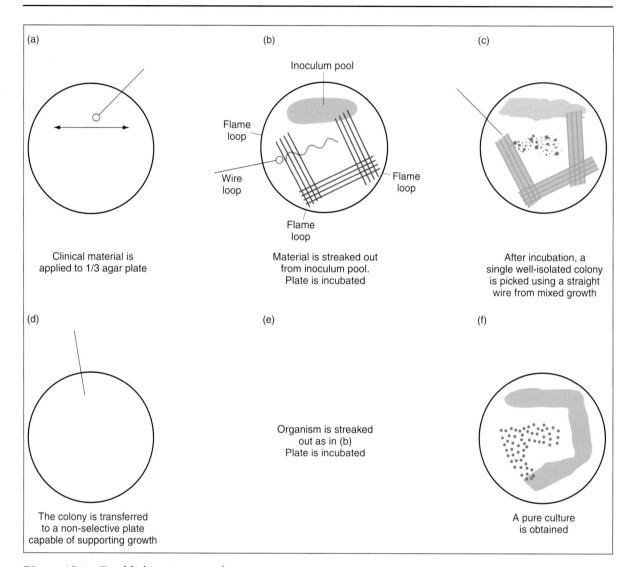

Figure 12.1: *Establishing a pure culture.*

of producing a meaningful report before retirement! However, experience in examining these plates, combined with knowledge of site sampled, clinical picture, likely pathogens and commensal flora will yield a reasonably accurate idea of the organisms present. This approach allows the bacteriologist to choose the initial range of tests that are likely to lead to rapid identification of the pathogen.

If this fails to confirm the most probable causal organism, the investigator must proceed with an open mind and widen the investigations. This method, termed the progressive method, requires the establishment of a few fundamental

characteristics of the organism, and from these, subsequent sets of tests are chosen according to tables until the organism is identified.

Finally, if all else fails, the blunderbuss method may be adopted where every conceivable test is done and compared with those listed in standard texts of systematic bacteriology. This is rarely necessary, but will be required, for example, to establish a new species.

Preliminary identification

The ability of bacteria to grow under aerobic or anaerobic conditions, their growth requirements, colonial morphology, effect on the medium (e.g. haemolysis on blood agar), motility in liquid medium, ability to form spores, and appearance and reaction on Gram stain allow a preliminary identification to be made. Subsequent application of a few simple, rapid tests will then indicate which further tests (if any) are required to complete identification.

The Gram stain is the most widely used differential staining procedure in clinical laboratories today. There are many modifications, but the principle is the same. A solution of crystal violet, followed by an iodine solution, is applied to a heat-fixed preparation of bacteria on a microscope slide. After washing, the preparation is exposed to a decolorizer (alcohol or acetone) for a few seconds before a red counterstain (e.g. safranin) is applied. Gram-positive bacteria are not decolorized by alcohol or acetone and stain purple. Gram-negative bacteria are decolorized, allowing the cells to take up the red counterstain. This reaction depends upon differences in the structure of the cell wall between Gram-positive and Gram-negative bacteria. The size and shape of the bacteria are also taken into account, e.g. round (cocci), rods (bacilli).

Not all bacteria can be isolated on solid media, nor stain with Gram stain. These are considered briefly at the end of the chapter.

The Bacteriologist's Toolbox

Like a master craftsman, the skilled bacteriologist selects the tools required to complete identification based on the results of colonial morphology and Gram stain. These tests may be grouped into the broad categories listed below. They may be performed sequentially or simultaneously, depending on the organism to be identified. They must be carefully controlled each time they are performed. Brief descriptions of the tests and their applications are given below.

Enzyme detection
Here, the ability of a bacterium to produce an enzyme is tested by exposing it to a substrate and detecting the resulting product. Common tests are listed below.

Catalase test
Catalase-producing organisms, when exposed to hydrogen peroxide, produce visible bubbles within 30 seconds. This test may help differentiate staphylococci which are catalase-positive from streptococci which are catalase negative.

Oxidase test
This tests for the presence of cytochrome oxidase. Oxidase-positive bacteria such as Pseudomonas can oxidize the reagent tetramethyl-p-phenylenediamine to a coloured product. Oxidase-negative Enterobacteriaceae cannot.

Urease
Certain species produce a powerful enzyme that splits urea to ammonia which can be detected by a colour change in a pH indicator. This test helps differentiate urease-positive Proteus mirabilis, a gut commensal, from urease-negative Salmonella and Shigella, important pathogens.

Coagulase test
Staphylococcus aureus possesses an enzyme that coagulates plasma in vitro. Other staphylococci are negative.

This list is not comprehensive. Many other tests exist, and these are often incorporated into commercial kits.

Antigen detection
Detection of cell antigens by specific antisera is used widely in bacteriology to speciate and type organisms. Two examples are given below.

Lancefield grouping
A cell wall group antigen is extracted from beta-haemolytic streptococci by an enzyme. The antigen is then detected by agglutination with antisera bound to latex particles.

'O' and 'H' typing
Cell wall (O) antigens and flagellar (H) antigens are detected on Gram-negative bacilli such as Salmonella by mixing suspensions of the organisms with specific antisera on a slide or in a test-tube. A positive reaction is noted by clumping of organisms.

149

Carbohydrate metabolism

The ability of an organism to utilize certain sugars such as glucose, oxidatively (aerobic) or fermentatively (independent of oxygen), or other carbohydrates, e.g. starch, is a useful characteristic commonly used in identification. The test requires a defined medium containing the carbohydrate and a detection system for the metabolic product, often a pH indictor.

Sugar utilization may be incorporated into primary isolation media such as MacConkey agar which differentiates lactose-fermenting Enterobacteriaceae from non-lactose fermenters, and thiosulphate citrate bile sucrose agar (TCBS) which identifies sucrose-fermenting *Vibrio cholerae* from other species. Other tests detect the ability of the organism to use a carbohydrate as a sole carbon source, e.g. citrate utilization.

Panels of carbohydrates are conveniently tested simultaneously in commercial kits.

Growth factors

Here, the absolute requirement of defined compounds for bacterial growth on a particular medium is utilized as an identification tool. For example, *Haemophilus* species differ in their requirements for two factors present in blood, X (haematin) and V (diphosphopyridine nucleotide), for growth on nutrient agar. Only *Haemophilus influenzae*, the most important pathogen, requires both.

Protein metabolism

Here, the ability of a bacterial species to metabolize a protein or an amino acid to a defined product is tested. Detection systems for the product and the need for a defined medium are similar to those required for carbohydrate utilization. For example, different species of the Enterobacteriaceae will vary in their ability to: (a) liquefy gelatin; (b) decarboxylate or deaminate amino acids; (c) produce hydrogen sulphide from sulphur-containing amino acids; (d) produce indole from tryptophan.

These tests are often performed in commercial kits.

Susceptibility tests

The susceptibility of a species to a compound may be used, not only to help decide on anti-biotic treatment, but also to aid in its identification. Two commonly used examples are given.

Optocin test Streptococcus pneumoniae is sensitive to optocin (ethylhydrocupreine hydrochloride). Other streptococci which resemble it on blood agar are not.

Metronidazole sensitivity

True anaerobes are almost always sensitive to this antibiotic. Aerobes which can grow anaerobically are invariably resistant.

Toxin production

This important characteristic may help differentiate pathogenic from non-pathogenic species. Examples:

Elek test

This test is used to differentiate toxin-producing (therefore pathogenic) strains of Corynebacterium diphtheriae, the cause of diphtheria, from non-pathogenic strains. A filter-paper strip containing diphtheria antitoxin is incorporated into a defined medium. The organism is streaked onto the agar at right angles to the strip. After incubation, precipitin lines representing antigen (toxin) – antibody (antitoxin) complexes may be seen.

Cytoxin

Here, a cytotoxin produced by strains of Clostridium difficile is associated with antibiotic-induced diarrhoea, and is detected by antitoxin neutralization in cell culture, or by commercial kits.

Molecular techniques

At the time of writing, few of these techniques have made the transition from research laboratory to routine clinical bacteriology. The polymerase chain reaction and gene probes have shown promise in the rapid identification of *Mycobacterium tuberculosis* in clinical samples. This slow-growing organism usually takes several weeks to isolate and identify by conventional methods. However, the high cost of these molecular methods at present limits their use to specialized reference laboratories.

IDENTIFICATION OF BACTERIA

Commercial identification systems
Identification of Bacteria of Medical Importance
Gram-positive cocci

Commercial identification systems

The development of commercial systems for the rapid identification of pathogenic bacteria has greatly simplified the life of the clinical bacteriologist. Prior to their introduction, each biochemical test had to be set up individually in a test-tube or glass bottle leading to impressive displays of laboratory glassware! The new commercial systems are easy to use and allow up to 20 biochemical tests to be performed simultaneously from a pure culture. The pattern of test results obtained is then compared with patterns derived from known bacteria held in a computerized data bank. Statistical tests are used to determine the likely identity of the clinical isolate. The data bank may also suggest additional tests if identification is in doubt.

The two most commonly used systems in the UK are the API system and Vitek, both made by BioMerieux (BioMerieux UK Limited, Basingstoke, England).

API identification system (Appareils et procedes d'identification)

This system consists of plastic cupules containing a variety of substrates and indicator chemicals held on a plastic strip. Each cupule comprises a different biochemical test. The addition of a standard inoculum of the test organism to each cupule in the strip results, after incubation, in a series of colour changes that can be read by the naked eye. The pattern of results obtained can be readily decoded by the data bank. Separate strips with different panels of tests exist for the identification of staphylococci, streptococci, coryneform bacteria, Enterobacteriaceae, anaerobes, and non-fermenting Gram-negative bacteria.

The Vitek system

This system employs a similar principle to API. The biochemical tests are performed in miniature wells encased in a plastic card of similar size and shape to a credit card. The wells are filled with bacterial suspension by vacuum suction. After incubation, the cards are read by a customized, computer-controlled reader. The range of cards produced is similar to the API range. The advantages of this system include its ability to perform antibiotic susceptibility testing, semi-automation requiring reduced operator time, and enclosed system for greater laboratory safety.

Both systems require strict adherence to the manufacturer's instructions if errors are to be avoided. Failure to start with a pure culture is a common source of error. This can be avoided by inoculating a purity plate from the suspension used to inoculate the card or strip. If the plate shows a mixed growth, the tests are repeated. Inexperienced bacteriologists often accept the results from these systems without question, regardless of how improbable they may be clinically. Experienced workers will interpret the results in their clinical context, and will confirm or repeat unlikely or unusual identifications.

Identification of Bacteria of Medical Importance

Gram-positive cocci

The ability of a Gram-positive coccus to produce catalase is a useful rapid test differentiating catalase-positive genera such as *Staphylococcus* and *Micrococcus* from catalase-negative genera, namely *Streptococcus* and *Enterococcus*. Subsequent identification proceeds according to Fig. 12.2.

Staphylococcus and Micrococcus

These catalase-positive genera characteristically produce cells arranged in clusters when grown in liquid medium. Staphylococci may be differentiated from micrococci by their ability to grow under anaerobic conditions.

Staphylococcus aureus, a common cause of skin, wound and lung infection, can be differentiated from other staphylococci which are skin commensals by its ability to coagulate plasma and produce a thermostable DNAase enzyme. Coagulase activity is detected within a few hours, providing a rapid, reliable identification. Coagulase-negative strains of staphylococci may be speciated by commercial kits such as API and Vitek.

Identification of Bacteria of Medical Importance
Gram-positive cocci

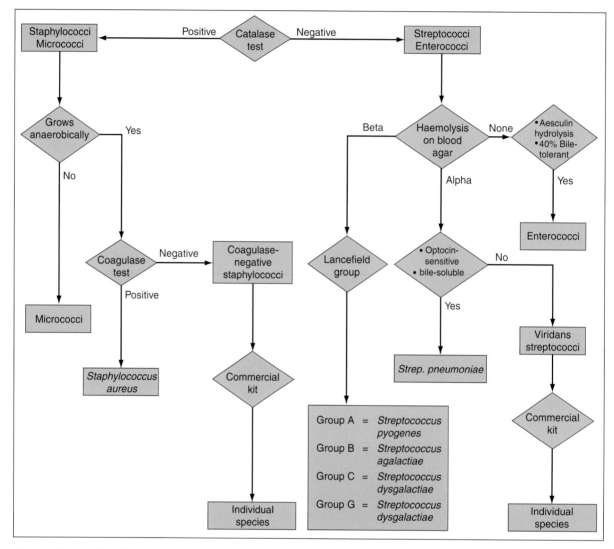

Figure 12.2: *Identification of aerobic Gram-positive cocci of medical importance.*

Streptococcus and Enterococcus

In liquid medium these catalase-negative genera produce cells arranged in pairs or chains. On blood agar, they produce colonies 0.1–1.0 mm in diameter after 24 hours incubation and the type of haemolysis produced around the colonies provides a useful initial classification.

Beta-haemolytic streptococci are best demonstrated in cultures grown anaerobically. Strains producing complete clearing of the medium (β-haemolysis) comprise several important pathogenic species which are differentiated by

Lancefield grouping. This can be performed by commercial tests in less than one hour. Generally, this is sufficient to complete identification, although commercial biochemical test kits may be used in cases of doubt.

Alpha-haemolytic streptococci Partial or α-haemolysis results in a greenish discoloration of the medium around the colony. The most important pathogenic species is *Streptococcus pneumoniae*, the pneumococcus. It is differentiated from other α-haemolytic species by its colonial appearance (draughtsman colonies), optocin sensitivity and solubility of its colonies in bile salt solution. Other α-haemolytic species are found as commensals in the upper respiratory tract, but may occasionally cause serious sepsis, e.g. subacute bacterial endocarditis. They may be identified by commercial kits.

The genus *Enterococcus* is typically non-haemolytic on blood agar, although individual strains can show α- or β-haemolysis. Enterococci, unlike the streptococci, can grow on medium containing 40% bile and hydrolyze aesculin, and these properties are used to

identify them in the clinical laboratory. They often carry Lancefield group D antigen, and may be speciated if required by commercial kits.

Gram-positive bacilli
The medically important genera are identified initially by their colonial morphology, spore forming ability and requirement for aerobic or anaerobic growth conditions (Fig. 12.3).

Bacillus and Clostridium
These spore-forming genera may be differentiated by catalase and conditions required

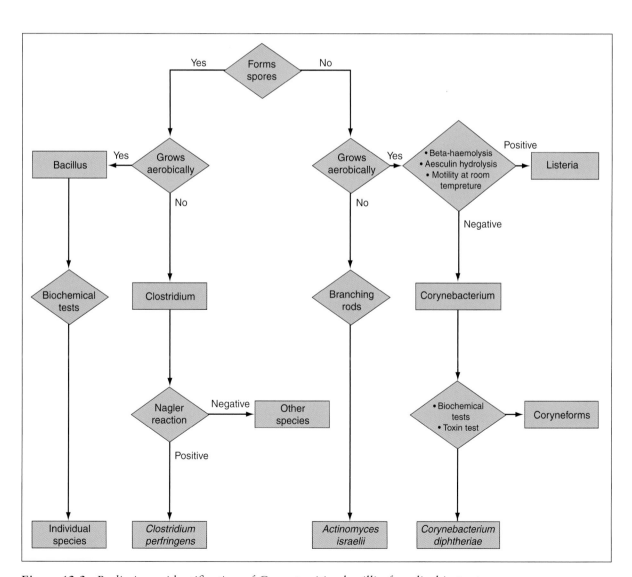

Figure 12.3: *Preliminary identification of Gram-positive bacilli of medical importance.*

Identification of Bacteria of Medical Importance

Gram-negative cocci

Aerobic Gram-negative bacilli

---

for growth. *Clostridium* species are catalase-negative and strict anaerobes, *Bacillus* are catalase-positive and can grow aerobically or anaerobically. *C. perfringens*, the cause of gas gangrene, is identified provisionally by the Nagler test which detects a specific enzyme, lecithinase, produced by this species. Both genera may be speciated by biochemical tests.

Listeria and Corynebacterium
These aerobic, non spore-forming genera can be confused on primary isolation media. *Listeria* show characteristic 'tumbling' motility in broth culture at room temperature but not at 37°C, can hydrolyze aesculin and are often β-haemolytic on blood agar. *Corynebacteria* comprise skin commensals, opportunist pathogens and several major pathogens, including *Corynebacterium diphtheriae*, the cause of diphtheria. They are isolated from throat swabs on selective media containing tellurite. Toxigenic strains of *C. diphtheriae* are detected by the Elek test.

Gram-negative cocci
There are three major human pathogens: *Neisseria gonorrhoea* (the gonococcus), the cause of gonorrhoea; *Neisseria meningitidis* (the meningococcus), a cause of septicaemia and meningitis; and *Moraxella* (formerly *Branhamella*) *catarrhalis*, a cause of chest infections. They must be distinguished from each other and other species which are common human commensals by growth characteristics and biochemical tests (Table 12.1). They are oxidase- and catalase-positive.

Aerobic Gram-negative bacilli
Simple growth requirements
Commercial systems have greatly simplified identification for this group. However, a few simple tests are still required to screen out commensal flora from potential pathogens, and to help choose the correct Vitek card or API strip (Fig. 12.4). The oxidase test is a useful preliminary investigation that takes seconds to perform. Oxidase-negative genera comprise many species that are commensals and pathogens of the gastrointestinal tract (Enterobacteriaceae). Lactose fermentation is usually noted on MacConkey agar which supports growth of these organisms on primary isolation. Non-lactose fermenters may be screened by a urease test or a commercial kit such as the Vitek EPS card for the possible presence of *Salmonella* and *Shigella*, which are then confirmed by further biochemical tests and O (*Salmonella* and *Shigella*) and H (*Salmonella* only) agglutination.

Oxidase-positive genera may be differentiated into those which ferment sugars, for example *Vibrio* and *Aeromonas*, and non-fermenters such as *Pseudomonas*. Different API strips and Vitek cards are available for fermenters and non-fermenters.

Table 12.1: Identification of aerobic gram-negative cocci of medical importance.

	NG	NM	CNS	MC
Acid from*				
Glucose	+	+	v	—
Maltose	—	+	v	—
Lactose	—	—	v	—
Sucrose	—	—	v	—
Grows on nutrient agar	—	—	v	+
Tributyrin**	—	—	—	+
DNase	—	—	—	+

v = Variable, depending on species
* = Test performed on serum-free medium
** = Detects ability of bacterium to split glyceryl tributyrate.

Identification of Bacteria of Medical Importance

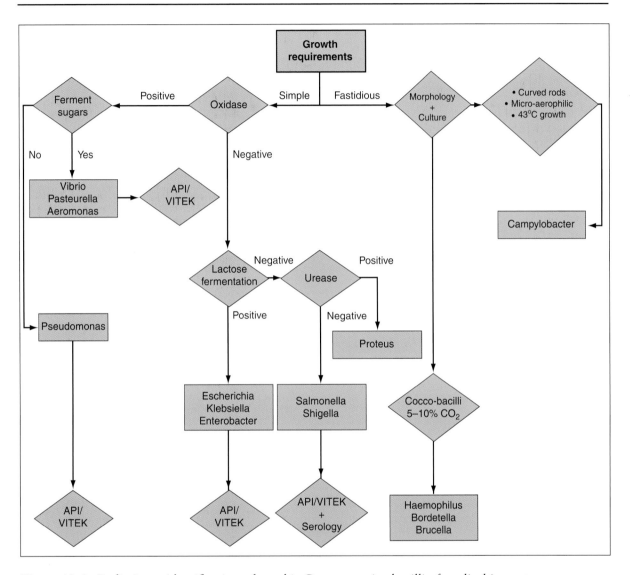

Figure 12.4: *Preliminary identification of aerobic Gram-negative bacilli of medical importance.*

Fastidious growth requirements

Within this group, *Campylobacter* species are most readily identified by morphology, and ability to grow in a microaerophilic atmosphere at 42°C but not in air at 37°C.

Haemophilus, *Bordetella* and *Brucella* are small, mainly non-motile Gram-negative bacilli which grow comparatively poorly on blood agar and poorly, or not at all, on MacConkey agar. This allows them to be readily differentiated from *Pseudomonas* and Enterobacteriaceae. They require enriched, blood-containing media for primary isolation, and the addition of 5–10% CO_2 to the atmosphere enhances growth.

Haemophilus species are commonly isolated from respiratory specimens. They are speciated by their requirement for X and V factors for growth on nutrient agar. *Bordetella* may be identified initially by agglutination with specific antiserum. *Brucella* may be speciated by susceptibility to the dyes fuchsin and thionin, requirement for CO_2 and H_2S production.

155

Identification of Bacteria of Medical Importance

Anaerobes

Other bacteria

Further Reading

Anaerobes

Strict anaerobes are differentiated by their inability to grow in the presence of oxygen and sensitivity to metronidazole, detected by a disc placed on the primary isolation plate. They may be speciated by commercial kits or by detection of their products of metabolism by gas liquid chromatography. However, this is rarely undertaken in clinical laboratories unless the anaerobe has been isolated from a sterile site, for example blood or soft tissue. Gram-positive genera include *Peptostreptococcus*, *Clostridium* and *Actinomyces*. Common Gram-negative genera include *Bacteroides* and *Fusobacterium*.

Other bacteria

There are many bacteria that stain poorly or not at all with Gram's stain. Genera which can be cultured on artificial media include *Mycobacterium* which requires special media (e.g. Lowenstein–Jensen) and stain (Ziehl–Neelsen), and *Mycoplasma* which has no cell wall.

Bacteria which are not routinely cultured on solid media include the spirochaetes, and the obligate intracellular pathogens *Rickettsia*, *Coxiella* and *Chlamydia*. Infections caused by these genera are usually diagnosed by serology or, in the case of *Chlamydia*, antigen detection.

Further Reading

Barron G I, Feltham R K A. *Cowan and Steel's Manual for the Identification of Medical Bacteria*. 1993; 3rd edn, Cambridge University Press.

Collins C H, Lyne P M, Grange J M. *Collins and Lyne's Microbiological Methods*. 1995; 7th edn, Butterworth-Heinmann Ltd, Oxford.

Murray P R, Baron E J, Pfaller M A, Tenover M A, Yolken R H. *Manual of Clinical Microbiology* 1995; 6th edn, A S M Press, Washington, US.

Spencer R C, Wright E P, Newsom S W B. *Rapid Methods and Automation in Microbiology and Immunology*. 1994; Intercept, Andover, UK.

Stokes E J, Ridgway G L, Wren M D W. *Clinical Microbiology*. 1993; 7th edn, Edward Arnold, London.

13 AUTOMATED TESTS IN BACTERIOLOGY

Paul C Boreland

'Automation: the use of automatic equipment to save mental and manual labour.'
The Concise Oxford Dictionary

Introduction

Although automated instrumentation was first introduced into the clinical microbiology laboratory almost thirty years ago, many microbiologists have been reluctant to fully embrace the concept. This has been due in part to a conservative attitude among microbiologists which perpetuates the use of methods for detecting growth which were developed at the end of the nineteenth century. Other relevant factors include the variety and complex nature of the specimens submitted to the laboratory, the greater complexity of microbiological tests, the difficulty in integrating an instrument into the existing laboratory regime, together with the fact that many of the earlier machines did not perform adequately. However, recent improvements in technology and bi-directional interfacing between instruments and laboratory computer systems have now made automation a practical and cost-effective alternative.

Automated equipment is now available for the detection of positive blood cultures, the antimicrobial susceptibility testing and identification of microorganisms, the screening of urine samples for bacteria and the identification and antibiotic susceptibility of *Mycobacterium tuberculosis* in clinical samples. The automated systems described in this chapter are not totally inclusive of all the systems currently on the world market but represent those most commonly encountered in clinical microbiology laboratories within the United Kingdom.

Blood Culture Systems

The rapid detection of septicaemia is one of the most critical tests performed in the clinical microbiology laboratory, and constitutes a major part of the workload. Consequently automated blood culture systems have been developed and refined over the past twenty-five years. The first semi-automated instrument

to be used, the BACTEC 460 (Johnston Laboratories Inc), detected radioactive carbon dioxide metabolized by microorganisms growing in a liquid medium with ^{14}C incorporated. This soon gave way to the non-radiometric BACTEC 660/730 using infrared detection of carbon dioxide.

Recently, several fully automated systems have been developed, each of which comprises three basic units: an incubator, a detector and a computer. The inoculated blood culture bottles or vials are placed in racks or in individually heated silos and may or may not be agitated. Each bottle is monitored continuously for growth every 10 to 15 minutes; and the computer analyzes the data by means of a predetermined algorithm and indicates when a culture is positive. When a positive bottle is identified, it can be removed from the system for isolation and identification of the organism. Importantly, unlike the older instruments, microbial growth is measured non-invasively. Most detection

Blood Culture Systems

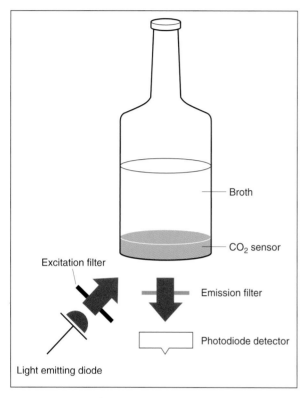

Figure 13.1: Schematic drawing of BACTEC 9240 blood culture bottle and carbon dioxide detector system.

methods are based directly or indirectly on the production of gases (mostly carbon dioxide) or the resulting pH changes, following growth of microorganisms in broth culture.

The **BACTEC 9120/9240** (Becton Dickinson) uses a pH-sensitive sensor containing fluorochemicals which respond to carbon dioxide, embedded in a matrix at the base of each culture bottle. Carbon dioxide, produced by microorganisms metabolizing nutrients in the culture medium, diffuses through the matrix causing a decrease in pH which is detected by the fluorochemicals. The instrument's photodetectors measure specifically the level of fluorescence emitted from the sensor every 10 minutes (Fig. 13.1). These measurements are interpreted by the computer software according to pre-programmed positivity parameters.

The **BacT/Alert** (Organon Teknika) culture bottles each have a colorimetric sensor bonded to the base, and separated from the growth medium by a semipermeable membrane. The

membrane is only freely permeable to carbon dioxide which, when produced by organisms growing, diffuses across the membrane, lowers the pH and initiates a change in colour of the sensor from green to yellow. This colour change is detected by reflecting light from a red light-emitting diode off the sensor onto a photodiode. The voltage signal produced is proportional to the intensity of the reflected light and thus the concentration of carbon dioxide in the bottle. The data obtained by the computer are plotted as a growth curve of reflectance units versus time.

The **Vital** (bioMerieux) uses a method of detection known as Homogeneous Fluorescent Technology (HFT) which is based on the changes in fluorescent molecules which are suspended in the blood culture broth. As organisms grow, the carbon dioxide they produce causes a decrease in pH which inactivates the fluorescent molecules. This reduction in the intensity of the fluorescence emitted is measured by projecting a beam of green light into the bottle, which is then returned as a beam of red fluorescent light and transported via optical fibres to a photon counter. The readings are interpreted by an algorithm in the computer software.

The **Sentinel** (Difco Laboratories Ltd) uses the principle of conductance by having in the base of each bottle two electrodes, one aluminium and one gold. When a culture bottle is placed in an individual silo within the instrument, the electrodes pierce a thin membrane and enter the growth medium. The bottle then acts as a simple battery with two dissimilar metals in an electrically conducting liquid generating a potential difference of 500 MV. As microorganisms grow they deplete the amount of available electron acceptors, for example oxygen, in the aerobic bottle, to remove electrons from the gold electrode. This has the effect of reducing the measured voltage between the two electrodes. The decrease and rate of decrease in voltage is measured every 15 minutes and from these measurements it can be determined whether the voltage has dropped sufficiently to indicate that the bottle is positive.

The **O.A.S.I.S.** (Oxoid Automated Septicaemia Investigation System: Unipath Ltd) is

The following labels appear in Figure 13.1: Broth, CO_2 sensor, Excitation filter, Emission filter, Photodiode detector, Light emitting diode.

based on the continuous monitoring of pressure changes resulting from the metabolic activity of microorganisms growing in a sealed culture bottle. The contents of the bottle are continually mixed by magnetic stirring, and positive or negative pressure changes occurring within the bottle headspace are expressed in the movement of a flexible septum which seals the bottle. This movement is monitored every five minutes by a computer-controlled high-resolution laser which scans across the septum. Measurements, corrected for barometric pressure, are taken of the septum height relative to reference points on the aluminium crimp, and used to plot a graph of septum displacement versus time. The rate of change of the septum displacement is analyzed by the computer, which signals microbial growth when the threshold rate is exceeded.

Antibiotic Susceptibility Testing and Identification Systems

The identification and antibiotic susceptibility testing of bacterial isolates are two of the most important tasks in the clinical microbiology laboratory. A number of instruments are currently available from semi- to fully automated. Most offer identification of organisms as well as antibiotic susceptibility testing and also a choice of conventional or rapid incubation and analysis times. Some instruments have strips which can be inoculated either automatically or manually, incubated externally and then placed in a reader which interprets colour reactions and growth end points. With fully automated systems, microdilution trays or cards are incubated within the instrument which continually monitors and interprets growth or biochemical reactions.

Each system requires an inoculum standardization step, usually performed using a densitometer to measure bacterial density which may be expressed in McFarland units. For the detection of colour changes or growth in liquid medium containing either substrates or dilutions of antibiotics, most automatic readers employ a combination of three methods of light measurement, namely: the transmission of light in four regions of the spectrum, colorimetry; the intensity of transmitted light which is inversely proportional to the amount of bacterial growth, turbidimetry; and the intensity of scattered light at 30° which is directly proportional to the amount of bacterial growth, nephelometry. Light measurements are easily converted into electrical impulses, and then quantified.

A few instruments use fluorogenic substrate hydrolysis to detect bacterial growth and can provide results within 4 to 5 hours. All of the systems are equipped with a microcomputer and software capable of interpreting results from the reader, producing algorithm-derived minimum inhibitory concentration (MIC) or breakpoint values, identifying organisms from a database containing several biocodes and performing statistical and epidemiological analyses.

The **ATB Expression** (bioMerieux) involves the use of strips with cupules containing either substrates for biochemical identification tests or dilutions of antibiotics. The breakpoint dilution test involving a high and a low concentration of antibiotic is performed in semi-solid medium thus paralleling the agar diffusion test. The strips may be inoculated manually or automatically with a solution of the isolate adjusted to the required bacterial density, followed by external incubation for up to 24 hours. Reading of the strips is automatic using both colorimetric and turbidimetric measurements, and the ATB Plus software which controls the reader interprets the results and gives an automatic identification of the organism or qualitative S,I,R (Sensitive, Intermediate, Resistant) results for a range of antibiotics.

The **Vitek** (bioMerieux) uses novel plastic reagent cards containing small quantities of growth medium and either antibiotics or biochemical test media in 30 test wells. Cards are available for the identification of several bacteria and yeasts, and a range of antibiotics as either S,I,R or MIC results. The system includes a filling and sealing module for the inoculation and hermetically sealing of the cards, and a combined incubator and reader in which the cards are held in a carousel and where biochemical colour changes and optical density are photometrically measured every hour. Results are usually available within 4 to 18 hours. Identification and antibiotic susceptibility of an organism are derived from computer analysis of the data.

The **Sensititre** (AccuMed International Ltd) detects bacterial growth by means of compounds known as fluorophores. They consist of different substrates such as peptides and esters linked to the fluorescing compounds, 4-methylumbelliferone (4MU) and 7-aminomethylcoumarin (7AMC). Normally these complexes are non-fluorescent but during bacterial growth specific enzymes are produced which cleave the substrates from the fluorophores allowing the 7AMC or 4MU to fluoresce under UV light. Susceptibility to a specific antibiotic is recorded as absence of fluorescence, that is, no growth, and resistance as fluorescence due to the enzyme production by actively growing bacteria. Results usually take only 4 to 5 hours but may require overnight incubation. The system comprises an inoculator, an incubator, a fluorimeter reading fluorescence at 450 μm and a computer. Tests are performed in wells in prepared microtitre trays and the software contains an algorithm which can interpret the signals and produce breakpoint or MIC results. The identification system works similarly, with only those biochemical tests that can produce fluorescence or are non-fluorescent being included. The organism is identified from a computer database.

The **Mastascan Colour** (Mast Laboratories Ltd) is a unique system which uses multipoint technology to inoculate agar dilution antibiotic susceptibility tests, both breakpoint and MIC, and biochemical identification tests. It consists of a scanner module containing a colour video camera, a multipoint inoculator and a microcomputer. Predosed, freeze-dried pellets of antibiotics are used to prepare breakpoint and MIC plates, and a range of culture media are used for bacterial identification. Agar plates are inoculated and incubated, and growth is seen as 19 or 36 macrocolonies. They are then placed in the scanner module and inspected at predetermined points by the video camera. The quantity of each of the three basic colours, red, blue and green, is sent as an electrical signal to the microcomputer which converts the signals to numbers. For breakpoint and MIC plates, where susceptibility or resistance is defined as growth or no growth, the three colour signals combine to produce the equivalent of a black and white signal. When biochemical identification agar plates are examined, details of the colours measured are used to define positive or negative results from the different microorganisms tested.

Urine Screening Systems

The investigation of urine samples for the presence of bacteriuria and pyuria represents a significant proportion of the workload and cost of running a clinical microbiology laboratory. Only 20 to 30% of these specimens yield clinically significant results, and consequently, various attempts have been made to automate the process in order to screen out negative urines. The requirement has been for an instrument which has the ability to detect bacteria and other particles in urine such as erythrocytes and leucocytes, can process specimens rapidly, and has a high negative predictive value. There are currently two such instruments which employ the technology of particle counting and fulfil these criteria.

The **Questor** (Difco Laboratories Ltd) is an automated single-channel impedance particle counter which distinguishes between microorganisms, red and white blood cells, and epithelial cells on the basis of their relative volumes.[4] When a urine sample is placed into a conductive electrolyte solution any particles in the urine will displace a volume of the solution equivalent to their own volume. In the instrument the diluted sample is passed through an orifice in a particle-counting probe which also contains two platinum electrodes, one internal and one external. The volume of the orifice is varied by a tapered spike being moved in and out automatically. This causes a 'filtration effect' where larger particles are deflected from the orifice thus preventing blockage (Fig. 13.2).

When particles are drawn through the orifice by vacuum and enter the electrical field, they displace their own volume of electrolyte and

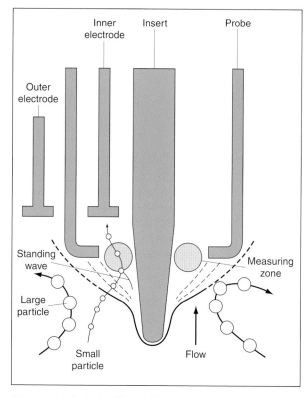

Figure 13.2: The filter effect.

cause changes in the impedance of the electrical current. These changes are detected as pulses, the height and area of each pulse being proportional to the mean spherical volume of a particular particle. Thus by passing a known volume of urine through the orifice, the number and size distribution of the particles present can be counted and reported. A histogram of the number of particles and their respective sizes (range 0.5 to 40 μm) is formed and analyzed by the computer software to give enumeration of the particles of different size bands.

The **UF-100** (Sysmex) combines flow cytometry together with impedance detection to directly identify and count cells and microorganisms in urine. Each urine sample is mixed with a diluent, and a two-part fluorescent stain with affinity both for DNA and RNA is added. The stained sample is then guided into a flow cell which is irradiated by a laser. The laser beams are scattered by the cells in the sample, and forward scattered light (fluorescent and non-fluorescent) which is proportional to the

cross-sectional area of the cells, is measured by a photodiode. The fluorescence emitted, which indicates the degree of nucleation of the cell, is measured by a photomultiplier. Using five signals of fluorescent and non-fluorescent height and width plus impedance measurements, the instrument differentiates the three-dimensional cell structures into their appropriate cell types and numbers, and counts numbers of organisms. The cell distribution can be displayed on scattergrams and histograms using the Adaptive Cluster Analysis computer software.

Identification and Antibiotic Susceptibility Testing Systems for Mycobacteria

The re-emergence of tuberculosis and the increasing incidence of outbreaks of multiple-drug-resistant strains of *Mycobacterium tuberculosis* has brought into sharp focus the need for automated systems for the rapid detection, identification and antibiotic susceptibility testing of mycobacteria. Most of the systems currently available have been developed from existing blood culturing technology and use similar instrumentation. All instruments have safety features designed to protect the operator and prevent environmental contamination.

The **BACTEC 460 TB** (Becton Dickinson) was the first semi-automated instrument used for the rapid detection of mycobacteria. It is a radiometric method using vials of Middlebrook 7H12 broth medium containing radiolabelled palmitic acid as the substrate and five antimicrobial agents to reduce contamination. Radiolabelled carbon dioxide is released into the headspace of the vial by mycobacteria in the inoculated specimen metabolizing palmitic acid. The radioactivity in the carbon dioxide is measured by a scintillation counter and converted to a growth index (GI) value. A GI value of 10 or more indicates the presence of mycobacteria. The *M. tuberculosis* (MTB) complex may be differentiated from other mycobacteria by inoculating an aliquot from a positive vial into a BACTEC vial containing nucleic acid phosphate (NAP Test). No increase or a decrease in the GI value indicates the presence of the MTB complex. The system may also be used for antibiotic susceptibility testing of MTB complex isolates.

The **BACTEC 9000 MB** (Becton Dickinson) uses fluorescence technology to detect mycobacteria growing in liquid culture medium. The culture vials contain a fluorescent sensor which responds to the concentration of oxygen present. Photodetectors in the instrument measure the level of fluorescence, which corresponds to the amount of oxygen consumed due to growth of the organisms. Vials are held in racks and are tested every 10 minutes by light-emitting diodes (LEDs) which activate the fluorescence sensors. Positive cultures are flagged by an indicator light on the front of the instrument and displayed on the monitor.

The **MB/BacT** (Organon Teknika) has an identical detection system to the BacT/Alert blood culture instrument. A sensor on the base of each culture bottle detects carbon dioxide as an indicator of microbial growth. The change in colour from green to yellow is continuously monitored by a reflectometer in the detection unit.

The **BACTEC MGIT 960** (Becton Dickinson) which is currently undergoing trials uses the Mycobacteria Growth Indicator Tube (MGIT). Growth within the tube is indicated by orange fluorescence under UV light. The system is fully automated, has a capacity of 320 tubes in each of three drawers and is designed to perform antibiotic susceptibility testing as well as growth detection.

Comment

It is inevitable that, in order to perform 'real-time' microbiological tests, that is, to send meaningful clinical diagnostic information from the laboratory to the physician, microbiologists must turn increasingly to automated instrumentation. This will also help to alleviate the pressure caused by shrinking budgets, staff reductions and an ever-increasing workload. The many advantages of automated tests include: the release of skilled staff from repetitive work to perform more demanding complicated tasks, thus enhancing the overall quality of the work of the laboratory; improved turnaround times; better standardization of tests by eliminating subjectivity and human error; and cost-effective performance of tests by screening out negative specimens which require no further processing. It is difficult to imagine the disappearance of the agar plate and wire loop after over a century of use; however the time may be swiftly approaching when they are not the first tools the clinical microbiologist reaches for.

Further Reading

Eyre A E. Blood cultures: a review of methodologies. *British Society for Microbial Technology Newsletter* 1995; **18**: 2–17.

Jorgensen J H. Recent developments in automated and rapid susceptibility testing methods. In Spencer RC, Wright EP, Newsom SWB, eds. *Rapid Methods and Automation in Microbiology and Immunology* 1994; Intercept Ltd, Andover, pp. 481–488.

Stevens M, Mitchell C J, Livsey S A, MacDonald C A. Evaluation of Questor urine screening system for bacteriuria and pyuria. *Journal of Clinical Pathology* 1993; **46**: 817–821.

Wellstood S A. Diagnostic mycobacteriology: current challenges and technologies. *Laboratory Medicine* 1993; **24**: 357–361.

Woods G L. Automation in Clinical Microbiology. *American Journal of Clinical Pathology* 1992; **4** (suppl. 1): 23–30.

14 BACTERIOLOGY MOLECULAR TECHNIQUES: SAMPLE PREPARATION AND APPLICATION

Richard E Holliman and Julie D Johnson

The Need for Molecular Methods

To justify the significant resources required to develop and perform molecular diagnostic methods, a bacterial infection must satisfy a number of basic criteria. Firstly the infection must represent a significant clinical problem in terms of numbers of cases, morbidity and mortality. Early diagnosis of the infection should improve the prognosis for the patient; usually specific, efficacious therapy will be available. Finally, the existing diagnostic approach, based on traditional methods of microscopy, culture and serology, should produce a sub-optimal performance. There is little clinical justification in developing a molecular based diagnostic method for a bacterial infection that can be readily identified and tested for antimicrobial susceptibility in the routine laboratory. The application of advanced molecular methods should be targeted on bacteria that are difficult to grow in culture, those that cannot be readily distinguished from similar non-pathogenic bacteria, those that cannot be reliably assessed for antimicrobial susceptibility and species that cannot be separated with sufficient discrimination by existing typing methods. This chapter will concentrate on molecular methods dealing with bacterial nucleic acids.

Sample Preparations

The success of any technique employed in studying bacterial nucleic acids initially relies upon the release and purification of the target nucleic acids (Table 14.1). As yet there is no universally accepted method for the preparation of clinical specimens but there are many interrelated factors which must be taken into account. Once the target organism has been

selected, the type of clinical specimen examined will be dictated by the pathogenesis of the disease. To maximize the chance of detection

Sample Preparations

Table 14.1: Sample preparations.
Key points

- Release and purification of target nuclei acids
- Consideration of pathogenesis of disease to determine specimen type
- Concentration of target organism
- Consideration of PCR inhibitors
- Minimal sample handling
- Robust protocols

the bacterial load within the specimen (the number of organisms per specimen volume) should be considered. Optimally, where the bacterial load is low, the largest convenient sample volume should be screened; however, molecular techniques often use volumes of <100 μl. Ultimately concentration of the target organism into a small volume is required. This will require a high level of concentration in specimens such as sputum for *Mycobacterium*

tuberculosis and blood for bacteraemia, but low levels in specimens such as urine for chlamydia in order to achieve the required sensitivity. Large sample volumes require complex target extraction techniques, such as ethanol precipitation and nucleic acid target capture, which result in decreased sensitivity of the assay employed. Large sample volumes may also contain higher levels of non-specific nucleic acid from extraneous DNA which may compromise the assay.

The specimen type and how it is processed during and after collection is of relevance. Specimens such as CSF, urine and sputum may contain inhibitors. Haem (at 0.8 μM) and its metabolic products are known inhibitors of DNA polymerases due to binding of haem and/or porphyrin to the amplification enzyme. Acidic polysaccharides, components of glycoproteins in sputum, are also inhibitory. Additional steps may be necessary for the removal of inhibitors from specimens such as sputum and blood compared to urine or CSF.

Amplification enzymes are also inhibited by reagents used in specimen collection such as

Table 14.2: Problem-solving in sample preparation.

Clinical context	Problem	Solution
Large volume samples	Large amounts of extraneous DNA compared to small processing volume	Stringent DNA extraction Maximize amplification sensitivity
Range of clinical specimen types	Variable levels of enzyme inhibition	Individualize extraction techniques
Chemicals used in specimen collection	Enzyme inhibition	Dilution Chelating agents Positive controls
Range of pathogens to be detected	Variable target stability	Rapid specimen processing Optimal storage/transport conditions
Partially treated patients	Presence of viable or non-viable pathogens	RT-PCR
Presence of clinical samples and previous amplification products in the laboratory	Contamination of samples generating false-positive reactions	Positive displacement/ plugged pipettes Dedicated pre and post PCR workstations Dedicated equipment

EDTA and heparin. If the target is present in abundance, dilution of the specimen may eliminate the inhibitory effect whilst maintaining the nucleic acid at a level at which the frequency of sampling zero copies is low. In contrast, enzymatic or chemical destruction of the nucleic acid will reduce the effective number of amplifiable nucleic acid targets. The target organism and the durability of its cell wall will have a significant effect upon the extraction procedure. For example, the cell wall of *M. tuberculosis* is particularly resistant to lysis whereas that of *Mycoplasma* species will lyse spontaneously.

It is also important to protect laboratory personnel employing molecular techniques when pathogens such as *M. tuberculosis* are the target organism. It may therefore be necessary to include sterilization steps within the extraction procedure. Minimal sample handling and robust protocols are required with the reduced requirement for specialized equipment. Sample preparation procedures contribute to the reliability of target detection within clinical specimens. If these are inefficient, false-negative or false-positive results may be generated (Table 14.2).

Nucleic acid targets may be either DNA or RNA, double or single stranded and must be stabilized against degradation once isolated. RNA is more difficult to stabilize than DNA. It is a requirement of the isolation of RNA that no contaminating DNA is present. Selective extraction or destruction of DNA or RNA allows one to target the appropriate nucleic acid. rRNA may be stabilized in chaotrope solutions for months at room temperature. Pathogens that have an RNA and a DNA stage in their life cycle are problematic. Reverse transcription polymerase chain reaction detects both unless steps are taken to destroy the DNA target. Amplification methods such as self-sustaining sequence replication (3SR) that are theoretically capable of using solely RNA templates should not amplify DNA unless a denaturation step is included as part of the extraction technique. It is important to determine whether single-stranded DNA actually interferes with this RNA-specific approach. Analagously, PCR would detect only DNA unless a reverse transcription step precedes the PCR. Amplification methods that target stable

nucleic acids can detect dead, dormant and replicating organisms. Detection of all forms of the organism may be advantageous when viability is rapidly lost during transport or storage or if the organism cannot be cultured. However, discrimination of dead from viable organisms would present a problem if nonviable or dormant organisms remain once active infection has cleared.

Once isolated the target must be placed into an aqueous environment compatible with amplification. Amplification enzymes are inhibited by many reagents used in molecular biology for the purification of nucleic acids including detergents such as sodium dodecyl sulphate (SDS) or chaotropes such as guanidinium hydrochloride used to solubilize cell membranes or inactivate nucleases. Additional steps must be taken to remove or neutralize such reagents. Quality control of reagents and equipment in clinical molecular biology techniques is of paramount importance. With techniques as powerful and sensitive as PCR the risk of false-positive reactions due to contamination and of false negatives due to reaction inhibitors have led to scrupulous avoidance procedures which make the technique relatively expensive and the domain of those who can afford to dedicate the necessary time, facilities and patience. Of particular importance in diagnostic microbiology is the use of insert controls for avoidance of false negatives e.g. intrinsic DNA controls of a low copy number of a control sequence can be spiked into the clinical specimen. If the control does not amplify it can be assumed that the specimen is inhibitory. Special equipment requirements include plugged tips or positive displacement pipettes, separate workstations, thermocyclers and detection based equipment. All require a large initial financial outlay. Molecular techniques are still, as yet, the tool of reference laboratories and research units although future developments may eventually lead to more general usage.

Current Practice

In the mid 1990s a limited number of bacterial infections are subject to molecular diagnostic

<u>Current Practice</u>
Respiratory tract
Soft tissues

methods in the course of routine clinical practice. A larger number have been investigated in the research laboratory and some of these may find a clinical role in the future. Routine laboratory methods are used in a number of distinct functions in the process of diagnosis; these comprise detection of the organism in a clinical sample, identification of the isolate, susceptibility testing and epidemiological typing. Molecular methods have been applied to each of these four functions and representative examples are listed in Table 14.3. From the clinical perspective, molecular methods are used in the diagnosis of bacterial infections of the respiratory tract, soft tissues, urogenital system, gastrointestinal tract and central nervous system.

Respiratory tract

A number of bacteria causing infection of the respiratory tract are difficult to grow or identify in culture. Consequently these infections are suited for the application of advanced molecular methods. *Mycoplasma pneumoniae* can be detected in throat swabs using PCR while *Legionella pneumophila* can be detected in deep lung secretions by PCR and DNA probes.

A single tube-nested PCR incorporating an EIA based detection system has been developed for the diagnosis of *Chlamydia pneumoniae* infection. Isolates of the *Mycobacterium avium–intracellulare* complex grown on slopes or in liquid media can be identified rapidly by hybridization with specific DNA probes. Molecular methods can be used to detect *Mycobacterium tuberculosis* in clinical samples, identify isolates grown *in vitro*, assess susceptibility and distinguish strains in epidemiological studies.

Soft tissues

Established methods for the identification of staphylococcal species are based on phenotypic characteristics. Such methods can be unreliable due to variable expression of these phenotypic factors. The 16S rRNA gene has conserved and variable regions. By designing PCR primers for specific sequences within the gene it has been possible to speciate staphylococcal isolates with greater accuracy.

Group A streptococci (*Streptococcus pyogenes*) isolates can be genotyped by analysis of the restriction enzyme pattern of 16S rRNA — a process known as ribotyping. The pyrogenic

Table 14.3:   Clinical application of molecular methodology.

Function	Bacteria	Conventional methods	Molecular methods
Pathogen detection	*Neisseria meningitidis*	Microscopy Culture on agar media Antigen detection	PCR amplification and DNA probing of amplification products
Identification of isolates	*Staphylococcus* species	Examination of phenotypic characteristics e.g. coagulase enzyme production	PCR amplification using species-specific primers for 16S rRNA gene sequences
Antimicrobial susceptibility	*Mycobacterium tuberculosis*	Culture on media containing antibiotics	Electrophoresis of PCR products to detect genetic differences associated with resistance
Typing	*Streptococcus pyogenes*	M protein serotyping	PCR amplification of 16S rRNA and examination of restriction enzyme fragments of the PCR products

exotoxin gene can be detected by PCR amplification. A further typing scheme is based on PCR amplification and restriction enzyme digestion of the virulence regulon, a gene cluster comprising virulence factors such as complement inactivating factor and antiphagocytic activity under the transcription control of a virulence gene.

Urogenital system

Chlamydia trachomatis can be detected in genital specimens by ELISA, immunofluorescence tests and DNA probes but these methods have proved to be less sensitive than conventional cultures. In contrast, PCR amplification appears to be more sensitive than chlamydia culture while retaining high specificity. In addition it can be applied to first pass urine samples, as well as to endourethral swabs.

The diagnosis of gonorrhoea remains based on isolation of the bacterium by conventional culture. However, DNA probing or amplification by PCR or ligase chain reaction may be of value when isolation is impractical due to difficulties in specimen transport or lack of immediate access to a laboratory with culture facilities. DNA probes to *Neisseria gonorrhoeae* have a sensitivity limit of approximately 10^3 organisms per sample. Precision of amplification methods may equal or even exceed that of culture but clinical experience is limited.

Gastrointestinal system

In general, molecular methods are of limited value for the diagnosis of gastrointestinal infection. Although conventional methods of microscopy and culture are relatively insensitive and time consuming, most patients require only supportive treatment and a specific diagnosis will often not affect management. A possible exception is Campylobacter infection where current identification methods are based on unreliable biochemical factors. Little is known of the epidemiology of this condition, partly due to the lack of a reliable typing scheme for clinical isolates. PCR primers specific for the genus *Campylobacter* and species within the genus C. *upsaliensis, helveticus, fetus, hyointestinalis* and *lari* are based on the conserved and variable regions of the 16S rRNA gene. Restriction enzyme digestion of the amplified products can be used to develop a typing scheme for following the spread of strains in outbreaks.

Central nervous system

DNA probes have not been able to provide a clinically useful level of sensitivity when used for the detection of bacteria in the CSF. DNA amplification methods have been more successful. PCR for *Neisseria meningitidis* in CSF samples has achieved levels of sensitivity and specificity of over 90% compared to conventional cultures. This technique may be of particular value when the patient has been given antibiotic therapy prior to lumbar puncture, and represents a significant advance over antigen detection methods. PCR has also been used to detect *Listeria monocytogenes* in immune suppressed patients with meningitis and *Treponema pallidum* in the diagnosis of symptomatic neurosyphilis. The sensitivity and specificity of these applications is not yet established.

Mycobacterium Tuberculosis

Tuberculosis represents an infection ideally suited to the application of molecular diagnostic methods and so will be discussed in greater detail. The infection causes significant morbidity and mortality as well as a threat to the public health, yet the prognosis is improved markedly by prompt diagnosis and the instigation of appropriate therapy. Traditional diagnostic methods are inadequate. Microscopy of sputum provides a valuable marker of infectivity but lacks sensitivity for the detection of the organism, more so when applied to other specimen types. Culture is slow, positive results often taking two to six weeks, as is subsequent susceptibility testing. Many patients are diagnosed on the basis of

<u>Mycobacterium Tuberculosis</u>

Methodology

Clinical diagnosis

Identification of isolates

Susceptibility testing

clinical and radiological evidence and receive empirical drug therapy prior to microbiological confirmation.

Methodology

The IS 6110 gene is a multiple copy DNA sequence often used as an amplification target. Other targets include the 65 kD heat shock protein, MPB 64 and 16S rRNA genes. Amplification is most often performed by PCR although the ligase chain reaction, transcription mediated amplification and strand displacement amplification show similar sensitivity with the same risk of false-positive reactions due to contamination. Commercial assays include the Gen-Probe single test transcription mediated amplification for rRNA which incorporates an acridinium ester-labelled DNA probe specific for *M. tuberculosis*. The Amplicor system is based on PCR amplification of the 16S rRNA gene followed by hybridation to a *M. tuberculosis*-specific oligonucleotide probe fixed to a microtitre tray well. *In vitro* assessment indicates that the Amplicor, Gen-Probe and IS 6110 gene amplification methods have comparable sensitivity and specificity.

Clinical diagnosis

Amplification methods can be applied to a range of clinical samples including sputum, bronchial lavage, pleural fluid, gastric aspirate, CSF, peripheral blood and biopsy tissue. The level of specificity is high in all specimen types but sensitivity is variable, reflecting numbers of bacteria per unit volume as well as inhibition of the amplification process. False-negative results due to amplification inhibition is a particular problem with samples of pleural fluid. Amplification methods have achieved sensitivity levels of approximately 85% when used to test sputum samples, placing PCR above microscopy but below culture. The positive predictive value of PCR approaches 100% in a smear-positive sample while the negative predictive value of PCR is of the order of 95% for smear-negative specimens. Consequently the smear- and PCR-positive patient is highly likely to have tuberculosis, while the smear- and PCR-negative patient is unlikely to be infected, although further

samples should be taken if clinical suspicion of tuberculosis is high.

Identification of isolates

When conventional culture produces a bacterial growth on a slope or in liquid media, specific DNA probes can be used to identify the isolate as can PCR methods. An identification of the organism can be available within one working day of testing the culture. A commercial DNA probe, Accuprobe, can identify isolates of the *M. tuberculosis* complex. Amplification of part of the hypervariable region of the 16S rRNA gene by PCR and sequencing the product also permits speciation of isolates.

Susceptibility testing

The recent spread of multiple drug-resistant strains of *M. tuberculosis* has given greater impetus to the drive towards rapid assessment of susceptibility. A novel approach to the determination of viability is to insert the gene encoding a luciferase enzyme from fireflies into a bacteriophage. When the phage infects a live bacterium the luciferase enzyme is synthesized and emits light. If, however, the bacterium is dead as a result of susceptibility to an antibiotic, no light is produced. An alternative approach is to detect genetic differences between drug-sensitive and resistant strains. These methods require a detailed knowledge of the genes responsible for resistance to each anti-tuberculosis agent. Changes in the nucleotide sequence of a gene can often be detected by differences in mobility of denatured, single stranded nucleic acid molecules on electrophoretic gel. PCR is used to amplify the region of interest and the product run on a gel against control sequences with and without resistance mutation. This method can detect 98% of rifampicin resistant *M. tuberculosis* isolates within two days of receiving the specimen. Resistance mutation can also be detected using specific probes under conditions of high stringency. To date, isoniazid resistance has been more difficult to detect reliably due to the larger number of genetic mutations involved as compared to rifampicin.

Typing

Conventional typing methods such as phage typing and serotyping have been of limited epidemiological value when applied to strains of *M. tuberculosis* due to low discrimination power. The repeated DNA sequence IS 6110 shows sufficient polymorphism to allow a typing scheme based on PCR amplification of the insertion sequence and Southern blotting of the restriction enzyme fragments. Strains carrying only a single copy of the insertion sequence cannot be separated by IS 6110 typing. Such isolates may be investigated using another repetitive element, the DR sequence. In each case the target gene consists of direct repeats separated by unique sequences. The variability of these unique sequences leads to different banding patterns after cutting with restriction enzymes, known as restriction fragment length polymorphism. The method developed to amplify and label DNA sequences in the DR region is known as spacer oligotyping or 'spoligotyping'.

Problems with Molecular Methods

Although molecular methods have led to advances in the diagnosis and management of infection, significant problems remain to be addressed. The resource requirements of these techniques are often greater than that of the conventional methods they seek to replace. Specialized equipment and reagents combined with the need for further operator training has limited the application of molecular methods in routine diagnostic laboratories. The clinical significance of the enhanced sensitivity of assays based on DNA probing and, in particular, DNA amplification may be uncertain. For example, a smear-positive sputum sample on routine microscopy must contain around 10^4 tubercle bacilli. Despite this relative lack of sensitivity, the findings are of great clinical value for predicting infectivity. In contrast, the significance of a positive PCR assay for *M. tuberculosis* performed on a sputum sample taken from a patient on appropriate therapy is limited as the organisms may be dead.

The danger of false-positive reactions due to carry-over in the performance of DNA amplification is well described. In contrast, the restricted test volumes used in these methods can result in false-negative results due to sampling error associated with non-uniform distribution of the pathogen in clinical specimens. Finally, first generation molecular methods were designed only to detect the presence or absence of a pathogen and gave no information as to the viability of the organism. Although later assays have corrected this defect they tend to be complex and more difficult to perform.

Future Application

Molecular methods are likely to be developed for other organisms which are difficult to grow in culture, such as *Brucella* and anaerobic bacteria, or conditions where antibiotic therapy has been given before specimens are taken for diagnosis, including meningitis, osteomyelitis and endocarditis. Rapid detection of antibiotic resistance would have immediate clinical application for vancomycin-resistant enterococci, methicillin-resistant *Staphylococcus aureus*, β-lactam-resistant pneumococci and Gram-negative bacteria resistant to multiple agents. Molecular methods may provide useful information as to the likely virulence of clinical isolates of coagulase-negative staphylococci and alpha-haemolytic streptococci. Genotyping may assist studies into the spread of antibiotic resistance and mechanisms of cross-infection in hospitals. Molecular methods have enjoyed an extended period of research interest; the future challenge will be to change their present reputation as being 'better for papers than patients'.

Further Reading

Clewley J. The work of the Molecular Biology Unit at Central Public Health Laboratory. *PHLS Microbiol Dig* 1996; **13**: 49–53.

Dilworth D D, McCarrey J R. Single step elimination of contaminating DNA prior to reverse transcriptase-PCR. *PCR Methods Applic* 1992; **1**: 279–282.

Mandell G L, Bennett J E, Dolin R (eds). *Principles and Practice of Infectious Diseases*. 1995: 4th edn, Churchill-Livingstone, New York.

Marshall B G, Shaw R J. New technology in the diagnosis of tuberculosis. *Br J Hosp Med* 1996; **55**: 491–94.

Persing D H, Smith T F, Tenover F C, White T J. *Diagnostic Molecular Microbiology Principles and Applications*. 1993: American Society for Microbiology, Washington DC.

15   OTHER TESTS IN BACTERIOLOGY

David Parratt

Introduction

Traditionally, diagnostic microbiologists have relied on culturing microorganisms, identifying them and inferring the significance of the grown organisms. The methods by which this is accomplished are covered elsewhere in this book but it is important to note that there are many infections in which the culture approach to diagnosis is not possible. This occurs for several reasons. For example, there are some microorganisms which cannot be cultured, such as the cause of syphilis, *Treponema pallidum*, or organisms which are difficult to grow such as *Legionella pneumophila*, the cause of legionnaires' disease. In addition, there are some organisms which are too dangerous to attempt to culture for routine diagnostic purposes, a good example being *Brucella abortus*. It is also interesting to note that *Brucella abortus* falls into the second of the categories also in that it is difficult to culture.

In these circumstances, the microbiologist will attempt to make a diagnosis by detecting the presence of the organism rather than by isolating it, and there are a variety of methods available to achieve this. These other methods are discussed below but it should be appreciated at this point that the diagnosis using these methods is almost always *inferred* and is rarely scientifically proven. For example, if we detect antigens of *Legionella pneumophila* in the urine of patients with pneumonia (see below), we can infer that this organism is causing an infection in the lung without actually proving that to be the case. Similarly, if we detect high levels of antibody to *Treponema pallidum* in a patient suspected of having syphilis, we infer that the patient is indeed infected.

A move towards more formal proof can sometimes be achieved using other tests if the test results are monitored over a period of time. For example, by measuring antibody during the patient's acute illness and again in convalescence, it may be possible to demonstrate that antibody has increased during this period of time and this is good evidence that the patient is actively responding to the presence of an active infection. The reverse argument of demonstrating a decline in antibody over time is more tenuous but can, on occasions, be helpful.

Tests for Antibody

The commonest tests are those grouped under the general term serology. Serology is the study of serum, which has been practised since the early days of diagnostic microbiology and is generally taken to mean the study of antibody

Tests for Antibody
Older tests

in the patient's serum. As indicated above, patients who are infected by bacteria will almost always produce antibody against that organism. Antibodies are proteins which occur in the serum (the cell-free compartment of blood) and which are complex molecules of different types (named immunoglobulins). They perform numerous useful defence reactions against invading microorganisms. There are five types of immunoglobulin in man but for general microbiological consideration and certainly for diagnosis only three of them, IgM, IgG and IgA, are of major relevance. These different types (called isotypes) of immunoglobulin have different properties. For example, IgM antibody is formed early in the course of infection and is a potent agglutinator of bacteria as well as being a strong activator of the biological system called 'complement'. IgG is found in many tissue fluids and this type of antibody will agglutinate, will activate complement and is good at precipitating bacterial toxins or neutralizing the attachment of bacteria to tissue cells. It also crosses the placenta and affords protection to the fetus. An additional important role of IgG antibodies is to assist the phagocytosis of bacteria by phagocytic cells such as polymorphonuclear leukocytes and macrophages. IgG antibodies are formed later than IgM antibodies and therefore it is common practice in many infections to measure both types of antibody in order to determine whether the infection is very recent or has been active for a longer time. Antibodies of IgA type are poorer at all of the activities mentioned above except for neutralization.

Serological tests for antibody can be broadly divided into older tests and current testing methods.

Older tests
Agglutination tests

Agglutination methods depend upon the ability of antibody in the patient's sample to agglutinate bacterial particles or artificially coated particles (e.g. latex) in suspension. A typical example of an agglutination test is the direct agglutination method for detection of antibody to *Brucella abortus*. A suspension of bacterial cells is added to a series of dilutions of the patient's serum contained in test-tubes. The tubes are incubated for an hour or longer, usually at 37 °C, and the result is then read. It is common with this kind of test to incubate overnight in order to detect the weakest agglutination. Agglutination is read by tapping the tubes gently to disturb the cells which will rise in the fluid either as aggregates or, in the case of negative controls, as a fine wispy suspension. Details of such procedures relevant to many different infections can be found in standard textbooks.

Agglutination tests are particularly likely to be positive when IgM antibody is present as it is a better agglutinator than the other immunoglobulin isotypes. However, IgM antibody does not always cause agglutination and false negatives can occur. An additional problem with agglutination tests is the so-called prozone effect where agglutination is not seen at the highest concentrations of antibody due to steric inhibition of the antibody binding sites and only becomes obvious when the sample is diluted.

Variations using a variety of 'artificial' particles are numerous; for example, latex particles can be coated with extracted antigens from organisms. Red blood cells (e.g. from sheep) can also be used as in the *Treponema pallidum* haemagglutination assay (TPHA) used for the diagnosis of syphilis. These coated particle tests have the benefit that they do not suffer from auto-agglutination, that is agglutination of the particles simply through protein adhesion effects, which is a frequent problem with bacterial suspensions.

A variant of the agglutination test is the indirect agglutination test which is similar to the Coombs haemagglutination test used in haematology. The rationale is that IgG antibody to a microorganism will attach to the organism but may not bring about agglutination and therefore there is a requirement to help the agglutination to take place using antihuman IgG. The test, therefore, is a two-stage procedure. During stage one, the patient's serum at various dilutions is mixed with a suspension of the organisms for varying periods of time, the bacterial suspension is then washed and a dilute solution of a second antibody such as rabbit antihuman IgG is then added. An example of such a test, infrequently used nowadays, is that described for the diagnosis of brucella infection.

Complement fixation tests

Complement fixation tests have two stages. In the first stage, the patient's serum diluted through a range is mixed with the organism or its antigens. A source of complement which is usually an aliquot of fresh guinea-pig serum is added and the mixture incubated. Antigen–antibody complexes formed between the bacteria and the patient's sample activate the guinea-pig complement and therefore remove it from the mixture. At the end of the incubation period, all the mixtures are removed to the second stage of the test, the reagents for which are pre-prepared from red cells of a suitable species which have been sensitized with antibody against the red cell antigens. Typically, one uses sheep red cells which are sensitized with rabbit anti-sheep red cell antibody so that the red cells are coated with antibody in the absence of complement. If complement is present in the first stage mixture, the sensitized red cells will lyse. Lysis therefore indicates that the patient's sample in the first stage of the procedure did not have any antibody present, whereas non-lysis indicates that antibody was present and that the complement was used up in that first stage.

Details of complement fixation tests which have been frequently used for many purposes, including the diagnosis of rubella infection and brucella infection, can be found in most standard textbooks of microbiology. There are many problems with complement fixation tests. Notably, complement activation as a function of antibody–antigen complexing is highly variable and it is therefore necessary to carry out these tests across wide ranges of antigen and antibody (patient's serum) concentrations. Typically a chessboard titration is required to make these tests really accurate. Further, it is not uncommon to find substances in serum which are inhibitory to complement.

Precipitation tests

This infrequently used method is generally non-quantitative. It relies on the principle that antibody, particularly IgG, will precipitate soluble

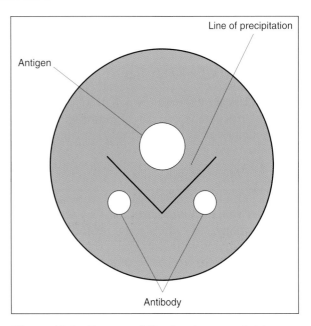

Figure 15.1: *Format of Ouchterlony precipitin test.*

antigen. The precipitation can be carried out in aqueous solution in test-tubes but it is more frequently performed by the Ouchterlony method. This uses a plate (Petri dish) containing 1–2% plain agar, with wells punched out which are filled to the brim with antigen (from the organism of interest) and antibody (patient's serum). The general format is shown in Fig. 15.1. Antigen and antibody diffuse towards each other through the agar and where they meet, a line of precipitation forms. Almost any antigen can be used provided it diffuses easily. Typically, this kind of test can be used with bacterial toxins such as those associated with tetanus and diphtheria. By using an antibody of known specificity, the identity of an unknown antigen can be determined. Although simple to perform, precipitation tests are difficult to quantitate and are very insensitive.

Newer tests

The principle of these tests is straightforward in that the patient's antibody in the serum binds to a substrate which is provided in the form of bacteria, or their products attached to a solid surface. After this, unwanted serum proteins are washed free from the substrate and a second antibody, usually raised in rabbits,

Tests for Antibody

Newer tests

---

sheep or goats, which is specific for human antibody and which is labelled with an appropriate marker is added in the second stage of the test. If the patient's antibody has attached to the substrate in the first stage, the second stage antibody will also attach. The marker, or label, varies but is usually something which is easily measurable. For example, in the fluorescent antibody technique, this label is fluorescein which can be visualized in ultraviolet light whereas in the ELISA, the label is an enzyme which can subsequently be made to act on a suitable substrate to produce a measurable colour change. It should be noted that the number of available labels is very large and includes radioactive labels, but the principle is the same for all of these tests.

Fluorescent antibody tests
A suspension of the organism is dried onto a microscope slide, fixed in acetone or ethanol and patient sera are added. Usually special Teflon coated slides are used which have ten 'spots' so that several specimens can be examined on a single slide. After incubation (usually 30 min) the slide is washed and anti-human immunoglobulin (IgG, IgM or IgA) is added which has been labelled with fluorescein. After further incubation and washing, coverslips are applied and the slide is examined under a UV microscope. If the specimen contains antibody to the test organism, that antibody will have attached to it, the labelled anti-immunoglobulin will have attached and the organisms will fluoresce bright green in the UV light. By using a series of dilutions of the patient's serum it is possible to quantitate the amount of antibody present.

There are several problems with these tests. For example, they are labour intensive and the reading of the end result is not always clear because of the subjectivity introduced by different observers. Further, the UV light causes the fluorescence to fade so observations must be fairly rapid. Generally, these tests work best for cell wall antigens as the antibodies will not usually penetrate into the organisms to detect internal antigens. The test is not easy to use for IgM antibody measurement. Despite these difficulties, fluorescent antibody tests have been very useful. As mentioned above, a good

example is the FTA used in the diagnosis of syphilis where the test is still regarded as the 'gold standard'.

Enzyme-linked immunosorbent assay (ELISA)
This extremely popular method, which is in principle similar to the fluorescent methods, uses inert substrates such as plastic to which are attached organisms or their antigens. Typically 96-well microtitre trays are used which can carry large numbers of samples as well as controls and which can be machine-washed, centrifuged if necessary and the results generated and analyzed by a reading machine. Many ELISAs are produced commercially. Samples are pipetted into the antigen-coated wells, incubated and washed, and anti-human immunoglobulin labelled with an enzyme is added. After further incubation and washing a substrate for the enzyme is added. There is a change in colour of the substrate if the enzyme is present and this can be machine read. The intensity of colour is proportional to the amount of antibody which is attached to the antigen. Therefore the method is fully quantitative. However, it is important to remember that this will only be true if there is an excess of antigen attached to the plate and an excess of anti-human immunoglobulin is provided in the later stages. These conditions are guaranteed in commercial kits but it is important with in-house ELISAs to attend to these details.

The anti-immunoglobulin used can be anti-IgM, anti-IgG, anti-IgA, etc. and therefore the test offers an easy route to determine the type of antibody present at different stages of infection. The most valuable aspect of this is the measurement of IgM as an early marker of acute infection.

ELISA methods are easy to use, cheap and have the benefit of semi-automation. They are therefore less labour intensive than many other serological methods. They have few problems, provided that the amount of reagent has been adjusted properly (see above). On a minor technical note, for in-house assays of this type, it is important to recognize that the outside rows of ELISA plates are frequently unreliable as adsorbents. This problem can be easily overcome by using only the inner rows.

Radioimmunometric methods

These were the forerunners of ELISA and the principle is exactly the same. Generally carried out in tubes rather than wells, the only significant difference is that the anti-immunoglobulin added is radio-labelled, usually with ^{131}I or ^{125}I. Because of the potential hazards from radioactivity, these tests are used infrequently nowadays although they do have greater sensitivity than ELISA and they may have a place in some research work where meticulous measurement is required.

Tests for Antigen

Tests for microbial antigen are becoming increasingly popular both in general microbiology and in virology. The main reason for this is that antigen will be present early in the course of infection and therefore its detection will provide useful clinical information. A good example is the detection of antigens from *Legionella pneumophila* in the urine of patients with legionnaires' disease. These tests are often positive when the patient is severely and acutely ill and at a time when other diagnostic procedures are not helpful.

There are, however, other good examples, one of which – the detection of antigens from *Neisseria meningitidis* in cases of septicaemia or meningitis due to this organisms – has been in use for many years. Originally, this method used a technique called counter-immunoelectrophoresis, which is a variant of precipitation methods discussed above. Essentially, serum from the patient is separated in an agar gel by passing an electrical potential through the gel, which causes human proteins and meningococcal antigen to migrate to different positions and to be separated. At the end of this stage a trough is cut longitudinally alongside separated proteins and antibody specific for the microbial antigen of interest is added to the trough. Diffusion of the antibody towards the separated proteins will detect the presence of the microbial antigen if it is there.

As with other precipitation methods, counter-immunoelectrophoresis is relatively insensitive, and most attempts to detect and measure microbial antigen now utilize ELISA systems. The modification required to the ELISA is to use antibody specific for the antigen of interest on the surface of the microtitre plate. This antibody, often a monoclonal antibody, is used to 'capture' antigen from the patient's specimen. In a second stage, antibody which is specific for the antigen and is enzyme labelled is added and the remainder of the test procedure carried out. It is generally accepted that the capture antibody and the detecting antibody should be different although the test will work with the same antibody on both sides of the 'sandwich'. Whether one uses monoclonal antibodies for both purposes or whether a polyclonal and a monoclonal are used is essentially a question of trial and error.

This kind of approach has been particularly useful for the diagnosis of viral infections such as HIV and the hepatitis viruses. For bacteria, there has been a tendency to try to simplify the methods using latex particles in an agglutination test, the particles being coated with antibody against the antigen of interest. Like all agglutination tests, these are relatively insensitive and have not proved to be as useful as initially thought possible.

On a technical note, where specimens such as urine or sputum are used for antigen detection testing, it is often necessary to remove 'inhibitors'. The nature of these inhibitors is not well established but, generally, heating the specimen to boiling point for two or three minutes is sufficient to remove them. This usually does not have any deleterious effect on the antigen. There will probably be improvements in ELISA methods for antigen detection in the coming years. Particularly, there should be a move away from the use of these tests to simply detect antigen towards full quantitation of antigen which the method is perfectly capable of achieving.

Antigen-specific Immune Complex Testing

Figure 15.2 shows a theoretical analysis of the events which happen in an infection. It indicates

175

Antigen-specific Immune Complex Testing

Methods using polyethylene glycol

Direct ELISA measurement

Tests utilizing binding agents for immune complexes

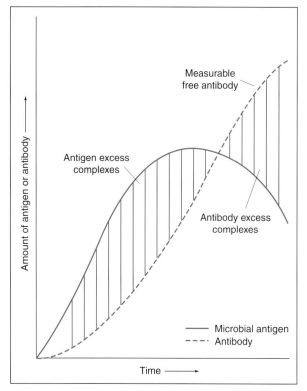

Figure 15.2: Diagram of the theoretical aspects of antigen and antibody interactions in an infection.

that the growth of a microorganism will produce increasing amounts of microbial antigen to which the infected host responds by producing antibody. Eventually, in a successful response the amount of antibody formed will suppress the growth of the organism. Several things are worth considering from this diagram. Firstly, at an early stage there is more antigen available for measurement than there is antibody. Secondly, free measurable antibody only appears late in the course of infection and, thirdly, throughout much of the infection, immune complexes are formed between antigen and antibody as represented by the hatched area on the diagram. As these immune complexes will contain antigens from the infecting organisms, their measurement provides a means towards diagnosis.

It has been known for many years that the majority of systemic microbial infections produce elevated levels of immune complexes in the patient's blood. This recognition has rarely been exploited diagnostically, probably

because the techniques for measurement of the complexes have in the past been difficult. In the last few years, methods for diagnosing HIV infection, pneumococcal pneumonia, infective endocarditis and Lyme disease using immune complex assay have all been described.

Some of the techniques used are discussed below:

Methods using polyethylene glycol
In these tests, complexes are precipitated from serum by the addition of polyethylene glycol. This works because the complexes have a different size from native immunoglobulin or antigen. The polyethylene glycol is allowed to work for several hours, usually overnight, and at the end of this time the serum sample is centrifuged vigorously and the precipitate removed for further analysis. The next stage of the test involves disrupting the complexes and detecting the antigen component. This can be done by heating (60°C for 30 minutes), by adding a low pH buffer (e.g. glycine/HCl), or adding a high molarity buffer such as 1 M phosphate. After disruption of the complexes, the antigen is assayed using one or other of the methods described above, e.g. ELISA.

Direct ELISA measurement
These tests usually use monoclonal antibodies specific for the antigens of interest, attached to the wells of microtitre plates and used as capture reagents. The patient's sample is added and complexes present are captured. In a second stage, enzyme-labelled anti-human immunoglobulin is added which will attach to any human antibody bound to the surface of the plate via an immune complex. This version relies on the high specificity of monoclonal antibodies to capture only the antigens of interest. It should also be noted that the diagnosis by this method is only *inferred*, not proven, in that it is argued that the patient's antibody cannot be present unless it is bound to the antigen which is captured on the ELISA plate.

Tests utilizing binding agents for immune complexes
There are many substances known to specifically bind immune complexes. For example, sepa-

rated and purified C1q (the first component of complement), rheumatoid factor (an antibody developed in some patients and directed against human IgG) and conglutinin (a bovine serum protein), all bind immune complexes. These substances can be attached to microtitre plates in the manner described for ELISA assays in general and thereafter these substances will capture any immune complexes present in the patient's sample, the nature of the complex then being determined by using an enzyme-labelled antibody against antigens of interest. Many of the reports on the use of this kind of assay are experimental at present but they offer speed and economy and are generally more sensitive than the other methods described above. They will probably become more frequently used in the future.

Chromatography Tests

As described above, the detection of antigen from microorganisms can be used as a marker of their presence in an infection. In the same way, the detection of metabolites from organisms has been used to signal the presence of the organism. The detection and identification of the metabolites is carried out by gas – liquid chromatography (GLC) or high – performance liquid chromatography (HPLC), although the former method accounts for the best-known diagnostic examples.

GLC is generally used to separate and identify volatile and non-volatile fatty acids by passing a sample through a suitable separating substance (e.g. Chromasorb) using a flow of carrier gas. Different fatty acids separate at different times. An early application was the identification of arabinitol in the serum of patients with systemic *Candida albicans* infection. It was thought initially that high levels of this metabolite were associated only with the infection but subsequent investigations proved that the measurement was an unreliable diagnostic marker. It is said that the presence of such organisms in pus and exudates can be determined directly although it is not common practice to use the method on routine specimens. More successful has been the use of the

method to identify and classify anaerobic bacteria, particularly Gram-negative organisms.

Breath Tests

These non-invasive tests have been used to detect *Helicobacter pylori*, now recognised as the cause of duodenal ulcers. *H. pylori* has a powerful urease enzyme which is able to hydrolyze ingested radioactivity-labelled urea to release labelled CO_2 which can be measured in exhaled breath. For the test two isotopes have been used: ^{13}C which is safer but more expensive than ^{14}C. The tests are semiquantitative and, as urea is distributed throughout the stomach, there is no sampling error. The sensitivity and specificity of these tests compare well with culture and histology. The tests may be used for diagnosis of *H. pylori* or monitoring response to management.

Future Developments

There are several challenges in the general area of serology. The first is to address the question of speed of results. A slow result (i.e. several days) is either of academic interest or useless in terms of diagnosing and treating a patient's infection. It will be clear that antigen or antigen-specific immune complex detection offers a faster route to diagnosis than antibody detection, and development of these assays is therefore desirable.

Further, both antigen and antigen-specific immune complex assays can be fully quantitative and, used properly with serial measurements, they should be able to assess the severity of any infection and the response to treatment. It is disappointing that these methods have usually been used qualitatively to date, and improvement in their performance will be more to do with a change in philosophy rather than a change of technology.

A real challenge for the future will be to apply some of the above methods to infections caused by commensal organisms. There are many instances, but the diagnosis and management of serious infection due to *E. coli* serves as a useful example. Conventional techniques are frequently unhelpful and PCR methods as used at present have little to offer because they will only identify the presence of the organism. The challenge is to know what the organism is doing.

The future is therefore one of increasingly sophisticated quantitation of antigen, whether free or complexed, and it is likely that immunosensors or their equivalents will participate in this development. Given that most serological methods depend on antigen–antibody interaction and that this takes place within minutes, it is surprising that most available tests take several hours and have to use separated serum. Methods which can quantitate microbial antigen inside five minutes, using whole blood or body secretions, are long overdue and their development offers a real challenge for the future.

Further Reading

General reference

Collee I G, Marmion B P, Fraser A G, Simmons A. Eds. *Mackie & McCartney's Practical Medical Microbiology* 1996; 14th ed. Churchill-Livingstone, Edinburgh and London.

Immune complexes

Henrard D R, Wu S, Phillips J, Wiesner D, Phair J. Detection of p24 antigen with and without immune complex dissociation for longitudinal monitoring of human immunodeficiency virus type 1 infection. *J Clin Microbiol*. 1995: 33(1): 72–75.

Odds, F C. *Candida and Candidosis*. 1988: 2nd edn, Ballière Tindall, London, p. 250.

16 CONTROL OF ANTIMICROBIAL CHEMOTHERAPY

Ian M Gould

Introduction

The modern age of chemotherapy can be said to have started over 100 years ago with the pioneering work of Robert Koch and others who described the germ theory of disease and allowed concepts to develop about magic bullets that would kill microbes while not harming the host. The first agents, heavy metal derivatives of mercury, antimony and arsenic, proved too toxic for general use but found a limited role in the treatment of syphilis. While great advances have been made in most areas of antimicrobial chemotherapy, derivatives of these early agents are still used for certain parasitic diseases such as leishmaniasis and sleeping sickness.

In the 1930s German industrialists and scientists worked together to create the first modern antimicrobials – the sulphonamides, which were derived from dyes. These were quickly followed by the discovery of naturally occurring antimicrobials (antibiotics) such as penicillin (in fact discovered in 1928 by Alexander Fleming but first used in a major way to treat infection during the Second World War). At first, penicillin was in such short supply that doctors would collect urine from treated patients to extract the 'miracle drug' to reuse in other patients.

Thus the era of chemotherapy, as we understand it, had begun and during the 1940s, 50s and 60s great leaps were made in discovering new antibiotics, learning to synthesize them and indeed designing and constructing totally new agents such as the quinolones.

The first principles of chemotherapy

As early as the 1940s it was realized that different antibiotics interacted with bacteria in different ways that might affect the optimum dosing regimen, and in the 1950s it became apparent that resistance to almost any antibiotic developed after prolonged use. The first clinical applications of these two founding principles of the science of chemotherapy were in the treatment of tuberculosis, a disease with an annual incidence and death rate both measured in millions.

The first principle of the control of therapy learned in those early days was the application of knowledge on the dose response (the pharmacodynamics) of the antimicrobial–microbe interaction which led to intermittent (twice weekly) treatment with rifampicin and isoniazid. This was feasible due to the prolonged suppressive effect of these antimicrobials on growth of the tubercle bacillus long after the drugs had been excreted from the body, and allowed more user-friendly treatment regimens leading to improved compliance. This prolonged suppression of growth is called the post-antibiotic effect.

Antibiotic resistance

General Principles of Laboratory Control of Chemotherapy

When the first antituberculous drug, streptomycin, was released it was found that the initial response led to relapse after a few weeks due to the surviving bacteria becoming resistant. In fact, it is now understood that simultaneous therapy with three active drugs (triple therapy) is essential for cure of tuberculosis without the risk of development of resistant strains. This is the second principle which is relevant to treatment of many infections with antimicrobials, and illustrates the need for primary testing of sensitivity of isolates as a guide to successful therapy. Routine use of clinical diagnostic laboratories for such sensitivity tests started at this time (late 1950s and early 1960s) and is now in extensive, worldwide use.

The issue of compliance with therapy is another important principle of the control of chemotherapy learned in those early days of treating tuberculosis and is particularly important for such diseases where cure depends on prolonged therapy (6–18 months). Unfortunately many of the sufferers of tuberculosis came from socially deprived backgrounds which made compliance with therapy difficult. It was soon learned that treatment was frequently unsuccessful in this situation, often due to the development of resistant organisms. Consequently, directly observed therapy became popular. Alternatively, urine from patients can be checked for the excreted drugs. These basic lessons had to be relearned recently in New York where cutbacks in social and medical services led to cessation of directly observed therapy and produced a large outbreak of multi-resistant tuberculosis with a high fatality rate.

Antibiotic resistance
Unfortunately, the very success of antimicrobial chemotherapy is leading to its downfall. Antimicrobials are seen by both doctors and patients as a panacea or cure-all such that antimicrobials are frequently used indiscriminately. This over-use is linked inextricably with resistance. Although technically available only on prescription in many countries, the majority of the world's population can purchase antibiotics legally or illegally. They are a multi-

billion dollar industry worldwide and there is a large black market in them. The socially deprived people of the Third World who need antibiotics more frequently because of their very high infection rates cannot afford the proper medical advice, laboratory tests or the full treatment courses necessary to eradicate infections. Hence antibiotic resistance is a particular problem in poorer countries, particularly in deprived inner city areas. Even in the rich countries of Western Europe and North America doctors frequently misuse antimicrobials and the last ten years has seen very worrying trends in resistance (see Table 16.1). For no obvious reason trends in antimicrobial prescribing are on the increase both in hospitals and in community medical practice and the increased consumption of antibiotics is being paralleled closely by increases in resistance (see Fig. 16.1 and Fig. 16.2).

General Principles of Laboratory Control of Chemotherapy

There are currently over 100 antibiotics licensed for clinical use in the UK and many more worldwide. The main role of the routine hospital-based diagnostic laboratory is to isolate the causative pathogen responsible for

Table 16.1: 1997 resistance levels (%).		
	UK	Southern Europe
Penicillin/pneumococci	5	50
Penicillin/meningococci	0	40
MRSA	5	75
Glycopeptide/enterococci	1	5
Ciprofloxacin/E. coli	2	15
Gentamicin/Pseudomonas	3	40
Ceftazidime/Klebsiella	1	20
Amoxycillin/Haemophilus	20	30
Amoxycillin/Moraxella	80	80
Ciprofloxacin/Campylobacter	1	40

General Principles of Laboratory Control of Chemotherapy

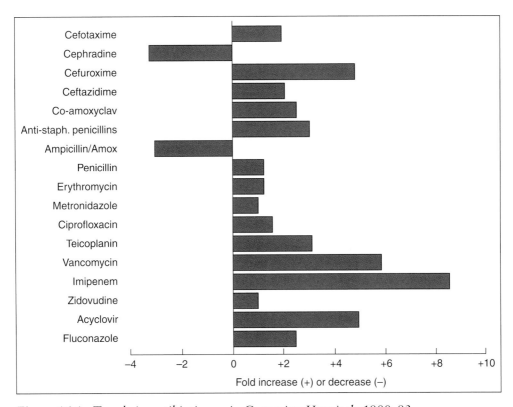

Figure 16.1: Trends in antibiotic use in Grampian Hospitals 1988–93.

disease in a specific patient from whom specimens are being processed and to test the isolate(s) for sensitivity to relevant antibiotics. Normally testing will only be performed on a limited, predetermined, battery of antibiotics which are clinically relevant for that patient's infection and which are thought to be active against the isolated pathogen.

The decision-making process about which antimicrobials will be tested is complex and should take into account factors such as site and seriousness of infection, method of excretion or metabolism of the antimicrobial, function of the patient's liver and kidneys, toxicity, available routes of administration, cost, need for combination therapy, proven clinical benefit, current treatment both with antimicrobials and non-antimicrobials, and drug interactions. Although there are over 100 licensed antimicrobials in the UK these are made up from only some dozen different drug classes and it is often appropriate to test just one representative agent from each class.

Often patients will have been started on treatment empirically, before culture and sensitivity results are available, but hopefully only after appropriate specimens have been sent to the laboratory for processing. Nevertheless it is still important to process specimens as quickly as possible in case treatment needs to be modified in the light of culture and sensitivity results, e.g. to a more potent or less toxic agent. Similarly, it is important to have good transport of specimens and good communication to enable advice to be obtained easily and results to be disseminated quickly. It is also useful for the laboratory to publish summaries of sensitivities of various organisms which will help doctors in choosing appropriate empirical therapy, and to take part in sentinel surveillance schemes to give early warning of the emergence of unusual or new resistant variants. This enables doctors and public health officials to use the information for appropriate treatment and also to contain the spread of new resistant variants which, in the modern world

General Principles of Laboratory Control of Chemotherapy

Sensitivity Testing

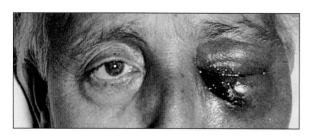

Figure 16.2: An example of a highly immunosuppressed patient, suffering Pseudomonas *skin and eye infection with bloodstream spread after receiving cancer therapy which reduced his body's defences against infection. This type of infection commonly killed patients in the past. Now treatment with modern antibiotics is often successful. However, such patients are increasingly common as modern medicine becomes more successful and more aggressive. Consequently more and more antibiotics are used, both in hospital and in general practice.*

of high speed travel can, and do, spread rapidly from country to country and continent to continent.

There are other ways in which the laboratory can usefully direct or control antimicrobial therapy. The most important is the measurement of blood and (occasionally) tissue levels of the drugs to ensure adequate therapeutic levels are being achieved in critically ill patients and to ensure that toxicity is minimized or prevented. This is not required in the majority of patients, only in those where it is thought necessary to use antimicrobials with a narrow therapeutic ratio, that is, agents where doses needed to be effective approach those that may be toxic to the patient. The use of such particularly toxic drugs should be reserved for those serious infections where the choice of active agents is limited, often through problems of resistance.

In critically ill patients it is sometimes useful to assess potential benefits of combination therapy in the laboratory to try to predict the most active regimens. These tests can be useful particularly in patients who are immunosuppressed or have infections such as endocarditis or meningitis when it is necessary to achieve killing of the microbe by the antibiotics in

order to cure the patient without the help of the host's immune system.

Sensitivity Testing

The concept of sensitivity testing has remained remarkably constant since it was first introduced on a wide scale almost 40 years ago. Of necessity, tests are simple to perform as the average clinical laboratory serving a population of 250 000 will perform such tests on tens of thousands of organisms per annum. Despite the simplicity of the tests they have proved remarkably useful over the years in guiding therapy. This is all the more surprising when one considers the complexity of individual cases where the microbe interacts with the host immune system in a set of conditions apparently remote from the test situation in the laboratory.

There are four methods of sensitivity testing in common use: disc diffusion (see Fig. 16.3), agar incorporation, broth macrodilution, and broth microdilution. The first is the one in most common use in the UK – in about 85% of laboratories it is the routine method. In this method, carefully controlled amounts of antibiotics are contained in paper discs which are placed on an agar plate surface previously inoculated with a carefully controlled number of the bacteria to be tested. Normally up to six antibiotics are tested per plate. The plates are incubated under strictly controlled conditions for 6–48 hrs depending on the rate of growth of the bacteria. The zones of inhibition of growth due to the diffused antimicrobial are measured and related to those of known sensitive and resistant control bacteria. Results are usually reported as simply 'sensitive' or 'resistant' based on knowledge about the specific pharmacokinetics of each antimicrobial including achievable concentrations of the drug at the site of infection. If this type of test is regulated very carefully then the actual concentration that is inhibitory to the bacterium (in the test conditions) can be calculated.

Alternatively, in agar dilution, pre-set concentrations of an antimicrobial are included in agar plates before they are poured and then, when

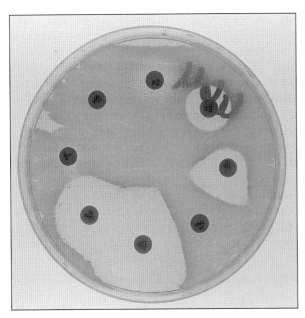

Figure 16.3: An example of disc sensitivity tests. This is the most common method of sensitivity testing used in the UK. The zone of inhibition of growth of the lawn of bacteria is determined by the concentration of antibiotic in each of the paper discs and the sensitivity of the bacterium. In this example the bacterium is completely resistant to four antibiotics. There are small zones of inhibition around two discs (the bacteria is still resistant) and large zones of inhibition around another two discs (sensitive). This example of a multiply-resistant organism is increasingly common. The odd, non-circular zone of inhibition of two discs is because the adjacent disc between them contains an antibiotic which is interacting with them, causing antagonism of action (cut off) and synergy (bell shape) respectively.

they have set solid the bacteria are 'spotted' on the surface. Up to 30 microbes can be tested to a single agent per plate. The lowest concentration of antimicrobial which inhibits visible growth of the bacteria after incubation is the minimum inhibitory concentration (MIC).

Broth dilution tests of antimicrobial sensitivity are carried out either in test-tubes (macrodilution) or in microtitre plates (microdilution). A carefully controlled inoculum of the test microbe is incubated with known concentrations of the antimicrobial. The chosen microbe, unlike in agar tests, can be a virus (if a cell line

is included) or certain fungi or protozoan parasites such as malaria parasites in addition to bacteria. The MIC is the lowest concentration inhibiting growth (as assessed by turbidity to the naked eye). Normally it is adequate just to assess levels of the antimicrobial which will inhibit growth, the host's immune system allowing cure by killing most of the microbes after they have been brought under control by the antimicrobial.

Unlike with agar tests, the minimum bactericidal concentrations (MBC) can be assessed by subculturing the inhibitory concentrations to look for any survivors. The lowest concentration with 99.9% kill of the original inoculum is the MBC. For complicated infections it can be important to establish such values for individual organisms and to make sure that such levels of activity are achieved in the patient.

Measurement of antimicrobial activity in the patient is most easily achieved by measuring the inhibitory or cidal activity of the antimicrobial in the patient's serum, usually taking samples before administration of a dose (the trough level) and approximately one hour after administration of a dose (the peak level). Distribution of the antimicrobial in the tissues is usually complete by then. Depending upon the pharmacodynamics of the antimicrobial and the disease state it may be important to achieve high inhibitory or cidal levels in the peak sample, e.g. for aminoglycosides such as gentamicin. In contrast the β-lactams are drugs where it is usually important to have activity during the whole dosing period due to their lack of post-antibiotic effect against many bacteria.

Tests on microbes other than bacteria
The sensitivity testing of microbes other than bacteria is, by comparison, in its infancy. Very little work had been done until recently, probably because of the relative absence of effective antimicrobials for many of these microbes. This meant that there was no alternative choice of therapy in the presence of resistance. There has, undoubtedly, also been a lack of perception of the problems of resistance. Now, however, there is an explosion of new agents, particularly antifungal and antiviral antimicrobials, in

Sensitivity Testing

Automation

response to increasing needs generated by new diseases such as acquired immunodeficiency syndrome (AIDS) caused by the human immunodeficiency virus (HIV). This disease not only requires antiviral therapy specific for the HIV virus but also therapy for many other viral, fungal, bacterial and protozoal infections to which the patients become more susceptible.

HIV patients are frequently given suppressive antimicrobial therapy over many months or years as, due to their severe immunosuppression, it is frequently impossible to eradicate the infecting microbes. This is a recipe for emergence of resistance analogous to the situation with tuberculosis, and lessons on the use of combination therapy to improve therapeutic efficacy and prevent emergence of resistance are having to be relearned for the proper treatment of HIV/AIDS patients.

Resistance is a particular problem in the treatment of the primary viral infection of AIDS where, by the time disease is clinically apparent, there is a huge viral load with the potential for many innately resistant mutants to exist that can survive the therapy and multiply. Now that many new anti-HIV agents are being made available, detection of these strains will be important in the future so that the best combination therapy can be individualized to each patient.

Recent developments have allowed the ascertainment of MICs both of bacteria and fungi on agar plates by the use of E tests® which contain gradients of antimicrobials on plastic strips, and, the inhibitory value can be read off after incubation in much the same way that zones of inhibition are measured in the classical agar disc diffusion test (see Fig. 16.4).

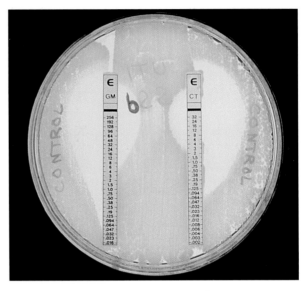

Figure 16.4: An example of E test® sensitivity. Graduated concentrations of an antibiotic are contained in each of the plastic strips. A control organism of known activity is plated on the outside of each strip and a test organism on the inside. In this case the test organism is very resistant. The minimum level of resistance (MIC) can be read off the strip.

routine procedure, but automated reading of inhibition zones in agar disc diffusion tests holds some promise.

Newer methods of sensitivity testing are much more susceptible to automation and indeed often require it. These include nephilometry, bioluminescence, impedance or conductance monitoring and flow cytometry. While these 'direct' methods can give rapid results (within one to two hours) on inhibitory and also perhaps cidal activity of antimicrobials, they are, at the moment, research techniques only.

Many serum levels of antimicrobials are routinely measured by automated methods such as EMIT® and TDX® which utilize enzymatic reactions and fluorescence, while new or experimental antimicrobial levels can be assayed by high-performance liquid chromatography (HPLC) or by traditional plate assay where the patient's serum or tissue specimen takes the place of the antibiotic-containing disc in the agar disc diffusion test and the lawn of organism is a sensitive control strain. The concentra-

Automation

As automation has become more widespread in laboratories, attempts have been made to adapt existing sensitivity testing methods. Broth microdilution tests are probably the most amenable for modification and pre-prepared plates are now available which can be read automatically by spectrophometry. Broth dilution has not proved popular in the UK as a

tion of drug in the serum (volume known) or tissue (weight known) and the size of the zone of inhibition can be used to calculate the concentration of drug.

Hospital Control and Clinical Liaison

The knowledge base acquired from working in the laboratory can be utilized to co-ordinate the work of various groups of people concerned with infection who work in the community and hospitals. These people include the infection control team of nurses and doctors and the public health physicians concerned with control of infection in the community. By giving early warning, outbreaks can be controlled more effectively. Hospital-acquired infection is very common (probably about 10% of patients admitted to hospital) so any advice on its prevention and update on the latest epidemic organisms can prevent a lot of infection and limit the inappropriateuse of antibiotics.

A knowledge of local sensitivity patterns is useful for all doctors to help them in the empirical treatment of infection although rapid communication of results is also important to guide antimicrobial therapy from a rational base. Most hospitals and some general practitioners have written antibiotic policies and the sensitivity data available from the local laboratory form a useful basis for designing these policies, allowing local recommendations for empirical treatment to be most appropriate. This is proven to save unnecessary exposure to antibiotics, some of them costly and toxic, and to improve patient outcome.

The laboratory should also be a platform for education of doctors and the public on improved use of antimicrobials. Very little on the subject is taught to undergraduates and yet it is a complex field with an ever-expanding number of drugs which it is increasingly difficult for the average doctor to use properly. A policy of limited sensitivity reporting, either reducing the number of agents reported to those seeming most appropriate (perhaps two or three) or not reporting any sensitivities to

isolates that are not clinically important, may be a further way of reducing antibiotic exposure. However, these strategies have not been properly assessed and rely heavily on appropriate information being given to the laboratory by the doctor submitting the specimens.

Anything that limits the improper use of these valuable and irreplaceable drugs should be encouraged. There are some suggestions that patients are now appreciating that resistance is a problem and are less demanding of antimicrobial therapy on consultation with their general practitioners. There certainly seems to be a public appetite for information on current problems and those that lie ahead.

Conclusion

Pasteur or Fleming would have no trouble orientating themselves in a routine hospital diagnostic laboratory in the 1990s. There has not been the great advances in test procedures that one might have imagined from knowledge of current work in genetics. This work, specifically in microbial genetics, has increased our knowledge base and understanding of resistant mechanisms tremendously and no doubt will have an impact on the way we test for resistance in the routine diagnostic laboratory in the next 10 or 20 years. Even now, larger laboratories can test directly by DNA probe for a small selection of resistant genes such as the *mecA* gene that turns *Staphylococcus aureus* into a superbug, resistant to all β-lactam antimicrobials. Similarly we routinely test for the presence of β-lactamase enzymes in some bacteria rather than assessing the phenotypic expression of these enzymes (which can be difficult by traditional sensitivity test methods). Certainly direct, genotypic tests are going to be much more widely used in the future as they tell us the potential resistance profile of an organism rather than simply what it is resistant to at the time of testing under the rather artificial experimental conditions of the laboratory.

This is an optimistic and, I believe, realistic view of the future role of the laboratory. However, one cannot help but be pessimistic about the potential of bacteria to become resistant to all antimicrobials unless we learn to use them much more carefully. The discovery of transposons, operons, regulons, synergons, etc. teaches us that microbes are supremely adaptable and usually at least one step ahead of humankind in the microbial–antimicrobial battle that we wage.

Further Reading

Garrett L. *The Coming Plague*. 1995: Penguin Books, Middlesex, UK.

Harold P Lambert & Francis W O'Grady. *Antibiotic and Chemotherapy*. London 1992: 6th edn, Churchill-Livingstone, London.

Kucers A. & N McK. Bennett. *The Use of Antibiotics*. 1987: 4th edn, Heinemann Medical Books, London.

Levy S B. *The Antibiotic Paradox*. 1992: Plenum Press, New York.

Lorian V. *Antibiotics in Laboratory Medicine*. 1986: 2nd edn, Williams & Wilkins, London.

SECTION 3
MICROBIOLOGY: VIROLOGY, MYCOLOGY AND PARASITOLOGY

17 MICROSCOPY IN VIROLOGY: APPLICATION AND SAMPLE PREPARATION

Marie M Ogilvie

Introduction

Light microscopy has played a significant role in virology from its earliest use in examination of stained cell preparations or sections of tissue. Today on the virology bench of many microbiology laboratories no microscope is to be found, since diagnostic work at a district general level is based on use of immunoassay kits for detection of virus antigen or antibody. Increasingly even in the specialist virus diagnostic laboratory microscopy is used less frequently as more sensitive methods of virus detection based on nucleic acid amplification by the polymerase chain reaction (PCR) are introduced alongside existing culture and antigen detection methods. However, in the remaining years of this millennium many microscopes are in daily use for diagnostic virology work, as cell cultures are examined for cytopathic effects due to virus growth and cells stained with fluorochrome-labelled reagents are screened for virus antigens.

Histopathology: Inclusion Bodies and Multinucleate Giant Cells

The histopathologist who examines fixed stained cell smears or tissue sections observes the characteristic morphological changes which are associated with the presence of specific virus infections. The best known of these distinctive features are *inclusion bodies* – accumulated virus particles (as in the classical Negri body of rabies) or excess proteins synthesized during virus replication, and *multinucleate giant cells*. The latter form as a consequence of fusion between the plasma membranes of adjacent cells, and are a feature of infection with enveloped viruses which possess a glycoprotein inducing pH-independent fusion at the cell surface: respiratory syncytial virus (RSV), and human immuno-

Histopathology: Inclusion Bodies and Multinucleate Giant Cells

Virology

Sample collection and transport

Sample processing and inoculation of cell cultures

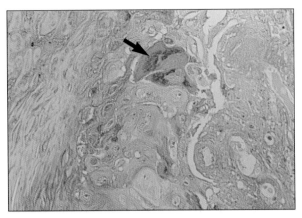

Figure 17.1: *Section of an herpetic skin lesion, stained with haematoxylin and eosin. A multinucleate giant cell is indicated by the arrow. [Courtesy of Dr K McLaren, Department of Pathology, University of Edinburgh.]*

deficiency virus (HIV), for example. Virologists use the term *syncytium* (from the Greek *syn* = together) for such a cell. Herpes simplex virus (HSV) and varicella-zoster virus (VZV) produce multinucleate cells *in vivo* and *in vitro* (in life and in glass, i.e. culture). Tzanck's name is still given to cell smears prepared by his method of scraping from the base of an ulcer or vesicle, stained and examined for the giant cells of herpes (HSV or VZV) (Fig. 17.1).

The well-known 'owl's eye' inclusion body seen in cells infected with cytomegalovirus (CMV) is an intranuclear inclusion surrounded by a clear halo, within a considerably enlarged (*megalic*) cell, but there is usually only one nucleus. CMV can produce multinucleate giant cells *in vivo*; these are of endothelial origin and their presence in the circulation signifies serious systemic disease. Evidence of the intracellular location of CMV is important in confirming the pathological significance of finding this virus, which simple virus isolation cannot always provide.

Virology

Success in the isolation of virus (by culture) or detection of viral antigens in cells from clinical material is very dependent on obtaining the correct sample, handling it appropriately, and using the range of cell cultures and immunofluorescent probes most suitable for detection of the virus(es) likely to be responsible for the patient's condition. Resources are not available for undirected screening for every possible virus, although inoculation of a range of cell cultures will allow any that can be cultured routinely to grow. Modern standard texts should be consulted for fuller details of the aspects discussed below and a new one gives a good introduction for the research worker.

Sample collection and transport

Many infections are relatively short with respect to the period of active viral replication once symptoms have developed, so that samples containing infectious virus and antigen-expressing cells are best collected within the first two to three days of illness. Material should contain cells from the affected site: epithelial cells from the back of the nose and throat, or from the base of an ulcer. Respiratory secretions may be collected from infants by suction up a fine catheter, or washed out in older subjects, but cells collected onto a swab should be placed in a virus transport medium. Any buffered isotonic fluid containing stabilizing protein can be used, to preserve infectivity and prevent cells drying out. Samples should *not* be frozen before processing, but transported to the virus laboratory as soon as possible, being kept chilled on ice or in a refrigerator if there is any delay. When the period between collection of a sample and its inoculation into cell culture is kept to a minimum the isolation rate is increased and virus is detected sooner. If it is not possible to inoculate appropriate cells within the same day, a sample may be held at 4°C overnight. Longer storage to maintain viability has to be at very low temperatures, usually in an ultrafreezer running at −70°C. (The commoner laboratory freezers running at −18 to −20°C are *not* suitable for virus preservation; considerable drop in infectivity occurs at that temperature.)

Sample processing and inoculation of cell cultures

Request forms accompanying samples should indicate clearly the nature of the current illness, the date of onset, the nature of the sample and the site from which it has been collected, and the age of the patient, in order that appropriate investigations may be undertaken. Sample processing for inoculation of cell cultures and/or preparation of cells for immunofluorescent staining is generally a standardized procedure according to the nature of the specimen. Cultures have to be examined for any *cytopathic effects* (CPE: the morphological change in cells resulting from virus replication) on a daily basis for the first five days after inoculation so as not to miss any signs, though later 'reading' of the tubes on alternate days is usually sufficient to catch the more gradual changes of slower-growing viruses like CMV and many adenoviruses.

Requirement for rapid diagnosis of virus infections

Few viruses can be identified in routine cell culture in less than three days – herpes simplex virus is the only regular one. For clinical management, control of infection within hospital wards, and specific antiviral therapy where available, the earliest confirmation of a clinical diagnosis or identification of an unsuspected infection is important. To this end, appropriate samples are examined directly for evidence of specific viruses, by immunofluorescence (IF) microscopy for respiratory, skin and other infections where infected cells are readily obtainable. Respiratory secretions must first be diluted and washed in a buffered saline to prepare respiratory epithelial cells (free of mucus) which can be deposited on slides. Several spots or wells are generally used, but a cytocentrifuge preparation is useful and quick if one is to test for a predominant virus first, as in an influenza epidemic or RSV season. Once air-dried, the slides are fixed by immersion in cold acetone for ten minutes. This ensures cells remain on the slide, retain antigenicity and are permeable to antibody, but in most instances have no residual infectivity.

Immunofluorescence

Virus diagnostic laboratories in the 1980s and 1990s have expanded their use of microscopy, particularly as an aid to rapid diagnosis of viral infections. The commercial availability of high-quality reagents in the form of monoclonal antibodies supports the application of immunofluorescence (IF) for a wide range of viral antigens. Specific antibody (or a pool of antibodies) conjugated to a fluorochrome dye may be applied to a cell preparation in a *direct immunofluorescence test* (DIF) for the target antigen. This is the most widely-used method for rapid diagnosis by light microscopy, particularly suitable for single samples as they arrive, but also applied to the daily influx of respiratory secretions from infants and children which constitutes a major part of the work of a virus laboratory serving a children's unit during the annual epidemics of respiratory disease.

The same reagents may also be useful for staining cells from cell cultures, either for *culture confirmation*, and *typing* in the case of HSV, or for screening for *early (pre-CPE) detection of antigens*, particularly useful for slower growing viruses such as CMV and adenoviruses. Examples of the range and applications are given below. Some *serological tests for viral antibodies* are still based on *indirect immunofluorescence*, commonly for antibodies to Epstein–Barr virus, human parvovirus (B19), or the newer human herpesvirus 6 (HHV6).

In virology the most commonly used fluorochrome dye is fluorescein isothiocyanate (FITC), which gives a bright apple-green fluorescence. It is helpful if a counterstain has been included so that contrasting negative background cells are visible (stained dull red if Evans blue dye is used). The appropriate antibody is applied to the well or slide bearing cells to be examined; a smear or deposit of cells direct from a patient, cells from a culture, or a shell vial coverslip. An incubation period (averaging 15 to 30 minutes) in a humid chamber permits antibody to react with any virus-specific antigen in the cells. Unbound excess antibody is removed by washing in buffered saline, before the slide is air-dried and mounted for viewing on a special microscope with a source of incident UV light. Mounting fluid consists of analytical-grade glycerol (50%) in phosphate-buffered saline at a pH optimum of 8.6 to maximize fluorescence. Fluorescence

THE SCIENCE OF LABORATORY DIAGNOSIS

Immunofluorescence

Respiratory viruses

Skin or mucocutaneous cell preparations

Cells from culture

Virus antigens produced early in growth cycle

fades rapidly on exposure to UV irradiation, so prolonged viewing is not advisable and photographic records should be obtained promptly when required.

Respiratory viruses

Direct immunofluorescence is now the commonest IF procedure in diagnostic virology for rapid detection of antigens, and may be the only test used to diagnose RSV infection in children, having become so reliable in experienced hands that parallel virus isolation is no longer considered necessary as a routine. Most infants become infected with RSV in their first winter season, and one in every hundred babies is admitted to hospital having developed the alarming condition of bronchiolitis. Since in the annual winter epidemic season RSV is by far the commonest respiratory pathogen in infants and children, a rapid test for RSV is a top priority. The characteristic appearance (intracellular globules staining apple-green) of a positive DIF test for RSV in respiratory cells in secretions from such an infant is shown in Fig. 17.2. There is specific antiviral treatment for RSV infection in those at special risk of serious disease, and the DIF test (or an equivalent enzyme-labelled one) is often required as an urgent or on-call procedure.

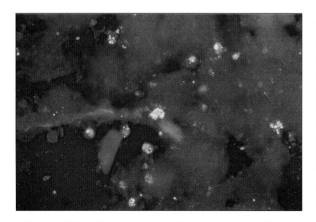

Figure 17.2: *Direct immunofluorescence stain of respiratory epithelial cells from an infant with acute bronchiolitis. Bright apple-green staining of cells labelled with fluorescent antibody to RSV indicate infection with that virus. (Uninfected cells counterstained with Evans blue dye appear dull red in contrast.)*

Skin or mucocutaneous cell preparations

Cells scraped from the base of vesicular skin lesions are frequently examined by DIF with antibodies specific to HSV-1 or HSV-2 or VZV (if it is not obvious clinically which infection is present). Since specific antiviral therapy is available, and herpes infections are serious in immunocompromised hosts, rapid diagnosis is important. To be effective, antiviral drugs have to be given as soon as possible, and the dosage varies according to which virus is to be treated. The contagious nature of VZV is also a problem for control of infection; approximately 10% of young adults have not had chickenpox and are at risk if exposed to VZV.

Cells from culture

This is very similar to DIF on patient cells. The benefits of rapid confirmation of a presumed CPE are clinical and save laboratory time and resources. As HSV-1 and HSV-2 have different associations and vary in their tendency to cause recurrent disease at different sites, it is useful to know the virus type, and this can be done with type-specific antibodies. Monoclonal antibody to common group-specific antigens present in adenoviruses (hexon antigen) or enteroviruses (VP1 antigen), can be used to confirm the CPE produced by members of these groups respectively.

Virus antigens produced early in growth cycle

When CMV was recognized as a serious pathogen in transplant recipients who would require antiviral therapy, it became essential to detect this virus much more rapidly than in the past. Gleaves (US) and Griffiths (UK) established the value of looking for the CMV early antigens that appear after a few hours, compared to the days it takes for viral DNA and later antigens and a CPE to appear. The term 'shell vial' came from the US, while in the UK the test was referred to as the DEAFF test (Detection of Early Antigen Fluorescent Foci). Early antigens of VZV are also sought occasionally. Wider use of the shell vial system has become popular in the US and in mainland Europe, where many laboratories use it for respiratory virus detection particularly. Our own experience has shown it to be very useful in that regard, for early detection of adenovirus eye

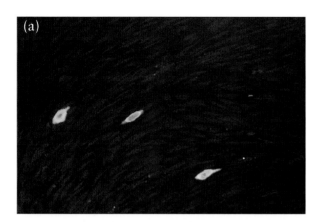

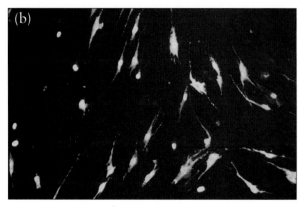

Figure 17.3: *DIF staining of infected HEF shell vial cultures 48 hours post-inoculation with (a) a conjunctival swab: stained with adenovirus group-specific monoclonal antibody;*
(b) a throat swab: stained with influenza A group-specific antibody, showing nuclear staining and no spread of infection outside original cells infected.

infections, and also for rapid and improved rate of isolation of varicella-zoster virus. Examples of shell vial IF are illustrated (Fig. 17.3).

Microscopic Examination of Cell Cultures

Although certain gross changes in cell culture are visible to the naked eye, as in the unfortunate case of turbidity or acidity due to growth of bacteria or fungi, microscopic examination is necessary before changes produced by virus growth can be detected. Serial observations are made over days and even weeks, and virus may have to be passed to fresh cultures for subsequent tests, so cultures are examined unstained. A rest holds the culture tube on the microscope stage while the whole area of the cell monolayer is carefully scanned at low power (using ×4 or ×10 objectives) with the substage condenser lowered. Focal areas of altered cells are then inspected at higher magnification. It is not difficult to notice the difference between a complete healthy cell monolayer (uninoculated control tube from same batch of cells) and one in which holes have appeared as infected cells round up and fall off, or groups of cells form large clusters, but it takes a good deal of experience and careful, regular observation to develop real expertise in recognizing the cytopathic effect produced by specific viruses in different cell cultures.

Cytopathic effects in routine cell cultures
Degenerative CPE: scattered areas with round, shrunken cells, which soon fall off the surface of the tube: – seen with enteroviruses such as poliovirus, and rhinoviruses.

Round, refractile, swollen cells in clusters: seen with adenovirus ('bunches of grapes' in HEp$_2$ cells) and herpes simplex. HSV grows very fast, starting in a few patches ('plaques') the day after inoculation and spreading throughout the monolayer by next day. Small syncytia are seen, especially with HSV-2.

Cytomegalovirus CPE: quite unique, progressing very slowly and exhibiting elongated foci of swollen (cytomegalic) cells in human fibroblast cultures.

Classical syncytial CPE: the hallmark of RSV growing in fresh HEp$_2$ cells (Fig. 17.4), but multinucleate giant cells are also seen with measles and VZV in sensitive cell lines. The features are different to the trained eye in each case.

(HIV is not cultured routinely, but its growth may be recognized by the appearance of syncytia in the mononuclear blood cell cultures, which grow in suspension, not as monolayers. The human herpesvirus type 6 (HHV6) was

193

Microscopic Examination of Cell Cultures

Non-cytopathic growth of viruses in cell culture

Further investigations of cytopathic agents

Into the Next Millennium

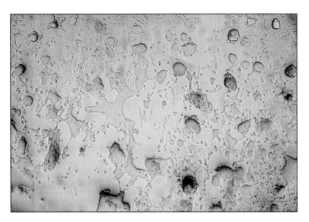

Figure 17.4: *Classical syncytial cytopathic effect of RSV growing in HEp₂ cell culture (unstained), five days post-inoculation of patient's respiratory sample.*

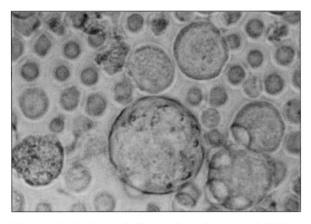

Figure 17.5: *Large balloon-shaped syncytial CPE (unstained) produced by human herpesvirus type 6 (HHV6) in suspension culture of lymphoblastoid (JJban) cell line.*

discovered in 1986 when it produced syncytial CPE in cultures of peripheral blood (Fig. 17.5) and on further examination turned out not to be HIV but a previously unknown herpesvirus.)

Non-cytopathic growth of viruses in cell culture

The virology microscopist is aware that there are some viruses which replicate in cell culture without producing obvious cytopathology. The best-known example is of influenza viruses growing in monkey kidney cells, where the presence of the virus may be revealed by

haemadsorption. A glycoprotein (haemagglutinin) coded for by the virus and inserted into the cell plasma membrane is able to attach to red blood cells added to the surface. In the earliest stages of any virus replication, when only single cells are infected, a CPE is not obvious, but viral antigens will be present.

Further investigations of cytopathic agents

The microscopist is not finished when a recognizable CPE is observed in an inoculated culture. Confirmation of the informed diagnosis is expected, and further identification may be indicated. The judgement of the microscopist, who will select the confirmation test based on the CPE, cell line, sample, and other factors, is critical in reaching a speedy diagnosis and saving resources. Confirmation and typing of HSV has already been mentioned. Adenovirus or enterovirus CPE can now be confirmed by IF of cells, but typing will require a *neutralization assay* because there are so many different types. This entails mixing aliquots of a well-grown isolate with separate pools of antisera covering common types, inoculating fresh cultures and observing which antiserum inhibits CPE i.e. has neutralized the infectivity of the virus. These typing exercises seldom affect clinical management, but are important for epidemiological studies.

Into the Next Millennium

The diagnostic virologist wishes to have the best of all approaches to identification of virus infections. Rapid detection is critical for the reasons outlined previously, and while IF microscopy may continue to be of use for individual samples, antigen-capture enzyme-immunoassays or immunofiltration, less subjective methods which can be automated could be used for screening larger sample numbers and culture-amplified fluids. Molecular amplification of nucleic acid by the polymerase chain reaction (PCR) can provide the most sensitive means of detection of an ever-increasing range of viruses. Parallel attempts at virus isolation will still be required in a laboratory offering a comprehensive service including epidemiological typing and antiviral susceptibility testing. Enhanced culture is used now, and there is a continuing search for sensitive cells particularly for currently non-cultivable viruses. The emerging area of genetic engineering of cells may provide novel approaches, such as enzyme-linked virus-inducible systems (ELVIS), already tested for HSV, which combine three strands – old and new – cell culture, antigen detection and recombinant DNA technology, including microscopy.

Acknowledgements

Thanks are expressed to the following in relation to figures used in this chapter:

Figure 17.1: photography by Dr K McLaren, Consultant Histopathologist, University of Edinburgh.

Figures 17.2–5: photography by AJ MacAulay FIMLS; CMLSO in Clinical Virology Laboratory, Department of Medical Microbiology, University of Edinburgh.

All figures: copies submitted were prepared by D Dirom, Department of Medical Illustration, Medical School, University of Edinburgh.

Further Reading

Lennette E H, Lennette D A, Lennette E T (eds). *Diagnostic Procedures for Viral, Rickettsial and Chlamydial Infections*. 1995: 7th edn; American Public Health Association, Washington DC.

Mahy B W J, Kangro H O (eds). *Virology Methods Manual*. 1996: Academic Press Ltd, London.

Olivo P D. Transgenic lines for detection of animal viruses. *Clinical Microbiology Reviews* 1996; 9; 321–334.

Simmons A, Marmion B P Rapid diagnosis of viral infections. In: *Mackie & McCartney Practical Medical Microbiology*, 1996; 14th edn: Collee J G, Fraser A G, Marmion B P, Simmons A (eds). Churchill-Livingstone, Edinburgh.

Zuckerman A J, Banatvala J E, Pattison J R (eds). *Principles and Practice of Clinical Virology*. 1994: 3rd edn; John Wiley & Sons, Chichester.

18 ELECTRON MICROSCOPY IN VIROLOGY

Hazel Appleton

Viruses are regarded as malign agents which cause disease and suffering. When visualized in the electron microscope, however, a variety of elegant structures is revealed. Viruses from different virus groups look different, and it is this characteristic morphology that is the basis for their identification by electron microscopy. Electron microscopy provides the means for very rapidly detecting and identifying viruses in material taken directly from patients (Table 18.1). This rapid diagnosis can facilitate the management and treatment of patients. It also has public health implications in the management of outbreaks and controlling the spread of infectious diseases in the community. In the long term it has a role to play in epidemiological surveillance of infectious disease. Unlike many diagnostic tests which select for one particular agent, electron microscopy is a catch-all method that can be used to detect any virus or mixture of viruses present in the sample. Use of electron microscopy has led to the discovery and identification of many new viral agents in recent years, and has been particularly useful in the diagnosis and study of viruses that cannot be readily cultured *in vitro*.

Methods

Negative staining
This is the most widely used method for diagnostic virology and entails staining the background of the virus rather than the virus itself. Specimen preparation is simple and results can be obtained rapidly. The technique, however, does rely both on there being sufficient numbers of virus particles present in the specimen (a minimum of 10^6 virus particles per ml specimen is usually required for detection), and on the structural integrity of the virus particles remaining intact so they can be recognized and identified. Enhanced sensitivity can sometimes be achieved by use of immune sera (immune electron microscopy). Viruses that do not stand out clearly against the background material,

e.g. parvoviruses and hepatitis B surface antigen, may be aggregated into clumps by mixing the sample with a specific antiserum and hence may be seen more easily. Alternatively, viruses may be attracted onto a grid by coating the grid with antiserum (solid

Methods

Thin sectioning

Scanning electron microscopy

Table 18.1: Viruses detected by electron microscopy

Specimens examined	Examples of viruses detected
Skin – vesicle fluids or scrapings of lesions[*]	Poxvirus – orf, molluscum contagiosum Herpesviruses – H. simplex, varicella-zoster Papillomavirus (human wart)
Faeces[*]	Gastroenteritis viruses – rotavirus, adenovirus, astrovirus, SRSV, calicivirus (Hepatitis A & E, enterovirus)
Serum	Hepatitis B Parvovirus B19
Urine	Polyomavirus BK (Cytomegalovirus)
Liver	Hepatitis B
Foetal liver	Parvovirus B19 (hydrops fetalis)
Brain	Measles virus (SSPE) Polyomavirus JC (PML) Herpesvirus
Tumour	Epstein–Barr virus
Laboratory cell cultures for rapid confirmation of identity of isolates[*]	Any virus that grows e.g. influenza, parainfluenza, measles, adenovirus, polyomavirus, enterovirus, herpesvirus, retrovirus (Exotic viruses e.g. Marburg, Ebola)

[*] Current main uses of electron microscopy in diagnostic virology

phase immune electron microscopy – SPIEM). Immune electron microscopy methods can be used for antigenic typing of viruses. When a virus is detected by simple negative staining it is identified as a member of a virus group or family, but it is not usually possible to differentiate between members of the group without further tests. For instance the herpes virus causing chickenpox (Herpes varicella-zoster) is identical in appearance to the herpes virus causing cold sores (Herpes simplex).

Thin sectioning

Thin sectioning electron microscopy is useful for examination of specimens where there is an insufficient number of virus particles present to be seen in negatively stained suspensions. Some viruses, such as retroviruses, have structures which are more easily identified in thin sections than in negatively stained preparations. Although enhanced sensitivity can be achieved, it is not a rapid technique and has limited application in a diagnostic laboratory. It is useful in studying the pathogenesis of infection, and can be used for confirmation of diagnosis in biopsy specimens and post-mortem specimens. Virus structures are resistant to cell lysis and poor tissue preservation, and positive results can be obtained from apparently unpromising material.

Scanning electron microscopy

Few diagnostic laboratories have access to a scanning electron microscope or even a scanning attachment to a transmission electron microscope. The scanning electron microscope is mainly used as a research tool for investigating virus attachment and pathogenesis, and so far has had little use in diagnostic virology. There has been some interest in solid phase immuno-assays using latex beads coated with specific antibody. Virus attaches to the beads and is coated with gold. The technique appears to offer little advantage over negative staining immune electron microscopy, and has the disadvantage that characteristic virus morphology is obscured and the reagents are expensive.

Uses of Electron Microscopy

Electron microscopy first came to prominence in diagnostic virology in the 1960s for the rapid diagnosis of smallpox. The skin lesions produced in smallpox and those caused by chickenpox can be clinically confusing. The alarming implications of smallpox infection made rapid differentiation of these infections essential. Skin lesions and particularly fluids from vesicles are normally rich in virus particles. By just mixing the sample with a drop of negative stain, the virus can readily be seen without the need for concentration. Smallpox is caused by a member of the Poxvirus family, and chickenpox by the herpesvirus varicella-zoster. Poxviruses and herpesviruses have very different morphologies and can readily be distinguished in the electron microscope (Fig. 18.1 and Fig. 18.2). The smallpox virus, variola, and the vaccinia virus used in the vaccine are indistinguishable, and further more complex tests were required to differentiate between these two, usually by culture on the chorioallantoic membrane of fertile hens' eggs which took three days. However the diagnosis of a herpesvirus infection avoided the need for all the public health measures that would have had to be activated if there was a possibility of a case of smallpox.

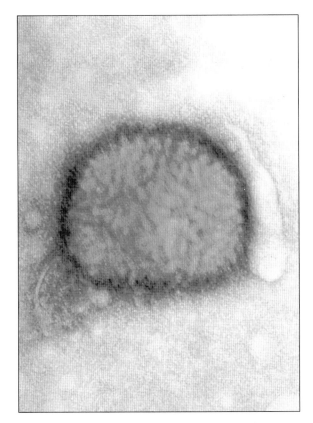

Figure 18.1: Vaccinia virus – a member of the Poxvirus family. ×180 000. [Micrograph courtesy of Mr A A Porter.].

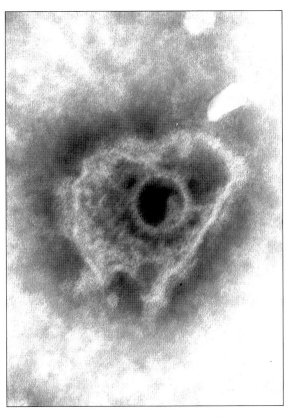

Figure 18.2: Herpesvirus from a skin lesion. ×180 000.

Skin Lesions

Electron microscopy has continued to have an important role in the rapid diagnosis of herpesvirus infection. It is particularly useful for immunocompromised patients, where the use of appropriate antiviral drugs can facilitate treatment. Furthermore, it can aid the management of patients on transplant units, where an outbreak of chickenpox could have very serious and sometimes fatal consequences. Although smallpox has been eliminated from the world, electron microscopy is still used in the diagnosis of two other poxvirus infections, orf and molluscum contagiosum, neither of which can be readily identified by other means. Orf is a zoonotic poxvirus infection acquired from sheep and molluscum contagiosum a human poxvirus that causes benign eruptions on the skin. These two particular poxviruses

have characteristic patterns on the surface of the particles, which allow specific identification of each by an experienced microscopist. Electron microscopy is also occasionally used for the detection of the human papillomavirus which causes warts.

Gastroenteritis

The discovery of viruses that cause gastroenteritis led to a massive expansion in the use of electron microscopy in diagnostic and public health laboratories in the 1970s and 1980s. Several different viruses can cause gastroenteritis and all were discovered by electron microscopic examination of faecal samples from patients. It was surprising that viruses could be visualized in such complex material, but in fact these viruses are excreted in vast numbers into

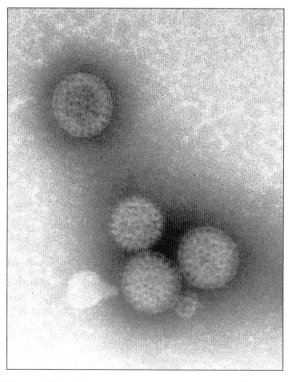

Figure 18.3: Rotavirus — a major cause of gastroenteritis in babies and young children. The typical 'spokes' can be seen around the particles. The centre particle has lost its outer capsid layer. ×180 000.

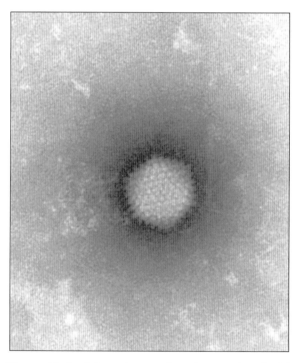

Figure 18.4: Adenovirus — largely associated with infections of the respiratory tract and the eyes. Two new adenoviruses are associated with gastroenteritis mainly infecting young children. ×180 000.

the intestinal contents and can readily be detected, if samples are collected at the appropriate time.

Gastroenteritis viruses do not grow in conventional cell cultures, and electron microscopy has remained the main method for their detection and identification. Some gastroenteritis viruses, such as rotavirus and adenovirus, have such distinctive morphologies that only one or two particles need to be seen for positive identification (Figs 18.3 and 18.4). Samples can be so rich in virus that no concentration is necessary. (Concentrations of 10^{12} particles/gram have been estimated.) It is often sufficient simply to emulsify a small sample of faeces in a drop of distilled water, mix with negative stain and place on a grid. For other gastroenteritis viruses, such as astrovirus and the Norwalk-like viruses, identification is more difficult, and more particles may have to be examined to make an accurate identification (Figs 18.5 and

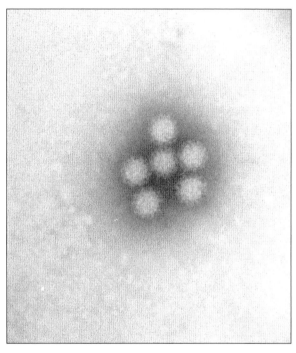

Figure 18.6: Small round structured viruses (SRSV) or 'Norwalk-like' viruses. These cause many outbreaks of viral gastroenteritis in the community. ×180 000.

18.6). It is usually necessary to concentrate the virus from the specimen in these cases.

Electron microscopy reports of the viruses detected in cases of gastroenteritis in England and Wales are collected by the Public Health Laboratory Service's Communicable Disease Surveillance Centre. This has enabled an epidemiological picture to be drawn up of the age groups affected by the different viral agents, the seasonal distribution, the pattern of excretion and modes of transmission. This information makes it possible to give appropriate advice on such factors as management of outbreaks, how long food handlers should be excluded from work and the optimum time for collection of specimens.

Rotavirus

The most well-known and readily identified of the gastroenteritis viruses is the rotavirus (named from the Latin word *rota* meaning wheel: the arrangement of capsomeres seen on the surface of the virus particles looks like the

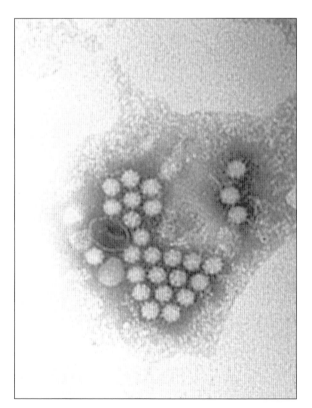

Figure 18.5: Astrovirus. The solid 5- or 6-pointed star can be seen on the surface of a few particles. ×180 000.

Gastroenteritis

Adenovirus

Astrovirus

SRSV

---

spokes of a wheel) (Fig. 18.3). Rotavirus is a major cause of gastroenteritis in babies and young children worldwide. In the UK and other developed countries, it is responsible for the largest number of admissions to hospital in this age group, and in underdeveloped countries it is estimated to cause about a million deaths a year. Infection mainly occurs over the winter months in temperate climates. Outbreaks are also seen among the elderly, presumably due to waning immunity.

Rotavirus was first found in thin sections of duodenal biopsies of children in Australia, but such invasive techniques are not necessary, as the virus can readily be seen in simple emulsions of faecal specimens. Commercial kits have been developed for detection of rotavirus using either an ELISA test or a latex agglutination test, and are now widely used in diagnostic laboratories. These kits, however, only detect the commonest type of rotavirus known as group A rotavirus. Other types of rotaviruses, particularly group C, also infect humans, although they are seen less frequently. Group C rotavirus infects all age groups and has been associated with a number of family and school outbreaks. In many laboratories, specimens are only examined by electron microscopy if the results of an ELISA or latex test are negative. Non group A rotaviruses have usually been detected when there is a discrepancy of a negative kit result and positive electron microscopy finding.

Adenovirus

The examination of faecal specimens from children with gastroenteritis led to the discovery of two new adenoviruses. Adenoviruses had long been associated with respiratory and eye infections, and are routinely isolated in cell cultures. The two new adenoviruses, designated types 40 and 41, are associated specifically with gastroenteritis and cannot readily be cultured. Electron microscopy has limitations and can only indicate the presence of adenoviruses (see Fig. 18.4) and not specifically types 40 and 41, for which further tests are required. Common respiratory adenoviruses are isolated from faecal specimens, but this is regarded as an incidental finding. Fluorescent tests for the aden-

ovirus group are now available as commercial kits, but electron microscopy remains the most usual method for detection of faecal adenoviruses. Like rotavirus, adenovirus types 40 and 41 mainly infect young children and occur during the winter months.

Astrovirus

Another virus associated with gastroenteritis is astrovirus, a novel virus, so named from the solid five-or six-pointed star seen on the surface of a proportion of particles (Fig. 18.5). Astroviruses account for around 1–2% of reports of gastroenteritis viruses in the UK. Infection mainly occurs in the very young, and outbreaks in newborn baby units have been described. Like rotavirus, outbreaks occasionally occur in the elderly. On very rare occasions foodborne transmission has been implicated. Detection is always by electron microscopy. Eight antigenic types have been identified. Typing is by immune electron microscopy.

SRSV

Small round structured viruses (SRSV) cause gastroenteritis in all age groups. They are also known as Norwalk-like viruses (Fig. 18.6). The first virus discovered in this group originated from an outbreak in the town of Norwalk in the United States and became known as the Norwalk agent. The term SRSV is used in the UK and relates to the appearance of the virus in the electron microscope. Virus particles measure 30–35 nm in diameter, have an amorphous surface and ragged outline. SRSV is responsible for many outbreaks in schools, hospitals and residential homes, and is possibly the most frequent cause of viral gastroenteritis in the community. Gastroenteritis viruses are usually transmitted directly from person to person via the faecal – oral route or in aerosol droplets. Occasionally some may also be transmitted via food or water and in these situations it is the SRSVs that are most frequently implicated. Since 1994 the number of general outbreaks of SRSV in England and Wales reported to the Communicable Disease Surveillance Centre has exceeded the numbers of reported outbreaks of salmonella infection. Unlike salmonella outbreaks, however, most SRSV outbreaks were due to person-to-person spread and very few were foodborne.

SRSV cannot be cultured and most diagnosis is by electron microscopy. However SRSV is only excreted in numbers sufficient for detection for about 48 hours after onset of symptoms and hence it is often difficult to obtain appropriate specimens. SRSVs tend not to be excreted in such great numbers as rotavirus and adenoviruses, and as they do not have such distinctive morphological features they are technically far more difficult to detect and identify. Furthermore, they infect older children and adults who are less likely to seek medical advice and be investigated. SRSV is believed to be grossly under-reported. Electron microscopy is not sensitive enough to be able to detect virus in food samples. In foodborne viral outbreaks the usual method of investigation is to detect virus in faecal samples from the patients and use epidemiological methods to link infection to a food source.

Molecular tests such as the polymerase chain reaction (PCR) are being developed. PCR assays for SRSV are only available in a few specialized laboratories at present, and they do not detect all strains of SRSV. Until commercial kits are available it is likely that most diagnosis will continue to be done by electron microscopy. More rapid results can be obtained by electron microscopy than PCR, but PCR is useful for epidemiological investigation by identification of strain variation. It is clear that there are several different antigenic types of SRSV, but antigenic diversity in this group of viruses is poorly understood. Comparisons of SRSV strains by immune electron microscopy have been made, and have resulted in a number of conflicting typing schemes. It is difficult to correlate these antigenic typing schemes with genotyping schemes.

Calicivirus

Viruses with the morphological characteristics of calicivirus have been associated with gastroenteritis outbreaks in nurseries and sporadic illness in all age groups. The viruses are identified by cup-like depressions seen on the surface of the virus particles, and are named from the Latin word *calix* meaning cup. On the

basis of their genomic arrangement, SRSVs have been classified as members of the Caliciviridae family. Although similar in appearance, the classic cup-like depressions are not seen on particles identified as SRSV. It is not clear, on morphological or biochemical grounds, whether these two groups should be identified separately. The differentiation of SRSV, calicivirus and also astrovirus by electron microscopy can be difficult and needs an experienced microscopist.

Hepatitis

Electron microscopy has had a major role in the discovery of the various viral agents of hepatitis. The virus causing hepatitis A was discovered in 1972 by immune electron microscopy of faecal specimens from patients involved in volunteer studies. It is identical in appearance to members of the Picorna virus family which includes the classical culturable enteroviruses (polio-, echo- and coxsackieviruses). Electron microscopy is not used diagnostically for hepatitis A, as it was quickly shown that most virus excretion occurs in the prodromal phase of illness. It was electron microscopy that revealed that the other enterically transmitted virus, hepatitis E, is a calicivirus, but this is antigenically distinct from the caliciviruses associated with gastroenteritis. Hepatitis E is not commonly seen in the UK, but it has been associated with large waterborne outbreaks in developing areas of the world. Infection is particularly severe in pregnant women. As with hepatitis A, electron microscopy has not been used routinely for diagnosis.

It is in the diagnosis of hepatitis B infection that electron microscopy has been most useful. Viral particles and viral antigens, particularly the hepatitis B surface antigen, are present in serum for prolonged periods. Diagnosis can readily be made if complete virus particles are detected, but often only 22 nm spheres of virus coat protein (surface antigen) can be seen. Surface antigen is difficult to distinguish from other background material in serum. To enhance sensitivity and ease identification the patient's serum is usually mixed with a specific antiserum in an immune electron microscopy test. Immune electron microscopy is not suitable for testing large numbers of specimens, and must be used selectively. Many other tests for hepatitis B are available commercially, and electron microscopy is rarely used now in diagnostic situations.

Brain

When antiviral drugs first became available for the treatment of herpes encephalitis, attempts were made to detect herpesvirus in negatively stained suspensions of brain material. Rapid and accurate diagnosis was important because early antiviral drugs were extremely toxic. Electron microscopy did not prove particularly sensitive, however, and was soon replaced by fluorescence microscopy and more recently by PCR techniques. Paramyxovirus helix of measles virus has been detected in thin sections of brain tissue from patients with subacute sclerosing panencephalitis. The first human polyomavirus, JC, was discovered in thin sections of brain tissue from patients with progressive multifocal leukoencephalopathy. Although electron microscopy was useful for establishing the aetiology of both these conditions, fluorescence technique and PCR assays are more sensitive for examining brain material.

Urine

Attempts to find viruses in urine samples have had mixed success. Electron microscopy was responsible for the discovery of a second human polyomavirus, known as BK virus. This virus commonly infects transplant patients and is excreted in urine. It is very slow-growing in cell cultures and electron microscopy has been extremely useful for diagnosis. PCR assays have been developed and are now the usual method employed diagnostically. Cytomegalovirus, a member of the herpesvirus group, is also excreted in urine, but has only rarely been detected by electron microscopy when very large numbers of virus particles

are present. The symptoms of both cytomegalovirus and BK virus infections can mimic organ rejection. Diagnosis of a viral cause results in better patient management, since inappropriate use of immunosuppressive drugs would actually prolong virus infection.

Virology Laboratory

Apart from its primary diagnostic role, electron microscopy has many other functions in a virology laboratory. The electron microscopist provides support in the development of new, alternative diagnostic tests. Electron microscopy is used for the rapid identification of viruses isolated in cell cultures, and can greatly reduce the time spent in trying to identify a cytopathic agent, especially when more than one type of virus is present. It is used when equivocal or even negative results are obtained from other tests. For instance, PCR assays for SRSV do not detect all strains and electron microscopy may provide positive results on PCR-negative samples. Conflicting results between tests for parvovirus B19 infection (e.g. a positive dot blot but a negative IgM result), may be rapidly resolved by electron microscopy. Laboratory confirmation of B19 infection may significantly affect the management of patients, particularly if immunocompromised or pregnant. Electron microscopy is also used to check viral antigens, such as measles virus and rubella virus, prepared for other tests. It is used for detecting naturally occurring viral contaminants of cell cultures, such as SV40 (Fig. 18.7).

Conclusions

The emphasis for electron microscopy in virology appears to be shifting more to research aspects, where it always has had an essential role. Electron microscopy is often used as a primary diagnostic method in the early stages after a virus is first discovered, but it does have some disadvantages. The initial cost of the equipment means that electron microscopy is not available in all laboratories. Furthermore, a satisfactory service requires highly skilled and

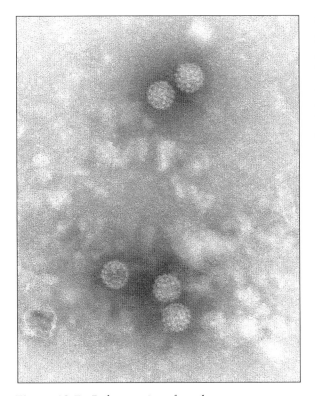

Figure 18.7: Polyomavirus found as a contaminant in a cell culture. ×180 000.

tion of infants with diarrhoea. It is the most rapid method for the diagnosis of vesicular lesions caused by viruses, and is of special relevance in the management of immunocompromised patients. Electron microscopy also has an important role in the rapid identification of viruses isolated from clinical specimens in cell culture.

Many new viruses have been discovered by the use of electron microscopy, particularly since the early 1970s. Electron microscopy still has a major contribution to make in the discovery and characterization of new viruses, alongside the recent advances in molecular virology. For instance, 40% of gastroenteritis infections still remain undiagnosed. There are hepatitis viruses and retroviruses that still require characterization by electron microscopy. Electron microscopy is being used to look for viruses in tumours. It will continue to be used for gaining an understanding of the pathogenesis of viral infections and the role of viral antigens, which could lead to the development of effective treatments and vaccines. Such studies are being aided by the development of improved and more rapid automated preparation techniques for thin sectioning and scanning. Recent advances in electron microscope design, such as environmental scanning microscopes that do not require lengthy, complex drying procedures, mean that not only can specimens be processed more rapidly and easily, but shrinkage and distortion of specimens is avoided. As microscopes continuously become more user-friendly, viral investigation by electron microscopy becomes easier.

experienced staff. Electron microscopy is labour intensive and is not suitable for examining large numbers of specimens. Consequently, if suitable alternative tests become available, electron microscopy tends to take on a more confirmatory role.

At present, electron microscopy is used widely for the detection of viruses in faecal specimens from patients with gastroenteritis, and is the front line method for the investiga-

Further Reading

Appleton H, Field A M. The electron microscope and public health virology. *Microscopy and Analysis*, 1990; **20**: 7–9.

Caul E O, Appleton H. The electron microscopical and physical characteristics of small round human fecal viruses: An interim scheme for classification. *J Med Vir*, 1982; **9**: 257–265.

Doane F W, Anderson N. *Electron Microscopy in Diagnostic Virology: A Practical Guide and Atlas*. 1987: Cambridge University Press.

Madeley C R, Field A M. *Virus Morphology*, 1988: 2nd edn, Churchill-Livingstone, Edinburgh.

Mortimer P P (ed). *Public Health Virology: 12 reports*. 1986: Public Health Laboratory Service, London.

19   VIRUS ISOLATION

William L Irving

Introduction

Virus particles consist of genetic material (nucleic acid) plus a small number of proteins – hence the derivation of Sir Peter Medawar's memorable quote that 'viruses are trouble wrapped in a protein coat'. Some viruses, in addition, possess a lipid envelope. There are no internal organelles, such as mitochondria, ribosomes, or Golgi apparatus. Viruses are therefore *obligate intracellular parasites*, that is, they can replicate only within living cells, usurping the host cell's energy-generating and biosynthetic machinery to do so. The isolation of viruses from clinical material thus presents a number of challenges quite distinct from those encountered in a bacteriology laboratory, where bacteria can be grown on inanimate media. The presence of living cells in one form or another is the first essential prerequisite for the successful growth of viruses. For many years, viruses were grown in fertile hens' eggs. An alternative is to use whole experimental animals. Whilst both of these techniques may still be of value in specialized circumstances, they have been largely replaced in routine laboratories by the use of cell cultures derived from a variety of tissues, grown in monolayers on glass or plastic surfaces (e.g. tubes or bottles). In this chapter, the practicalities of running a tissue culture laboratory for the isolation of viruses will be discussed, and the advantages and disadvantages of this approach to the diagnosis of virus infection highlighted.

Choice of Cell Cultures

The first step in the replication cycle of any virus is that of attachment to its target cell. This is a very specific process, involving precise interaction between a ligand on the surface of the virus and a receptor on the surface of the target cell. Thus, not all viruses will infect and grow in all cell types – cells which lack the appropriate receptor for a particular virus will be resistant to infection by that virus. This creates a problem for the diagnostic laboratory. To provide a comprehensive service for the isolation of all possible viruses would require the availability of a multitude of different cell types. In practice, most laboratories will run only two or three different cell types, each of which will support the growth of as broad a range of viruses as possible. The most commonly used cell cultures are listed in Table 19.1, which also indicates which viruses may grow in each. Although this list includes many of the common viruses encountered in clinical practice, some important viruses (e.g. human immunodeficiency virus – HIV, the hepatitis viruses, the viral causes of gastroenteritis including rotaviruses and enteric adenoviruses,

Epstein–Barr virus – EBV) clearly are missing, as are several others. The isolation of some of these viruses can be achieved by use of particular specialized cell culture techniques. HIV and EBV can be grown in human peripheral blood lymphocytes, and some of the hepatitis viruses will grow in primary hepatocyte cultures or hepatoma-derived cell lines. However the difficulties involved in the provision of a regular supply of these more specialized cultures means that isolation of these viruses is usually restricted to reference or research laboratories. Yet other viruses (e.g. the human papillomaviruses, hepatitis C virus) are so exacting in their requirements for growth that isolation in cell culture has proved to be virtually impossible. Diagnosis of infection with these viruses must of necessity rely on approaches other than cell culture.

Preparation of Cell Cultures

The efficient functioning of a diagnostic virology laboratory requires the availability of (i) stock cells grown up on a large scale, and (ii) mature cells in small numbers ready and waiting in a receptacle (usually a tube, but tissue culture plates are an alternative) ready for inoculation with appropriate clinical material, as and when that material arrives in the laboratory. As these tubes are used up, they are replaced by fresh tubes prepared from the stock cultures.

All of the standard cell types listed in Table 19.1 grow as adherent cells rather than as cell suspensions. This means that they will attach themselves to a flat surface (usually plastic tissue culture flasks) and then multiply and divide, provided that the culture medium contains the necessary nutrients, until the whole surface is covered. At this point, most cells will stop dividing due to contact inhibition. This process is known as *growing to confluence*. Once a cell sheet is confluent, the cells can be stripped off the surface, diluted in culture medium, and poured back into a number (e.g. three or four) of new flasks, where they will then once again grow to confluence. This process is known as *passaging* of cells, and in this way, the number of cells available can be expanded rapidly. Alternatively, the cells from a confluent flask may be distributed in small numbers into a rack of tissue culture tubes which, once the cells have settled down and reached confluence, will then await inoculation with clinical material.

Cells differ in their ability to be passaged repeatedly. *Primary cultures*, ie those established directly from tissue (e.g. monkey kidney cells) do not survive more than two or three passages *in vitro*. This is a major drawback to their use, as a continual supply of fresh

Table 19.1: Commonly used cell cultures.	
Type of culture	*Viruses capable of growth*
Primary/secondary cultures	
Monkey kidney cells	Influenza viruses, parainfluenza viruses, enteroviruses, mumps virus
Semi-continuous cell lines	
Human embryonic fibroblasts	Herpes simplex virus (HSV), varicella-zoster virus, cytomegalovirus, enteroviruses, adenoviruses, rhinoviruses
Continuous cell lines	
Vero cells (derived from monkey kidney)	HSV, mumps virus
HEp-2 cells	Respiratory syncytial virus, adenoviruses
HeLa cells	Adenoviruses

primary cultures is expensive and inconvenient. By comparison, tumour cell lines (eg HEp-2 cells, HeLa cells) are able to divide indefinitely when passaged *in vitro*, and are therefore referred to as *continuous cell lines*. In between these two extremes, diploid cells derived from human embryonic tissue (e.g. human embryonic fibroblasts) can be grown successfully for 30 or 40 passages before finally petering out, and are therefore known as *semi-continuous cell lines*.

Cells are cultured in tissue culture flasks under sterile conditions. Preparation is often done in laminar flow cabinets, but can be performed on an open bench with a bunsen burner and appropriate aseptic technique. The medium added to the flasks must be isotonic and of suitable pH, and is usually based on physiologically balanced salt solutions. The exact composition of the medium may vary according to cell type: detailed recipes are available in practical guidebooks. It is useful to add an indicator dye to enable recognition of cell metabolism by colour change (healthy and growing cells produce an acid medium). For growth, essential amino acids and protein are necessary, and these are usually provided in the form of serum derived from fetal calves. Antibiotics are often added to the growth medium as an added precaution against bacterial or fungal contamination, the main sources of which are waterborne bacteria, yeast from the carbon dioxide source, and mycoplasma species from contaminated reagents or from the operator. The latter will severely reduce the ability of the cells to support virus growth.

Once confluence is reached, cells can be stripped using physical means with a sterile rubber scraper (known as a 'rubber policeman'), or, more usually, by treatment with trypsin and EDTA, which disrupt the binding of cells to the plastic surface, and cause the cells to round up and detach. The cells can be counted in a haemocytometer at this stage, and the appropriate volume for resuspension calculated. However, with experience, a rough guess of the necessary volume will suffice.

If the cells are not to be passaged further, e.g. those in tubes ready for inoculation, then once they have reached confluence, the growth medium is replaced by maintenance medium, the difference being that in the latter the concentration of serum is reduced dramatically. Confluent cells in tissue culture tubes in maintenance medium will survive for several days, but eventually they will slowly decay despite medium changes, at which point they must be discarded.

Cells being propagated for virus investigations may, when surplus to requirements, be preserved as seed pools frozen in liquid nitrogen. With renewed need or in the event of bacterial contamination of cells in use, frozen cells may be rapidly thawed and fresh cultures prepared.

Clinical Specimens for Virus Isolation

There are no restrictions on the nature of clinical material that can be inoculated into cell culture for virus isolation. Fluid samples (e.g. cerebrospinal fluid – CSF, saliva, urine, vesicle fluid, nasopharyngeal aspirate, bronchoalveolar lavage fluid, blood, diarrhoeal faeces) can be sent to the laboratory in a sterile container, and added to appropriate tissue culture tubes either neat or after dilution in maintenance medium. Swabs (e.g. conjunctival, throat, base of ulcer, cervical, rectal) must be broken off into viral transport medium (isotonic fluid plus antibiotics to inhibit bacterial overgrowth), as viruses will not survive on dry swabs. After vortexing the bottle to release as much cellular material as possible from the swab into the medium, the transport medium is inoculated onto the cell sheets. Tissue biopsies (e.g. brain, bowel) should also be placed in viral transport medium. The tissue can be finely minced and both cellular and supernatant material inoculated into culture.

Identification of Virus Growth

Once a clinical specimen has been inoculated into cell culture tubes, the tubes are incubated

Identification of Virus Growth

Cytopathic effects

Passaging of viruses

---

under conditions which most resemble those from where the material was obtained. Most cultures are held at 37°C, but some viruses, most notably those from the upper respiratory tract, will grow better at a slightly lower temperature, e.g. 33°C, and in the presence of 5% carbon dioxide. Cultures may be slowly rotated on a roller drum, which improves the aeration of the cell sheet, or held stationary. The challenge for the microbiologist is now to determine whether or not a given cell culture contains cells in which a virus is replicating. There are a number of options available to achieve this goal.

Cytopathic effects

When viruses replicate within cells, the cells may undergo morphological changes e.g. swelling due to alteration of membrane permeabilities, shrinkage due to cell death, or giant multinucleate cell formation due to the presence of a fusion protein encoded by the virus. These changes in cellular morphology, visible under the light microscope, are referred to as a 'cytopathic effect' (CPE), and viruses which induce these changes are said to be cytopathogenic. Thus, the presence of a virus within a cell culture may be determined by regular examination (e.g. every other day) of the culture under the low power lens of a light microscope for the development of a CPE.

The exact appearance of a CPE is variable, according to which virus is responsible, and in which cell type it is occurring. The cells may balloon in size, shrivel up, or fuse into syncytia. The effect may be widespread throughout the whole cell sheet, or may be much more focal in nature. It may be seen predominantly, if not exclusively, at the edge of the sheet rather than in the middle. The speed of development of the CPE may vary from as short as 18 hours to as long as four weeks. Taking all of these factors into account, plus the clinical details relevant to a particular specimen, a trained virologist will be able to make a definitive diagnosis of which virus is present in the culture through light microscopy observation of the CPE alone. Thus, a CPE originating from a vesicle swab consisting of ballooning cells appearing after 24 hours of culture and thereafter spreading

rapidly to destroy the whole cell sheet is highly likely to be due to herpes simplex virus. In contrast, a vesicle swab causing a CPE to appear only after 10 days in culture, in only two or three foci of swollen cells in the centre of the sheet which spread slowly over the next several days is likely to be due to varicella-zoster virus. Illustrations of CPEs characteristic to specific viruses are shown in Fig. 19.1.

Passaging of viruses

Virus replication within a cell sheet is not the only cause of a visible CPE. Material inoculated onto the sheet may be toxic, a problem especially frequent with faecal samples, or contamination with other microorganisms may occur, despite all the precautions taken. If there is any doubt as to the origins of a CPE, a simple way to distinguish between a virus as opposed to a toxic effect is to attempt to passage the putative virus. The cells remaining in the cell sheet are scraped into the culture supernatant, and a few drops of the resultant material inoculated into a fresh tissue culture tube. If there was indeed a virus in the original culture, then not only will the CPE reappear within the new tube, but the speed of development should be much enhanced, as the amount, or titre, of virus will have increased significantly following viral growth in the first culture. If however, the original CPE arose due to some toxic component of the specimen, then this will have been diluted in the second tube, and the subsequent CPE should develop more slowly and less extensively, if at all.

Passaging of viruses is useful for two other reasons. Firstly, some viruses may not produce a visible CPE when first grown in culture, even though replication is indeed taking place. However, on repeated passaging in the same cell substrate, a CPE may become apparent following adaptation of the virus to growth in that particular cell type. The process of passaging viruses from apparently normal-looking cells is known as 'blind' passage, presumably because at that stage, the virologist is unable to see evidence of the presence of virus. The identification of rubella virus growing in rabbit kidney cells may require several such blind passages. Secondly, passaging of viruses is a good

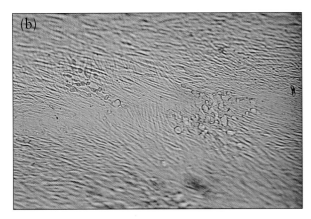

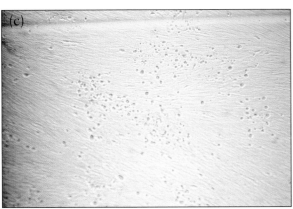

Figure 19.1: Cytopathic effects. (a) A normal cell sheet of fibroblasts. The cells have grown to confluence, and are spindle-shaped.
(b) Some of the cells are rounded up and swollen. This appearance in discrete foci separated by normal-looking cells is typical of the cytopathic effect induced by cytomegalovirus (c) Several cells all over the cell sheet have rounded up to give a 'flick-drop' appearance. This is the characteristic appearance of a rhinovirus-induced CPE.

method of increasing the amount of virus available for further studies, such as neutralization assays (see below).

Confirmation of virus isolation

In most instances the type of virus in a cell culture can be determined with reasonable certainty by observation of the characteristics of the CPE present in the cell sheet, as outlined above. However, there are instances where confirmation of virus identity may be required, e.g. if the CPE is atypical, does not passage well or is absent, or alternatively, when more information about the particular strain of virus is required. This can be achieved by use of electron microscopy, antigen detection, or neutralization assays.

The process of cell culture acts as a means of increasing viral titre to a sufficient level to allow visualization by electron microscopy (EM). Thus, provided there is access to an EM, most problems associated with atypical or unusual CPEs can be resolved rapidly by appropriate EM examination of the cells or culture supernatant.

Cells infected with a particular virus will express antigens derived from that virus on their surface. These antigens can be detected by staining with antibodies. Thus, the specific identity of a virus growing in cell culture may be determined by staining the cells with a panel of appropriate monoclonal antibodies, suitably labelled with an immunofluorescent tag. Cells can either be scraped off and sucked out of the tissue culture tubes, and then dried onto a glass slide, or, if it is known in advance that antigen detection will be necessary, the cells can be grown on a flat surface such as a coverslip within the tissue culture tube, which can then subsequently be retrieved and stained. Antigen detection will allow distinction between, say, influenza A and B viruses, or parainfluenza 1, 2 or 3 viruses, which all produce a similar CPE.

Neutralization assays are used most commonly to distinguish between the various enteroviruses which grow in culture, or for serotyping adenoviruses. In principle, virus isolated in culture is distributed into a series of tubes, and to each tube a different antiserum is added (e.g. anti-polio-1, anti-polio-2,

Identification of Virus Growth

Adaptations of cell culture

anti-polio-3 to tubes 1, 2, and 3 respectively). Following incubation of virus plus antiserum for one hour, the mixtures are added to individual tissue culture tubes, and the appearance of CPE monitored over the next few days. The occurrence of a typical CPE in tubes 1 and 3, combined with the absence of a CPE in tube 2, would indicate that the original virus was poliovirus type 2.

Adaptations of cell culture

Virus isolation by cell culture is usually much slower than bacterial isolation on inanimate media. The fastest growing virus, herpes simplex virus, may produce a CPE after 24 hours, but most viruses require several days (or even weeks) to do so. This is a considerable disadvantage! Thus, various modifications of cell culture have been introduced, with the aim of speeding up the process. Two such modifications which have been widely adopted by diagnostic laboratories are those of haemadsorption and detection of early antigen fluorescent foci.

Some viruses (e.g. the influenza and parainfluenza viruses, mumps virus) possess a haemagglutinin (i.e. a protein which binds red cells). Infected cells will express this molecule on their surface. Thus, if red cells are added to a cell culture tube in which such a virus is replicating, they will become adherent to the cell sheet, a phenomenon known as *haemadsorption* [see Fig. 19.2(a)]. Haemadsorption is demonstrable (by gently rotating the culture tube) for some days before a CPE has become evident. The exact nature of the haemadsorbing virus can be determined by staining with monoclonal antibodies, as described above (antigen detection).

The *detection of early antigen fluorescent foci* (DEAFF test) was developed specifically to accelerate the detection of cytomegalovirus (CMV) in tissue culture. In essence, DEAFF is an adaptation of antigen detection, where the antigens to be detected are selected as those which appear early (within 24 to 72 hours) in the replication cycle of the virus (hence 'early antigens'). Thus, clinical material is inoculated onto a cell sheet grown on a coverslip, or other flat surface (a type of culture known as a shell

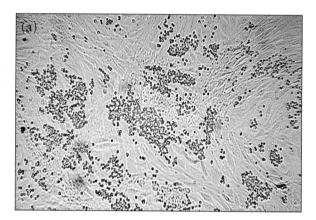

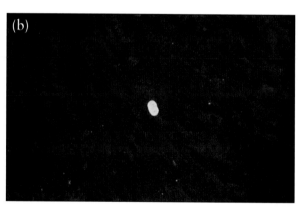

Figure 19.2: Adaptations of cell culture. *(a) Haemadsorption. The cell sheet (primary monkey kidney) is normal, i.e. no visible cytopathic effect has yet developed. However, many cells within the sheet are expressing a virally-encoded haemagglutinin on their surface, as the red cells, here seen as small dots overlying the cell sheet, have become attached to the sheet. (b) The DEAFF test. The cell sheet is stained with a fluorescently-labelled anti-CMV monoclonal antibody. A single nucleus is seen shining bright apple-green under UV light, indicating the presence of CMV in this cell. All the cells (seen here counterstained with Evan's blue dye) are morphologically normal.*

vial). There is a centrifugation step (700 *g* for 1 hr) which increases the infectivity of the cell sheet by virus. After 48 hours, the sheet is washed, and stained with a fluorescently-tagged monoclonal antibody directed against a CMV-early antigen. The coverslip is then examined under UV light. A positive result is indicated by the presence of fluorescent nuclei

Table 19.2: Potential viral isolates from clinical material.

Clinical specimen	Viruses which may be isolated in routine cell culture
Vesicle fluid or swab	Herpes simplex virus (HSV); varicella-zoster virus
Nasopharyngeal aspirate (NPA) and/or throat swab	Respiratory syncytial virus; influenza A and B viruses; parainfluenza viruses 1–4; adenoviruses; rhinoviruses; enteroviruses; HSV; cytomegalovirus (CMV)
Faeces	Enteroviruses; adenoviruses
Cerebrospinal fluid	Enteroviruses; mumps virus
Urine	CMV; mumps virus; adenoviruses
Conjunctival swab	HSV; adenoviruses
Blood (buffy coat)	CMV

in isolated cells (i.e. foci), which appear morphologically normal [see Fig. 19.2(b)]. This technique has been extended to other slow-growing viruses; for example, adenoviruses can be detected long before any CPE is evident by staining with antibodies against early adenovirus antigens.

Conclusions

The isolation of viruses in tissue culture remains an important technique for the diagnosis of virus infections. In theory, a single virus particle within a clinical specimen can be grown in cell culture, and thereby expanded by many orders of magnitude, allowing accurate detection and characterization. The high degree of sensitivity and specificity inherent in virus isolation are the 'gold standards' against which new techniques should be measured. The methodology is appropriate for a wide range both of clinical specimens and different viruses (Table 19.2). On rare occasions, its use results in the identification of unexpected, or even previously unidentified viruses – HIV and the human herpesviruses 6 and 7 are the latest in a long list of viruses first discovered in cell culture.

The two major drawbacks to this approach are that not all viruses can be grown in culture, and some viruses are rather slow-growing. The development of new types of cell culture able to support an ever-widening array of viruses may overcome some of the former problem, whilst there is a variety of adaptations of cell culture which can speed up the process of virus identification.

Further Reading

Landry M L, Hsuing G D. Primary isolation of viruses. In: *Clinical Virology Manual*. Specter S, Lancz G J (eds). 1986; Chapter 3, 31–52.

Lenette E H, Schmidt N J (eds). *Diagnostic procedures for viral, rickettsial and chlamydial infections*. 7th edition, 1996. American Public Health Association, Washington DC.

Smith R D, Sutherland K. The cytopathology of virus infections. In *Clinical Virology Manual*. Specter S, Lancz G J (eds). 1986; Chapter 4, 53–70.

20 SEROLOGICAL TESTS IN VIROLOGY

Goura Kudesia

Introduction

Antibodies are produced by the immune system in response to various infections and serology is the science of measurement of these antibodies in the serum. Conventionally the term serology also includes the study of serum for antigen and by extension of this definition any test involving an antigen and antibody reaction is defined as a serological test. Serological tests take advantage of the fact that most viral and many bacterial, fungal and parasitic infections elicit good antibody responses. These tests have been used for diagnosis of viral diseases or other diseases where the organisms are not easily isolated, such as toxoplasmosis and syphilis. In virus infections like hepatitis B, where there is a prolonged viraemic phase, similar techniques can be used to detect viral antigen. This chapter, although mostly confined to virus serology, will also consider other serological tests presently used in the virology laboratories for the diagnosis of infectious diseases and will deal with the principles, techniques, interpretation and future of these tests.

Principles

The antibody classes most useful for measurement are the IgM and IgG. The measurement both of secretory and serum IgA antibody may also be useful but is technically more demanding and therefore not used routinely in diagnostic laboratories. The initial antibody to be produced after primary infection is of IgM class and generally becomes detectable from one to two days after onset of symptoms and remains detectable for 6 to 12 weeks. Specific IgG antibody begins to rise at one to two weeks and remains detectable for many years, if not lifelong, after the infection. Virus-specific IgG antibody alone is therefore associated with past infection and in most cases denotes immunity to future infection. On the other hand, as the virus-specific IgM antibody is generally undetectable after three months, its presence indicates a recent infection. The measurement of virus-specific IgG and IgM antibody in a single serum sample can therefore aid in the diagnosis and help distinguish recent from past virus infection. Many techniques like enzyme-linked immunoassay (ELISA or EIA), immunofluorescent assay (IFA) and radioimmunoassay (RIA) have been developed to measure specific IgG and IgM. These techniques can also be used for antigen detection. They have similar principles whereby the antibody reaction with antigen is detected by addition of a second antibody directed against human immunoglobulin. The anti-immunoglobulin is labelled with fluoresceine (IFA), enzyme (ELISA) or radioisotope (RIA) (Fig. 20.1).

The IgG or IgM class of antibody produced may also have different functional properties, that is they may be complement fixing, haemagglutinating or neutralizing. The antigens present on the virus determine the functional property of the antibody produced in response, so only those viruses (for example rubella, measles or influenza) that possess haemagglutinin antigen will elicit haemagglutinating antibodies. The knowledge of the anti-genic structure of viruses can be utilized for devising suitable serological tests such as the complement fixation (CF), haemagglutination (HA) or haemagglutination inhibition (HAI) tests. These tests detect both IgG and IgM class of antibody at the same time. Serial dilutions of the serum can be made to determine the titre of the antibody present. Paired acute and convalescent serum samples are required to make a diagnosis of recent infection, a fourfold or greater rise in antibody level being diagnostic.

Techniques

Serological techniques can be divided on the basis of the complexity of test. The most simple are those where the presence of antibody is shown by a simple interaction with antigen (precipitation or agglutination tests). Next are those which involve indicator systems to detect the antibody–antigen reaction (neutralization or complement fixation). The most complex tests involve the use of a second labelled antibody system (ELISA or IFA).

Precipitation

Ouchterlony's double diffusion (DD) method can be used to detect either antibody or antigen. In the first case a known antigen is used and in the second case an antibody of known specificity is used. The antibody and antigen diffuse towards each other in agarose gel and a line of white precipitation indicates a positive reaction. Counter-immunoelectrophoresis (CIE) specifically directs the movement of antigen and antibody towards each other in an electric field and hence is more rapid than DD. CIE was the method originally used in the detection of hepatitis B surface antigen. These methods have mostly been replaced by much more sensitive techniques, although some laboratories still use them for fungal antibody tests.

Haemagglutination and haemagglutination inhibition (HA and HAI)

The haemagglutinin possessed by certain viruses such as influenza, rubella and measles viruses has the property of agglutinating red

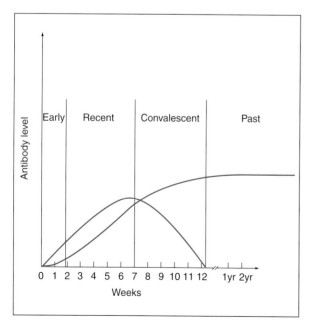

Figure 20.1: IgM and IgG response in early, recent, convalescent and past infection.

blood cells (RBC) of selected species. HA tests are most commonly used with influenza viruses. Influenza A and B agglutinate human group O, guinea-pig and chicken RBCs at 4 and 20°C whereas influenza B in addition agglutinates fowl RBCs. HA tests are therefore useful in the detection and titration of viral antigen. HAI utilizes the presence of haemagglutinin on the virus to detect antibody. The test is based on the principle that specific antibody combines with the haemagglutinin and inhibits HA. Serial dilutions of patient's serum are allowed to react with a specified amount of haemagglutinin and appropriate indicator RBCs are then added. If specific antibody is present it will block the haemagglutinin and a positive reaction is therefore shown by the absence of haemagglutination. Where specific antibody is absent the viral haemagglutinin is free to agglutinate the indicator RBCs (negative reaction). In the past HAI tests were used extensively to establish immune status and to diagnose recent rubella virus infections. The HAI is however complicated by the fact that the serum needs prior treatment to remove non specific inhibitors and has therefore been replaced by more sensitive and specific techniques for the diagnosis of rubella. HAI, though, is still used by reference laboratories for the identification and typing of influenza viruses. HA techniques can also be used for viruses which do not possess haemagglutinin. This is achieved by coupling the viral antigen to the surface of RBCs by a coupling agent such as tannic acid. When mixed with serum containing specific antibody, the RBCs are agglutinated because of the viral antigen bound to their surface (indirect or passive HA). Indirect HA has been used for the detection of antibody to toxoplasma. However, because of the instability of RBCs, inert carrier particles such as latex are now being used.

Latex agglutination (LA)

Polystyrene latex micro-particles sensitized or coated with viral antigen agglutinate when mixed with patient serum containing specific antibody. The antigen-coated latex particles are mixed with patient's serum on a glass slide or in a microtitre well. A visible agglutination pattern appears if specific antibody is present.

These tests are in wide use in virus laboratories because of their speed, simplicity and ease of use. Currently good LA tests are available for rubella, toxoplasma and cytomegalovirus. LA tests are used both for screening of a single serum sample to establish immunity and paired sera to diagnose a recent infection.

Complement fixation (CF)

Patient serum, after inactivation at 56°C for 30 minutes to destroy indigenous complement, is added to a known amount of viral antigen and rabbit complement. If antibody and antigen reaction has occurred then the complement is activated or 'fixed' or bound. An antigen and antibody detector system, in the form of sheep RBCs sensitized with rabbit antibody to sheep RBCs (haemolysin), is then added. If complement has been 'fixed' by the first antigen and antibody reaction, the sheep RBCs are not lysed, indicating a positive reaction and presence of specific antibody in the serum. A negative reaction is indicated by haemolysis of sensitized sheep RBCs by complement. The CF test is a quantitative test. The serum is diluted serially and the level of antibody expressed as a reciprocal of the highest dilution of the serum giving rise to haemolysis of 50% of the sensitized RBCs. A fourfold rise in titre or seroconversion between an acute and convalescent sample is diagnostic. This technique requires considerable expertise and is labour intensive but the serum can be tested against multiple antigens on a single occasion using the same indicator system. CF tests are done only in specialist virology laboratories and are still the tests of choice for the serological diagnosis of respiratory viral and atypical bacterial infections.

Neutralization

The interaction of specific antibody with virus neutralizes infectivity and prevents infection of a susceptible living host system by that virus. A major disadvantage of these tests is that a living host system either in the form of cell culture or animals is required and hence many of these tests have been replaced by other techniques. Neutralization tests are still in use for the detection of poliovirus antibody and certain toxins such as that of *Clostridium difficile*.

Techniques

Enzyme-linked immunosorbent assays (ELISA)

Enzyme-linked immunosorbent assays (ELISA)
This is the most popular serological test in current use. There are many variations in methodology but all involve the attachment of antigen to a solid phase which is generally a polystyrene or polyvinyl plate or bead. Patient's serum is added and, after an appropriate length of time to allow the antibody to bind to the antigen on the solid phase, non-specifically bound material and excess serum is removed by washing. An anti-human immunoglobulin labelled by conjugation with an enzyme (conjugate) is then added. The conjugate binds to the antibody in the antigen and antibody complex. Excess conjugate is then washed off and presence of the bound labelled anti-human immunoglobulin is detected by the addition of a suitable substrate for the labelling enzyme. If appropriate reactions have occurred then the substrate is converted to a light-absorbing product and appears coloured. In the absence of antibody no colour is produced. The intensity of the colour is directly related to the amount of antibody bound to the antigen. The colour change can be measured by the naked eye or read by a spectrophotometer to give the exact strength of reaction. The enzyme–substrate systems in common use are horseradish peroxidase (HRP) and o-phenylene diamine (OPD), and alkaline phosphotase and p. nitrophenyl phosphate. To adapt the test for detection of antigen, the solid phase is coated with antibody specific to the antigen to be detected. A second labelled antibody is then added to detect any antibody and antigen complex on the surface of the solid phase. Depending on the sequence of reaction, ELISAs are divided into direct, indirect, capture or competitive assays. Fig. 20.2 explains some of the differences between these assays. The assays are specific for IgM or IgG, depending upon whether anti-human IgM or IgG immunoglobulin is used as the second antibody. For a detailed review the reader is referred to Booth J.

ELISA is a very sensitive technique because a small quantity of enzyme can process a large amount of substrate. False-negative IgM results may occur in the presence of high levels of specific IgG which compete for the antigen on the solid phase. This can be avoided by removing the IgG prior to testing of the sample. Non-specific reactions in the IgM assay may also occur because of the presence of rheumatoid factor (RF). RF factor of the IgM class binds to new antigens exposed due to configurational changes on the Fc region of the specific IgG molecule when it binds to the antigen on the solid phase. IgM RF cannot be distinguished from virus specific IgM, but RF can be removed by adsorption with aggregated IgG prior to testing for IgM. Capture assays for IgM are preferred as they are not affected by RF or

Figure 20.2(a), (b) and (c): Different ELISA formats
(a) Indirect ELISA
1. Coat solid phase with viral antigen.
2. Incubate with patient's serum. Specific antibody present attaches to antigen bound to solid phase.
3. Add enzyme labelled anti-IgG or IgM.
4. Add substrate, colour change if reaction is positive.
(b) Capture ELISA
1. Coat solid phase with anti-IgG or IgM.
2. Incubate with patient's serum. All IgG or IgM present is captured onto solid phase.
3. Add antigen, this will bind to any captured specific antibody.
4. Add enzyme labelled antiviral IgG.
5. Add substrate, colour change if reaction is positive.
(c) Competitive ELISA
1. Coat solid phase with antigen.
2. Add patient's serum and enzyme labelled specific antibody. Specific antibody competes with the conjugate for attachment to solid phase.
3. Add substrate. Positive reaction is shown by no colour in (a) as conjugate has been blocked by specific antibody. Negative reaction is shown by colour in (b) as enzyme labelled antibody has not been blocked.

<u>Techniques</u>

Enzyme-linked immunosorbent assays (ELISA)

Immunofluorescence (IF)

specific IgG in the patient's serum. ELISAs have the advantage of being objective, can be easily automated and do not require great technical expertise. They are rapid tests and most assays can be completed within two to three hours. Most, if not all, microbiological laboratories are equipped to perform ELISAs, which are in extensive use for screening and serological diagnosis of HIV, viral hepatitis, rubella, cytomegalovirus, Epstein–Barr virus, varicella-zoster virus, measles, mumps, toxoplasma, *Chlamydia trachomatis*, etc.

Immunofluorescence (IF)

In the indirect IF for detection of antibody, virally infected cells or bacterial antigen are fixed to wells on Teflon coated glass slides, patient's serum is added and the antigen and

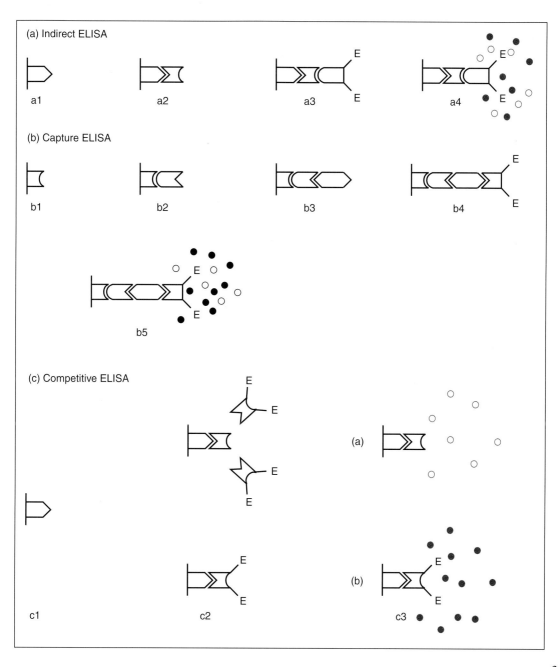

Radioimmunoassays (RIA)

Western blot (WB) or line immunoassay (LIA)

<u>Interpretation and Use of Serological Tests</u>

Diagnosis of acute infections

---

antibody reaction is detected by the addition of anti-human immunoglobulin labelled with fluorescein dye (fluorescein isothionate). The reaction is read under a fluorescent light microscope, positive reactions being indicated by typical apple-green fluorescence. Indirect IF tests for the detection of IgM and IgG antibody to cytomegalovirus, Epstein–Barr and varicella-zoster viruses have been in use for many years. False-positive reactions due to the expression of receptors on infected cells, to which non-virus specific antibody of IgM class may bind, is a problem. IF also requires specialist equipment such as a fluorescence microscope and is subject to operator bias in reading. Therefore they have mostly been replaced by ELISAs for antibody detection. The availability of good quality monoclonals, on the other hand, to a variety of viral antigens has made direct IF the method of choice for the detection of antigen in various tissues and samples. Infected material is fixed on the glass slide with the help of acetone or alcohol and stained with fluorescein-labelled monoclonal antibody directed against the antigen under test. Direct IF is used widely for the rapid diagnosis of respiratory viruses by testing of epithelial cells from nasopharyngeal aspirates for respiratory syncytial, influenza A and B, parainfluenza 1, 2 and 3 and adenoviruses.

Radioimmunoassays (RIA)
These have the same principles as ELISAs. RIA tests use a radioisotope label instead of an enzyme label. Because of the short shelf life of the radiolabel and special radioactivity disposal requirements, they have been replaced by ELISAs.

Western blot (WB) or line immunoassay (LIA)
This provides a highly specific and sensitive tool for detecting and characterizing antibodies to microorganisms by virtue of their binding to antigens that have been affixed to nitrocellulose membranes. For WB, semi-purified viral or bacterial proteins are separated by electrophoresis on a polyacrylamide gel and then electrophoretically transferred to a nitrocellulose membrane. In LIA the viral antigens produced by recombinant molecular techniques or artificially synthesized (synthetic peptides) are attached directly to the nitrocellulose membrane. The nitrocellulose membrane is incubated with patient's serum to allow antibody to bind to the antigens fixed on the membrane. Enzyme–labelled anti-human immunoglobulin is then added on a principle similar to that of ELISA. Appropriate washing steps are included. On addition of substrate, antigen bands, to which specific antibody is present, become visible.

The technique is unique in that antibody to single viral or bacterial proteins or antigenic epitopes can be detected, hence making the test very specific. They are used extensively as confirmatory tests for HIV and hepatitis C virus and for the diagnosis of Lyme disease.

Interpretation and Use of Serological Tests

Diagnosis of acute infections
Serologic studies contribute significantly to the diagnosis of infectious diseases. Normally a serologic confirmation requires examination of a serum sample taken immediately after onset of illness (acute) and a second sample one to two weeks later (convalescent). A fourfold rise in antibody or seroconversion from negative to positive antibody status between acute and convalescent sample indicates acute infection. New technologies for the detection of specific IgM and IgG, however, enable the laboratory to make a diagnosis or rule out a suspected infection on a single serum sample. For this ELISAs are used extensively by microbiology laboratories. If neither IgM nor IgG is detected then the patient has not been exposed to the organism or the sample was taken too early. As IgM antibody to most viruses can be detected within one week of onset of symptoms, a sample taken at this time, if negative for viral IgM, is sufficient to rule out recent infection. Specific IgM can normally only be detected for six months. As IgG will only be present later, a positive IgM reaction, with or without the presence of specific IgG, indicates recent infection.

SEROLOGICAL TESTS IN VIROLOGY

Interpretation and Use of Serological Tests
Detection of antibody to verify immunity
Transplanted and immunosuppressed patients
Screening for blood, organ and tissue donation

Specific IgG remains positive for life, therefore the presence of IgG alone, with a negative IgM, indicates a past infection and in most cases immunity from further infection to that specific organism. It is clear that the test selection and interpretation of the result depends on the clinical condition and date of onset of symptoms, which should therefore always be communicated to the laboratory.

Detection of antibody to verify immunity
Verification of immunity to infections is required in many clinical situations such as post-vaccination, pre-employment, pregnancy, pre-transplant or in immunosuppressed patients who may come in contact with infections. Tests to detect protective antibody have to be sensitive and require testing for specific IgG. Viral specific IgG ELISA, IFA or total antibody tests such as latex agglutination are used.

Post-vaccination seroepidemiological surveys to establish seroconversion and immunity after vaccination to measles, mumps, rubella and hepatitis B have formed a vital part of evaluation of the effectiveness of vaccination programmes. Automatable sensitive ELISAs have made mass post-vaccination screening feasible. Antibody to hepatitis B is expressed in international units and this ability to quantitate allows the clinician to decide on the timing of the follow-up boosters.

Immunity to rubella and hepatitis B is a pre-requisite for employment for many health care workers. Immunity to other infections such as varicella-zoster virus, measles and mumps is also desirable, especially for those working with children or immunocompromised patients, both to protect themselves and to prevent spread of infection to susceptible patients. Those who are susceptible to varicella-zoster infection and who are exposed to chickenpox should be excluded from work, to avoid exposing susceptible patients to the infection.

During pregnancy, screening to detect protective antibody to rubella is offered to all patients, susceptible patients being vaccinated post-partum. It is also recommended that all patients be screened for hepatitis B virus and hepatitis B immunization is given to babies of infected mothers to prevent vertical transmission of infection. HIV screening for at-risk mothers enables specific drug treatment of the mother during pregnancy and labour to reduce the risk of vertical HIV transmission. Screening for antibody to other organisms such as varicella-zoster, toxoplasma and cytomegalovirus enables the clinician to advise susceptible patients about how to avoid infection. All of these screens require a simple IgG ELISA test or latex agglunitation. However in case of recent contact with an infection, IgM assays have to be performed in addition to ensure that the IgG detected is from a past and not a current infection.

Transplanted and immunosuppressed patients
These patients are particularly prone to developing cytomegalovirus (CMV) infections. CMV antibody-negative patients who are given an organ from a CMV-positive donor require prophylaxis to prevent development of primary CMV infection. In addition donor-acquired toxoplasma infection is a serious problem in heart transplant recipients, so all donors and recipients are screened for antibody to toxoplasma and negative recipients of a heart from toxoplasma antibody-positive donors are given prophylaxis. Immunosuppressed patients are also screened for common infections such as chickenpox, herpes simplex and measles as they may suffer from severe disease if exposed to them.

Screening for blood, organ and tissue donation
Many organisms, especially blood-borne viruses, can be transmitted via blood and blood products, organ and tissue transplantation. It is essential that blood be screened for these prior to transfusion. In the United Kingdom all blood is screened for HIV, hepatitis B, hepatitis C and syphilis. In the case of HIV and hepatitis C virus, the presence of antibody signifies current infection and screening for viral antigen is not necessary. Blood destined for immunosuppressed patients is also screened for CMV. Because of the importance of discarding infected blood, only the most sensitive tests are used. Donations found to be positive are then subjected to confirmatory tests by specialist reference laboratories. To cope with the volume of screens required, Blood Transfusion Laboratories have automated ELISA systems for microbiological

screening of blood. Organ and tissue donors are subjected to similar screening procedures.

Diagnosis of congenital infection

As maternal IgG crosses the placenta into the fetus, the presence of specific viral IgG in neonatal blood does not necessarily indicate infection. The persistence of IgG antibody beyond six months of age indicates congenital infection as maternally derived antibody should disappear by then. The presence of specific IgM at or soon after birth indicates congenital or vertical infection as the IgM class of antibody does not cross the placenta.

Future of Serology

The ability to semi or fully automate ELISAs has made these tests available to a vast number of laboratories. The older tests were technically demanding and limited to only a few specialist laboratories. The explosion in ELISA technology along with awareness of the importance of virus infections in many vulnerable groups of patients has made serology a mainstay of virus diagnosis. Many of these tests have been adapted for the testing of urine and saliva samples. As these are non-invasive samples they are preferred for children and other groups such as intravenous drug abusers where it is difficult to obtain blood samples. Serological diagnosis by testing of saliva is now available for measles, mumps and rubella. Large scale serosurveillance of HIV infection is being done by testing urine and saliva. Techniques to measure avidity of IgG antibody have been developed to aid in the timing of infection by serology. Antibody of low avidity is produced initially after primary infection, whereas high avidity antibody is produced after reinfection or recrudescence. Antibody avidity tests have been invaluable in the management of rubella and Toxoplasma infections in pregnancy by helping to establish the timing of infection. Serology is now firmly established for the diagnosis of infections, especially viral diseases. Newer technology means that many of the routine diagnostic tests can now be performed by general microbiology or other non-specialist laboratories.

Further Reading

Booth J C. The use of the enzyme-linked immunosorbent assay (ELISA) technique in clinical virology. *Recent Advances in Clinical Virology*, Waterson A P (ed) 1983; Churchill-Livingstone: 73–98.

James K. Immunology of infectious diseases. *Clinical Microbiol Review* 1990; 3(2): 132–152.

Parry J V, Perry K R, Mortimer P P. Sensitive assays for viral antibodies in saliva: an alternative to tests on serum. *Lancet* 1987; 2: 72–75.

Thomas H I J. Specific antibody avidity studies in clinical microbiology: past, present and future. *PHLS Microbial Digest* 1995; 12(2): 97–102.

21   AUTOMATED TESTS IN VIROLOGY

Roger P Eglin

Introduction

Diagnostic testing in clinical laboratories has evolved over the past 50 years from manual operation of tests such as examination of blood films and simple chemistry assays using techniques requiring relatively large quantities of blood, serum or plasma. The 1960s saw the development of the multichannel analyser for clinical chemistry and the introduction of electronic counting methods, e.g. Coulter counter. The continued development of such automated testing began to concentrate on improvements in the quality and consistency of results and to reduce both the times taken for assays and the volume of sample required for each assay. Although sophisticated automated systems have been in routine use in other areas of pathology for the past 20 years, microbiology and particularly virology laboratories used traditional testing methods. For virology these were based around cell culture and virus isolation with antibody tests using reagents produced largely in house. Enzyme immunoassays (EIAs) were introduced in the 1970s and their commercial developments have allowed progress to be made towards automation. Impetus was given to the development of such equipment by the requirement of the Blood Transfusion Service (now National Blood Authority) to screen blood donations for a limited but steadily increasing range of blood-borne virus infections. This began with HBs antigen in the 1970s, then followed anti-HIV in 1984, selective anti-CMV in the 1980s and anti-HCV in 1991. The great expansion in the range of commercial EIAs in the 1980s extended the use of standard protocols and encouraged manufacture of automated systems. It is only since the early 1990s that a range of such equipment has been developed specifically for the diagnostic virology laboratory. A wide range of routine diagnostic assays is now in the repertoire of these automated machines. The assays available are based around the EIA technique. The early systems were developed for the screening tests most frequently requested, i.e. HBs antigen, anti-HBs, rubella IgG and *Chlamydia trachomatis* antigen. After the initial rush to market a variety of automated equipment in the early 1990s, the marketplace has now become more stable. It has become possible to identify different classes of machines and to identify the type of workload that is most appropriate to each of the classes of instrument. Working definitions of the type of automation to be discussed are as follows.

Liquid handling processor (LHP)

An LHP (a) completes the preparation of a microtitre plate containing appropriately diluted samples and test-specific controls using a worksheet to identify the samples and protocols specific to the test required; and (b) completes the separation of serum from a blood clot and so prepares a serum store from blood samples received.

Automated EIA processor

An automated EIA processor (a) completes an EIA with only the supply of samples and reagents specific to that test; and (b) completes an EIA with only the addition of a microtitre plate containing appropriately diluted samples and reagents specific to that test.

The equipment may then be subdivided into the following classes:

Random access/batch testing

EIA processors are generally designed for specific tests on specimens which have been accumulated as a batch and are identified by a specific worksheet. Some processors are also able to run tests on single specimens, to allow response to urgent clinical demand. These single tests require control calibrators for the test in addition to the test sample. It may be possible to interrupt the current testing to run the urgent specimen or it may be introduced at a convenient time between batches of other tests. These random access machines require manufacturer-specific test modules or use of controls that are permanently on board to operate the test.

Single tube format/microtitre plate format

Some processors operate by sampling the specimen tube directly and perform all subsequent operations as single tube tests, e.g. VIDAS, E7001. Other processors accept single tube specimens but set up the test using microtitre plates. This plate format may still be manufacturer-specific, e.g. Amerlite, or may allow any standard EIA-based microtitre plate to be used.

Manufacturer-specific test system/accept any microtitre assay

The manufacturer's processing system is unique and use of the processor dictates that all the tests to be used must also be purchased from that manufacturer, e.g. VIDAS, AXSYM, Amerlite. Other processors have been designed to handle any microtitre-based EIA and the choice of manufacturer for each test to be used lies with the laboratory and may be decided by the performance characteristics of the test. Some examples of current equipment available in each class are given in Table 21.1.

How Automation Works in the Diagnostic Laboratory

In order to discuss this topic, it is necessary to make the following assumptions: firstly, that the laboratory uses a diagnostic software programme for handling its patient database; secondly, that specimens are given unique identity by means of a bar-coding system with labels on the associated request form, primary blood tube and stored serum sample; and thirdly, that the laboratory is using an automated system comprising an LHP and microtitre-based EIA processor.

Following reception of the specimen and request form in the laboratory, the first two stages in processing often occur simultaneously.

Worksheets

A set of tests is ordered which is appropriate to the clinical details and date of onset stated on the request form. This set of tests is logged on to the computer and leads to the creation of test-specific worksheets, which may then be called off as required according to the daily planning sheet for the automated system.

Serum separation

After centrifuging the primary blood tube, to spin down the blood clot, the serum is separated by the LHP or manually into a storage tube, which is labelled with the same bar-code identification as the primary blood tube.

Preparing the microtitre plates for the assay

If a random access system is in use then the serum storage bottle will be loaded directly onto the system and the required dilutions

Table 21.1: Which automated equipment is most appropriate?

Type of machine	Advantages	Disadvantages
Random access – manufacturer-specific tests	Rapid testing of single samples. Requires a full set of control samples once/month. Does not require full set of controls for each test, uses calibrators. Wide range of assays available covering several disciplines. Share costs with other users of machine (biochemistry, immunology).	Daily throughput may be small, e.g. 300/day. Total lab. throughput in a normal working day may be >400 samples. Premium paid for same single commercial supplier of both test modules and equipment. Limited range of infectious diseases tests may be available. If used as a core lab. facility, can the current test runs really be interrupted?
Batch testing – 2 or 3 microtitre plate-based system	May also include sample dispensing. May be able to run any microtitre-based system.	May be manufacturer-specific tests, e.g. Amerlite (chemiluminescence). Is a full range of infectious diseases tests available? May only achieve 3 batched runs in a normal working day. Careful scheduling of test runs may be required.
Open access microtitre plate-based system	Uses any EIA-based microtitre plate assay. Capable of accepting next test plate at any time.	May require separate sample dispensing equipment.
Sample dispensing system	Allows flexibility of unlabelled or unlinked sample handling. Can be used for other purposes, e.g. sample aliquots for serum store into bottles/microtitre plates, CFT, SRH	Costs may be increased.

How Automation Works in the Diagnostic Laboratory

made by the machine. The LHP should be able to identify sample tubes or primary blood tubes in racks or carousels. It will check that all the samples on the current worksheet are present and then proceed to make appropriate dilutions of the serum into wells, following the specific protocol. The plate will be bar-coded to allow positive identification and selection of the correct protocol by the software. This will then allow the software to order the appropriate reagents for the specific EIA. It should also add the appropriate standards, both those supplied by manufacturers and laboratory 'in house' samples, and calibration samples as necessary to allow quality control (QC) of the test run. These QC specimens will be dispensed into wells designated in the protocol. The system will flag up any samples for which it has failed to collect liquid.

EIA processor
The plate is identified by bar-code and the software identifies both the correct worksheet and the correct protocol associated with that test run. The machine checks that the requested EIA reagents have been placed correctly in the system and the volumes of these on board reagents are checked by weight. This checking includes the wash buffer, test reagents and ensures that there is sufficient spare volume in the waste bottle. The first step, which is part of the quality control monitoring of the system, is to take a spectrophotometric reading of the plate to check that a specimen has been added to each of the expected wells. A well with a discrepant optical density (OD) reading identifies where no sample is present. The processor starts the EIA and follows the protocol stored in the software. If an open access system is in use, then the processor will recalculate the time slots for the assays already in process and fit in the new plate to start processing as soon as possible. The start time will be displayed together with a warning if the time delay before starting the assay exceeds the default time for the system. Generally EIAs which use incubations at room temperature are avoided because, although the incubation periods are often longer than those with 37°C incubations, the first incubation reactions start immediately the diluted sample is dispensed into the wells. Incubations at 37°C or 40°C allow a fixed start time and this is necessary for the open access machines. The EIA protocol followed by the processor should include monitoring after each step requiring addition of liquid reagents and also monitoring of the wash heads after each operation to ensure that all the wells have been washed correctly. The readout from each liquid addition monitoring should be displayed as the EIA proceeds and any errors detected flagged up immediately. If an open access machine is in use then each batch of test reagents should be added when requested by the processor.

Data handling
The final optical density (OD) readings, taken on completion of the assay, are transferred automatically to the system software for manipulation by the data reduction package. This package will, depending on the type of assay, either (a) calculate the cut off value from the controls and apply it to the sample OD values, in which case the results will be expressed as positive, negative or equivocal for each specimen, or (b) generate a standard curve from the controls and apply it to the sample readings in which case the results for the samples will be expressed as units per ml.

The software also checks that the manufacturer's calibrators and standards which have been included in the run are in range and flags up any discrepancies. If the calibrators have acceptable values then the stored standard values are applied to the sample ODs for the current test run. After validation of the displayed results by the experienced technician, the results are transferred automatically to the worksheet. This worksheet may be printed for hard copy storage, and contains all the necessary information to track back the details of the assay should any problems be discovered at a later date. These details include for both assay plate and associated reagents, the type, batch number, expiry date of the plate and reagents, date of assay, worksheet requester, assay performer and results validator. From the worksheet the results are automatically transferred to the individual patient records in the laboratory database.

Automated Tests in Virology

Should the Laboratory Automate?
Analyse the current laboratory business
Which type of equipment to choose?

The software will also perform the required internal quality control checks on the run by: (a) updating the 20 rolling averages for the control samples and flagging any discrepant results; and (b) updating the Shewhart charts[1] with the new control results. It then applies the associated rules to check that the run is valid and may be released. Any results which are found to be out of range by these criteria will be flagged up for immediate action.

Should the Laboratory Automate?

The above describes the operation of an automated system within the laboratory. Prior to this, the decision must be made to move to an automated system for EIA testing. The preparative work involved in reaching this decision is considerable and includes several analytical steps. It will also involve major changes in work patterns in the laboratory and the staff must be involved in this development project to achieve new ways of working. The next section describes some of the important factors to be considered during this review process.

Analyse the current laboratory business

This includes the range of viruses, types and number of tests undertaken by the laboratory. Review the current turnaround times for results required by the contracted service level agreements. Is there room for improvement to meet clinical demands for more timely results? Is random access testing a realistic option for small numbers of any test which are currently batched to 1 or 2 runs a week? If large volumes of some screening assays are identified, are these tests currently EIA-based and if not, can the test be moved successfully to EIA with no loss of quality and perhaps an improvement in sensitivity and specificity (Fig. 21.1). Decide how to batch the regular screening tests to 1 or 2 runs a day (around 30 tests is usually the minimum number per batch, for economic reasons), is a daily run required, is a same-day result service provided? Define the requirement for one-off urgent or on-call testing and estimate how many could fit into the normal runs without delaying the result unduly (Fig. 21.2).

Which type of equipment to choose?

Primary laboratory (district general hospital laboratory) undertaking routine screening of a relatively small number of samples can choose a small dedicated machine; make use of the

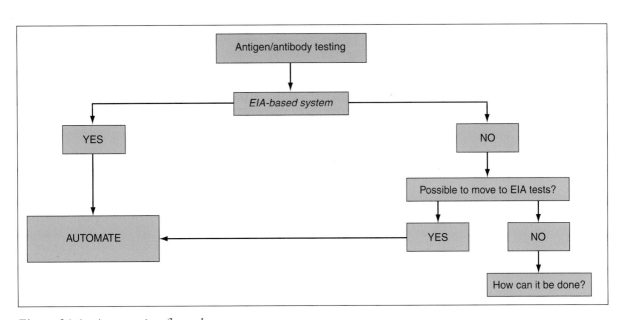

Figure 21.1: Automation flow chart.

Should the Laboratory Automate?

Quality issues

Financial considerations

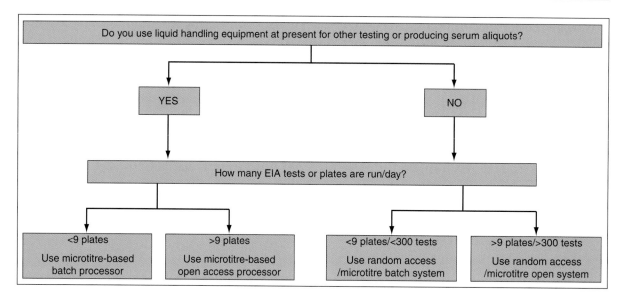

Figure 21.2: Which type of equipment to choose?

infectious diseases range of tests on the large pathology department analyser; and underwrite the cost of equipment by running a screening test on the machine to be used for random access, e.g. antibiotic assays.

Secondary laboratory (teaching hospital laboratory, large referral laboratory) undertaking a wide range of tests on a large number of samples: requires a large throughput of specimens daily and provides a wide range of tests; consider batch runs, decide how many runs per day are required, most EIAs are completed within three hours. This allows two runs in the normal working day plus one run overnight. For a three plate system this equates to nine plates per day. Open access systems will complete eight test plates every five hours.

The final choice of equipment requires detailed comparison of their performance, mechanics, quality systems and software and lies beyond the scope of this chapter.

Quality issues
The transfer to an automated system will realize a number of benefits to the laboratory. The system removes subjectivity from all aspects of the procedures used. The runs will be completed reproducibly and follow the proto-

col exactly on every occasion. Variations in the protocols will only occur when the protocol is amended by the system manager. This standardization will improve the reproducibility of assays, as judged by the CVs of standards.[2] The automated system ensures positive identity of the sample throughout the testing and allows the laboratory to approach the standards already demanded of the NBA laboratories. This security of identity resides with the barcoding of all specimens and all EIA plates throughout the system. The monitoring of liquid additions and washing stages confirms that all steps of the protocol have been successfully achieved. It allows identification of the point of breakdown in the system in the event of a test run failing the quality control validation. Automated transfer of the worksheet from the laboratory diagnostic software to the automated system software and return of the validated results directly to the patient database removes transcription errors completely. Turnaround times for testing may be reduced with the results produced in a time frame that is effective in assisting with patient management.

Financial considerations
Changing work practices allows increased numbers of tests per member of staff. This

AUTOMATED TESTS IN VIROLOGY

Should the Laboratory Automate?
Improve the competitive position of the laboratory
Other Developments in Automation
Conclusions
Further Reading

leads to greater income generation, either by fewer staff with the original workload or, if staffing levels do not change, then extra new work can be introduced, driven by customer demands. Increasing the number of tests spreads the staff costs over a large number of specimens and helps to reduce the direct costs per test. The more testing the automated system completes, the lower the overhead per test for capital depreciation of the system and annual maintenance charges. The choice between outright purchase rather than leasing or reagent rental must be made and it will depend largely upon the type of equipment required and the financial position of the laboratory at that time. If it is decided to use a manufacturer-specific system then the premium to be paid should be estimated by costing routine EIAs for the same testing. If random access equipment is required, the expected number of samples requiring this urgent treatment should be estimated and a current routine screening test identified that can be run on this equipment to defray the costs, e.g. antibiotic assays on an AXSYM.

Improve the competitive position of the laboratory

Acquisition of an automated system in the laboratory allows for repositioning the role of the laboratory within the pathology department. It should be possible to become the core facility for the provision of EIA-based testing within pathology and cover a large range of testing for virology, bacteriology, immunology and biochemistry. A significant improvement in some turnaround times for results should be achieved. The laboratory is well placed to undertake evaluation work for new test developments and for field trailing tests before they reach the marketplace. The laboratory stores a large range of samples for all routine tests and can offer completely reproducible testing following protocols that have been set up and trialed by the commercial company.

Other Developments in Automation

This chapter has discussed the automation of antibody and antigen EIAs for which there is now a wide choice of equipment. The next testing area which is expected to be automated is the nucleic acid amplification assay and specifically the PCR assay. It is already possible to use automated systems which run batches of PCR amplifications and detections automatically. In the next year or two it is anticipated that the extraction of nucleic acids from relatively clean samples such as serum and plasma will be automated and this will then give a totally automated system from sample to result.

Conclusions

Automation is the only solution to maintaining a cost-effective laboratory. There is downward pressure from all sides on the finances of the laboratory, ranging from cost reductions expected year on year in contracts to the ever-increasing demands for more testing and for an increasing range of new tests. It is essential that old technology is not clung to unnecessarily. New systems are available and re-engineering of the laboratory to make best use of these systems is the way forward. This entails getting the confidence of the staff in making these changes. They need to see the benefits of implementation of new systems and the emergence of completely new areas of work, e.g. viral load, that are continuing to appear at an unprecedented rate. In order to cope with these major changes it will be essential to invest in the staff in terms of retraining and learning new skills.

Further Reading

Costongs G M, van Oers R J, Leerkes B, Janson P C. Evaluation of the DPC IMMULITE random access immunoassay analyser. *European Journal of Clinical Chemistry and Clinical Biochemistry* 1995; **33**, 887–892.

Westgard J O, Hunt M R, Groth T. A multiShewhart chart for quality control in clinical chemistry. *Clinical Chemistry* 1981; **27**, 493–501.

22 MOLECULAR TECHNIQUES IN VIROLOGY

Paul E Klapper

Introduction

The application of molecular biological techniques in virology has been remarkable both for the speed with which these techniques have been developed and introduced and for the variety of the methodologies. Even more dramatic has been the way in which these new technologies have: revolutionized the diagnosis of viral infection, have led to the discovery of new viruses, the production of new, more potent vaccines for the prevention of infection, the development of new methods for treatment of infection, the rapid identification of drug resistance, and the active monitoring of the efficacy of therapy. Individual patients have benefited from the improved accuracy and speed of diagnosis afforded by molecular biological methods through the earlier application of specific antiviral chemotherapy. Rapid, accurate diagnosis has reduced unnecessary testing and in some instances allowed the replacement of an invasive diagnostic procedure with a less invasive, more accurate and reliable diagnostic test. An example is in the diagnosis of herpes encephalitis — a severe infection of the brain caused by herpes simplex virus — where polymerase chain reaction testing of CSF has now replaced brain biopsy as the 'best method' of diagnosis.

Direct Hybridization

Direct hybridization methods for the detection of nucleic acid sequences were widely applied in diagnosis but their relative lack of sensitivity when compared to methods involving amplification of target nucleic acid sequences has meant that in most instances their use has been restricted to situations where sensitivity is not the pre-requisite. Examples are in the rapid detection and genotyping of an organism where a sample contains an abundance of the specific nucleic acid, as in cell cultured virus, or in biopsy material (for example, papillomavirus

identification and genotyping using nucleic acid isolated from a tissue biopsy). Both homogeneous and heterogeneous solution (liquid) and solid phase (e.g. 'slot-blot' and 'dot-blot') hybridization techniques may be used. Hybridization techniques are now widely used in conjunction with nucleic acid amplification procedures. Techniques of sample preparation are essentially the same as those used in nucleic acid amplification procedures (see below).

Restriction Fragment Length Polymorphism (RFLP)

RFLP is a powerful tool for the study of viral pathogenesis, for the study of virus transmission, and for developing genotypic rather than serological classification of viruses. The technique can be used to compare viruses isolated at different times and/or from different body sites to aid the understanding of an infection. An example would be comparison of strains of herpes simplex isolated at peripheral sites with virus isolated from brain in an attempt to define the source of a patient's encephalitic illness. Alternatively, RFLP may be used during the investigation of an outbreak of virus infection, for example an epidemic of adenovirus kerato-conjunctivitis centred on an eye hospital (Fig. 22.1). Here, RFLP analysis of different viral isolates can give a clear indication of the source, or sources, of infection and provide information to enable the control of infection and prevention of future outbreaks. RFLP is also valuable in classification of viruses. Viruses are frequently subgrouped and classified according to phenotypic, serologically identified, differences. RFLP analysis can often enable more objective, rapid and clear-cut differentiation of viruses than serological typing, particularly for groups containing large numbers of serotypes.

Polymerase Chain Reaction (PCR)

The PCR was the first of the methods of nucleic acid amplification to be described and is the most widely applied and researched of these techniques. Several commercially produced assays using this technology are now available and a variety of instrumentation, ranging from

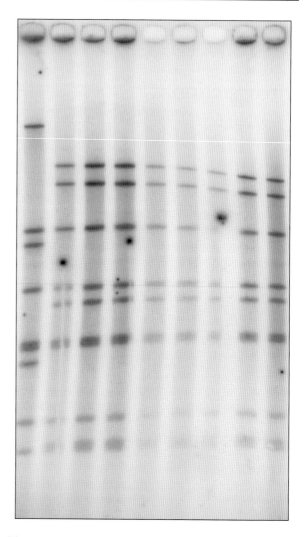

Figure 22.1: Autoradiograph showing an analysis of isolates of adenovirus type 8 collected during an outbreak of epidemic keratoconjunctivitis. Virus strains were propagated in Graham 293 cell cultures and DNA was labelled by the addition of ^{32}Phosphorus to cell culture medium. Viral DNA was extracted from cell culture lysates by proteinase-K digestion and phenol/chloroform extraction and ethanol precipitation. DNA was then digested with a restriction enzyme and the digest analysed by gel electrophoresis and autoradiography. The restriction pattern produced by the isolate run in lane 1 is clearly different to that produced by the isolates in lanes 2 to 9, indicating that the virus in lane 1 was from a different source to those analysed in lanes 2 to 9. The restriction fragments produced by digestion of the same DNAs with other restriction enzymes allow these isolates to be genotyped as adenovirus type 8. [Autoradiograph courtesy of Mr A S Bailey.]

a microcapillary system enabling thermal cycling to be completed within 15 to 20 minutes, through to automated equipment to allow unattended thermal cycling and product detection, is now available.

PCR has been applied widely in diagnostic virology. Whilst a very large number of techniques have been described on a research basis, fewer are actually applied in the routine laboratory. For day-to-day use a technique must be robust, that is, it must be reproducible, capable of being run by different operators while producing assays of similar sensitivity and specificity with 'wild type' viruses. One of the many potential pitfalls of the test is to develop an assay with well-characterized laboratory strains and not thoroughly test the assay with sufficient numbers of viruses to ensure that the full spectrum of strains of virus capable of causing disease are identified by the assay. A careful clinical evaluation must always be performed before the assay is applied to ensure that cases are not being missed.

Major uses of PCR
a) to diagnose infection
PCR has brought about a revolution in diagnosis particularly for viruses which are not readily cultured *in vitro*. Hepatitis C virus, an RNA virus found to be a major cause of post-transfusion hepatitis, can be rapidly identified using reverse transcription PCR. In viral meningitis, the application of enterovirus PCR to CSF enables prompt definition of the cause of aseptic meningitis in children, where previously diagnostic tests were very inefficient.

b) to assess response to chemotherapy
The application of PCR in the diagnosis of encephalitis has now been extended to the management of disease with monitoring of the efficiency of antiviral chemotherapy being accomplished by PCR of CSF collected post-treatment to ensure clearance of viral DNA in response to therapy.

c) to allow genotyping via RFLP or Southern blot (or ELISA) hybridization
An example of the important application of genotyping aided by PCR can again be found in hepatitis C infection. Analysis of PCR products by RFLP or hybridization with genotype-specific oligonucleotide probes (particularly within the 5′-non-coding region of the virus' genome) has led to the identification of different genotypes of the virus and to the definition of genotypes correlating with disease severity and resistance or susceptibility to treatment.

d) to monitor effects of therapy
Quantitative PCR has also been applied to monitoring of the efficacy of treatment in several diseases. A large increase in the use of quantitative techniques has occurred in monitoring AIDS chemotherapy. The rapid mutation of HIV means that drug resistance develops rapidly. Measurements of changes in the amount of virus circulating in plasma — monitored by quantitative PCR — are important in signalling the development of drug resistance.

e) to identify specific genomic mutations (e.g. those conferring resistance to antiviral chemotherapy)
The development of drug resistance can often be linked to specific point mutations in certain regions of the viral genome. PCR amplification followed by RFLP or specific hybridization with mutation-specific oligonucleotides can be used in rapid identification of the emergence of drug resistance.

Sample preparation
Type of sample
The range of samples which may be investigated is large and may, depending upon the virus and the stage of the infection, produce different results according to the clinical specimen investigated. The choice of methodology depends upon ease of use, efficiency (for example, recovery of virus from a CSF containing 100 or less viral genomes per ml needs to be more efficient than a method of extracting virus from vesicular fluid which may contain several million virus particles) and the final amplification technique to be used. Alternatives to extraction of total nucleic acids are to select virus from a sample and then extract nucleic acid from virus. Methods employing virus capture by antibody have been used. However,

Polymerase Chain Reaction (PCR)

Internal controls

Table 22.1:	Known inhibitors of Taq polymerase.
• Haem	• Urea
• Protein	• Polyamines
• EDTA	• Polysaccharides
• Heparin	• Calcium alginate
• Phenol	• DNAase or RNAase

whilst these methods work well when large numbers of the organism are present (e.g. with virus cultures) in 'real' clinical specimens their less than 100% efficiency in capture of virus reduces overall sensitivity. The same criticism may be levelled at methods in which virus nucleic acid is selected from a mixture of nucleic acids by hybridization of the viral nucleic acid before amplification.

Inhibitors

It is known that several substances are capable of inhibiting the activity of the thermostable enzymes used in the amplification reaction (Table 22.1) and thus methods aim to remove these inhibitors from the sample. Sample preparation methods show differences in the efficiency of removal of different inhibitors, thus the exact method employed depends upon the sample to be analysed. Protein can be denatured by simple boiling of the sample; degraded by digestion with proteinase-K — an enzyme with broad capability to degrade proteins; or removed by extraction with organic solvents (for example phenol and chloroform extraction followed by ethanolic precipitation of nucleic acids). The choice of method depends upon the sample to be investigated. Simple boiling often suffices for CSF specimens, proteinase-K treatment may be adequate for investigation of throat swabs, while protein-rich fluids such as serum may require extraction with organic solvents after proteinase-K digestion. Other inhibitors such as the urea found particularly in urine may require the use of partitioning and precipitating reagents such as polyethylene glycol or ion exchange methodologies. The choice of sample preparation method can also be affected by the genome of the virus to be detected. RNAases are much more prevalent in the environment than DNAases, thus sub-

stances such as guanidinium isothiocyanate which inactivates RNAases are often used in extraction of RNA, RNA being collected by precipitation with isopropanol.

Not all PCR techniques show the same sensitivity to inhibitors. Nested PCR techniques appear to be more robust than single round PCR techniques in this respect. The amplification reaction is a complex physico-chemical process and as yet probably only a small number of the range of potential inhibitors of enzyme activity have been identified. In addition to enzyme inhibitors there are further, incompletely understood, inhibitors affecting the physics and the chemistry of the reaction. Notwithstanding these potential difficulties, careful work has evolved – for individual sample types – robust and reliable methods of sample preparation.

Internal controls

A major advance in improving the reliability of PCR has been the introduction of internal controls. These are molecules which are either added to the sample prior to processing of the sample or, more usually, added to the amplification reaction 'cocktail' to which the sample will be added. The internal control molecule is a short length of nucleic acid which has the same primer binding regions as the target nucleic acid but produces an amplicon which is either longer or shorter than that produced by the target virus' nucleic acid; or produces a molecule which has a different inter-primer binding region nucleotide sequence to that employed by the standard amplicon. In the latter case the internal control amplificate can be distinguished from the target sequence by RFLP or hybridization (Fig. 22.2). The sequence will always be amplified provided no inhibitor for the amplification has been added to the reaction cocktail. The use of internal controls is increasing and has revealed that many of the previously accepted methods of sample preparation are in fact inadequate. False negative reactivity and partial inhibition, leading to reduced sensitivity, can be avoided by the use of these controls. The development of internal controls has also allowed the development of reliable methods for the quantitation of PCR.

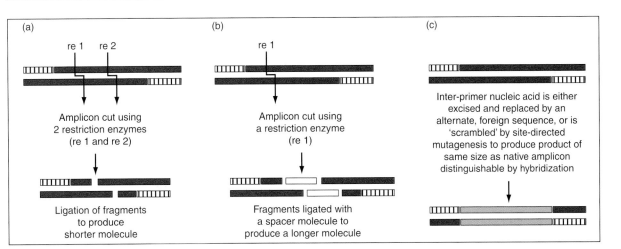

Figure 22.2: *Methods of producing an internal control molecule*

(a) *A small amount of DNA is excised from the amplicon by digestion of the amplicon with two restriction enzymes (or a single enzyme capable of cutting twice within the amplicon). The fragments are then ligated and re-PCR'd. The shortened molecule can then be added to reaction cocktails to provide an internal control molecule. Target and internal control amplification can be distinguished by size differences.*

(b) *An amplicon is lengthened by ligation of a 'spacer' oligonucleotide after cutting the amplicon with a restriction enzyme. The lengthened molecule is used as an internal control molecule and distinguished by size difference from the amplicons produced by the target DNA.*

(c) *Inter-primer nucleic acid is either replaced by foreign (i.e. non-target) DNA or the inter-primer DNA of the amplicon is 'scrambled'. The new amplicon is of the same size as that produced by the target nucleic acid but can be distinguished by hybridization.*

Amplification

Both single and nested PCR techniques are used. The nested PCR techniques are generally accepted as providing more sensitive detection of nucleic acid than single round PCR techniques. However, single round PCR techniques, particularly those in which methods of product detection are applied, achieve the same sensitivity as nested PCR techniques. In routine application the single PCR is less labour intensive than the nested PCR and less vulnerable to false positive reactivity through carryover contamination. In a conventional nested PCR, after the first round of amplification, the reaction tube is opened and a sample is transferred to a second reaction tube containing new primers. This opening of the tube can result in the liberation by aerosolization of a large number of amplicons which can then become templates for future PCRs. Care in laboratory design and a great deal of technical skill is required to minimize this possibility. One tube methods of nested PCR (e.g. the guanine-cytosine 'clamp' methods) have been devised to circumvent the need to open tubes after the first round of amplification.

RNA viruses require a pre-treatment step in which RNA is converted to cDNA by the action of a reverse transcriptase enzyme. The cDNA then serves as a template for PCR amplification. The thermostable enzyme rTth is now available to accomplish both reverse transcription and DNA polymerization within the same reaction tube by the use of a bicine buffer which provides (at different temperatures) optimum reverse transcriptase activity and alternately optimum DNA polymerase activity.

Often it is desirable to detect more than one organism in a clinical sample, thus 'multiplex' PCRs have been devised to allow the detection of a number of different targets within a clinical sample. An example is in eye infection. A patient presenting with symptoms of keratoconjunctivitis may be suffering herpes simplex virus, adenovirus or *Chlamydia trachomatis* infection. To diagnose infection three separate, expensive, time-consuming PCR tests would be required which in turn may consume limited supplies of a precious sample. Instead, the addition of primers for each organism to a reaction cocktail (together with careful re-optimization of reaction components and thermal cycling parameters) allows detection of each of the organisms within the same test. A further example is in neurological disease in AIDS patients. A very wide number of organisms can infect the CNS in AIDS. Large volumes of CSF would be required to allow PCRs to detect all possible organisms. By exploiting homologies and also differences in sequences found within the DNA polymerase gene of herpesviruses it has been possible to devise PCR tests to detect all of the human herpesviruses within a single reaction tube. A first round common amplification reaction amplifies the DNA polymerase and a second round selection differentiates the individual viruses by an ELISA based hybridization using specific oligonucleotide probe sequences (Fig. 22.3). This rapid single tube detection system achieves the speed of specific diagnosis which is so important for the early application of antiviral chemotherapy.

Detection
Detection of the products of amplification is most easily achieved by electrophoresis followed by ethidium bromide staining and UV illumination. However, if more information than the production of an amplicon of defined molecular size is required then hybridization techniques (Southern blotting or solution hybridization) can be used. A number of commercial assays are now available which utilize a simple-to-perform ELISA-type test for product detection. The oligonucleotide probe sequences are either immobilized on a microtitre plate or membrane, or they are reacted in solution and then entrapped on microtitre plates or magnetizable particles to effect separation of hybrids from the other reaction components.

Automation is now becoming available for PCR. A machine automating both thermal cycling and production detection (via a magnetic particle based ELISA) is now available. Further development is expected to enable sample preparation to also become a part of the automated process.

Alternative Nucleic Acid Amplification Methodologies

A number of alternative nucleic acid amplification methodologies have been developed, some of which, as in PCR, result in amplification of the target nucleic acid and some of which result in the amplification of a probe binding to the original target nucleic acid. At the time of writing three methodologies are generally available as commercial products: the gapped ligase chain reaction (LCR) developed by Abbott Laboratories; the nucleic acid sequence-based amplification (NASBA) developed by Organon Teknika; and the branched DNA (bDNA) signal amplification assay developed by the Chiron Corporation. All of these assays utilize a high degree of automation. For clinical laboratories automation is an immediate attraction since it simplifies the introduction of the new technology.

In situ PCR

The generic term *in situ* PCR encompasses PCR *in situ* hybridization and its equivalents for detection of RNA viruses or mRNA transcripts – reverse transcription *in situ* PCR and reverse transcription PCR *in situ* hybridization. Further developments are in progress involving alternative amplification methods such as *in situ* LCR or signal amplification in situ (bDNA). The technology enables the detection of specific nucleic acid sequences within a single cell and this ability has great potential in the study of viruses which establish latent or slow and persistent infection. In contrast to the situation in acute virus infection, in latent or persistent infection virus-infected cells comprise only a small fraction of the total number of cells in the tissue or tissue fluids under examination. Thus

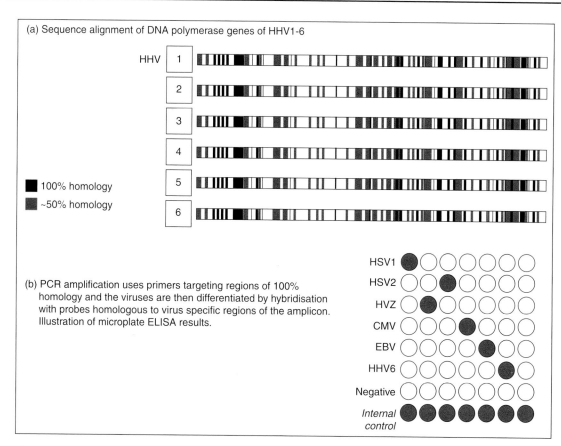

Figure 22.3: *Alignment of sequences of the DNA polymerase gene of each of the human herpesviruses showing regions of complete, partial or no homology. Detection and differentiation of the different viruses is accomplished by a PCR amplification using primers designed to bind to regions of 100% sequence homology followed by denaturation of product DNA and hybridization in a microplate ELISA with oligonucleotide probe sequences exploiting sequence dissimilarity.*

conventional *in situ* hybridization methods may not reveal infection. The techniques provide important tools for the study of viral pathogenesis. In addition they provide powerful procedures for the examination of archival postmortem specimens, opening an extensive avenue for review of diseases of unknown aetiology.

Sample preparation is of great importance for these techniques. The objective of sample preparation is to provide within single cells a discrete reaction chamber to contain the PCR reaction. Cells, either in suspension or fixed to some form of solid phase support, are rendered sufficiently permeable so that oligonucleotide primers and other reaction components may diffuse into the cell. The permeation is con-

trolled so that the products of amplification are retained within the cells upon thermal amplification and tissue morphology is retained so that meaningful histopathological interpretations can be made. Typical pretreatments are to fix cells or tissue in formalin or paraformaldehyde and affix the cells or tissue to glass slides using (for example) Denhardt's solution (dewaxing and rehydration is necessary for paraffin wax-embedded tissues). Tissues or cells are then digested with a carefully optimized low concentration of proteinase-K over 60 minutes to prepare for *in situ* PCR. A number of alternatives have been described including detergent, chemical denaturant, or microwave pre-treatments.

Discovery of 'New' Viruses

A new and exciting phase in the diagnosis of infection has begun with the identification of the agents responsible for a wide variety of diseases, and long suspected to have an infectious cause. Perhaps the first agent identified solely through the use of a molecular biological approach was hepatitis C virus. Despite enormous research effort the identity of this agent remained elusive until 1989. Nucleic acid was extracted from a pool of chimpanzee plasma known to transmit the infection. The extracted nucleic acid was inserted in plasmids capable of protein expression when transfected in bacteria. These bacterial 'expression libraries' were then screened with sera from patients recovering from non-A non-B hepatitis. Reactive samples were used to construct a further yeast expressed plasmid to produce a protein which could be used to develop an ELISA for antibody detection. This ELISA, and its progressive refinements, showed that the new agent – hepatitis C – was the major (but not sole cause of) post-transfusion hepatitis. The methodology – complementary cDNA library screening – has also been applied in the discovery of a further cause of post-transfusion hepatitis, hepatitis G virus.

The speed with which a novel agent can now be defined is illustrated by the identification of the agent responsible for a severe, frequently fatal, acute respiratory disease in a remote part of the south-western United States. Between May and June 1993 thirteen deaths associated with an acute form of adult respiratory distress syndrome with unusual and distinctive pathology, were reported. First autopsies were performed on 14th May 1993 and by 4th June 1993 the agent responsible – a new, previously unrecognized member of the Hantavirus group was defined as the cause. Initial serological studies had shown the serum of patients cross-reacted with known hantavirus antigens. PCR primers were designed based upon consensus sequences within the G2 protein coding region of the M segment of the genomes of known hantaviruses and used in reverse transcription nested PCR to amplify a short sequence of the viral genome from autopsy tissues. The vector for this novel virus was rapidly identified – *Peromyscus maniculatus*, the deer mouse – and methods for the control of infection were rapidly deployed. Similar technology, known as 'consensus sequence based PCR', has been used in the identification of the cause of cat-scratch disease (and in immunocompromised patients, bacillary angiomatosis), a newly recognized bacterium *Bartonella henselae*, and in identifying the cause of Whipple's disease, a new Gram-positive actinomycete, *Tropheryma whippelii*.

One of the newest and perhaps most robust method of identifying a new agent, since it requires no prior knowledge of an agent's class, is 'representational difference analysis' (Fig. 22.4). In this technique PCR is used to enrich DNA present in diseased tissue but absent from healthy tissue of the same patient. The DNA is first digested using a restriction enzyme. PCR primers are then ligated to the DNA and the DNA is non-specifically amplified. As PCR preferentially amplifies fragments of 150 to 1500 bp, restriction fragments within this size range are enriched. To identify unique – disease specific – sequences a subtractive hybridization process is applied. Using this technology a new herpesvirus, human herpesvirus 8, has been identified in Kaposi's sarcoma and in a rare subset of AIDS-related, body cavity-based lymphomas.

Summary

The explosion of applications of molecular biological techniques in virology and in particular in diagnostic virology which has occurred since 1989 continues to gather pace. In diagnostic virology molecular biological procedures are likely to supplant many of the currently accepted methods for diagnosis including virus isolation in cell culture, many serological diagnostic tests, and even current 'rapid' diagnostic tests such as immunofluorescence, ELISA and electron microscopy. The application of automation will reduce the technical complexities of testing, while improving reliability and reproducibility. Already the wider application of technologies is leading to a reduction in cost

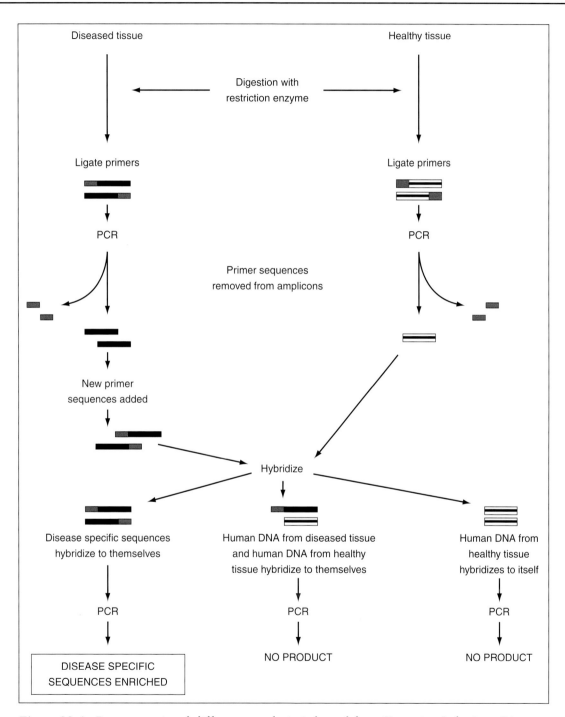

Figure 22.4: *Representational difference analysis (adapted from Emerging Infectious Diseases 1996; 2:159–167).*

of procedures involving nucleic acid amplification and cost per test is likely, in time, to reduce to the current costs of ELISA proce- dures. Whilst PCR presently dominates, alterna- tive amplification techniques will 'catch up' and the virus laboratory of the future is likely to apply a range of different techniques each optimized for the diagnosis of individual virus infections. In addition to this the virus laboratory will become much more involved in disease management, advising on changes in drug therapy and dosage as a consequence of the development of tools for monitoring 'viral load' and the identification of drug resistance.

Further Reading

Chang Y, Cesarman E, Pessin MS *et al*. Identification of herpesvirus-like DNA sequences in AIDS-associated Kaposi's sarcoma. *Science* 1994; **26**: 1865–1869.

Cinque P, Cleator G M, Weber T, Monteyne P, Van Loon A M et al. The role of laboratory investigation in the diagnosis and management of patients with suspected herpes encephalitis: a consensus report. *Journal of Neurology, Neurosurgery and Psychiatry* 1996; **61**: 339–345.

Di Domenico N, Link H, Knobec R, Caratsch T, Weschler W, Loewy Z G, Rosenstrans M. COBAS AMPLICOR[TM]: Fully automated RNA and DNA amplification and detection system for routine diagnostic PCR. *Clin Cham* 1996; **42**: 1945–1923.

DNA Technology and rapid diagnosis of infection. *Lancet* 1989; **ii**: 897–898.

Houghton M. Hepatitis C viruses. In: *Fields Virology*, 3rd edn 1996. Eds: Fields B N, Knipe D M, Howley P M et al. Lippincott-Raven Publishers, Philadelphia.

Katzenstein D A, Hammer S M, Hughes M D *et al*., for the ACTG 175 Virology Study Team: The relationship of virological and immunological markers to clinical outcomes after nucleoside therapy in HIV-infected adults with 200 to 500 CD4 cells per cubic millimeter. *N Eng J of Med* 1996; **335**: 1091–1098.

23 OTHER TESTS IN VIROLOGY

Alex W L Joss

This chapter includes a description of techniques which are outside the remit of most viral diagnostic laboratories but are of great general interest: prion disease, antiviral susceptibility and cell mediated immunity.

Detection of Prion Infection

Prions are classed as a separate infectious entity because most research workers believe they lack any nucleic acid and consist solely of *protein-aceous infectious* (prion) particles. They belong in this section for several reasons: they are subviral in composition; historically, they were termed slow virus infections; and minority opinion still maintains that they are really viruses, 'nemaviruses'. They cause brain disease, transmissible spongiform encephalopathy (TSE), whereby accumulation of prion protein results in nervous tissue vacuolation and neurodegeneration manifesting clinically as slowly progressive dementia, ataxia, sleep and eating disorders, leading inevitably to death. Diseases include: scrapie in sheep; BSE in cattle; and four types of human disease, Gerstmann–Straussler–Scheinker disease (GSS), fatal familial insomnia (FFI), Creutzfeldt–Jacob disease (CJD), kuru, plus a fifth if the variant CJD (vCJD) associated with the BSE epidemic is included (Fig. 23.1). Before considering the question of diagnosis, it is essential to understand some of the background and theoretical mechanism of the infectious process as then the difficulties inherent in diagnosis can be appreciated.

The essence of prion disease is the corruption of the α-helical conformation of a normal, essential neuronal membrane protein (PrP^c) to a protease-resistant β-sheet conformation (PrP^{Res}), the deposition of which leads to neurological degeneration (Fig. 23.1). The proposition that protein alone (PrP^{Res}) can induce this change is supported by *in vitro* evidence, but the definitive experiment to prove that corrupted PrP^c is able to propagate 'infection' in a new host has yet to be done.

Of the human prion diseases, GSS and FFI arise from various point mutations in the PrP^c gene which are genetically transmitted within families (Fig. 23.1). CJD arises sporadically, again with evidence of point mutation, or perhaps also over-expression of the PrP^c gene. The infectious aspect of CJD is its proven iatrogenic transmission, from dural or corneal grafts or pituitary hormone extracts, and the possibility of accidental infection when handling brain tissue. Kuru, recognized as the consequence of cannibalistic practices in Papua New Guinea, more easily fits the picture of an infectious process. Similarly, artificial cannibalism of ovine or bovine brain leads to BSE infection, and subsequent ingestion of BSE-infected neural tissue probably produced vCJD which is histologically and epidemiologically distinct from CJD. Interspecies transmission occurs more readily the more closely related the PrP^c of the recipient is to that of the source. Ovine and bovine PrP^c only differ at seven residues, whereas bovine and human PrP^c differ by 30

Detection of Prion Infection

Diagnosis

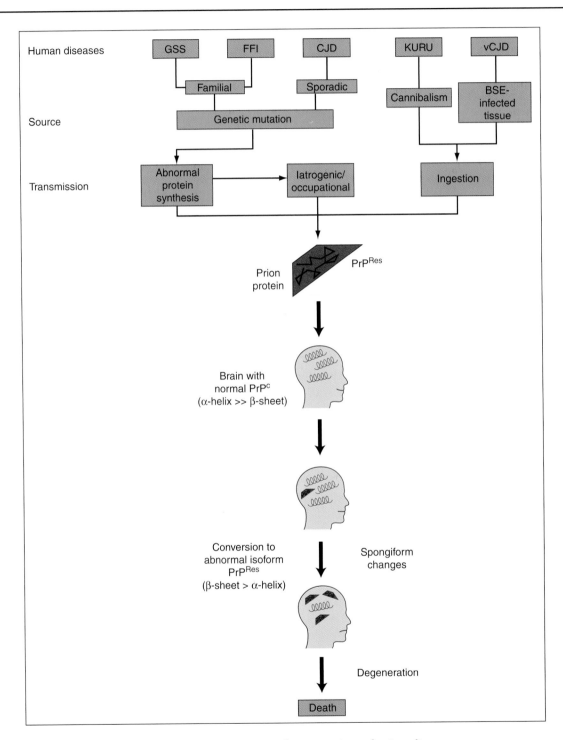

Figure 23.1: *Mechanisms for transmission and progression of prion disease.*

residues. Nevertheless, all TSEs with the exception of FFI have been transmitted experimentally to a range of species.

Diagnosis

The characteristics which make diagnosis so difficult are the disease site, the closeness of the

242

pathogen to its host equivalent, and its apparent lack of nucleic acid. Brain is unlikely to be biopsied when therapy remains unavailable unless to exclude other treatable diseases, and small samples may be falsely negative. Clinical signs of CJD, which usually occur in older age, are not diagnostic, but may be more so in a younger person, as with vCJD. Electroencephalography is generally regarded as useful, although not specific. Periodic sharp wave complexes and reactivity to external stimuli or drugs are prominent observations. Physiological measurements are generally unhelpful.

Histology
A definitive diagnosis of prion disease requires evidence of PrP^{Res} deposition, in human brain itself, or after transmission to animal brain. Congo red stained amyloid plaques, loosely packed PrP synaptic deposits, spongiform changes, neurofibrillary tangles and subcortical gliosis are all histological features consistent with the diagnosis. However, all of these features are shared in varying degrees with other neurodegenerative disorders, as for example amyloid plaques in Alzheimer's disease. They can be related specifically to prion disease using immunohistochemistry.

Prion-specific antibody is not easy to produce but polyclonal rabbit antisera have been raised: against purified amyloid plaque cores from human brain or CJD-infected mouse brain; and against synthetic peptides equivalent to the altered sequences in human prion. Formalin-fixed paraffin wax-embedded tissue can be tested but pretreatment with a protein denaturant is essential to enhance immunoreactivity.

Formic acid is the simplest and most effective denaturant, but may be superseded by 'hydrolytic autoclaving' to 121°C for 10 minutes in an appropriate concentration of hydrochloric acid. Prion deposition is then identified by binding specific antibody which is visualized by reaction with an enzyme-labelled (biotin–streptavidin or peroxidase–antiperoxidase) or fluorescent conjugate. Different prion strains produce varying proportions of the two principal pathologies, amyloid plaques (GSS, kuru) or punctate synaptic deposits (CJD), while human vCJD and BSE-infected macaque monkey brains yield abundant florid cortical plaques intersperced with vacuoles in a daisy-like pattern.

Electron microscopy
Tubulofilamentous particles, often over 1 μm long, are diagnostic features seen in impressions of moistened freshly cut brain tissue, touched on to electron microscope grids and negatively stained with phosphotungstic acid. These are distinguishable from the neurofibrillary filaments seen in Alzheimer's disease. It has been suggested, from protease and nuclease digestion evidence, that the filaments are tri-layer 'nemavirus' particles, composed of prion fibrils enclosed successively in non-host single-stranded DNA and protein. Electron microscopy diagnosis may fail due to random sampling of uninfected tissue, but it can find positive evidence of infection in animals before other histological changes become apparent.

Culture
Apart from FFI, prion 'infections' can be confirmed by passage in mice or hamsters. Diagnosis is slow, requiring at least 60 days to demonstrate characteristic histology in inoculated brains, and longer than a mouse lifetime for some slower growing strains. Transmission success can be low, but BSE crosses the species barrier more easily and may be transmitted orally. Human prions can be expressed in tissue culture (e.g. Chinese hamster ovary cells) but no cytopathic effect is evident. Cell-free *in vitro* culture, if it can be so described, has been developed in which radio-labelled PrP^c was converted to PrP^{Res} in two days on exposure to unlabelled scrapie prion. However, the latter had to be purified and added in fifty-fold excess, suggesting the technique requires refinement to have diagnostic applications.

Immunoblotting
Rapid diagnosis, within one day, can be achieved on small brain samples by immunoblotting. Proteinase K-digested tissue, separated on polyacrylamide SDS gels and electrophoretically transferred to nitrocellulose membranes, yields three bands of 16–31 KDa, representing non-, mono-, and diglycosylated PrP^{Res}, which react

with prion-specific antiserum. Their size and intensity ratios can distinguish VCJD from CJD. These are not found in Alzheimer's disease and normal PrPc is fully digested by proteinase K. CJD in humans is usually only detectable in brain or spinal cord, but the ability to detect VCJD in tonsilar tissue should facilitate preclinical diagnosis.

Nucleic acid technology
How far these techniques will succeed depends on the evolution of the protein-only versus 'nemavirus' controversy. Nemavirus proponents have prepared a probe from scrapie-infected brain extract which reacts with a 1.2 *kilobase* DNA band from scrapie, BSE and CJD brain tissue but not normal brain. If confirmed this might provide a sensitive method of detecting infection. Failing this, it could still be possible to diagnose inherited prion disorders by polymerase chain reaction specific to mutated PrPc genes.

Tests in other tissues or body fluids
All the methods discussed so far are performed on brain tissue. Diagnosis would be simpler on more accessible material. The lack of serological techniques is a major gap in the potential for the diagnosis of prion disease. An indication of the immune system's ignorance of the difference between prion and normal PrPc is the absence of any inflammatory infiltration of infected brain. This contrasts with the position in another neurodegenerative disorder, multiple sclerosis, when a strong autoimmune response is mounted against myelin basic protein. The fact that PrPc is found in tissues outside the brain, even on the surface of T-lymphocytes, is thought to account for this immune tolerance. Immunoblotting on cerebrospinal fluid has identified two abnormal polypeptides in TSE patients. Although also found in patients with Herpes encephalitis, they may yet be diagnostic when distinguishing prion from Alzheimer's disease. Urine or blood are other suggested target fluids, especially the latter using assays based on a monoclonal specific to PrPRes epitopes to identify 'infected' white cells.

In conclusion, current diagnostic methods for prion disease are slow, invasive and often achieved only at autopsy. Although the nature of the disease severely limits the usual approaches to diagnosis, there has been progress in devising reliable methodology. However, any evidence that vCJD is more than a rare, passing phenomenon will provide urgent impetus for more rapid and available techniques.

Antiviral Susceptibility Tests

Antiviral susceptibility assays are not yet regularly carried out in many routine virology laboratories. Tests take several days or weeks to perform and are therefore only likely to benefit patients who require lengthy therapy. They are more likely to occur in laboratories dealing with large numbers of immunocompromised patients, perhaps to monitor human immunodeficiency virus (HIV) antiviral resistance, or to identify resistant herpes group viruses in such patients. In practice, decisions to change antiviral therapy are based often on empirical evidence of resistance, i.e. failure to respond clinically (Fig. 23.2). Another commonly used approach is to measure surrogate markers of emerging resistance, such as failure of viral antigen or nucleic acid levels in blood to fall in response to therapy. True susceptibility assays are of two categories: phenotypic, which measure the effect of the antiviral on virus growth *in vitro*; or genotypic, which directly detect the presence of mutants which confer resistance.

Phenotypic assays
Phenotypic assays provide the definitive proof of antiviral resistance. They measure the antiviral concentration required to inhibit either the overall cytopathic effect (CPE) of virus growth on culture cells or specific stages of viral metabolism, namely DNA or protein synthesis. Virus has first to be propagated in tissue culture, a step which itself can confound the result by altering the proportion of resistant mutants subsequently tested. Tests are therefore done preferably on isolates which have been passaged a few times. HIV is often isolated from peripheral blood mononuclear cells

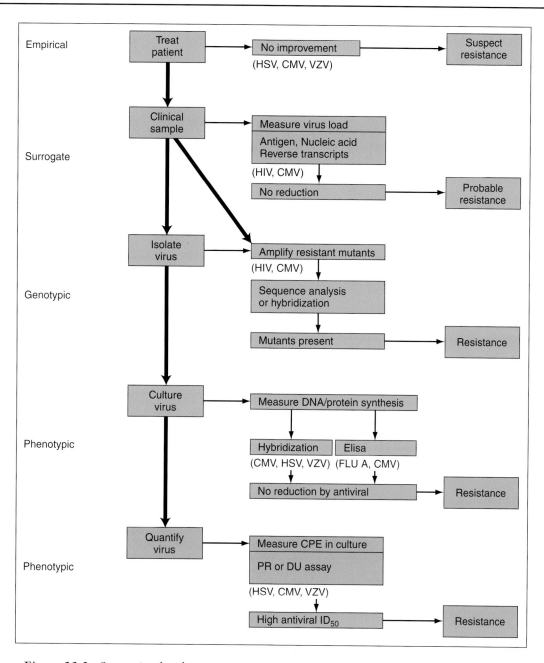

Figure 23.2: *Strategies for determining antiviral resistance.*

(PBMC) by co-culture with a lymphoblastoid cell line, another added complication.

Plaque reduction (PR) assays

When cell monolayers are seeded with diluted virus in conditions which limit virus movement, i.e. under a solid agar or cellulose overlay, or liquid containing antiviral immunoglobulin, each virus plaque forming unit (pfu) produces a discrete CPE plaque. Addition of serially diluted antiviral together with fixed titrated amounts of virus (15–500 pfu) allows measurement of antiviral susceptibility as the concentration which causes 50% plaque reduction

Antiviral Susceptibility Tests

(ID_{50}). PR assays only detect resistant strains which constitute more than 20–25% of the isolate. Lower proportions may be detected using a 90% plaque reduction threshold, but ID_{90} measurements are less accurate than ID_{50}.

PR assays have the advantage of using relatively inexpensive routine culture techniques. Disadvantages are the volumes of reagents, media and virus used and time required to standardize cell, virus and antiviral concentrations and to manually count plaques in replicate cultures. Overall test time is at least two weeks. The virus to cell ratio must be optimized to avoid generating falsely high or low susceptibility estimates when ratios are respectively too low or too high. Appropriate controls should include tests on reference susceptible and resistant virus strains. Herpes simplex (HSV) susceptibility testing can be speeded up by prescreening isolates in parallel with titrating their infectivity. Three days incubation of serial viral dilutions, with and without acyclovir at 1.5 times the accepted resistance threshold concentration, gives preliminary identification of resistant and susceptible strains.

PR assays are the gold standard for detection of HSV, cytomegalovirus (CMV) and varicella-zoster (VZV) resistance. Accepted resistance thresholds have been established: 2 μg/ml for acyclovir, 100 μg/ml for foscarnet and for ganciclovir a three- to fourfold increase in ID_{50} compared to pretherapy. An HIV PR assay measures reduction of syncytial plaques on adherent monolayers of HT4-6C cells, a HeLa line expressing human CD4 receptor. Results correlate well with those of similar assays in lymphoblastoid cells. However, the lengthy procedures involved and low isolation rates, frequently as low as 30%, make HIV PR assays less useful clinically than more rapid genotypic assays.

Dye uptake (DU assays)

The semi-automated technology of a DU assay suits laboratories with a higher throughout and avoids the tedium and subjectivity of plaque counting. Similar principles apply, testing constant virus concentrations against serial dilutions of antiviral, but the CPE after two to three days incubation is measured spectrophotometrically. The amounts of neutral red dye absorbed by surviving viable cells, in one hour, then eluted into buffered alcohol, produce optical density readings which are inversely proportional to CPE and virus titres. They can be read and computed automatically to ID_{50} values. Because liquid overlays are used, ID_{50} estimates are higher than in PR assays and resistance thresholds are therefore raised, e.g. from 2 to 3 μg/ml for acyclovir. Dye pH is critical, otherwise erroneous readings may result from dye precipitation. The technique, in microtitre plates, requires less reagents and will detect resistant strains constituting only 3–9% of a total isolate. However, PR assays more accurately predict clinical failure due to resistance.

DNA synthesis assays

Viral DNA synthesis in culture cells can be quantified by hybridization with specific radio-labelled DNA probes. Antiviral ID_{50} is measured as the concentration which causes a 50% reduction in the signal from bound probe. In the commercial Hybriwix assay, DNA is released at the end of a defined period of virus growth in the wells of the kit cell culture plate using lysis buffer, transferred by capillary action to nylon 'wicks', dried on and hybridized with ^{125}I-labelled probe. After washing, bound probe is counted in a gamma counter. In an alternative dot blot assay, DNA after viral growth is transferred and dried on to nitrocellulose filters, then hybridized with ^{32}P-labelled probes. These assays are faster than PR assays, producing results in four to six days, and have been used to detect resistance in HSV, CMV and VZV strains. Drawbacks are their cost and the short shelf-life of the probes.

Acyclovir resistance in HSV or VZV strains may be confirmed by demonstrating the mechanism of resistance. Most resistant strains show mutation in the thymidine kinase (TK) gene, which makes them unable to phosphorylate and activate acyclovir. TK deficiency can be measured in radiolabel incorporation assays in appropriate cell lines, as a reduced signal on plaque autoradiography, using either ^{125}I-iododeoxycytidine or ^{14}C-thymidine. A reduced ability to incorporate these nucleosides corre-

OTHER TESTS IN VIROLOGY

Antiviral Susceptibility Tests
Genotypic assays
Conclusions
Cell Mediated Immunity
Proliferation assays

lates well with inability to phosphorylate acyclovir.

Protein synthesis assays

For some viruses, growth can be monitored by the appearance of readily identifiable virus proteins in culture cells. The best example is influenza A haemagglutinin which can be detected on canine kidney monolayers 18 hours after infection, using monoclonal antibody in an enzyme-linked immunosorbent assay (ELISA). Resistance to amantadine or rimantadine is demonstrated as a failure to reduce ELISA optical density readings, i.e. haemagglutinin synthesis, except at high antiviral concentrations. This assay clearly discriminates resistant from susceptible strains, more successfully than PR assays, and is the method of choice for influenza A. Similar assays are available for HSV, VZV and CMV, detecting early or late proteins.

Genotypic assays

When point mutations within specific virus genes are known to confer antiviral resistance, they can be assayed directly, either in virus isolates or in clinical specimens, usually blood. Four HIV reverse transcriptase gene mutations, which confer azidothymidine resistance, are detected in this way, usually by polymerase chain reaction (PCR) amplification, followed by sequence analysis or hybridization with specific probes. Mutations in CMV phosphotransferase or DNA polymerase genes, and influenza A transmembrane protein gene, have also been linked with antiviral resistance, thus providing targets for genotypic assays. The advantage of this approach is its directness, avoiding the need to isolate, grow and quantify virus. It is not just technically faster; resistance mutants may be identified in blood before resistant virus is isolated. Disadvantages are cost, technique sophistication and the inability to detect resistance when the specific mutation(s) are unknown.

Conclusions

In clinical practice, decisions to change antiviral therapy on empirical or surrogate marker evidence are likely to continue. However, there is still a place for *in vitro* susceptibility testing to confirm resistance. Acyclovir-resistant HSV strains become latent infrequently, but when they do recur foscarnet is indicated as first-choice therapy. CMV or HIV resistance may display focal heterogenicity, e.g. resistant CMV retinal isolates concurrent with sensitive systemic isolates, which will influence treatment strategy. In HIV infection, confirmation of high level azidothymidine resistance is a poor prognostic sign. Recent years have seen rapid innovation in antiviral therapy and screening potentially useful compounds has obviously relied on good susceptibility assays. The introduction of more new antivirals, the assessment of combined therapy and investigation of conflicting data on *in vitro* and *in vivo* resistance should all increase demand for this methodology.

Cell Mediated Immunity

An effective cellular immune response is important in overcoming viral infection, yet routine laboratory investigations centre almost exclusively on the humoral response. Cellular immunity tests are much less amenable to large throughput than are serological tests. Apart from research studies, these tests are reserved for investigations of deficiency, such as failure to overcome herpes group infections. The measurement of CD4 markers in HIV infection is technically an investigation of cellular immunocompetence, but typical *in vitro* assays assess two aspects of lymphocyte function, ability to recognise virus using proliferation assays and ability to destroy infected cells, using cytotoxicity assays.

Proliferation assays

Patients' fresh peripheral blood lymphocytes (PBL) in culture medium are stimulated to proliferate by external activators, mitogens such as phytohaemagglutinin (PHA) or, more specifically, viral antigens. Several days incubation are required, at the end of which proliferation is measured as the amount of radiolabelled thymidine incorporated into DNA in the last few hours, quantified by liquid scintillation counting of acid precipitated, washed cells. Tests compare the response of patient T-lymphocytes to a particular virus to that of unstimulated (negative) or PHA-stimulated (positive) controls. Assays are done at least in triplicate and, when done on serial dilutions of PBL, estimate the number of circulating T-lymphocytes that recognize virus antigen, the responder cell frequency. Individual purified antigens or crude infected cell extracts can be assessed.

Cytotoxicity assays

Cytotoxicity assays can be performed on a variety of different leucocyte populations, antibody-dependent killer cells, non-specific natural killer cells, monocytes, but it is the cytotoxic T-lymphocyte (CTL) response that is most relevant in this context. These can be enriched from the PBL fraction by adsorption–elution procedures using monoclonal antibodies or flow cytometry. The test again involves several days culture, but this time to measure their effector activity on virus-containing target cells. Target cells should be histocompatible with patients' CTL and may be fibroblasts, B-lymphocytes, macrophages or tumour cells expressing viral antigens following either infection, transfection or pulses with viral peptides. Activity of CTL is measured by the release of radioactive chromium from labelled target cells over a short period at the end of the incubation. Tests involve replicate cultures, usually of serially diluted CTL, and measure the number of effector cells killing a specific percentage of a predetermined number of target cells. Data analysis is complex, and a well-controlled test protocol, with appropriate statistical methology, is essential. Active CTL should be detectable in patients with acute, persistent or reactivated viral infection.

In summary, these tests do not fit easily into the operational schedules of a routine diagnostic laboratory. They are time-consuming, use radioactivity, have all the maintenance problems of the most complex in-house methods and require a regular supply of control PBL, from volunteers. Properly controlled cytotoxicity assays should monitor day-to-day variation in results on cryopreserved high and low toxicity control CTL, and these in turn should be controlled using fresh CTL from volunteers, matched to patients for age, sex and time of collection. Normal ranges should be established from a large group of volunteers. The scale of requirements for controls relative to the infrequency of patient tests calls for specialist expertise. It is in such a setting that research is likely to be carried out, on efficacy of new viral vaccines and questions such as the contribution of impaired cell-mediated immunity to prolonged CMV excretion or the precise defects which lead to AIDS progression. Nevertheless, individual patients with severe recurrent HSV, VZV or EBV infections also require investigation to reveal the precise dysfunction in cellular immunity, and to suggest and monitor treatment strategies. Simpler, more widely adaptable CTL assays would make such investigation easier and probably more common.

Further Reading

Arvin, A M. Cell-mediated immunity to Varicella-Zoster Virus. *J. Infect. Dis.* 1992; **166**(Suppl 1), S35–41.

Kimberlin, D W, Spector, S A, Hill, E L, Biron, K K, Hay, A J, Mayers D L et al. Assays for antiviral drug resistance. *Antiviral Research* 1995; **26**, 403–13.

Narang, H K. Scrapie – associated tubulofilamentous particles in human Creutzfeldt–Jacob disease. *Res. Virol.* 1992; **143**, 387–95.

Safrin, S, Elbeik, T, Mills, J. A rapid screen test for in vitro susceptibility of clinical Herpes Simplex Virus isolates. *J. Infect. Dis.* 1994; **169**, 879–82.

Tateishi, J, Kitamoto, T. Developments in diagnosis for prion diseases. *Brit. Med. Bull.* 1993; **49**, 971–9.

24 MYCOLOGY

David W Warnock

Introduction

Among the 50 000 to 250 000 species of fungi that have been described, fewer than 500 have been identified as human pathogens. With few exceptions, these organisms are found in the environment and human infections are acquired through inhalation, ingestion or traumatic implantation. Human mycoses can be divided into three broad groups: superficial, subcutaneous or systemic.

The superficial mycoses are infections limited to the outermost layers of the skin, the nails and hair, and the mucous membranes. The principal infections in this group are dermatophytosis and candidosis. The aetiological agents of these diseases are dependent on the living host for their survival, but differ from one another in the manner by which this is achieved. The aetiological agents of dermatophytosis (the dermatophytes, *Microsporum* and *Trichophyton* species) depend on person-to-person spread for their survival, while the aetiological agents of candidosis, of which *Candida albicans* is the most important, are normal commensals of the gastrointestinal tract. These organisms do not produce disease unless some change in the host lowers its natural defences. In this situation, endogenous infection results in superficial or systemic infection.

The subcutaneous mycoses are infections involving the dermis, subcutaneous tissues and bone. Among the infections in this group are chromoblastomycosis, mycetoma and sporotrichosis. These diseases are most common in tropical and sub-tropical regions and are usually acquired as a result of the traumatic implantation of organisms that are found in the environment. The disease may remain localized at the site of implantation or spread to adjacent tissue. More widespread dissemination of the infection, through the blood or lymphatics, is uncommon, and usually only occurs if the host is in some way debilitated.

The systemic mycoses are infections that usually originate in the respiratory or gastrointestinal tracts, but may spread to many other organs. The organisms that cause these diseases can be divided into two distinct groups: the true pathogens and the opportunists. The first of these groups consists of a small number of organisms, such as *Histoplasma capsulatum*, that are able to invade the tissues of a normal host with no recognizable predisposition. Apart from histoplasmosis, the principal infections caused by members of this group are blastomycosis, coccidioidomycosis and paracoccidioidomycosis. The second group of pathogens, the opportunists, contains a much larger number of less well-adapted organisms, such as *Aspergillus fumigatus*, that are only able to invade the tissues of a debilitated or immunocompromised host. Apart from aspergillosis, the principal infections caused by members of this group are candidosis, cryptococcosis and mucormycosis. With the exception of candidosis, which is usually acquired from the patient's own endogenous reservoir, most systemic fungal infections are acquired from the environment rather than as a result of person-to-person spread.

As with other microbial infections, the diagnosis of fungal infection depends upon a combination of clinical observation and laboratory investigation. Superficial and subcutaneous fungal infections often produce characteristic lesions which suggest the diagnosis, but laboratory tests are essential where this is not the case, either because the clinical signs mimic those of other conditions or because the appearance of lesions has been altered by previous treatment. In most situations where systemic fungal infection is entertained as a diagnosis, the clinical presentation is nonspecific and can be caused by a wide range of infections, underlying illnesses, or complications of treatment.

The successful laboratory diagnosis of fungal infection depends in major part on the collection of adequate specimens for investigation. It is also dependent on the selection of appropriate microbiological and serological test procedures. These differ from one mycosis to another, and depend on the site of infection as well as the presenting symptoms and clinical signs. Interpretation of the results of laboratory investigations can sometimes be made with confidence, but at times the findings may be unhelpful or even misleading.

Laboratory methods for the diagnosis of fungal infection remain based on three broad approaches: the microscopical detection of the aetiological agent in clinical material; its isolation and identification in culture; and the detection of an immunological response to the pathogen or some other marker of its presence, such as a metabolic product. The search for more rapid methods of diagnosis is important because the earlier treatment is started, the better the prognosis.

Microscopic Examination

Fungal cells are much larger and easier to detect than bacterial cells on microscopic examination of clinical material. In some instances, microscopic examination will permit a tentative or definitive diagnosis to be made, long before growth is apparent in culture. In other instances, observation of fungal elements in a clinical specimen is more significant than isolating the fungus in culture, particularly if the organism is a common contaminant.

Although fungal cells are larger than bacterial cells, these organisms are often present in much smaller numbers in clinical specimens. For this reason, it is often essential to increase the concentration of fungal elements in a specimen before it is examined. Fluids and secretions should be centrifuged and the deposit retained for mycological investigation. Other specimens, such as sputum, must be digested before centrifugation.

There are several methods of preparing specimens for microscopic examination. Gram-stained smears are often used to investigate fluids and secretions (Fig. 24.1), but is is possible to detect fungal elements in these and other specimens without staining them. This can be done by mounting the material in 10–30% potassium hydroxide (KOH) solution, which clears the specimen without damaging the fungal cells. To highlight the fungal elements, specific stains can be incorporated into the KOH solution.

Direct microscopic examination of clinical material is most useful in the diagnosis of superficial fungal infections. The simplest method of preparing dermatological specimens

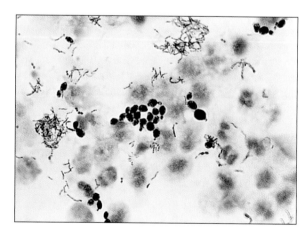

Figure 24.1: *Gram-stained smear of peritoneal drain fluid showing clusters of budding yeast cells and numerous much smaller bacterial cells.*

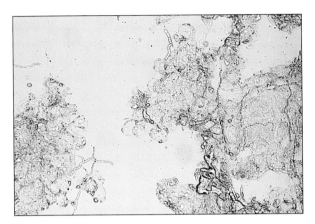

Figure 24.2: Unstained potassium hydroxide preparation of skin demonstrating the presence of branching dermatophyte hyphae some of which are fragmenting in arthrospores.

for microscopic examination is to digest them in KOH solution (Fig. 24.2). Recognition of fungal elements in skin scrapings, hair or nail clippings will often provide some indication of the mycosis involved, whether it be dermatophytosis or candidosis. Unlike cultural methods, which often require one to two weeks of incubation, microscopic examination can permit the correct treatment to be initiated much earlier.

In certain situations, direct microscopic examination of fluids or other clinical material can establish the diagnosis of a subcutaneous or systemic fungal infection. Instances include the detection of encapsulated *Cryptococcus neoformans* cells in cerebrospinal fluid, or *Histoplasma capsulatum* cells in peripheral blood smears. More often, however, only a tentative diagnosis of deep fungal infection can be made on the basis of microscopic examination. Nevertheless, this is often sufficient to allow the instigation of antifungal treatment pending the outcome of other investigations.

The detection of fungal elements in histopathological specimens is one of the best methods of diagnosing subcutaneous and systemic fungal infections. The ease with which a fungal pathogen can be recognized in tissue is dependent in part on its abundance, but also on the distinctiveness of its appearance. There are a number of special stains for detecting and

highlighting fungal cells, but specific identification of organisms is often difficult. For instance, the detection of non-pigmented, branching, septate mycelium is indicative of aspergillus infection, but it is also characteristic of a number of less common organisms. Likewise, the detection of small, budding fungal cells seldom permits a specific diagnosis. Tissue-form cells of *Histoplasma capsulatum* and *Blastomyces dermatitidis*, for instance, can appear similar and may be confused with non-encapsulated *Cryptococcus neoformans* cells.

Immunochemical staining procedures can permit the specific identification of fungal elements in histopathological sections. These methods have been applied to the diagnosis of a number of systemic fungal infections, including aspergillosis, candidosis and mucormycosis. Immunochemical staining can facilitate the identification of atypical fungal elements and the detection of small numbers of organisms.

Culture

Isolation in culture will permit most pathogenic fungi to be identified. Most of these fungi are not fastidious in their nutritional requirements and will grow on the media used for bacterial isolation from clinical specimens. However, growth on these media can be slow and development

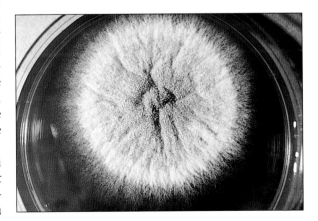

Figure 24.3: Typical culture of Aspergillus nidulans *on glucose peptone agar. Note the powdery appearance of the colonial surface due to the presence of enormous numbers of spores.*

251

of the spores and other structures used in
fungal identification can be poor. For these
reasons, most laboratories use a specific
medium, such as glucose peptone agar, to
isolate fungi (Fig. 24.3). To suppress bacterial
growth an antibiotic, such as chloramphenicol
or gentamicin, is added to the medium. If dermatophytes are being isolated, cycloheximide
(actidione) is often added to the medium as
well, but media without this selective antifungal agent must be used if other fungi are
included in the differential diagnosis.

The optimum growth temperature for most
pathogenic fungi is around 30°C. Material
from patients with a suspected superficial
fungal infection should be incubated at
25–30°C, because most dermatophytes will not
grow at higher temperatures. Material from
subcutaneous or deep sites should be incubated
at two temperatures: 25–30°C and 37°C. This
is because a number of important fungal
pathogens, including *Histoplasma capsulatum*
and *Sporothrix schenckii*, are dimorphic and
the change in their growth form, depending on
the incubation conditions, is useful in
identification. At 25–30°C these organisms
develop as moulds on glucose peptone agar, but
at higher temperatures on an enriched medium
(such as brain heart infusion agar), these organisms adopt a unicellular budding growth form.

Many pathogenic fungi grow slowly and cultures should be retained for at least two weeks,
and in some cases up to four weeks, before
being discarded as negative. In most cases,
however, positive culture results are obtained
within one week, and *Aspergillus fumigatus*
and *Candida albicans*, for instance, are
obtained within one to three days.

Should an isolate be identified as an unequivocal pathogen such as *Trichophyton rubrum* or
Histoplasma capsulatum, then the diagnosis is
established. If, however, an opportunistic
pathogen such as *Aspergillus fumigatus* or
Candida albicans is recovered, then its isolation
may have no clinical relevance unless there is
additional evidence of infection (such as its
detection on microscopic examination).
Isolation of opportunistic fungal pathogens
from sterile sites, such as blood or cerebrospinal fluid, often provides reliable evidence

of significant infection, but their isolation from
material such pus, sputum or urine must be
interpreted with caution. Attention should be
given to the amount of fungus isolated and
further investigations undertaken.

Many unfamiliar moulds have been reported
to cause lethal systemic infection in immunocompromised patients. No isolate should be
dismissed as a contaminant without careful
consideration of the clinical condition of the
patient, the site of isolation, the method of
specimen collection, and the amount of organisms recovered.

Although culture often permits the definitive
diagnosis of a fungal infection, it also has some
limitations. Failure to recover the organism
does not negate the diagnosis as this may be
due to inadequate specimen collection or
delayed transport of specimens. Incorrect isolation procedures or inadequate periods of incubation are other important factors.

Identification

Once isolated in culture, moulds and dermatophytes (filamentous fungi) are identified on
the basis of their macroscopic (colonial) and
microscopic morphological characteristics.
Macroscopic characteristics, such as colonial
form, surface colour and pigment production,
are often helpful in identification, but it is
essential to examine slide preparations of the
culture under a microscope. If well prepared
these will often give sufficient information on
the form and arrangement of the spores and
spore-bearing structures for identification of
the fungus to be accomplished (Fig. 24.4). If
spores are not found in slide preparations, cultures often cannot be identified.

Yeasts (unicellular, budding fungi) are
identified on the basis of their morphological
and biochemical characteristics. Useful morphological characteristics include the colour of
the colonies, the shape of the cells, and the
presence of a capsule around the cells. Useful
biochemical tests include the assimilation and
fermentation of sugars, and the assimilation of
nitrate. A number of simple rapid tests have
been devised for the identification of some of

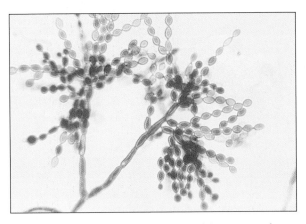

Figure 24.4: *Lactophenol cotton blue stain of* Cladophialophora carrionii *showing the characteristic long branching chains of spores by which this organism is identified.*

the most important human pathogens. Foremost amongst these is the serum germ tube test for *Candida albicans* which can be performed in less than three hours. For those organisms which are germ tube negative, identification can be made using one of the modern commercial systems, such as API 20 C (BioMerieux) or AUXACOLOR (Sanofi Diagnostics Pasteur). However, it is essential to examine the morphological characteristics of all isolates under the microscope if species with identical physiological profiles are to be distinguished.

In the past, unequivocal identification of *Histoplasma capsulatum* and *Blastomyces dermatitidis* took up to six weeks, requiring prolonged incubation and sometimes repeated sub-culture to reveal their characteristic dimorphism. With the introduction of commercial DNA probes (Accuprobe, Gen-Probe Inc), cultures of these organisms can now be identified in less than one hour. It remains to be seen whether similar tests will replace traditional methods of identifying other moulds.

Serological Tests

Serological tests often provide the most rapid means of establishing the diagnosis of a systemic fungal infection. Most tests are based on the detection of antibodies to specific fungal

pathogens, although tests for fungal antigens have been developed. For some infections, such as histoplasmosis and coccidioidomycosis, the tests are reliable, but for others the results are seldom more than suggestive or supportive of a fungal diagnosis. It is often more helpful if sequential tests can be performed, so that rising levels of antibodies may be detected.

Tests for antibodies have an established diagnostic use in the different forms of aspergillus infection that occur in the non-compromised individual. In contrast, these tests have proved much less helpful in diagnosing aspergillosis in neutropenic cancer patients and transplant recipients. Often, this is because patients fail to produce antibodies owing to their underlying condition or its treatment. Testing for antibodies to *Candida albicans* has also proved unhelpful in diagnosing patients with systemic candidosis, but this is because the somatic antigen preparations that are commonly used do not distinguish the antibodies formed during systemic infection from those produced during superficial colonization or infection.

Testing for fungal antigens in biological fluids is the method of choice for the rapid diagnosis of cryptococcosis and similar tests have been devised for a number of other systemic fungal infections, including aspergillosis, candidosis and histoplasmosis. In the case of cryptococcosis, a number of LPA and ELISA tests have been marketed for the detection of capsular antigen of *Cryptococcus neoformans* in serum, urine and cerebrospinal fluid specimens. These tests produce occasional false-positive and false-negative results, but permit the diagnosis to be made in over 90% of infected patients.

The major circulating antigen in systemic candidosis is mannan, a heat-stable cell wall polysaccharide. Unlike the capsular antigen of *Cryptococcus neoformans*, this is rapidly cleared from the circulation, necessitating frequent sampling if a positive result is to be obtained. In the case of aspergillosis, a galactomannan antigen has been detected in serum and urine of infected patients. However, as in candidosis, the antigen is short-lived and frequent testing of patients is essential. Moreover, the antigen often does not appear until too late in the course of the infection for treatment to affect the outcome.

Detection of Metabolic Products

Several gas–liquid chromatographic methods have been devised for the detection of fungal metabolites in biological fluids, but these have not had a significant impact on the diagnosis of systemic fungal infection. Among the fungal products that have been investigated as potential markers for infection are the aspergillus metabolite, D-mannitol, and the candida metabolite, D-arabinitol. Increased concentrations of the latter have been detected in the serum of patients with systemic candidosis, but elevated levels are also found in uninfected patients with renal failure.

Future Developments

Molecular biological techniques have had an enormous impact on the diagnosis of viral and bacterial infections, but have not been devel-oped to a similar extent for fungal infections. However, DNA-based methods are being developed for the detection of fungal pathogens in clinical specimens. In most cases DNA has been detected following *in vitro* amplification using the polymerase chain reaction (PCR). Species-specific primers have been designed for a number of organisms, including *Aspergillus fumigatus*, *Candida albicans* and *Cryptococcus neoformans* and several have been applied to detect fungal DNA in clinical specimens, including blood, bronchoalveolar lavage fluid, urine, and cerebrospinal fluid. PCR amplification with universal primers, common to all fungi, has also been used in attempts to detect fungal DNA in clinical specimens.

Molecular techniques have also been found to be useful for discrimination of strains of particular organisms. Among the methods that are now being used for typing of *Aspergillus fumigatus* and *Candida albicans* strains are restriction endonuclease analysis, Southern hybridization analysis and random primer PCR fingerprinting. Molecular typing methods have also been applied to a limited extent to a number of other fungal pathogens, including *Cryptococcus neoformans*.

Further Reading

Campbell C K, Johnson E M, Philpot C M, Warnock D W. *Identification of Pathogenic Fungi*. 1996: Public Health Laboratory Service, London.

Evans E G V, Richardson M D (eds). *Medical Mycology: A Practical Approach*. 1989: IRL Press at Oxford University Press.

Kibbler C C, Mackenzie D W R, Odds F C (eds). *Principles and Practice of Clinical Mycology*. 1996: John Wiley and Sons, Chichester.

Kwon-Chung K J, Bennett J E. *Medical Mycology*. 4th edn. 1992: Lea and Febiger, Philadelphia.

Richardson M D, Warnock D W. *Fungal Infection: Diagnosis and Management*. 2nd edn. 1997: Blackwell Science, Oxford.

25　PARASITOLOGY

Robert W A Girdwood

Introduction

In the context of this publication diagnostic parasitology can be defined as the demonstration of evidence of the presence of protozoan or metazoan organisms which live in or on human beings or other animals (the hosts). The evidence may be direct or indirect. Direct evidence is usually achieved by the examination of samples from the putative host such as faeces, urine, blood and other tissues for a stage of the parasite or a portion of the parasite. Indirect evidence can be obtained by demonstrating characteristic inflammatory responses, parasite products or specific antibodies in the putative host. The direct demonstration of a parasite stage in a host sample, e.g. a helminth ovum in a sample of faeces, is usually incontrovertible evidence of infection but the possibility of specimen contamination must always be considered. Conversely, a failure to demonstrate ova in a faecal sample does not necessarily exclude a diagnosis as it takes time for parasites to mature in their hosts and produce the looked for stage, or the parasite stage may be scanty or intermittently present in the samples examined. Indirect evidence of infection such as demonstration of antibodies must also be treated with caution especially because of the possibility of cross-reactions with other parasites. It is for these reasons that a detailed knowledge of parasite life cycles, modes of transmission and times taken for the various stages to be completed is a prerequisite for a soundly based diagnostic approach. This knowledge is required to decide what samples to examine and what tests are most appropriate in relation to the possible time of exposure to infection and the disease manifestations, if present.

The cornerstone of most diagnostic parasitology is based on morphology and morphometrics. Thus although in microbiological terms the transmissive stage (i.e. ova, cysts, oocysts and larvae) tend to be relatively large – in the order of tens to hundreds of microns – the conventional transmitted light microscope remains the most important diagnostic tool. Similarly, although most adult worms and most arthropod parasites (or vectors) are macroscopic, microscopy is usually required to detect the often subtle morphologic features necessary for species identification. In this latter instance a low magnification stereomicroscope is most useful.

Microscopy

The conventional transmitted light microscope providing total magnifications of ×100, ×400 and ×1000 is the parasitologist's basic instrument. Because an accurate measurement of the

Microscopy

Wet mounts

size of protozoan cysts and helminth ova is so important, an accurately calibrated eyepiece graticule is essential. Transmitted light microscopy requires that the specimen to be examined is sufficiently transparent to allow light to pass through it and provide adequate definition of morphology. This means that the samples have to be thin, in the order of microns, and when relatively opaque have to be rendered more transparent by clearing agents. When the parasites themselves have a refractive index similar to that of the sample containing them they require to be differentially stained so that the stain(s) used are taken up preferentially by the parasites. Less frequently the surrounding tissues or medium can be stained and the contained parasites remain unstained: this is negative staining. An alternative approach is to use different illumination systems such as dark ground, phase contrast or differential interference contrast (Nomarski) microscopy.

Wet mounts

In parasitology the most frequently examined sample is the wet mount where a few drops of the specimen or a suspension of the specimen are placed on a microscope slide, covered with a coverslip and examined at total magnifications of ×100 and ×400. The specific details of the preparation of the specimen will depend on the number of parasites likely to be present in the sample relative to the presence of contaminating or obscuring material. Thus, while direct examination of unconcentrated drops of blood or urine or saline suspensions of faeces may be useful, concentration of the sample is usually necessary because the parasite is present in small numbers relative to the volume of the specimen requiring to be examined. Transparent fluids such as urine can be scrutinized by centrifugation and examination of a wet mount of the resuspended deposit or by filtration and similar examination of the residue. Faecal material presents a more complex problem in that scanty parasites may be present in a mass of opaque and obscuring debris. Techniques of selective concentration are employed where parasite ova and cysts are concentrated and separated from the faecal debris or *vice versa* (Fig. 25.1). Such techniques

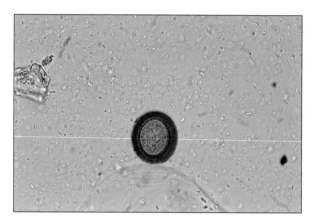

Figure 25.1: *Ovum of* Taenia *sp. Formal–ether concentrated faecal suspension.* ×400.

use flotation and/or centrifugation where the difference between the densities of the parasite stages (ova, cysts, oocysts and larvae) and the contaminating debris are exploited by using various suspending media of different specific gravities. Depending on the technique used the clean, concentrated sample to be examined microscopically will be taken from the centrifuged deposit, the interface between suspending media of differing specific gravities or the surface meniscus from flotation. Examples of such techniques include Ridley's formol-ether differential flotation/centrifugation, sucrose gradient concentration and zinc sulphate flotation. The same principles are used for the detection of parasite cysts and ova in environmental samples such as water, soil, sludge and sewage. In such samples the parasites are often even more scanty and further concentration techniques such as anti-parasite antibodies attached to magnetized particles are being evaluated.

Parasites in the bloodstream are present at low concentration and, again, techniques which involve concentration of the parasites and allow the examination of larger volumes of blood are employed. Thus detection of microfilariae which, although relatively large (200–300 microns) tend to be very scanty, invokes these techniques by either (1) filtration of a large volume of anticoagulated blood through a membrane filter which retains the microfilariae and allows the smaller cellular components of blood to pass through with sub-

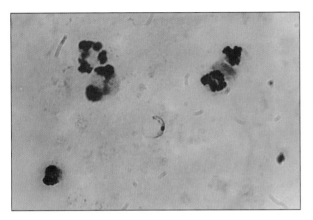

Figure 25.2: *Trypomastigotes of* Trypanosoma rhodesiense. *Romanowsky stained thin blood film.* ×400.

sequent staining, clearing and microscopy of the filter or (2) lysis of the erythrocytes in a large volume of blood (about 5 ml) and the sedimentation of any contained microfilariae which are examined in a wet mount of the resuspended deposit.

Films and smears

Films and smears are used widely to detect parasites in samples of blood, bone marrow and faeces. Blood samples for the detection of protozoan parasites such as malaria and trypanosomes are usually examined as Romanowsky stained thin or thick films (Fig. 25.2). Thin blood films, one cell thick, are fixed prior to staining and, because of this, retain the morphology of the erythrocytes and, in the case of malaria, the contained intracellular parasites. With thick films the erythrocytes are lysed prior to staining and fixation, thus the final preparation reveals only leukocytes, platelets and parasites. The advantage of the thick film is that more material can be examined but the disadvantages are that important morphological changes in the erythrocytes produced by the malaria parasite cannot be detected and parasites can be confused with platelets. Bone marrow smears stained with a Romanowsky stain are used to detect intracellular leishmania.

Fixed and stained faecal smears are required for the examination of protozoan trophozoites. Such techniques are necessary because trophozoites rupture in unfixed material and visual-

ization of the fine details of nuclear structure and intracytoplasmic inclusions is required for the species identification of amoebae. Iron haematoxylin, trichrome and Giemsa stains are widely used for these purposes. In addition stained faecal smears are used to detect *Cryptosporidium* spp. oocysts and microsporidial spores.

Less frequently, stained impression smears from tissue biopsy or necropsy material are employed to diagnose *Leishmania* spp. and *Pneumocystis carinii* infections.

Histopathology

Conventional tissue sections can provide diagnostic information for the parasitologist either by revealing characteristic or specific tissue responses to the infection or by demonstration of the parasite (protozoan) or sections of the parasite (metazoan). Here again micrometry is important and, in the context of examining histological sections of worms or their ova, due cognisance of shrinkage due to fixation and alterations to dimensions if sections are other than truly cross-sectional or sagittal must be made. Special stains are frequently employed to accentuate certain components of the parasite sections but description of their use is beyond the scope of this chapter.

Fluorescence

The ability of materials to become luminous when viewed with ultraviolet light is utilized in diagnostic parasitology in three ways: autofluorescence, fluorochrome staining and fluorochrome labelling. Autofluorescence refers to the intrinsic property of the organism or a component of the organism to fluoresce and is exemplified by the blue appearance of *Cyclospora* spp. oocysts when viewed in unstained wet mounts under ultraviolet light. Fluorochrome staining refers to the direct staining of the organism or a component of the organism with the fluorochrome. The apple-green fluorescence produced by *Cryptosporidium* spp. oocysts when stained with auramine phenol is an example of this method. Fluorochrome labelling usually involves immunological methods in which parasite-specific antibodies (polyclonal or monoclonal) are conjugated to a fluorochrome such as fluorescein isothiocyanate, and used to enhance the detectability of parasites in clinical material. The success of this technique depends largely on the specificity of the antibody used to bind the fluorescent label to the parasite. Examples of useful assays include the detection of structurally damaged *Giardia duodenalis* cysts in faecal samples and the detection of *Entamoeba histolytica* trophozoites in tissue sections of abscesses. Indirect methods which use fluorescence microscopy and the specific parasite as a fixed substrate to detect antibodies in serum are described briefly in the serology section below. The incorporation or exclusion of fluorochromes is being advocated increasingly as a surrogate method of determining viability and therefore potential infectivity of cysts or oocysts isolated from environmental samples. Thus the exclusion of propidium iodide and the inclusion of 4,6-diamidino-2-phenylindole (DAPI) by *Cryptosporidium* spp. oocysts is currently under evaluation in these circumstances.

Electron Microscopy

With the exception of microsporidial infections electron microscopy has little place in diagnostic parasitology. Although alternative diagnostic procedures are being developed, transmission electron microscopy of faeces, intestinal biopsies and other tissues is the definitive if somewhat inconvenient technique for diagnosing infections with these organisms, primarily because they are small (1–2 microns), intracellular and stain poorly.

Culture

A very basic form of culture is employed for the diagnosis and speciation of nematode larvae such as hookworms and *Strongyloides* spp. While strongyloides larvae are voided in the faeces of the host and ova are not usually present, the converse is true of the hookworms *Ancylostoma duodenale* and *Necator americanus* where ova only are voided in fresh faeces.

As the ova of the latter two are morphologically indistinguishable, speciation can only be effected by creating conditions in which ova hatch and develop into distinguishable third stage larvae. In addition the motility of the larvae of all three species is utilized to facilitate collection. This is particularly useful in the diagnosis of strongyloidiasis where larvae present in faeces may be scanty and do not concentrate well when conventional techniques such as formol-ether are used. The conditions which pertain in the natural transmission of these parasites are recreated in the Harada–Muri (or similar) technique. Here faecal material is smeared on filter paper strips, the lower ends of which are suspended in a well of distilled water contained in sealed test-tubes and incubated at 28°C for about ten days. Under these conditions the hatched hookworm larvae and the strongyloides larvae migrate down the filter paper to be collected in the water. The larvae are then speciated by detecting morphological differences. It should be noted that no replication of parasites occurs in this 'culture' technique.

In vitro culture of clinical material for diagnostic purposes is used relatively infrequently in parasitology compared with the other microbial disciplines. This is because protozoans and metazoans have more complex metabolic requirements which in the majority of cases cannot be met in current *in vitro* culture systems. Nevertheless true replicative cultural methods have a limited role in diagnostic parasitology where alternative methods are used but have other limitations. Thus Robinson's culture system for the isolation of *Entamoeba histolytica* as a diagnostic technique is fairly cumbersome and insensitive but it offers the advantage, when successful, of yielding trophozoites for isoenzyme analysis. *Zymodeme* determination of isolates can distinguish between pathogenic and non-pathogenic strains – a discrimination which is not yet possible by microscopy. Similarly, *in vitro* culture of biopsy material is used widely in the diagnosis both of cutaneous and visceral leishmaniasis, frequently as an adjunct to direct microscopy of a suitably stained portion of the same material. The advantage of microscopy is that it is quick and if positive, diagnostic, but this is offset by the frequent paucity of parasites. Culture is relatively slow – days to weeks – but has the advantage when positive of yielding viable organisms which can be speciated by molecular, serological or enzyme analysis and in addition can be used for drug susceptibility testing. It must be emphasized again that negative culture results do not exclude the diagnosis. Increasingly with the sophistication of *in vitro* culture techniques parasites are propagated in axenic culture so that the parasites, fractions prepared from them or their metabolic products can be harvested, purified and characterized for use in immunological diagnostic procedures. Two basic examples of the use of cultural methods for immunodiagnostic purposes are, firstly, *in vitro* culture of *Entamoeba histolytica* trophozoites which are harvested, attached to microscope slides and used as antigen in the indirect fluorescent antibody test for amoebiasis. Secondly, the maintenance of hatched second stage *Toxocara canis* larvae *in vitro* and the harvesting, concentration and standardization of the excretory/secretory products they produce for use as antigens in an ELISA test for the detection of circulating toxocara antibodies.

Animal Infection

The inoculation or feeding of clinical material into susceptible species of laboratory maintained experimental animals was the mainstay of all disciplines of diagnostic microbiology. A diagnosis was established by the sacrifice of the animals after an appropriate incubation period and the demonstration of the organism or the characteristic pathology produced by it in the organs or tissues by conventional microscopic and histological techniques. Increasingly, alternative diagnostic methods are being used but animals are still required either for the maintenance of parasites for use as antigens when there are no *in vitro* culture techniques available or for the production of anti-parasite antibodies used in diagnostic tests. It seems likely that in the former instance the use of construct antigens or the development of tissue culture techniques will reduce further this requirement.

Xenodiagnosis

This unusual method falls somewhere between culture and animal inoculation and utilizes a natural vector or intermediate host in the parasite's life cycle to concentrate the parasite and thus make it more readily detectable. The classic example of xenodiagnosis uses one of the insect vectors of *Trypanosoma cruzi* to facilitate the diagnosis of Chagas' disease (South American trypanosomiasis). Laboratory reared (parasite free) nymphal stages of the reduviid bugs are allowed to feed on the patient and are sacrificed some four weeks later. The contents of the hindgut are expressed, stained and examined microscopically for *trypomastigotes*. This almost unique example of xenodiagnosis acknowledges that parasites are extremely scanty in the peripheral blood of the host and the reduviid bugs are extremely efficient vectors.

Serology

Serodiagnosis is generally less reliable than the more direct microscopic methods because of the problems of cross-reactivity (poor specificity), low sensitivity and, frequently, the inability to distinguish between past and current infections. Of the three major groups of serological assays – i.e. detection of antibody, detection of antigen and the detection of immune complexes – it is the first category which is most widely used in diagnosis. Such serological techniques are usually employed when material for direct examination for the presence of the parasite is not available. Thus, generally, serological tests for the diagnosis of intestinal parasites would not normally be recommended because specific diagnosis by the demonstration of ova or cysts in the usually readily available faeces would be the method of choice. Conversely, in tissue invasive parasitic diseases such as echinococcosis, toxoplasmosis or toxocariasis the demonstration of circulating antibodies may be more productive than tissue biopsy examination. The interpretation of serological results in relation to the stage of the disease produced by the parasite (acute or chronic) can be improved by determining the immunoglobulin class and isotype involved in the antibody response. Greater sensitivity and specificity of the test can in some instances be achieved by immunoblotting. Similarly, better characterization of antigen preparations using, for example, monoclonal antibodies can achieve the same goal. Because antibodies can persist for years following infection and following successful treatment, the detection of parasite antigen in clinical material is, in theory, more attractive because the presence of antigen must indicate current or very recent infection. Examples of the value of this approach are the use of the ELISA technique to detect filarial antigen in the serum, urine and hydrocoele fluid of patients with *Wuchereria bancrofti* infections (where in the chronic stages microfilariae are difficult to demonstrate in the peripheral blood) and in the serum and urine of patients with *Onchocerca volvulus* infections. A potential additional advantage of antigen detection is that quantification of circulating or excreted antigen may correlate with worm burden and by extrapolation symptomatology and transmissibility. The detection of immune complexes is not yet sufficiently specific for diagnostic purposes but dissociation of these complexes to detect the antigen and/or antibody components is a more promising approach.

Molecular Methods

The use of DNA probes and the PCR technique has proliferated throughout all fields of microbiology in the last twelve years. While this is

Table 25.1: Some advantages and disadvantages of the major approaches used in diagnostic parasitology.

Method	Advantages	Disadvantages
Microscopy	Fast (for individual specimen) Direct visualization of parasite Positive result usually definitive	Requires skilled microscopist Requires relatively numerous parasites i.e. negative result does not exclude diagnosis Slow for mass screening
In vitro culture	Detects only viable parasites Provides isolates for further characterization, sensitivity testing and antigen preparation	Slow Only available for limited number of species/strains Negative culture does not exclude diagnosis
Animal infection	As above	As above Expensive
Serology	Simple Fast Can be used for mass screening	Lack of standard reagents (antigens) Difficult to differentiate between past and present infection False positive results due to cross-reactivity
Xenodiagnosis	Simple Cheap Specific	Low sensitivity Very limited application Slow ?Unpleasant
Molecular methods	Fast Sensitive Can detect live and dead parasites Direct detection of parasite	Expensive Detects live and dead parasites False-negative from PCR inhibitors False-positives from contamination

true in parasitological research where such techniques now predominate, in the fields of diagnostic parasitology the role of molecular methods remains limited at present. The main advantage of nuclear acid based detection methods is their sensitivity. Thus in diagnosis it is only when the parasite burden is low that these techniques can improve on the more conventional approaches. South American trypanosomiasis is a good example where in the chronic stage of the disease parasitaemias are so low as to be beyond the limit of detection by conventional microscopic methods (see xenodiagnosis above). Also in this disease, because of its endemicity, serodiagnosis not only lacks specificity but cannot distinguish between *infection* past or present and current disease status. Specifically, a conserved mini repeat sequence of kinetoplast DNA minicirclets used as a probe followed by PCR amplification has proved more sensitive and specific than microscopy, xenodiagnosis or serology. Molecular methods can also be valuable diagnostically where more conventional approaches are jeopardized by changes in the host. A prime example is the problem of diagnosing toxoplasmosis in the immunocompromised host. *Toxoplasma gondii* has a worldwide distribution with a high incidence of subclinical infection. Diagnosis of infections past or present is usually made by assaying the various classes of specific antibody. In the immunocompromised host latent infection can progress to potentially fatal disease and because of the immune deficiency serodiagnosis is unhelpful. PCR assays targeting the B1 gene or the P30 gene have been applied to brain biopsy, bronchial lavage and cerebrospinal fluid samples, with promising results.

Antigen production either by hybridization or recombinant DNA technology is beginning to provide potentially useful specific and sensitive diagnostic reagents and the use of molecular techniques to detect parasite-bearing vectors is a further example of the exciting promise of molecular research. However, enthusiasm for the real potential of such techniques must be tempered by awareness of the disadvantages of relative expense and the problems of false-positive results due to contamination of samples.

The main diagnostic procedures with some of their advantages and disadvantages are summarized in Table 25.1.

Further Reading

Basic Laboratory Methods in Medical Parasitology. 1991: World Health Organisation, Geneva.

Cook, G C, ed. *Manson's Tropical Diseases* 1996: W. B. Saunders Company Ltd, London.

Fleck, S L, Moody, A H. *Diagnostic Techniques in Medical Parasitology* 1988: Wright, London.

Gillespie, S H, Hawkey, P M, eds, *Medical Parasitology – A Practical Approach*. 1995: Oxford, University Press.

Kettle, D S, ed. *Medical and Veterinary Entomology*. 1995: CAB International, Wallingford.

SECTION 4
HAEMATOLOGY

26 BLOOD CELL AND BONE MARROW MORPHOLOGY

Supratik Basu

Peripheral Blood Morphology

Cell morphology is an essential part of any haematological investigation. Cell morphology is best assessed by examining a well-spread, well-stained film. A blood film may be made from non-anticoagulated (native) blood, obtained either from a vein or a capillary, or from EDTA anti-coagulated blood. A well-made film is evenly spread and has a tongue-shaped edge. Once made, the film should be rapidly air dried and then fixed in absolute methanol for 10 to 20 minutes.

Staining
All films once fixed should be stained as soon as possible. Blood and bone marrow films are stained by Romanowsky dyes consisting of a mixture of methylene blue and eosin. Methylene blue stains acidic components e.g. nuclei and cytoplasmic RNA blue, while eosin stains basic components such as haemogloblin red. A popular Romanowsky stain is May–Gruenewald–Giemsa stain. In certain situations, such as differentiating various types of leukaemias, special stains are employed (see Table 26.5).

Technique for examination of film
Films should first be examined under a low magnification, in order to get an idea of the quality of preparation, number, distribution, and staining of red cells, leukocytes and platelets. A low magnification is also best suited to detect the presence of abnormal precipitates and agglutination. Once a satisfactory low-power examination has been made, a suitable area of the film should be examined in greater detail under higher power or an oil immersion objective.

Red cell morphology
In health, red cells vary little in size and shape. The majority of red cells are round and smooth and have a diameter within a narrow range (mean $\pm 2SD$) of 6.0–8.5 μm with a central pallor. Examination should be made in a part of the film where red cells are well-spread and do not touch each other. Less than 10% of the red cells should be oval in shape. A very small percentage (less than 0.1%) may be contracted

Peripheral Blood Morphology

Red cell morphology

Table 26.1:   RBC abnormalities.

Terminology	What it means	Associated conditions
Anisocytosis	Greater variation in size than normal.	Non-specific feature. Pronounced in severe anaemia
Anisochromia	Dual population of cells. Some, but not all, RBC stain palely.	Iron deficiency being treated, or transfused. Combined hematinic deficiency
Acanthocytosis	Small cells with regular, multiple spiky projections.	Post-splenectomy (Hyposplenic), McLeod phenotype, α-β lipoproteinaemia, starvation
Auto-agglutination (Fig. 26.2)	Irregular clumping of red cells.	Cold agglutinin diseases, autoimmune haemolytic anaemia
Basophilic stippling (Fig. 26.3)	Deep blue small inclusions in RBC. Best seen under oil immersion.	Lead poisoning, pyrimidine 5' nucleotidase deficiency, myelodysplasia, megaloblastic anaemia, unstable haemoglobin disease, thalassaemia
Crenated cells	RBC showing evenly spaced blunt projections.	Artefact, hypothyroid, old age, renal failure
Elliptocytosis	Oval or elliptical cells.	Megaloblastic anaemia, iron deficiency, myelofibrosis, hereditary elliptocytosis/ovalocytosis
Howell Jolly bodies (Fig. 26.4)	Darkly staining, round, dot-like inclusion within cells (nuclear remnant).	Hyposplenism of any cause, megaloblastic anaemia
Hypochromia (Fig. 26.5)	Pale red cells (MCH <27 pg)	Iron deficiency anaemia, thalassaemia, sideroblastic anaemia
Macrocytosis (Fig. 26.6)	Large cells (MCV >100 fl)	Megaloblastic anaemia, myelodysplasia, hypothyroid, aplastic anaemia, liver disease
Microcytosis (Fig. 26.5)	Small cells (MCV <75 fl)	See hypochromia
Nucleated RBC (Fig. 26.7)	Presence of red cells with nuclei.	Any severe anaemia, myelofibrosis, severe haemolysis, thalassaemia (post-splenectomy), marrow infiltration. Normal in cord blood, large numbers found in haemolytic disease of newborn
Poikilocytes	Red cells with abnormal shape.	Any anaemia, specially associated with abnormal erythropoiesis, e.g. thalassaemia, myelofibrosis
Polychromasia	Presence of red cells staining bluish grey. These are reticulocytes.	Haemolysis, blood loss, extramedullary erythropoiesis
Rouleaux (Fig. 26.8)	Stacking of RBC in columns.	Some degree is normal, myeloma, macroglobulinaemia, chronic infection, and inflammation

Table 26.1: *continued*

Terminology	What it Means	Associated Conditions
Schistocyte (Fig. 26.9)	Fragmented red cells.	DIC, carcinoma, micro-angiopathic haemolytic anaemia (MAHA)
Sickle cell (Fig. 26.10)	Thin, elongated crescentic, cells.	Sickle cell diseases
Spherocytes (Fig. 26.7)	Small densely staining cells with no central pallor.	Hereditary spherocytosis, ABO haemolytic disease of newborn, autoimmune haemolytic anaemia
Spur cell	Cells with irregular, sharp projections.	Liver disease, pyruvate kinase deficiency
Stomatocytes	Cells with slit-like mouth at centre.	Hereditary stomatocytosis, alcoholism, artefact
Target cells (Fig. 26.11)	RBC with central dense staining area and disease, rim of haemoglobin at the periphery, with clear ring in between these two.	Haemoglobinopathies e.g. HbCC, SC liver disease
Tear-drop cells (Fig. 26.12)	Self-explanatory (type of poikilocytosis).	Myelofibrosis, thalassaemia

or fragmented. In premature and normal infants this proportion may be higher (0.3–5.6%). (For normal peripheral blood morphology see Fig. 26.1.)

Abnormalities of RBC morphology
A complete description of all normal variations and abnormalities is not possible in this small chapter. For this a detailed atlas should be consulted. Some common abnormalities affecting the red cells with their associated disorders are listed in Table 26.1.

White cell morphology
Normal peripheral blood leukocytes are classified as polymorphonuclear leukocytes and mononuclear cells. The latter term refers to lymphocytes and monocytes. In a blood film monocytes and neutrophils are concentrated at the edge and at the end of the film. Vital information is obtained by scanning the film for abnormal forms and numbers at a lower magnification. Detailed study of granulation and nuclear and cytoplasmic morphology is then best done under oil immersion or a higher power of magnification.

Normal morphology
The normal white cells are of five types.

Neutrophils: The mature neutrophil measures 12–15 μm in diameter. The cytoplasm is acidophilic with fine granules. The nucleus with clumped chromatin is divided into two to five distinct lobes by filaments which are dense hetero-chromatin. In females, some neutrophils have a drumstick-shaped nuclear appendage linked to the nucleus by a filament. This represents an inactive X chromosome (Fig. 26.1).

Eosinophils: These are slightly larger than neutrophils, being 12–17 μm in diameter. The nucleus is usually bilobed. Eosinophil granules are spherical, larger, coarse and reddish orange in colour (see Fig. 26.13).

Basophils: Basophils are similar in size to neutrophils. The nucleus is obscured by purple-black, coarse granules.

Peripheral Blood Morphology

White cell morphology

Table 26.2: WBC abnormalities.

Terminology	What it Means	Associated Conditions
Atypical lymphocytes (Fig. 26.14)	Large lymphocytes with basophilic cytoplasm. Often wraps around red cells.	Viral infections, drug reactions
Auer rods	Rod-like red inclusion in immature cells (blasts).	Myeloid leukaemias
Blast cells	Immature primitive cells.	Leukaemias
Döhle bodies (Fig. 26.15)	Blue cytoplasmic inclusions in neutrophil cytoplasm.	Infection, inflammation
Hypogranular neutrophils	Neutrophils with abnormal and reduced granulation.	Myelodysplasia
Leucoerythroblastic	Presence of nucleated red cells and early granulocytes in blood.	Marrow infiltration, myelofibrosis, acute haemolysis
Leucocytosis	White cell count more than $11 \times 10^9/1$.	Infection, inflammation, leukaemia
Lymphocytosis	Lymphocyte count >4 × 10⁹/1 in adults. >7 × 10⁹/1 in children.	Chronic lymphatic leukaemia, lymphoma in leukaemic phase. Pertussis, viral infection
Neutrophilia	Neutrophils >7.5 × 10⁹/1.	Infection inflammation, leukaemoid reaction, chronic myeloid leukaemia
Pelger–Huët anomaly	Neutrophils with two unsegmented lobes (bilobed).	Myelodysplasia, myeloid leukaemia, hereditary form
'Shift to left'	Presence of early myeloid cells.	(see Neutrophilia)
'Shift to right'	Neutrophils five or more lobes.	Megaloblastic anaemia
Smear cells	Smudged, degenerating lymphocytes.	Chronic lymphatic leukaemia
Toxic granulation (Fig. 26.16)	Neutrophils with coarse purple granules.	Infection, inflammation
Turk cells/plasmacytic cells	Reactive lymphoplasmacytic cells.	Severe bacterial, viral infection, rarely plasma cell leukaemia

Lymphocytes: These are 10–16 μm in diameter. The smaller lymphocytes (10 μm) which predominate have a scanty cytoplasm and a round nucleus with condensed chromatin. About 10% of the lymphocytes are larger, have more abundant cytoplasm and less condensed nuclear chromatin. Lymphocytes may have a small number of granules containing lysosomal enzymes (azurophilic granules). Occasional larger cells with more abundant cytoplasm have quite prominent azurophilic granules. These are called large granular lymphocytes.

(For normal lymphocyte morphology see Fig. 26.1).

Monocytes: These are the largest cells with a diameter of 12–20 μm. The nucleus is irregular and lobulated. Cytoplasm is plentiful with a greyish-blue colour. Fine azurophilic granules can be seen. The cell outline is often irregular and the cytoplasm may also be vacuolated (Fig. 26.1).

Delay in making films with EDTA blood gives rise to sequestrine changes. This shows as vacuolation of nucleus and cytoplasm. It first affects the monocytes and then the neutrophils.

Table 26.3: Platelet abnormalities.

Abnormality	What it Means	Associated Conditions
Large platelets	Platelets of above average size.	Immune thrombocytopenia, 'giant' platelets of Bernard–Soulier syndrome
Platelet clumping	Clumping of platelet in film, giving rise to low platelet count.	Anticoagulant related, poorly collected specimen, partially clotted specimens, small clumps normal in fresh films
Thrombocytopenia	Low platelet count of $<150 \times 10^9/1$.	Immune thrombocytopenia (ITP), marrow aplasia, or infiltration, myelodysplasia, hypersplenism
Thrombocytosis (Fig. 26.17)	High platelet count $>500 \times 10^9/1$.	Infection, inflammation, myeloproliferative states

Abnormalities of WBC morphology

Some common abnormalities affecting the leukocytes are listed in Table 26.2.

Platelets

Normal platelets measure 1–3 μm in diameter. They contain fine granules which are either dispersed or concentrated in the centre. A rough guess can be made of their number while examining a film. In EDTA anticoagulated blood platelets generally remain separate. In fresh films they are often clumped. A poorly collected specimen can cause a spuriously low platelet count. Some common abnormalities of platelets are listed in Table 26.3.

Examination of Bone Marrow and Bone Marrow Morphology

The distribution of haemopoietic marrow is age-dependent. In neonates, haemopoietic marrow occupies almost all of the bone marrow cavity. Haematopoiesis occurs in virtually all bones. With age, haemopoietic marrow contracts and is replaced by fatty marrow. In young adults haemopoietic marrow is confined to the skull, spine, ribs, clavicle, sternum, pelvis and proximal portions of the long bones. However, haemopoietic marrow can expand in response to increased demand.

Examination of bone marrow

Bone marrow should be examined for morphology by both aspiration biopsy and a trephine biopsy. Bone marrow aspirations are commonly carried out from the sternum, the iliac crest or the medial surface of the tibia in babies up to the age of 18 months. Special aspiration needles are available for this procedure. Aspiration specimens are suitable for fine and detailed cytological examination when spread properly on a slide. Aspiration marrow is also suitable for flow cytometric studies, karyotypic analysis and other molecular studies, and also for bone marrow culture studies.

Trephine biopsies are best and easily done from the iliac crests. Special trephine biopsy needles are available for this purpose. Trephines are essential for a proper histological and cellularity assessment. Cellularity of the marrow can, however, also be assessed by examining the fragments of aspirated marrow. Cellularity decreases steadily with age, with an accelerated decline above the age of 70. Trephine biopsies are always performed when a 'dry tap' or a dilute sample is obtained by aspiration. This often happens when a marrow is fibrotic, hypercellular or abnormally infiltrated with disease. Aspiration and trephine biopsies should be regarded as complementary procedures.

Bone marrow morphology

Once marrow has been aspirated it should be spread into films as described above. Bone

269

Examination of Bone Marrow and Bone Marrow Morphology

Bone marrow morphology

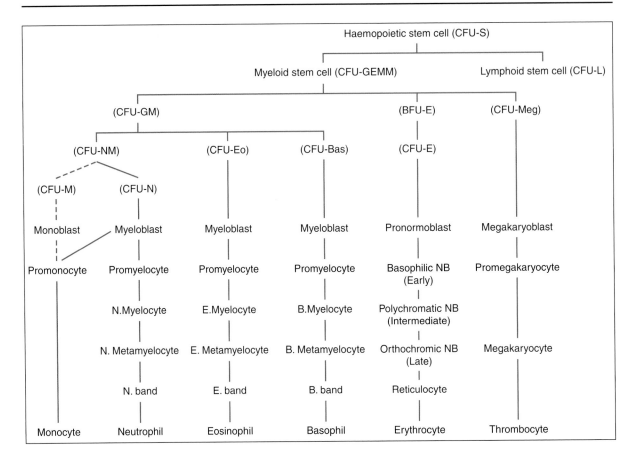

Diagram A: Diagrammatic representation of haematopoiesis. CFU-S, colony forming unit – spleen; CFU-GEMM, colony forming unit granulocyte, erythroid, macrophage, megakaryocyte; LSC (CFU-L), lymphoid stem cell (colony forming unit – lymphoid); CFU-GM, colony forming unit – granulocyte; BFU-E, burst forming unit – erythroid; CFU-Meg, colony forming unit – megakaryocyte; CFU-NM, colony forming unit – neutrophil, monocyte; CFU-Eo, colony forming unit – eosinophil; CFU-Bas, colony forming unit – basophil; CFU-E, colony forming unit – erythroid, CFU-M, colony forming unit – monocyte/macrophage; CFU-N, colony forming unit – neutrophil; N, neutrophilic; E, eosinophilic; B, basophilic; NB, normoblast.

marrow films, after staining, should be scanned under low objective (×10) for overall cellularity, distribution of haemopoietic cells, presence of abnormal clusters of non-haemopoietic cells, megakaryocyte numbers and morphology. Maturation of erythroid and myeloid components, their relative proportions and abnormal patterns of maturation (e.g. megaloblastic or dysplastic) should then be noted. The normal myeloid to erythroid ratio (M:E ratio) is 2.5/1 to 8/1. Ideally, a differential count (myelogram) of at least 200 nucleated cells should be done. This is important if abnormal infiltration with leukaemia, myeloma, or lymphoma is sus-

pected. Children have a large number of small lymphocytes. This number decreases with age. In adults about 5–15% of nucleated cells are lymphoid. Other cells to look out for are megakaryocytes, plasma cells, macrophages and mast cells. Both their number and morphology are important. Parasites are often best found in macrophages.

A Prussian blue stain of the marrow should be made for assessing iron stores and distribution. The entire haemopoietic marrow originates from a totipotent haemopoietic stem cell in the marrow. A simple diagrammatic representation is given in Diagram A.

Normal Erythropoiesis

The earliest recognizable erythroid precursor, the pro-normoblast, develops progressively and differentiates into a normal erythrocyte. In this process it acquires a rising haemoglobin content and gradually loses its cytoplasmic basophilia, as well as its nucleus. This entire process is arbitrarily divided into three stages: early normoblast, intermediate normoblast and late normoblast. Late normoblasts do not divide but lose their nucleus by extrusion and give rise to a marrow reticulocyte. These spend up to two days in the marrow before entering the peripheral blood where they make up less than 1% of the red cell population. Reticulocytes have a characteristic bluish-grey staining property and are best demonstrated and counted by a supravital stain. Mature red cells survive about 120 days before destruction in the reticulo-endothelial system. Normal erythropoiesis and haematopoiesis are illustrated in Diagram B.

Some Common Disorders Mainly Affecting Erythropoiesis

Megaloblastic anaemia

This arises from a deficiency of either vitamin B_{12} or folic acid. Principally due to defective formation of thymidylate, DNA synthesis in the S phase of the cell cycle is slowed down. Nuclear division is thus retarded, and nuclear cytoplasmic synchronization in development is affected. Apart from erythroblasts most proliferating cells are affected including gut mucosa, granulocytes and platelet precursors. The megaloblastic marrow is hypercellular. Erythropoiesis is left-shifted with increase in cell size and opening up of the nuclear chromatin network system. Premature haemoglobinization with loss of nuclear cytoplasmic developmental synchronization is common (megaloblastic features). Parallel changes in granulocyte precursors include the presence of giant myelocytes or metamyelocytes and multilobated neutrophils (right shift). Megakaryocytes also show nuclear hypersegmentation.

Peripheral blood shows the presence of macrocytes and right-shifted neutrophils (Figs 26.6 and 26.18).

Haemolytic anaemias

Haemolytic anaemias (excessive destruction of red cells) of any cause show compensatory marrow erythroid hyperplasia. The M:E ratio is reduced with normoblastic hyperplasia and obliteration of fat spaces. Apart from this common shared feature, further helpful diagnostic clues are best obtained from peripheral red cell morphology, and appropriate supplementary laboratory investigations for haemolysis.

Aplastic and hypoplastic states

These disorders commonly present with anaemia, leukopenia and thrombocytopenia, e.g. pancytopenia. The causes can be variable but are often idiopathic. Pancytopenia in some cases can become progressively severe. The anaemia is often normochromic and normocytic with undetectable reticulocytes in peripheral blood. The marrow is poorly cellular with a predominance of fatty spaces. A relatively higher proportion of lymphocytes and plasma cells can be found. Marrow aspirate is acellular and a definitive diagnosis is best made by trephine biopsy. Hypoplasia can affect one lineage only, as in pure red cell aplasia when the red cell lineage is predominantly altered.

Myelodysplastic syndromes

This is a group of morphologically heterogeneous conditions which are consequent on an acquired myeloid stem cell disorder leading to abnormal proliferation and disorderly maturation of one or more lineage of haemopoietic cells. It is characterized by ineffective haematopoiesis, which causes peripheral blood cytopenia and a propensity for leukaemic transformation. The FAB (French, American and British) classification subdivides myelodysplastic syndromes into several subgroups. *Morphologically the marrow shows dysplastic features affecting all three lineages.* Erythroid dysplasia is evidenced by ragged haemoglobinization, abnormal and irregular nuclear morphology, and cytoplasmic bridging. In a

271

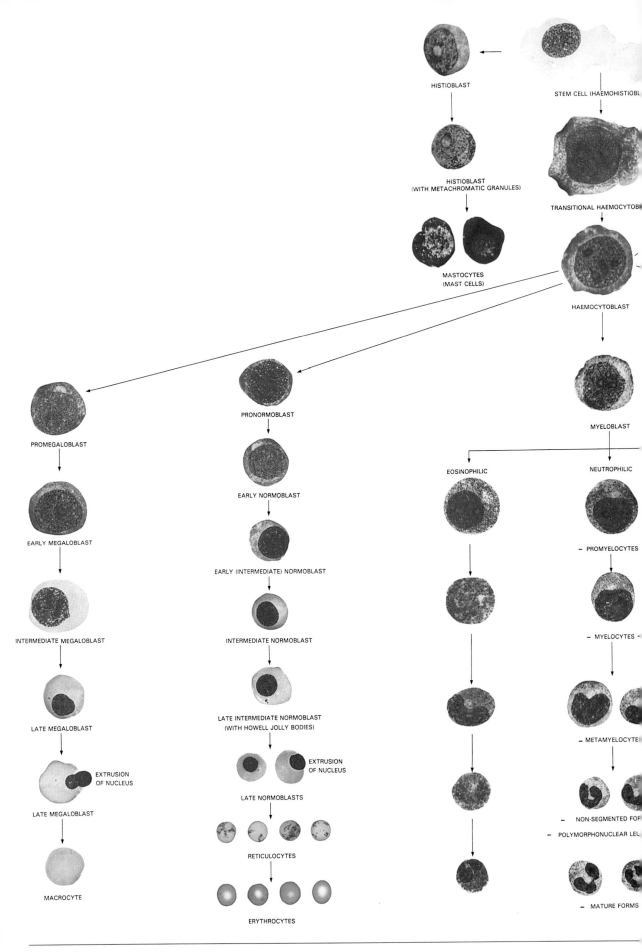

Diagram B: Maturation chart. Reproduced with permission from Churchill Livingstone, 'Atlas of Haematology'

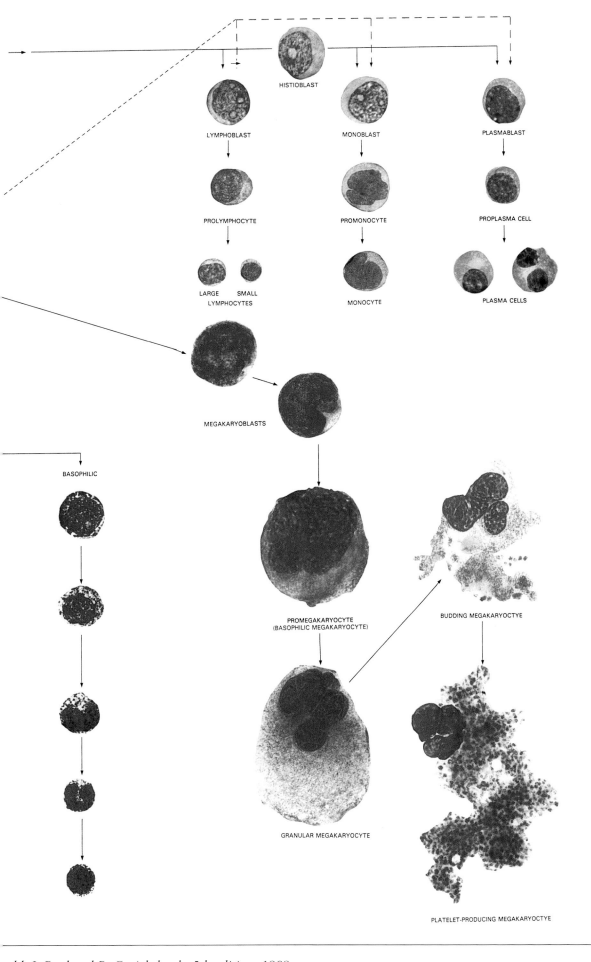

HISTIOBLAST

LYMPHOBLAST

MONOBLAST

PLASMABLAST

PROLYMPHOCYTE

PROMONOCYTE

PROPLASMA CELL

LARGE SMALL
LYMPHOCYTES

MONOCYTE

PLASMA CELLS

MEGAKARYOBLASTS

BASOPHILIC

PROMEGAKARYOCYTE
(BASOPHILIC MEGAKARYOCYTE)

BUDDING MEGAKARYOCTYE

GRANULAR MEGAKARYOCYTE

PLATELET-PRODUCING MEGAKARYOCTYE

nald, J. Paul and B. Cruickshank. 5th edition, 1989.

Some Common Disorders Mainly Affecting Erythropoiesis

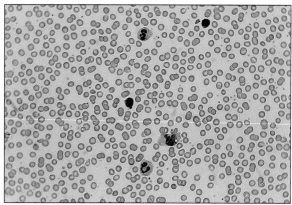

Figure 26.1: *Normal peripheral film showing neutrophil, lymphocyte, monocyte.*

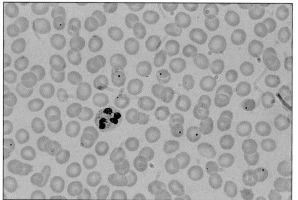

Figure 26.2: *Auto-agglutination of red cells.*

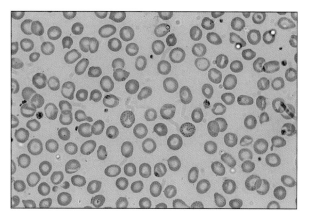

Figure 26.3: *Basophilic stippling of red cells.*

Figure 26.4: *Howell Jolly bodies.*

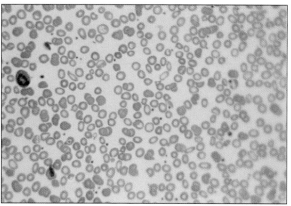

Figure 26.5: *Hypochromic, microcytic red cells.*

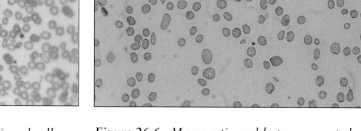

Figure 26.6: *Macrocytic and hypersegmented neutrophils.*

Some Common Disorders Mainly Affecting Erythropoiesis

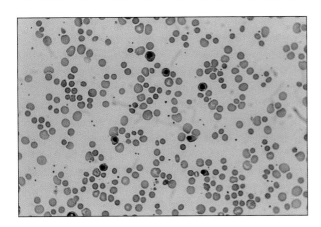

Figure 26.7: *Spherocytes with nucleated RBC in auto-immune haemolytic anaemia (AIHA).*

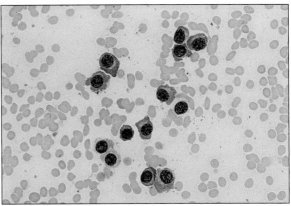

Figure 26.8: *Rouleaux with abnormal plasma cells in myeloma.*

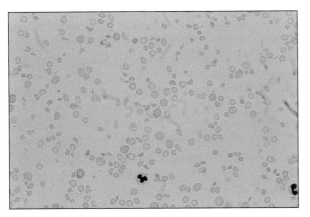

Figure 26.9: *Fragmented RBC in microangiopathic haemolytic anaemia (MAHA).*

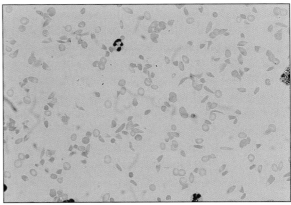

Figure 26.10: *Sickle cell disease.*

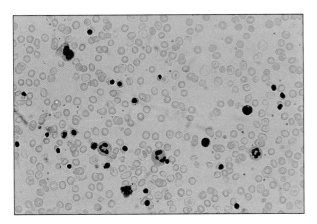

Figure 26.11: *Thalassaemia with nucleated red cells.*

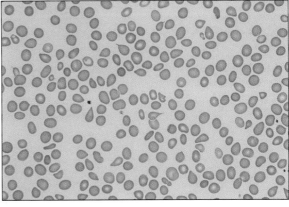

Figure 26.12: *Tear-drop cells in myelofibrosis.*

particular subgroup, known as *sideroblastic anaemia*, the red cell precursors show the presence of abnormal siderotic granules (Prussian blue stain) arranged in a ring fashion around the nucleus of the erythroblast (Fig. 26.27). Common peripheral red cell changes include anisocytosis, poikilocytosis, macrocytosis and, quite often, the presence of hypochromia or a dimorphic blood picture. Corresponding changes in white cell series include neutropenia and the presence of *hypogranular* neutrophils in peripheral blood with pseudo-Pelger changes. Similar abnormalities can also be detected in granulocyte precursors in marrow.

Thrombocytopenia is common. Bone marrow megakaryocytes are often smaller than normal and show abnormal morphology (micromegakaryocytes). Certain subtypes of MDS e.g. chronic myelomonocytic leukaemia (CMML) show characteristic monocytosis with an abnormal morphology. Myelodysplasia is a pre-leukaemic process and can terminate in acute leukaemia. Characteristic cytogenetic changes are often found in a high proportion of cases.

Polycythaemia

Primary proliferative polycythaemia (PRV or PPP) is clinically characterized by high haemoglobin, high haematocrit, high red cell count and mass. The white cell count and platelet count are often elevated and splenomegaly is common. The bone marrow shows obliteration of fat spaces with trilineage hyperplasia. Chromosomal changes can also occur. The transition to the myelofibrotic state can occur in up to 15–20% of cases. When this happens the trephine shows increased reticulin and marrow fibrosis. 'Tear-drop' poikilocytes and leukoerythroblastic features appear in peripheral blood. Terminal transformation to acute myeloid leukaemia or a myelodysplastic state can also occur.

Secondary polycythaemia is a condition which affects the red cell series only without showing leukocytosis or thrombocytosis. This happens most commonly in chronic cardiovascular or pulmonary diseases causing decreased oxygen saturation which, in turn, causes compensatory polycythaemia. Morphologically erythroid hyperplasia predominates without a parallel increase in other lineages.

Anaemia of blood loss and iron deficiency

Chronic blood loss can cause iron deficiency anaemia. The peripheral red cells show hypochromia and microcytosis with pencil cells. Erythropoiesis in the marrow is hyperplastic. The erythroblasts are often small and poorly haemoglobinized, with irregular and ragged outline (micronormoblasts). The Prussian blue stain fails to show any storage iron. A condition called anaemia of chronic disease (resulting from inflammation or chronic infection) can give a similar blood picture. In these conditions the marrow shows an increase in storage iron. Intra-erythroid iron stores are, however, reduced.

Erythroleukaemia

This is a form of acute myeloid leukaemia where the erythroid lineage is predominantly affected. The erythroid precursors are usually markedly abnormal with bizarre nuclear lobulation. Erythropoiesis can also be megaloblastic or sideroblastic. Prominent red cell abnormality may be found in peripheral blood including many circulating nucleated red cells.

Leucoerythroblastic anaemia (including idiopathic myelofibrosis)

This condition is characterized by the presence of 'tear-drop' poikilocyte, nucleated red cells and early granulocytes in peripheral blood. This picture can arise when marrow is infiltrated with metastatic tumour or foreign tissue, or when the marrow is fibrosed. Prominent marrow fibrosis can be the primary manifestation of a myeloproliferative state. This is called primary idiopathic myelofibrosis. The marrow shows an increase in reticulin and extensive fibrosis. Bone marrow aspirate is difficult or unhelpful in this condition. A trephine biopsy should always be performed and is diagnostic.

Normal Myelopoiesis and Megakaryopoiesis

The earliest recognizable cell of the granulocyte series is a myeloblast, which gives rise to a sequence of promyelocyte, myelocyte, metamyelocyte, stab cell and mature neutrophils

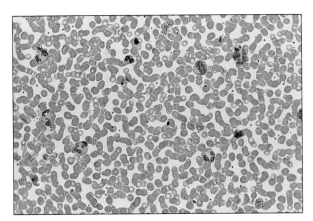

Figure 26.13: Eosinophils.

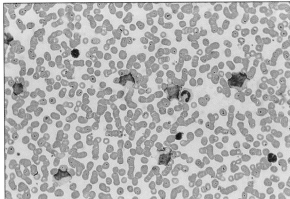

Figure 26.14: Atypical lymphocytes in infectious mononucleosis.

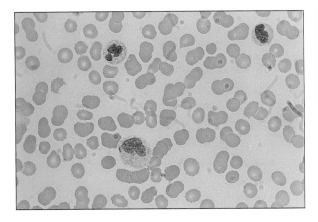

Figure 26.15: Döhle body in neutrophil.

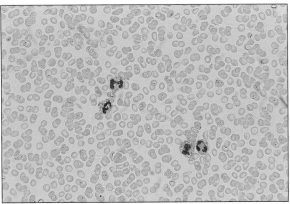

Figure 26.16: Toxic granulation in neutrophils.

(Diagram B). From the promyelocyte onwards, specific granules (neutrophilic, eosinophilic, basophilic) become increasingly conspicuous in the cytoplasm and differentiate the common neutrophil granulocytes from the less common eosinophilic and basophilic precursors. Monocytes and their precursors, monoblasts and promonocytes, are only present in small numbers in normal marrow. In abnormal states, notably in leukaemia, they can become very conspicuous.

Megakaryocytes are easily recognized in the marrow by their large size and nuclear lobulation. With maturation the cytoplasm fragments and gives rise to platelets. Megakaryoblasts are smaller and can be very similar to myeloblasts in appearance.

Common Disorders Predominantly Affecting Myelopoiesis and Megakaryopoiesis

Acute myeloid leukaemia

In acute myeloid leukaemia the bone marrow is infiltrated with primitive myeloblasts numbering more than 30% of the total myeloid cell lines. Myeloblasts are often present in the peripheral blood as well. The myeloblasts are primitive cells showing an open nuclear chromatin pattern and a nucleolus. Cytoplasmic granulation and Auer rods may or may not be present (Figs 26.19 and 26.20).

Common Disorders Predominantly Affecting Myelopoiesis and Megakaryopoiesis

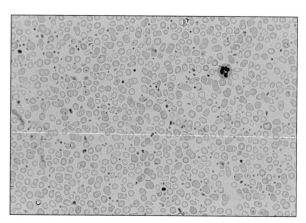

Figure 26.17: Raised platelet count in essential thrombocythaemia with some large forms.

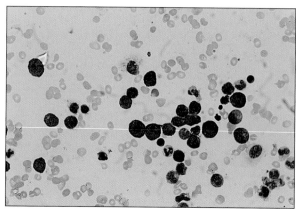

Figure 26.18: Megaloblastic bone marrow.

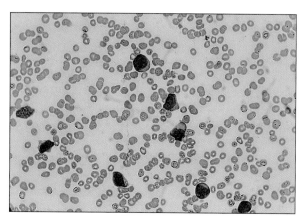

Figure 26.19: Acute myeloid leukaemia.

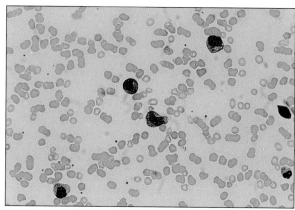

Figure 26.20: Acute promyelocytic leukaemia.

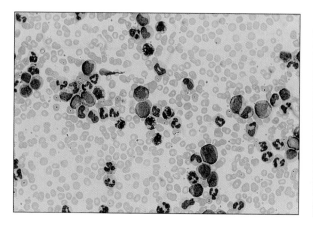

Figure 26.21: Chronic myeloid leukaemia.

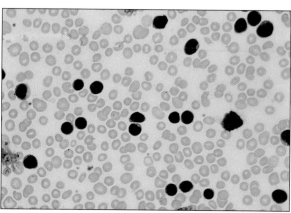

Figure 26.22: Acute lymphocytic leukaemia.

Common Disorders Predominantly Affecting Myelopoiesis and Megakaryopoiesis

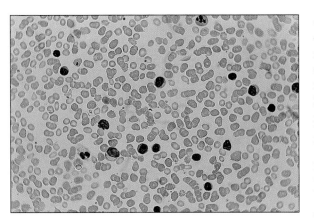

Figure 26.23: Chronic lymphocytic leukaemia.

Morphologically, acute myeloid leukaemia has been subdivided into various subtypes by the FAB group, depending on the degree of differentiation and the nature of predominant cells in the marrow. Sometimes primitive myeloblasts and monoblasts are difficult to differentiate by Romanowsky stains, and may not be easily distinguished from lymphoblasts. Special cytochemical stains are sometimes used in this situation (Tables 26.4 and 26.5). Recently, cytochemistry has been superseded by immunophenotyping (see Chapter 32). Acute myeloid leukaemia is a malignant disease. Chromosomal changes are readily demonstrable in 50% of cases. Clinically the patient often presents with anaemia, low platelet count, bleeding and infection. Circulating blasts are commonly found in peripheral blood. Bone marrow testing is mandatory and diagnostic.

Table 26.4: French-American-British (FAB) classification of acute myelocytic leukaemias.

	Category	Morphologic Criteria (bone marrow)
M1	Myeloblastic without maturation	≥90% of myeloid-line cells are blasts.
M2	Myeloblastic with maturation	30–89% of myeloid-line cells are blasts, >10% are promyelocytes to PMN (often dysplastic), <20% are monocytes.
M3	Promyelocytic	Hypergranular promyelocytes with heavy to dust-like granules, often Auer rods; nucleus often bilobed; microgranular variant may occur.
M4	Myelomonocytic	30–80% of myeloid-line cells are myeloblasts plus maturing neutrophils; >20% of myeloid-line cells are monocytic lineage. In addition, >5000/μl monocytic cells in peripheral blood.
M4	With eosinophilia	As above, with ≥5% abnormal eosinophils that may have unsegmented nucleus and both eosinophilic and large basophilic granules.
M5	Monoblastic, monocytic	>80% of myeloid-line cells are monoblasts, promonocytes, or monocytes; in M5a, 80% of myeloid-line cells are monoblasts; in M5b, <80% are monoblasts, and remainder are promonocytes and monocytes.
M6	Erythroleukemia	≥50% of bone marrow cells are erythroid precursors; ≥30% of non-erythroid myeloid-line cells are blasts.
M7	Megakaryocytic	Blasts in marrow or blood are identified as megakaryocytic lineage; if marrow inaspirable, biopsy shows large numbers of blasts, frequently with increased numbers of megakaryocytes and reticulin.

PMN: polymorphonuclear leukocytes

Common Disorders Predominantly Affecting Myelopoiesis and Megakaryopoiesis

Table 26.5: Special stains and assays used in classifying acute leukaemias.

| | | Stain | | |
| | Peroxidase or | | Esterases | |
Leukaemia	Sudan black B	Specific[a]	Nonspecific[b]	PAS[c]
AML-M1	+	+	—	—
AML-M2	+ to +++	+	—	—
AML-M3	+++	+++	—	—
AML-M4	++ to +++	+ to +++	+ to +++	—
AML-M5	+	—	+++	—
AML-M6	—	—	—	+++
AML-M7	—	0 to ++	0 to ++ (punctate)[d]	++ (punctate)
ALL	—	—	—	+++
Normal neutrophils	+++	+++	—	+++
Normal monocytes	+	—	+++	+++
Normal lymphocytes	—	—	—	±

[a] α-naphthol AS-D chloroacetate.
[b] α-naphthyl acetate esterase and α-naphthyl butyrate esterase.
[c] Periodic acid–Schiff.
[d] Megakaryoblasts negative for α-naphthyl butyrate esterase.

Chronic myeloid leukaemia

This is a stem cell disorder which is characterized by a high leukocyte count and the presence of granulocyte precursors, notably myelocytes and metamyelocytes, along with numerous circulating neutrophils. The marrow shows hypercellularity with granulocytic hyperplasia, frequent eosinophilia or basophilia (Fig. 26.21). Megakaryocytic hyperplasia with a raised platelet count is also common. The distinctive chromosomal abnormality is the presence of the Ph chromosome (Philadelphia chromosome). This is a reciprocal translocation between parts of the long arm of chromosome 22 and the long arm of chromosome 9, t(9:22) (q34:q11). This results in the transfer of the *abl* oncogene from 9q to a site on 22q, known as the breakpoint cluster region (BCR). Transformation to acute leukaemia (AML or ALL-like state) occurs after a variable length of time. This is the so-called blast crisis, the median interval being about three to four years.

Reactive changes in granulocytes and monocytes

In infective and inflammatory states the WBC count increases above 11×10^9/l. Neutrophils show a shift to the left with toxic granulation. Some circulating myelocytes and occasional myeloblasts may also be seen. Marrow shows a myeloid hyperplasia with predominance of promyelocytes and myelocytes. The overall picture can, in severe cases, resemble a leukaemic process and is sometimes called a 'leukaemoid reaction'. The clinical background of the patient, immunophenotyping, chromosomal study and clonality studies may be needed to separate this condition from leukaemia.

Myelodysplastic states

This heterogeneous group of disorders has been mentioned earlier (see page 275). Severe myelodysplastic states, particularly those involving trilineage dysplasia, can progressively show an increasing proportion of blasts in the marrow and, ultimately, transform to acute myeloid leukaemia. A special subcategory known as chronic myelomonocytic leukaemia (CMML)

BLOOD CELL AND BONE MARROW MORPHOLOGY

Megakaryocyte and Platelet Disorders
Lymphocytes, Plasma Cells and their Disorders
Common disorders affecting lymphocyte and plasma cell lineage

shows features of both dysplasia and a myelo-proliferative condition. This is characterized by the presence of peripheral blood monocytosis of $>1 \times 10^9/l$. The monocytes are often abnormal in morphology. Associated dysplastic features are also present in the red cells and other white cells.

Megakaryocyte and Platelet Disorders

Thrombocytopenia
A low platelet count of $<150 \times 10^9/l$ can be due to increased peripheral consumption (immune or non-immune) or decreased marrow production of platelets, i.e. marrow aplasia or infiltration. In idiopathic thrombocytopenic purpura (ITP), anti-platelet antibodies cause an increased reticuloendothelial destruction of platelets. In ITP or other consumptive states, the bone marrow shows a normal to increased number of megakaryocytes. Platelet production disorders are best diagnosed by a bone marrow test. Here the megakaryocytes may be absent, diminished, or show dysplastic morphology. The bone marrow aspirate also shows the presence of an abnormal infiltration.

Thrombocytosis
A persistently raised platelet count of over $1000 \times 10^9/l$ occurs in essential thrombocythaemia. Essential thrombocythaemia (ET) is a myeloproliferative disease predominantly involving the megakaryocyte lineage. The presence of large platelets or even megakaryocyte fragments is also characteristic of this disorder. Marrow aspiration can be difficult as it may clot readily before spreading. Bone marrow trephine shows hypercellularity with a conspicuous increase in the count of megakaryocytes, which are often atypical in morphology. An associated increase in reticulin or fibrosis of the marrow is also common. Reactive thrombocytosis (due to infection or inflammation) can sometimes cause a similar picture and can be, at times, difficult to differentiate from essential thrombocythaemia by morphology alone (see Fig. 26.17).

Lymphocytes, Plasma Cells and their Disorders

Morphological variations in both lymphocytes and plasma cells cover a much wider range than among granulocytes. In infections, particularly viral infections, lymphocytes show activated or immunoblastic features with cytoplasmic basophilia and the appearance of nucleoli. Children often have relative lymphocytosis. This diminishes with age. Plasma cells typically have more abundant basophilic cytoplasm with an eccentric nucleus showing clumped chromatin ('clock-face' appearance). Cytoplasmic inclusion of immunoglobulins can sometimes be seen.

Common disorders affecting lymphocyte and plasma cell lineage
Acute lymphoblastic leukaemia (ALL)
This is a monoclonal neoplastic disease arising from lymphoblastic precursors of lymphocytes. It accounts for about 85% of all acute leukaemias below the age of 16. Abnormal lymphoblasts are often present in peripheral blood associated with anaemia and a low platelet count. The bone marrow shows abnormal infiltration with lymphoblasts which have a higher nuclear cytoplasmic ratio than a typical myeloblast. The FAB (French, American and British) group have classified acute lymphoblastic leukaemia into three morphological subtypes (see Table 26.6). A pure morphological distinction between a lymphoblast and an undifferentiated myeloblast can be difficult in some cases. Flow cytometry and special stains are very helpful in this situation (see Table 26.5 and Fig. 26.22).

Chronic lymphocytic leukaemia (CLL)
This disease is uncommon before middle-age and its incidence increases with age. Typically it presents with peripheral lymphocytosis, lymphadenopathy and hepatosplenomegaly. The peripheral blood and bone marrow show the presence of many monomorphic small mature-looking lymphocytes. Smear cells are characteristically found in this disorder. CLL cells have also a distinctive immunophenotypic profile (Fig. 26.23).

Lymphocytes, Plasma Cells and their Disorders

Common disorders affecting lymphocyte and plasma cell lineage

Table 26.6: FAB classification of acute lymphocytic leukaemia.

Cytology	L1	L2	L3
Cell size	Small	Large	Large, homogeneous
Nuclear chromatin	Homogeneous	Variable	Finely stippled
Nuclear shape	Regular	Irregular	Oval to round
Nucleoli	Rare	Present	1–3
Cytoplasm	Scanty	Moderate	Moderate, vacuolated
Cytoplasmic basophilia	Moderate	Variable	Intense
Incidence in children	85%	13%	2%
Incidence in adults	35%	63%	2%
Immunologic markers	Early B or thymic T	Early B or thymic T	Differentiated B (SIg positive), Burkitt type leukaemia/lymphoma

SIg: surface immunoglobulin

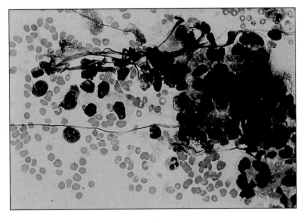

Figure 26.24: Metastatic carcinoma cells.

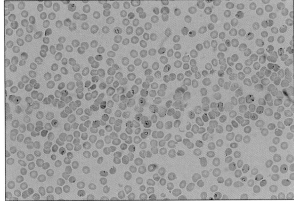

Figure 26.25: Malaria parasites in blood.

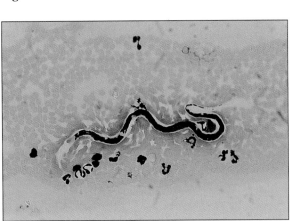

Figure 26.26: Microfilaria in blood.

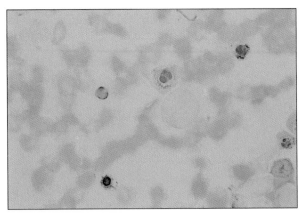

Figure 26.27: Sideroblasts.

Myeloma

This is a disease characterized by clonal, neoplastic growth of plasma cells. Patients present with paraprotein, hypercalcaemia, lytic bone lesions, anaemia and renal failure. Bone marrow, which is diagnostic, shows the presence of abnormal plasma cells in large proportion (>30%) (Fig. 26.8).

Lymphoma

Lymphomas are a complex, heterogeneous group of clonal neoplastic diseases, predominantly arising from lymph nodes but which can also involve peripheral blood or bone marrow. Lymphoma is a disease with many subtypes. The neoplastic cells can be small and can look similar to small lymphocytes (low grade lymphoma). On the other hand some lymphoma cells have very immature, large blast-like morphology (high grade lymphoma).

Hodgkin's disease (HD), classified as a type of lymphoma, is characterized by the presence of Reed–Sternberg cells.

Non-haemopoietic Cells and Parasites in Blood and Marrow

A bone marrow aspirate and trephine is a useful test to detect metastatic carcinoma cells, especially in the presence of a leuco-erythroblastic blood picture (Fig. 26.24).

Malaria parasites are best detected in peripheral blood film. Uncommonly microfilaria can also be found (Fig. 26.25 and 26.26).

Expertise and confidence in cell morphology come with practice. For a more exhaustive review on this subject, see reference 3.

Further Reading

Bennet J M, Catovsky D, Daniel M T, Flandarin G, Galton D A G, Gralnick H R, Sultan C. Proposal for classification of myelodysplastic syndrome. *British Journal of Haematology* 1982; 51:189.

Bennet J M, Catovsky D, Daniel M T, Flandarin G, Galton D A G, Gralnick H R, Sultan C. Proposal for classification of acute leukaemias. *British Journal of Haematology* 1976; 33: 451.

Hayhoe F G J, Flemans R J. *A Colour Atlas of Haematological Cytology*, 3rd edn 1992: Wolfe Publishing Ltd, London.

Holfbrand A V, Pettit J E. *Clinical Haematology*; 2nd edn 1994: Sandoz Atlas, London.

27 PRINCIPLES OF AUTOMATED CELL ANALYSIS

Carl Holland

The automation of haematological investigations has been commonplace in most laboratories for almost 30 years. In today's environment of increasing workloads, shortages of qualified laboratory personnel, and requirements for even greater productivity and efficiency within at best a static budget, laboratory managers look towards greater automation of their departments in an endeavour to meet the requirements of the service. Undoubtedly the major developments in haematology have taken place in the area of electronic blood cell counting with the automated full blood count (FBC) being the backbone investigation to all haematology laboratories' workload. These counters began life as semi-automated instruments accepting pre-diluted blood that was sampled, analysed on single channels, and the parameters displayed. Today we are offered fully automated multi-parameter haematological analysers capable of handling huge numbers of specimens at high speed, with accuracy and precision that could never be achieved by manual methods. These machines produce multi-parameter red cell indices, white cell counts with full differentials, platelet parameters, lymphocyte subsets, reticulocyte enumeration and blood smear production, all from a single analysis. These analysers may now be linked to sample transport systems allowing concurrent analysis of haematology, chemistry, coagulation, urinalysis and immunochemistry, all operated from a single remote computer terminal.

In this chapter I propose to provide an overview of automated cell analysers, past, present and future, and to consider the principles employed in their operation.

Automated Cell Counters

The last 30 years have seen a revolution in automated cell counting, with each new model delivering more parameters at greater speed with less operator involvement in their routine

functioning. In addition a new breed of compact instrument requiring minimal operator training to operate, calibrate and maintain has been produced for use in clinics and general practitioner surgeries, providing instant haematological screening for patients. All cell counters have been designed around two major methods of cell enumeration. The first uses electrical aperture impedance and the other employs laser light scatter and flow cytometry.

Aperture Impedance Counters

This widely used method was invented by F W Coulter in 1956 and became known as the 'Coulter principle' of cell counting. Coulter later set up Coulter Electronics Ltd to produce and develop the system. This principle is also used in variations by Sysmex (Toa Medical Electronics), Cell-Dyn (Abbott Diagnostics Division) and Argos (Roche).

Cells are suspended evenly by mixing in an electrolyte solution. Two platinum electrodes are placed in this electrolyte but completely separated except for a small orifice linking the two. Current thus passes freely from one electrode to the other through the orifice. The cell suspension is drawn through the aperture at a constant rate by a pneumatic supply. Cells are poor conductors of electricity, therefore as they pass through the orifice there is a demonstrable fall in the electrical current flow. The magnitude of the change in current is directly proportional to the volume of the cell passing through the orifice. The number of electrical pulses generated by cells passing through in a set volume of electrolyte is proportional to the number of cells in the suspension. Electronic gating allows the analyser to ignore pulses above or below a certain threshold value, thus eliminating the counting of debris. These gates can be adjusted, enabling the enumeration and

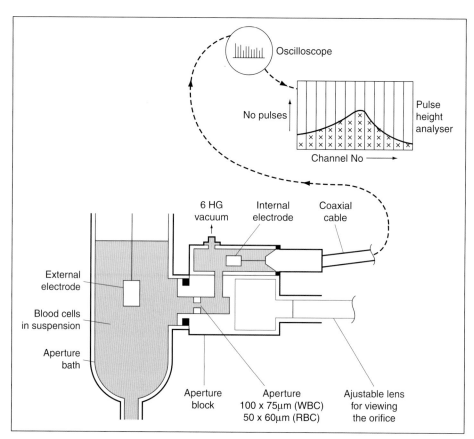

Figure 27.1: *Aperture impedance principle of the Coulter STK-S.*
[By permission of Coulter Electronics.]

Aperture Impedance Counters
Red cell count
White cell count
Haemoglobin

sizing of red blood cells, white blood cells and platelets (see Fig. 27.1).

Red cell count

Blood is diluted in an isotonic electrolyte. This dilution contains red cells, white cells, and platelets. Electronic gating separates the platelets from the total cell count and as the red cell count vastly exceeds the white cells in *normal* samples, their presence has a negligible effect on the total red cell count. It must be remembered that counts from samples containing markedly raised white cell counts such as leukaemic samples must be corrected to allow for their presence to avoid falsely raised counts being obtained. In addition to this, several other important issues must be dealt with before an accurate red cell count and red cell size can be obtained.

Coincidence

If two or more cells enter the aperture sensing zone simultaneously during a cycle, the resistance change created in this situation generates a single high amplitude pulse. As a consequence of this, the cell count is falsely low. This phenomena can be corrected for statistically as its occurrence is predictable for any count value.

Recirculation

As cells pass through the orifice they will often swirl around and sometimes re-enter the sensing zone of the aperture causing the cell to be counted twice. This is eliminated by the various manufacturers by blocking the recirculation of cells within the aperture.

White cell count

Blood is diluted in the electrolyte before a lysing agent is added that bursts the red blood cells but leaves the white blood cells intact. In the process the cytoplasm is stripped from the nucleated cells and therefore only the nucleus is counted as it passes through the orifice. It should be noted that nucleated red blood cells will also be counted as white cells and the count must be corrected manually for their presence.

Haemoglobin

As the lysing agent is added to the cell suspension and the red cells rupture, a modified Drabkins reagent converts all haemoglobins to the stable form cyanmethaemoglobin (HiCN). The sample then enters a cuvette where the haemoglobin is measured spectrophotometrically at the optimum wavelength of absorption by haemoglobin 450 nm. The greater the absorption of light the greater the haemoglobin concentration. High white cell counts will increase the turbidity of the haemoglobin sample and consequently give a falsely raised haemoglobin. In these cases the white cells must be removed, usually by centrifugation prior to analysis.

Mean cell volume (MCV) is measured from volume pulse heights. It is a mean result and does not take into account degrees in variation of cell volume known as anisocytosis. The result is expressed in femtolitres (f).

Haematocrit (HCT) represents the volume of whole blood taken up by red blood cells, and is calculated from:

Red cell count (RCC) × Mean Cell Volume (MCV)

The result is expressed as a percentage of the total volume (%).

Mean cell haemoglobin (MCH) is calculated from:

Haemoglobin (Hb)/Red Cell Count (RCC)

The result is expressed in picograms (pg).

Mean cell haemoglobin concentration (MCHC) is calculated from:

Haemoglobin (Hb)/Haematocrit (HCT)

The result is expressed in grams per decilitre (g/dl).

Red Cell Distribution Width (RDW) is a measure of variation in red cell size (anisocytosis). The RDW is derived from the RBC histogram and is expressed as a percentage coefficient of variation. It is important to trim the RBC histogram to remove erroneous signals caused by doublets, triplets and red cell agglutinates on the right (high volume) side of the histogram, and platelet clumps, large platelets and electrical interference on the left-hand side (low volume) of the histogram. This data manipulation is achieved by locating the channel containing 20% of the modal height channel on either side of the mode and calculating the coefficient of variation.

Platelet count is derived from the platelet histogram. The threshold is set at 2 and 20 fl to exclude electronic interference and small RBCs from interfering with the count. Platelet indices such as mean platelet volume (MPV), platelet crit (PCT), and platelet distribution width (PDW) are calculated in the same manner as the red cell indices.

Optical Flow Systems

Two companies dominated the market with cell counters utilizing this principle, Technicon Instruments Corporation with their range of Technicon instruments and Ortho Diagnostics with their ELT counters. Today this technology is provided chiefly by Technicon.

The principle of operation relies on monochromatic laser light that is focused onto an optically clear flow cell. The cells are isovolumetrically sphered and fixed after dilution and passed through the flow cell. As an individual cell passes through the flow cell, laser light is scattered at high and low angles. Photomultiplier tubes collect the scattered laser light and convert it to an electrical impulse. Light scattered at high and low angles simultaneously measures the cell volume and optical density (haemoglobin concentration) of each cell. The isovolumetric sphering of the red cells ensures accurate MCV measurement and ensures that differing orientation of the red cells in the flow cell do not give erroneous results. Each pulse that is registered by a passing cell is proportional to its size and therefore the sum of the pulse heights is equivalent to the haematocrit (HCT). This system supplies the same red cell and platelet parameters as the aper-

ture impedance methods, but in addition is capable of producing measurements of cellular haemoglobin concentrations (CHCM). This is the first measurement of haemoglobin variation in individual cells and hence is the first measurement of red cell anisochromia. White blood cells are subjected to cytoplasmic stripping with only basophils remaining intact. The white cells are counted and differentiated by size and nuclear lobularity. This, together with peroxidase staining, made the Technicon system the first to produce a full five-population differential. This will be discussed in detail later.

Red cell histograms are produced by both types of cell counters giving information on dual (dimorphic) cell populations, and help to identify red cell fragmentation and agglutination. The Technicon system also produces a red cell cytogram known as the 'Mie Map'. Cell size and red cell haemoglobin are plotted on the X and Y axes to create characteristic cell populations for red cell disorders, helping to differentiate iron deficient haemopoiesis from beta-thalassaemia trait (see Fig. 27.2).

Leukocyte Differentials

The usefulness of the leukocyte differential has been argued fiercely for many years. It is, however, here to stay and is now performed with almost every full blood count entering the haematology laboratory, due to dramatic developments in blood cell counters.

The standard 100-cell differential count that is performed on the standard wedge preparation has several limitations: non-random distribution of white cells at the edges and brush borders of slides, and the statistical limitations of the 100-cell differential whereby much greater precision would be obtained if more cells were counted. However, when this is done manually it becomes laborious and time-consuming. This has led to a demand for a rapid screening of the white cell differential.

Pattern recognition systems

These were the first instruments to analyse the white cell differential, of which the best known was the Geometric Data 'Haematrak' analyser.

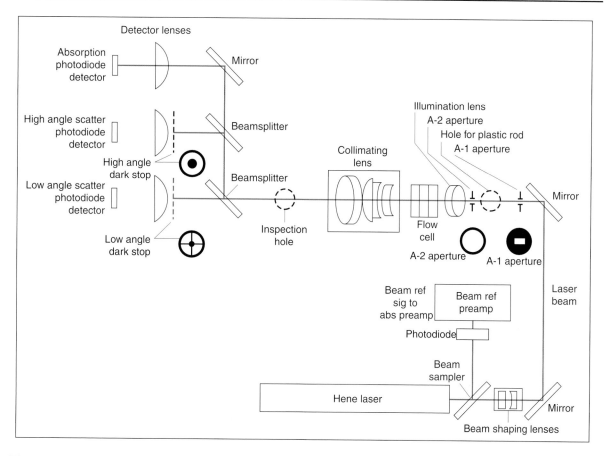

Figure 27.2: *Laser optical system of the Technicon H3 Analyser. [By permission of Bayer Corporation.]*

Conventionally stained blood smears are scrutinized by a microscope and a motorized microscope substage. White cells are counted and recognized by computer generated 'fingerprints'. Up to 100 smears an hour can be analysed and any cells the system fails to identify are stored for review by a suitably qualified member of staff at a later stage. This system has recently been totally revised by Coulter Electronics with their Micro 21 system. This fully automated walk-away microscope allows up to 52 prepared slides to be loaded. It then searches, analyses, stores and displays up to 170 white blood cells in addition to red cell morphology and platelet estimation. The system analyses colour, shape, size, texture, density, and nuclear/cytoplasm ratio of cells before producing full colour reports or transmitting to the review station for review by a staff member.

Light scattering and cytochemistry

This methodology was introduced by the Technicon Corporation and began with the Haemalog D and H6000 systems. The principle utilized flow cytometry and three white cell channels for identification and enumeration of the different cell types: channel 1 measured monocytes using esterase staining and measurements of cell size; channel 2 measured neutrophils, eosinophils and lymphocytes by staining for intracellular peroxidase; and channel 3 measured basophils using an alcian dye.

These analysers were capable of screening up to 10 000 white blood cells and hence the degree of precision was greatly enhanced in comparison with the manual 100-cell differential. Further development of the systems led to the Technicon H1, H2 and most recently the H3 analysers. With these systems red cells are lysed and the

Leukocyte Differentials

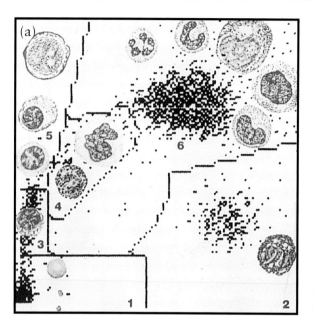

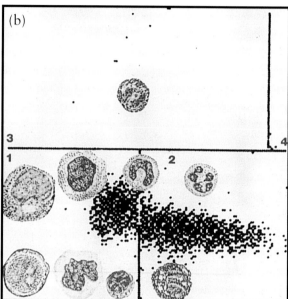

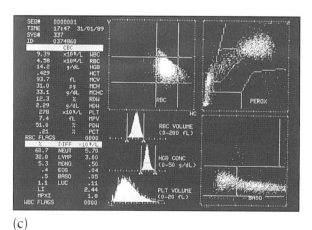

(c)

Figure 27.3: (a) Peroxidase leukogram. 1 Red cell debris and platelets. 2 Eosinophils. 3 Lymphocytes. 4 Monocytes and basophils. 5 LUC (large unstained cells). 6 Neutrophils.(b) Basophil/lobularity analysis. 1 Mononuclears. 2 PMNs – neutrophils and eosinophils. 3 Basophils. 4 Debris. (c) Normal report. [By permission of Bayer Corporation.]

white cells fixed and then stained for myeloperoxidase activity. The cells are passed one at a time through an optical channel comprising a tungsten light source past two detectors. Detector one measures dark field illumination and measures scattered light that has hit the stained cells and bounced off. The other detector measures the degree of staining of each cell by analysing the absorbance of the light. Cell size and peroxidase staining allows differentiation of neutrophils, lymphocytes, monocytes and eosinophils by the use of cell cluster analysis that is produced when light scatter information is plotted against absorption, giving what is known as a cytogram (see Fig. 27.3).

The system also produces the mean peroxidase index (MPXI) of the neutrophils which provides useful information of cell activity in conditions such as infection or myelodysplasia. Basophils are measured using the basophil/

lobularity channel. White cell membranes and cytoplasm are stripped from the nucleus by the use of a surfactant. Basophil membranes are resistant to this action and remain intact. When the cells are passed though the laser light the low angle scatter (0–5°) that measures cell size, the basophils are discriminated by their greater size and enumerated. High angle scatter (5–15°) measures the lobularity of the cell. The lobularity index provides information on the number of immature 'left shifted' neutrophils. The systems are capable of providing approximately 100 full blood counts with differentials per hour.

Volumetric differentiation

This method provides an automated screening differential. White cells are differentiated by their differing pulse heights when measured by aperture impedance methodology. The white cells undergo cytoplasmic shrinkage prior to analysis. This allows white blood cells to be separated according to their volumes into three populations: small cells = lymphocytes, medium cells = monocytes, eosinophils and basophils, large cells = neutrophils. This three-population differential provides a rapid white cell screen identifying abnormalities that may require further investigation.

VCS technology

V.C.S. technology has been pioneered by Coulter Electronics Ltd to provide a five-population differential. This is determined using a combination of three different measurements of each cell, these being cell volume, conductivity, and light scatter. A maximum of 8192 white cells are counted and categorized into one of the five cell types. The white cells are analysed in their near native states with no staining or stripping of cell membranes or cytoplasm. The white cells are focused by a fluidic stream to provide a constant target for the laser, which is focused onto the optically clear flow cell through which the cells are passed one at a time. *Volume*: this is measured using the standard aperture impedance method as described previously. *Conductivity*: reflects the cell's internal nuclear structure. Electromagnetic waves of high frequency pass through the cell where information is translated

about the nuclear to cytoplasm ratio, nuclear density and granularity. *Light scatter*: measures the characteristics of the cell surface as well as granularity and lobularity of each cell. Laser light striking the white blood cells as they pass through the flow cell results in reflection, refraction and absorption of the laser light which is collected by detectors and converted to electrical signals that are interpreted by computer processors and plotted on a three-dimensional channel plot, producing characteristic cell clusters that can be categorized (see Fig. 27.4).

Several other systems utilizing laser light and a flow cell to produce a full five-population differential include *MAPSS technology* (multi-angle polarized scatter and separation of white cells). Cells are diluted and hydrodynamically focused in a fast-moving fluid stream into the flow cell. As the cells enter the laser beam they scatter light in all directions. The intensity of the scattered light is measures at four angles. (a) Forward angle light scatter measures cell size. (b) Narrow angle light scatter (7–11°) is a measurement of the cell structure and complexity. (c) Orthogonal light scatter (70–110°) is a measurement of the internal granularity and lobularity. (d) Ninety degree depolarized scatter (70–110°) separates eosinophils from neutrophils by the ability of eosinophilic granules to cause polarized orthogonal laser light to depolarize. These four measurements are carried out on 10 000 white blood cells in each sample and has been developed by the Abbott Diagnostics Cell-Dyn system.

Toa Medical Electronics Sysmex systems utilize radio frequency (RF) and direct current (DC) measurements. RF measurements discriminate granulocytes, lymphocytes and monocytes, while eosinophils and basophils are enumerated in a separate DC measuring channel after pre-treatment of a sample aliquot.

Morphology Flags

In addition to providing multiple parameters on red cells, white cells and platelets, all manufacturers of modern cell counters provide morphology flags. These alert the operator of the analyser that microscopic examination of the

Morphology Flags

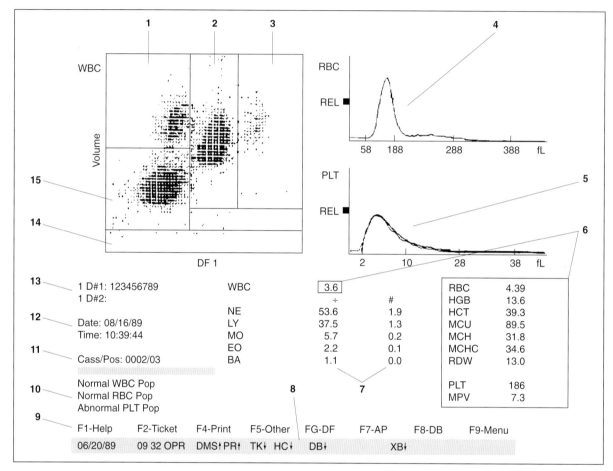

Figure 27.4: Coulter VCS Scatterplot (DF1) showing cell population discrimination. [By permission of Coulter Electronics.] 1 MO population. 2 NE population. 3 EO population. 4 RBC histogram. 5 PLT histogram. 6 CBC parameter results. 7 WBC differential percent and number results. 8 Status line. 9 Option line. 10 Condition field. 11 Cassette label. 12 Date and time the sample was analysed. 13 Two sample identification fields. 14 WBC threshold. 15 LY* population.

* The BA population is located in a third dimension in the upper right quadrant of the LY population.

blood may be required. By inputting the normal ranges for the measured parameters the analyser will produce morphological comments that interpret any deviation away from the normal range. These can be downloaded straight onto the final printed report. In addition 'Suspect' flags are also generated when the instrument's evaluation of scatterplots and histograms indicate the possible presence of an abnormal subpopulation. Examples of suspect flags include platelet clumps, nucleated RBCs, atypical lymphocytes and blast cells, all of which will require manual verification. Thus

the report produced by the analyser provides numerical as well as interpretive reporting.

On all of the manufacturers' 'flagship' analysers, samples loaded onto the systems are automatically mixed, auto-sampled, and barcode read at a sample rate of at least 100 samples per hour. Data storage functions allow the operator to review, sort, edit and print out data at any time. These results can be printed onto graphic or line printers or can be interfaced to bidirectionally communicate with a host computer for even further systematization. Automatic simple and effective quality control systems for storage, calculation and presentation of quality control data are inbuilt into the systems. Sophisticated computer-driven functions such as Start-up, Shut-down, Maintenance and Error messages, as well as future on-board modems that will allow interrogation of the analyser by engineers from the manufacturer's headquarters, will ensure the operation of these machines is as trouble-free as possible.

Reticulocyte Counting

A recent development has been the incorporation of reticulocyte analysis into multi-parameter blood cell counters, with all manufacturers providing analysers with on-line reticulocyte analysis in addition to the FBC and white cell differential. The ribosomes and rough endoplasmic reticulum present in the reticulocyte is stained with either new methylene blue stain, acridine orange, thiazole orange or Auromine-O. Using light scatter and volume measurements the larger stained reticulocytes are separated from the smaller unstained mature erythrocytes. More than 30 000 red cells are analysed per specimen giving excellent precision and accuracy compared to manual reticulocyte counts. The results are reported in absolute numbers and percentages in about one minute.

Lymphocyte subsets
This analysis was first carried out on a blood cell counting machine by the Technicon H1 using an immunoperoxidase reaction. Whole blood is incubated with specific monoclonal antibody that binds to the surface of specific lymphcytes. A second biotinylated antibody is added that binds to the monoclonal antibody. Finally an avidin–peroxidase reagent is added that binds to the biotin. Peroxidase is then stained for, with the labelled lymphocytes giving a positive result.

Coulter Electronics have adapted their VCS technology to analyse lymphocyte subsets, separating T-helper from T-suppressor lymphocytes in less than five minutes. The method uses

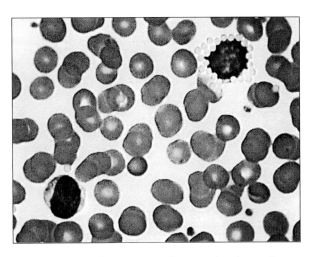

Figure 27.5: Blood smear showing binding of monoclonal antibody coated latex spheres to a CD4 positive lymphocyte.

lyophilized latex spheres coated in monoclonal antibody specific for the antigen on the lymphocyte surface. The beads are then mixed with blood in a safe closed system, where the spheres bind to the surface of the cells. These cells carrying the spheres give differing volume, conductivity and scatter characteristics compared to unbound lymphocytes. These are isolated and enumerated as an absolute count, percentage and as a CD4/CD8 ratio. This gives the operator the opportunity to monitor the cellular immunity of patients infected with HIV without even taking the cap off the bottle, thus protecting the health and safety of staff members (see Fig. 27.5).

Automatic slide-making capabilities
Slide-making facilities including staining were provided by the Technicon H-6000 in the early 1980s. However it is only recently that automatic blood smear preparation has been incorporated into cell counting analysers. The main advantage of these systems is safety, avoiding the need to expose staff to an open blood sample. There is no requirement to sort out the samples requiring smears. The systems will make slides upon demand or according to computer driven criteria set by the department, depending on the FBC and DIFF results. Each smear is labelled with a barcode label copied from the primary tube. Unfortunately

the analysers do not stain the slides but this may well become a future development.

Total Clinical Laboratory Automation

Systems have recently been installed in Japan and America that completely break down the dividing walls between haematology, biochemistry and immunology. These systems are totally automated, performing sorting of samples with barcode labelling. Centrifugation and aliquoting of specimens is performed, and all secondary tubes are barcoded accordingly. The specimens are then loaded onto haematology and chemistry analysers by a sample transport system that links all analysers together. Manual sample handling is eliminated, reducing infection risks and freeing laboratory personnel to concentrate on other laboratory functions.

The process begins with inputting of specimen information from the host computer into the system. Barcode readers identify the sample and the tests required. The sample is moved along transport lanes in single file to the main analysers, where they are picked out, analysed and then returned to the transport lane to be transported to another analyser or to be filed in a refrigerated storage unit for easy retrieval at any time. The whole system is driven from a remote computer and can pinpoint any sample's position in the laboratory at any time. Time spent hunting for individual samples is eliminated. Such complex systems are not cheap, but for large university hospital laboratories these systems can analyse several thousand samples a day with a minimal workforce (see Fig. 27.6).

Automation has come a long way in 30 years from the single channel analysers accepting single pre-diluted samples to the 'all singing, all

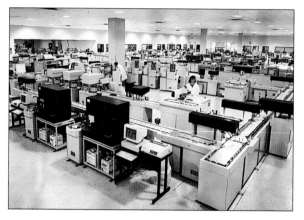

Figure 27.6: *Total clinical laboratory automation at Ciba Corning Laboratories, St Louis, USA. [By permission of Coulter Electronics.]*

dancing' total laboratory systems. Spiralling workloads, shortages of qualified staff and increasing pressure for a '*stat*' service will only conspire to ensure that automation at this level is here to stay.

Acknowledgements

I would like to express my gratitude to the following organisations for their cooperation and help in compiling this chapter.

Coulter Electronics Ltd, Northwell Drive, Luton, Beds. LU3 3RH

Bayer Plc, Diagnostics Division, Bayer House, Strawberry Hill, Newbury, Berks. RG14 1JA

Abbott Diagnostics Division, Abbott House, Norden Rd, Maidenhead, Berks. SL4 4XF

Sysmex (Toa Medical Electronics), Sunrise Parkway, Linford Wood East, Milton Keynes, Bucks. MK14 6QF.

Further information and literature is available by contacting the above companies.

28 METHODS FOR THE IDENTIFICATION OF THE HAEMOGLOBINOPATHIES

Anne Sermon

Introduction

The haemoglobinopathies and thalassaemias are the most common inherited genetic disorders. The molecular defects are located in the globin genes and affect the synthesis of haemoglobin in the developing erythrocyte. They manifest clinically as haemolytic anaemia and inheritance is autosomal recessive. The mutations which produce a haemoglobinopathy are diverse; the study and characterization of the human haemoglobin gene is used as an example to demonstrate most of the known types of genetic mutation. The clinically significant defects are found in the α and β genes, but the mutations may affect any of the globin-producing genes. The resulting abnormalities give rise both to qualitative and quantitative abnormalities of haemoglobin synthesis. Haemoglobinopathies result from the production of a structurally abnormal variant haemoglobin. The thalassaemias arise from the reduction in the rate of synthesis of one or more of the types of globin chains.

Point mutations, leading to amino acid substitutions, account for the majority (90%) of the globin gene defects and are typical of haemoglobinopathies and β thalassaemia. Gene deletion is the common cause of α thalassaemia. There are currently over 670 Hb variants which can be divided broadly into the following groups: (1) clinically silent; (2) thalassaemic haemoglobins; (3) unstable haemoglobins; (4) altered oxygen affinity; (5) miscellaneous atypical effects e.g. Hb S.

Haemoglobin S is the most common clinically significant variant Hb and in the homozygous state, Hb SS and in combination with Hb C or β thalassaemia trait, produces severe health problems in populations with high gene frequency. Tissue hypoxia secondary to acute sickling results in painful and potentially fatal crisis. The genes for Hb S and the thalassaemias are found world-wide. Hb S is commonest in Africa, Saudi Arabia, and the Mediterranean Basin. Screening, is therefore, aimed at those ethnic populations at risk of carrying these genes.

Screening Techniques

Current screening methodology allows rapid detection and accurate identification of the clinically significant haemoglobin disorders as well as their heterozygous states. These techniques can also be applied reliably in the screening of neonates to detect unexpected disease as well as carrier states. It is possible to assess genetic risk through the identification of carriers and offer prenatal diagnosis in the fetus. Policies are established in most laboratories for the screening services for adults and neonates. Techniques for antenatal diagnosis are more complex and are normally carried out in National Centres for molecular diagnosis.

Preliminary investigations should comprise information about the patient's ethnic background and clinical history, a full blood count and film analysis. Samples from patients targeted for screening should then channel through a flexible protocol of laboratory investigations which include electrophoresis, sickle solubility, Hb A_2 and F measurement, and ferritin levels. Diagnosis of the majority of the common trait states i.e. α and β thalassaemia, Hb S, C, D, and E, can usually be achieved by assessment of these results.

More sophisticated techniques, such as isoelectric focusing and high pressure liquid chromatography, which were found previously only in specialist centres, are becoming more widespread. These procedures are ideally suited to the automation of mass screening, being highly sensitive and cost-effective for this purpose.

Laboratory Diagnosis of Haemoglobinopathies and Thalassaemias

Full blood count
The majority of the trait states have no specific morphological features and the FBC may well show no abnormality. The red cell indices are important indicators in the assessment for thalassaemia trait which is characterized by hypochromic microcytosis, a normal haemoglobin and a normal or raised RBC count. An MCV of <80 fl and an MCH of <27 pg is indicative of possible thalassaemia, but these delineators may vary slightly from one laboratory to another, according to the principle of automated measurement and therefore the normal ranges assigned by the laboratory. For our purposes, a cut-off of <80 fl will certainly detect the β thalassaemia traits, and most of the mild α thalassaemia traits. The ferritin level should be determined in those samples which show microcytosis, to exclude iron deficiency. The FBC from patients who are clinically symptomatic may show the features of decompensated anaemia of variable degree, or even polycythaemic indices in haemoglobins with altered oxygen affinity.

Blood film analysis
The red cell morphology is significant in the identification of sickle cells in any of the genetic combinations of sickle cell disease. Target cells are characteristic of haemoglobins C and E and thalassaemia trait which also features microcytosis and basophilic stippling (see Chapter 26). In more severely affected patients, the red cell morphology may reflect the features of haemolytic anaemia with the presence of nucleated red cell precursors, schistocytes, poikilocytes, anisocytosis and polychromasia.

Detection, Identification and Quantitation of Haemoglobinopathies

The principles of detection, identification and quantitation of haemoglobins are based on the physical separation of haemoglobins in solution, according to their charge. The amino acid substitutions in most variants introduce a change in overall surface charge, which is integral to their detection. A limitation of these techniques, therefore, is that variants with the same overall surface charge cannot be distinguished from Hb A.

Detection and identification
Electrophoresis

Basic screening methodology relies on the migration of a charged molecule (Hb) in an electric field toward a cathode or anode. The strength and polarity of the charge is determined by the pH of the buffered environment. The rate of migration is governed by the pore size of the supporting medium and the magnitude of the charge on the molecule.

Cellulose acetate is a commonly used medium, being inexpensive and having an indefinite shelf life; agar is a widely used alternative. The pH for preliminary screening is alkaline, fixed at pH 8.4–8.9 with tris-EDTA-borate, or tris-barbitone buffers. At this pH, most haemoglobins are negatively charged and will migrate from the cathode toward the anode. Many variants separate from Hb A under these conditions, enabling visible detection which can be made more obvious by staining with a protein-specific dye e.g. Ponceu S or Amido black. The pattern of migration, marked by reference controls, can then be compared to a variant map to give probable identification. Fixed pH techniques are relatively insensitive to the discrete separation of groups of variants with similar charges. At pH 8.4, two groups of common variants, haemoglobins S, D and G and haemoglobins C, E and O Arab, comigrate. This makes distinction between the variants in each group impossible without further investigation. A differential change in charge in the haemoglobins can be induced by changing the buffer to acid. This alters the rate and characteristic pattern of migration. Under these conditions (citrate agar pH 6.3), the relative mobilities at both acid and alkaline pH are cross-referenced on variant maps, which allows a confident identification e.g. at pH 6.3, Hb C will become distinct from Hb E and O Arab, and Hb S will separate from Hb D and G. The identity of some variants will remain unresolved, and may be established with further analysis by more sensitive techniques e.g. IEF or HPLC. Some cases, usually rare, will require definition of the exact mutation at molecular level.

Sickle solubility

The sickle solubility test is a simple, inexpensive screen for the presence of haemoglobin S. A positive screen does not distinguish between homozygotes and heterozygotes and should have a sensitivity down to approximately 20% Hb S concentration. This test is most useful where a rapid screen is required, prior to general anaesthetic, in a patient whose haemoglobinopathy status is unknown. The detection of Hb S is based on its relative insolubility when deoxygenated and the subsequent deformation of the RBC membrane into the classic sickle shape. In the test-tube, deoxygenation is induced by sodium dithionite with trace saponin added. If Hb S is present, then the deoxy form polymerizes to form the classic tactoid crystals. A positive test retains the opaque appearance of sickled RBCs in suspension, whereas the deoxyhaemoglobin in negative samples gives a clear haemoglobin solution. There are six other rare variants which also have sickling properties so this screen is not unique for Hb S, rather for 'sickling' haemoglobins. The identity should always be confirmed by electrophoresis. Conversely, a variant band which migrates in the position of Hb S should always be confirmed with a sickle solubility.

This screen is insensitive to very low levels of Hb S such as those found in newborns and, therefore, is not useful as part of a neonatal screen. However, it can be used to detect the Hb S gene in individuals where electrophoresis is not available as a first line of investigation, e.g. Third World countries.

Isoelectric focusing (IEF)

Isoelectric focusing is a highly sensitive and much more sophisticated form of electrophoresis and is based on the separation of haemoglobins according to their isoelectric point. Low molecular weight carrier ampholytes with a range of isoelectric points are incorporated into polyacrylamide gel or agar, to create a pH gradient. For the purposes of haemoglobin separation, a pH range of 5.5–8.5 is used. As the haemoglobins migrate through the gradient, they become neutral at their isoelectric point (pI) and stop migrating i.e. they become focused

Detection, Identification and Quantitation of Haemoglobinopathies

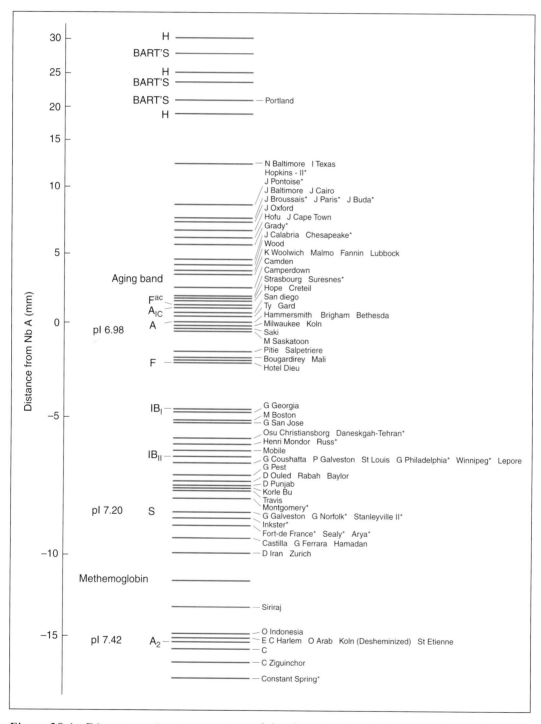

Figure 28.1: Diagrammatic representation of thin layer isoelectric focusing of normal haemoglobins and several haemoglobin structural variants. IB₁ and IB₂ are ferrous–ferric hybrids of Hb A. [Courtesy of Dr Yves Beuzard.]

at their pI. Since the pI is specific to the surface charge on a molecule, even haemoglobins with a very small differential charge (0.01) will separate discretely. On precast gels, the Hbs focus reproducibly in the same place, thereby offering much greater certainty of identification on a single separation. Due to the increased sensitivity of IEF, even variants which are present in very small concentrations can be resolved e.g. Constant Spring, A2 variants, H, Bart's. This techniques is, therefore, also suited to the cord blood screening of neonates (Fig. 28.1).

Quantitation

Quantitation of haemoglobin fractions is essential in (1) the further characterization of some variants i.e α chain variants, Hb E; (2) the diagnosis of compound haemoglobinopathy syndromes; (3) the distinction between α and β thalassaemia trait and the HPFH disorders (hereditary persistence of foetal haemoglobin). Estimation of haemoglobin fractions can be achieved by a variety of techniques including separation of the variant by electrophoresis followed by elution, microcolumn chromatography, HPLC, radial immunodiffusion and ELISA.

Microcolumn chromatography

Microcolumn chromatography is principly used for determining the percentage of Hb A_2 for the detection of β thalassaemia trait but may also be modified for the quantitation of major fractions e.g. Hb S percentage in the management of patients on exchange transfusion, or the further investigation of possible compound heterozygotes for a haemoglobinopathy and coexistent thalassaemia.

The principle of separation is dependent on adsorption and binding of charged haemoglobin molecules onto a resin with a polar side-chain. On the addition of a developer buffer to the column, the bound protein is displaced by stronger charged buffer ions, hence the term ion exchange chromatography. Displaced haemoglobins are subsequently washed from the resin in the eluate. Estimation of the percentage concentration of the fraction is then measured against a diluted total by optical densitometry. DEAE cellulose (diethylaminoethyl) is an anion

exchange resin which is paired with a glycine-KCN or tris-HCl buffer pH 8.3.

Levels of Hb A_2 <1.6% indicate α^0 thalassaemia trait; 1.6–3.5% comprises normal range and α^+ thalassaemia; while levels of 3.5–6.5% indicate β thalassaemia trait.

Measurement of haemoglobin F

Haemoglobin F comprises <1% in normal adults and is mildly raised in approximately 50% of β thalassemia traits. Hereditary persistence of fetal haemoglobin and $\delta\beta$ thalassaemia are a heterogeneous group of disorders, which are identified and classified according to the total Hb F percentage and by the distribution of Hb F in the RBC population, as established by a Kleihauer stain. The assay of total Hb F may be achieved by radial immunodiffusion, ELISA and HPLC techniques. The more widely used method was first introduced by Betke and is based on the selective denaturation of other haemoglobins by alkali to isolate haemoglobin F, which is resistant. A dilute lysate solution is subject to a fixed incubation of two minutes with NaOH which oxidizes all other fractions. The resulting methaemoglobins are precipitated with a saturated salt solution which also neutralizes the oxidation. Haemoglobin F, which remains in solution, can be separated from the precipitate by filtration or preferably by high speed centrifugation. The proportion of the Hb F fraction is calculated by optical densitometry against a total haemoglobin dilution.

An Hb F level of <1% constitutes the adult normal range; 1–5% is found in up to 50% of β thalassaemia traits; 5–20% is characteristic of $\delta\beta$ thalassaemia trait, and some HPFH; 20–45% is characteristic of pancellular African type HPFH.

High pressure liquid chromatography (HPLC)

HPLC combines detection, identification and quantitation of haemoglobins in a single technique and is eminently suited to screening large numbers of samples quickly, accurately and cheaply. The principle of separation remains the same as that of microcolumn chromatography, although the resin has a polyaspartate side-chain i.e. is a cation exchanger and the

<u>Detection, Identification and Quantitation of Haemoglobinopathies</u>
Detection of RBC inclusion bodies
Detection of unstable haemoglobins

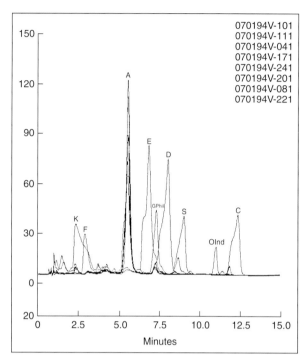

Figure 28.2: HPLC chromatogram overlay plot of the common variants.

fluid phase is a Cl⁻ ion. The analysis is automated with an autosampler injection onto the column and a pump which exerts a constant pressure of elution buffer onto the top of the lysate (Fig. 28.2). This controls and regulates the elution time. The sensitivity of the separation is vastly increased through the use of two buffers which differ in ion concentration and/or pH. Haemoglobin fractions are sequentially eluted from the column by the creation of an elution gradient achieved by mixing the two fluid phases. This enables the separation of previously unresolved variants i.e. D and G, and E and O. The optical density of the eluates is measured directly, as they pass from the column, by a photodetector and plotted continuously to create a chromatogram (Fig. 28.2). Identification is achieved by comparison of the retention times to those of known variants. Major and minor components can both be quantitated accurately by integrating the area under each peak. Very little, if any, further analysis is required, if only to cross-reference the characteristics of rare variants against secondary electrophoresis techniques.

Detection of RBC inclusion bodies

The redox reaction of supravital stains can be used to stain red cell inclusion bodies, formed from haemoglobin derivatives. This property is useful in the further characterization of haemoglobin disorders.

Haemoglobin H is formed from the excess β_4 tetramers in α thalassaemia and is detectable by electrophoresis, when present in significant quantities, in Hb H disease. Intracellular Hb H is soluble but very unstable and is precipitated by incubation with brilliant cresyl blue. The precipitate attaches to the RBC membrane to give a typical 'golf ball' appearance to the RBCs, with multiple stained bodies. Hb H inclusions are present in one to two cells per 1000 in α thalassaemia trait and can be difficult to detect microscopically. They are much more numerous and obvious in Hb H disease.

Heinz Bodies (see unstable Hbs) are not visible on a standard Romanowsky stained film, but are detectable as large, round and usually single intracellular precipitates following incubation with methyl violet. Their presence is often detected only in acute haemolysis and may not be obvious if splenic function is intact, or the stain is performed on very fresh blood.

Detection of unstable haemoglobins

Molecular instability in haemoglobin arises from amino acid substitution in the haem binding groups, the $\alpha\beta$ contact areas and in the interior of the haem pocket. These defects confer weakness in the haem–globin contacts and in the overall tetrameric and helical structures. This introduces a reduced tolerance to physiological stress with a tendency to the irreversible oxidation of haem iron and intracellular precipitation in the form of Heinz bodies. There are over 180 unstable haemoglobins and congenital Heinz body haemolytic anaemia (CHBA) varies widely in severity, depending on the nature and the position of the defect.

Electrophoresis may not be particularly helpful in the diagnosis of unstable haemoglobin disease, since the majority of these mutations show no change in the net charge of the molecule. Instability is detected using two denaturation screens based on exposure to a solvent and precipitation by heat. The samples should be fresh and a cord blood may be used as a positive control. Hb F has a relative intolerance to heat and hydrophobic stress compared to normal adult haemoglobin.

The heat instability test

This screen subjects haemoglobin to incubation at 50°C. This exerts further stress on already weakened internal van der Waals bonds, causing the subunits to dissociate more readily than normal.

Isopropanol stability test

Incubation with isopropanol induces hydrophobic stress. Isopropanol is more polar than water which weakens the hydrophobic bonds allowing water to enter the haem pocket, facilitating the oxidation of haem iron.

In both screens, normal haemoglobin remains in solution whilst unstable variants are detected by variable flocculation and precipitation.

Molecular Analysis

The standard screening techniques described above are adequate for the detection and characterization of the common mutations, but are limited in the unresolved identification of rare variants and the specific definition of the thalassaemia defects. The identification of the precise molecular lesion is essential for the purposes of genetic counselling, prenatal diagnosis and clinical management. This is achieved by analysis of genomic DNA extracted and amplified from peripheral blood leucocytes or from chorionic villus samples (CVS) for prenatal diagnosis.

Recent rapid progress has been made in the development of diagnostic techniques for DNA analysis. A detailed description of these and their applications are beyond the scope of this chapter (see Chapter 50). However, a brief outline is given on the technique which has revolutionized molecular DNA analysis, polymerase chain reaction (PCR).

Polymerase chain reaction

PCR is primarily applied to the detection of point mutations, deletions and DNA polymorphisms. This technique amplifies a region of the DNA of interest, simply and rapidly, and is particularly appropriate to prenatal diagnosis, since it requires only a very small sample which can be obtained by CVS at about 12 weeks gestation.

The principle of PCR involves the synthesis of DNA using synthetic primers (short single-stranded DNA sequences) which flank the DNA region of interest and a thermostable DNA polymerase (Taq polymerase). The enzymatic amplification of large quantities of DNA permits direct visualization of stained DNA fragments in an agarose gel. A single base substitution can be identified by the change in DNA fragment sizes following digestion of the PCR product with restriction enzymes that recognize specific DNA sequences. Southern blot analysis can also be applied to the detection of point mutations but takes up to a week to process and requires the use of radioisotopes. PCR analysis is possible within 24 hours when testing for a specific mutation, e.g. Hb S.

New techniques have been developed, based on PCR, that allow testing for specific mutations, without the use of restriction enzymes. One such technique is ARMS (amplification refractory mutation system) using allele specific primers. Here, two different primers are used, one complementary to the normal allele and the other to the mutant allele, i.e. they differ at the site of mutation only. The primers yield a PCR product if the primer and the DNA sequences are complementary. Thus, the normal and mutant primers will amplify the normal and mutant alleles respectively. Using this technique, the patient's DNA can be tested for a specific gene mutation e.g. Hb S. Primers have been synthesised for β^A, β^S, β^C α^0, α^+ and approximately 120 of the β thalassaemia genotypes. In β thalassaemia, a limited number of defects have been found to be prevalent in specific populations. The ethnic origin of the patient will determine a particular set of primers to be used first in analysis, with a high probability of positive identification in the first screen. The PCR based techniques mentioned above are used when screening for specific mutations or deletions. However, upon exclusion of the common molecular lesions, the putative mutation can be identified by directly sequencing the gene, using PCR. If the mutation still remains undefined and prenatal diagnosis is sought, this can be achieved using restriction fragment length polymorphism (RFLP) linkage analysis, using a DNA marker close to the mutant gene and so trace its inheritance in a family.

PCR is an extremely powerful technique enabling the development of DNA analyses from being a purely research tool, to providing a diagnostic service and the investigation of haemoglobinopathies have been at the forefront of this revolution.

Acknowledgement

Grateful thanks to Jaspal Kaeda FIBMS, PhD (Leukaemia Unit, Imperial College School of Medicine, Hammersmith Hospital, Du Cane Road, London) for his help with PCR.

Further Reading

Basset P, Beuzard Y, Garel M C, Rosa J. Isoelectric focussing of human haemoglobins : its application to screening, to characterisation of 70 variants and to study of modified fractions of normal haemoglobins. *Blood*, 1978; **51**, 971.

Betke K, Marti H R, Schlicht L. Estimation of small percentage of foetal haemoglobin. *Nature*, 1959; **184**, 1877.

British Committee for Standards in Haematology. Guidelines for the fetal diagnosis of globin gene disorders. *Journal of Clinical Pathology*, 1994; **47**, 199.

British Society for Haematology: Guidelines for Haemoglobinopathy Screening. *Clin Lab Haem*, 1988; **10**, 87–94.

Cao A, Rosatelli M C. Screening and prenatal diagnosis of the haemoglobinopathies. In *The Haemoglobinopathies. Baillière's Clinical Haematology*. Higgs D R, Weatherall D J. (eds). 1993; **6**, 263. Baillière Tindall, London.

Carrell R W, Kay R A. A simple method for the detection of unstable haemoglobins. *Br J Haem*. 1972; **23**, 615–19.

Cook A, Raper A B. The solubility test for Hb S: a cheap and rapid method. *Med Lab Technology*, 1971; **28**, 373–6.

Efremov G D, Huisman T H J. The laboratory diagnosis of the haemoglobinopathies. *Clin Haematol*, 1974; **3**, 542–3.

Galanello R, Ruggeri R, Addis M, Paglietti E, Cao A. Haemoglobin A2 in iron deficiency B thalassaemia heterozygotes. *Haemoglobin*, 1981; 5 613–618.

Grimes A J, Meisler A. Possible cause of Heinz bodies in congential Heinz body haemolytic anaemia. *Nature*, 1962; **194**, 190–1.

Grimes A J, Meisler A. Dacie J V. Congenital Heinz body anaemia. Further evidence on the cause of Heinz body production in red cells. *Br J Haem*. 1964; **10**, 281–90.

ICSH: Recommendations for selected methods for quantitative estimation of Hb A2 and for Hb A2 reference preparation. *Br J Haem*. 1978; **38**, 573–8.

International Committee for the Standardisation in Haematology. Simple electrophoretic system for presumptive identification of abnormal haemoglobins. *Blood*, 1978; **50**, 1058.

International Committee for Standardisation in Haematology. Recommendations for a system for identifying abnormal haemoglobins. *Blood*, 1978; **52**, 1065.

Itano H A. Solubility of naturally occurring mixtures of haemoglobins *Arch Biochem Biophys*, 1953; **47**, 148–59.

Kaeda J, Vulliamy T. DNA techniques in haematology. In *Practical Haematology*. Dacie J V, Lewis S M (eds) 8th edn, 1995; p. 529. Churchill Livingstone, London.

Further Reading

Marengo-Rowe A J. Rapid electrophoresis and quantitation of haemoglobins on cellulose acetate. *J of Clin Path*, 1965; **18**, 790.

Milner P F, Gooden H M. Rapid citrate-agar electrophoresis in routine screening for haemoglobinopathies using a simple haemolysate. *Am J Clin Path*, 1975; **64**, 58–64.

Molden D P, Alexander N M, Neeley W E. Fetal Hemoglobin: Optimum conditions for its estimation by alkali denaturation: *Am Jour Clin Path*. 1981; vol. 77, **5**, 568–72.

Old J M, Thein S L, Weatherall D J, Cao A, Loukopoulos D. Prenatal diagnosis of the major haemoglobin disorders. *Molecular Biology and Medicine*. 1989; **6**, 55–63.

Ou C N, Rognerud C. Rapid analysis of haemoglobin variants by cation exchange HPLC. *Clin Chem*, 1993; vol. 39, 5, 820–4.

Pearson H A, O'Brien R T, McIntosh. Screening for thalassaemia trait by electronic measurement of mean cell volume. *N Eng J of Med*, 1973; **288**, 351–3.

Righetti P G, Gianazza E, Bianchi-Bosisio A, Cossu G. Conventional isoelectric focussing and immobilised pH gradients for haemoglobin separation and identification. In Huisman THJ (ed). *The Haemoglobinopathies: Methods in Haematology*, 1986: vol 15, pp. 47–70. Churchill Livingstone, Edinburgh.

Roberts B. (ed). British Committee for Standardisation in Haematology. Guidelines for the investigation of the α and β thalassaemia states. *Journal of Clinical Pathology*, 1994; **47**, 289.

Saiki RK, Walsh PS, Levenson CH, Ehrlich HA. Diagnosis of sickle cell anaemia and β thalassaemia with enzymatically amplified DNA and non-radioactive allele-specific oligonucleotide probes. *New Eng Jour of Med*, 1988; **319**: 537–541.

Williamson D. Red Cell disorders: The Unstable Haemoglobins. *Blood Reviews*, 1993; **7**, 146–163.

Wood W G, Stamatoyannopoulos G, Lim G, Nute P E. F cells in the adult: normal values and levels with hereditary and acquired elevations of Hb F. *Blood*, 1975; **46**, 671.

29 SPECIAL VON WILLEBRAND FACTOR INVESTIGATIONS

Mohammad S Enayat

Introduction

von Willebrand disease (vWD) was first described by Erik von Willebrand in 1926 in several members of a large family from Åland archipelago in Finland. In 1953, an association between decreased factor VIII (FVIII) procoagulant activity and vWD was identified, leading to some confusion concerning the nature of the protein responsible for haemophilia A and vWD. A better understanding of the immunology and the molecular structure of vWF and FVIII in the late 1970s led to gene mapping and cDNA cloning of these two separate factors in 1989.

vWD is the commonest of the congenital bleeding disorders with a heterogeneous phenotype. It results from quantitative (type 1 and 3) or qualitative (type 2 variants) defects of vWF in plasma and/or platelets. This large multimeric glycoprotein ($10-20 \times 10^6$ kD) has two major roles in haemostasis, acting as carrier and proteolytic protector of FVIII and as the mediator of platelet adhesion to the subendothelium after vessel injury. vWF is synthesized in the endothelial cells and megakaryocytes by a ~ 9 kb mRNA transcription resulting from a 180 kb gene on the telomeric end of the chromosome 12 at 12p12 → pter (Fig. 29.1). Localization studies using a cDNA probe from the midportion of vWF has identified not only the authentic gene on this chromosome, but also a pseudogene sequence on chromosome 22 at 22q11 to 23. This pseudogene is 21–29 kb long with DNA corresponding to both exons and introns of the region encoding exons 23 to 34 of the authentic gene. vWF gene has 52 exons spanning approximately 178 kb, encoding a translation product of 2,813 amino acid (aa) precursor (pre-pro-vWF) with large internal repetition of homologous domains. The propeptide (763 aa) and the mature subunit (2,050 aa) of vWF is composed of repeating domains in the following order: D1–D2-D'-D3-A1-A2-A3-D4-B1-B2-B3-C1-C2. Before secretion, vWF undergoes an extensive post-translational processing including D1–D2 propeptide cleavage followed by glycosylation and multimerization. Several functional domains (see Fig. 29.1) have been identified in vWF and most of the mutations responsible for various types of vWD have been mapped to these regions.

Results from phenotypic and genotypic tests form the basis of the diagnosis and classification of vWD. However, as more details have emerged from these types of tests, more refined diagnosis but complex classification have regularly been put forward. A revised classification of vWD was published in 1994, but it has already been modified and as more mutations responsible for each type of vWD are identified, a newer classification based on functional defect and mutation is proposed.

Phenotypic Tests

Multimeric analysis of vWF

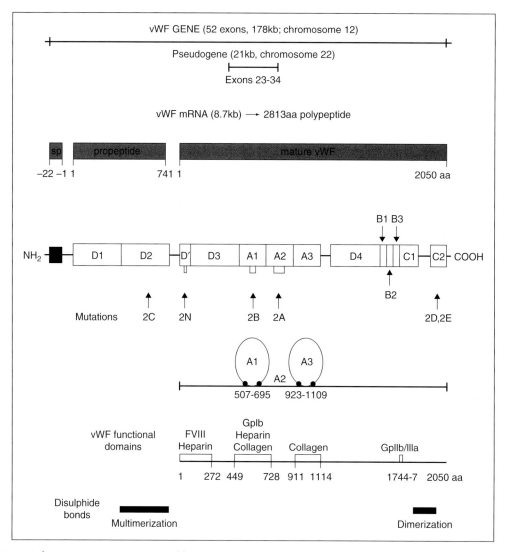

Figure 29.1: *Schematic representation of human vWF gene. From top to bottom: structural features of vWF gene, pseudogene and cDNA; locations of signal peptide (sp), propeptide and mature vWF; the lettered boxes denote regions of internally repeated homologous domains; the approximate locations of the cluster of mutations responsible for different types of vWD; A1 and A3 disulphide loops and the positions of the functional domains; positions of disulphide bonds responsible for dimerization and multimerization vWF.*

In this chapter, three special phenotypic tests which are now used for the diagnosis and classification of vWD are described. These are multimeric analysis of vWF:Ag, for differential diagnosis of all types of variant vWD; ristocetin-induced platelet aggregation, for diagnosis of type 2B vWD; and finally, vWF/FVIII binding assay for diagnosis of type N 'Normandy' vWD. Although it is not long since the vWF gene was identified, genotypic tests have now been introduced and a brief methodology of some approaches for mutation detection are also described.

Phenotypic Tests

Multimeric analysis of vWF

In 1981 a non-reducing SDS-gel electrophoresis for high resolution of vWF:Ag multimers was reported by Ruggeri & Zimmerman. This original method has since been modified and improved by others, but the principle of the method has remained the same. The modifications include variations to the actual method, the type of media in which the protein is separated and semi-automation, different types of antibodies and methods of visualization of the multimer bands. All of these methods are used for identification of qualitative abnormalities vWF:Ag, such as those seen in variant or type 2 vWD, where there is loss of high and/or intermediate molecular weight multimers. For comprehensive multimer analysis of vWF:Ag used in diagnosis and classification of type 2 vWD, both plasma and platelet vWF:Ag should be examined in a range of (1–2.2%) agarose gel concentrations. The method described here is Enayat & Hill's modification of the method original Ruggeri & Zimmerman method. This is a SDS-agarose gel electrophoresis using a discontinuous buffer technique. The multimer bands visualization is by autoradiography using a ^{125}I-labelled mono- or polyclonal anti-vWF antibody.

Gel preparation

A sandwich set made of a piece of gel bond film (Flowgen) covering one glass plate and separated from a second glass plate by a 1 mm thick U-shaped plastic spacer is used for preparing the gels. The running gel (agarose type VII LGT, Sigma) is poured in between the glass plates and after it has set, the top glass plate is removed and a 3 cm strip from the top of the gel is cut away and is replaced with stacking gel made up of 0.8% agarose (SeaKem HGT (P) Agarose, Flowgen Instruments Ltd). The sample wells are cut out in the stacking gel. Samples to be tested are incubated for 30 minutes at 56°C in a buffer containing bromophenol blue dye to monitor molecular migration and sodium dodecyl sulphate (SDS) for complete dispersion of vWF molecules and providing a negative charge to all the multimers.

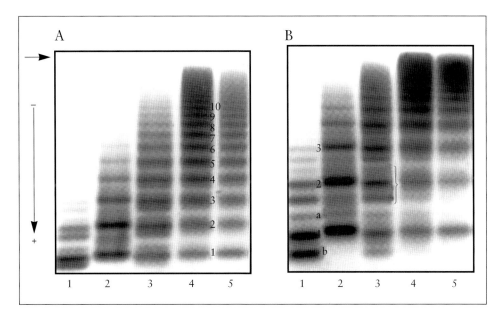

Figure 29.2: *Autoradiographs of different patterns seen in plasma vWF: Ag multimers from type 2A (lane 1), 2D (lane 2), 2B (lane 3), normal (lane 4) and type 1 vWD (lane 5); electrophoresed in 1.2% (panel A) and 1.8% (panel B) agarose gels. The triplet for band 2 is marked by a bracket and the satellite bands 'a' and 'b' can best be seen in the band 1 of plasma from type 2A vWD (lane 1). Arrow at the top of the gel points to the line between the stacking and separating gels. Direction of electrophoresis is from top to bottom.*

Phenotypic Tests

Multimeric analysis of vWF

Ristocetin-induced platelet aggregation assay

Electrophoretic conditions

Each electrophoresis instrument has to be optimized for this method but, in general, electrophoresis is initially carried out rapidly at 2.0 mA/cm for the samples to move out of the wells into the stacking gel. The empty wells are filled with molten stacking gel and electrophoresis is carried out at lower rate of 1.0 mA/cm overnight. When electrophoresis is completed, the gels are fixed in isopropanol solution, pressed dry and washed in 10% rabbit serum solution. Autoradiography is performed by incubating the gels overnight in ^{125}I-labelled anti-human vWF antibody (DAKO Ltd). After thorough washing to elute out unreacted antibody, the gels are dried and autoradiograph plates are produced using X-ray films and kept at –70 °C for two to five days prior to development.

Interpretation of the results

Autoradiography is an extremely sensitive method and by varying the amount of exposures, different autoradiographs with different intensities can be obtained from the same gel. Normal vWF:Ag pattern in plasma shows the full range of the multimer bands of von Willebrand factor. These are made up of high, intermediate and low molecular weight multimers (Fig. 29.2), and each multimer band is composed of a triplet band, the main central and two faint but equally stained satellite bands (a and b). The best spread of vWF:Ag multimers is seen in medium resolution (1.3–1.5%) agarose gel. The loss of high molecular weigh multimers is best investigated in low resolution (1.0–1.4%) agarose gels (Fig. 29.2A) and the triplet band abnormalities in high resolution (1.8–2.0%) agarose gels (Fig. 29.2B). Therefore, for a full multimeric analysis two to three different gel concentrations should be used. This is not an easy technique and each run can vary from another and needs individual optimization of electrophoretic conditions. vWF: Ag multimer bands from normal platelets are different to those seen from plasma. Much larger multimers are present in platelet than in plasma and the multimeric organization is also different (Fig. 29.3). Smaller multimer bands appear to be made up of a doublet and the central bands migrate less

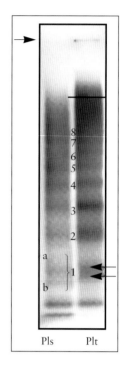

Figure 29.3: Autoradiograph showing different multimer patterns seen in normal plasma (Pls) and platelet (Plt) vWF: Ag, electrophoresed on 1.4% agarose. Arrow at the top of the gel points to the sample application wells. Two small arrows at the bottom point to the doublet band pattern best seen in 1.4% agarose. Note the presence of very high molecular weight multimers in platelet sample.

than the corresponding multimers in plasma (type 2A vWD and its mutations?).

Ristocetin-induced platelet aggregation assay

One of the major functions of vWF glycoprotein is to promote platelet adhesion to the subendothelium at the site of vascular injury through interaction with glycoprotein Ib in the platelet membrane – glycoprotein Ib–IX receptor complex. This functional domain mapped to the A1 domain of vWF plays an important role in primary haemostasis. Defects in this domain result in an increase in the affinity of vWF for platelet glycoprotein Ib. However, this does not cause thrombosis but, paradoxically, causes bleeding. This rare phenotype of variant type 2 vWD is referred to as type 2B and its characteristic functional abnormality is detected by the ristocetin-induced platelet aggregation assay (RIPA). The antibiotic ristocetin induces binding of vWF to platelet glycoprotein Ib in platelet-rich plasma (PRP), and the degree of platelet agglutination with different concentrations of ristocetin forms the basis of this assay. Aside from this abnormality, 2B vWD is also characterized by selective absence of the high molecular weight multimers (HMWM) in plasma which is identified by multimeric analysis of vWF:Ag. In fact, patients with type 2B vWD can synthesize a full range of vWF multimers, as shown by normal multimeric vWF:Ag multimer patterns in platelets and endothelial cells, but the HMWM are cleared from the circulation because of the increased affinity of the abnormal vWF for the platelet glycoprotein Ib receptor.

RIPA methodology described here is a modification of the original work described in 1977. Ristocetin (Paesel-Lore) is reconstituted in tri-buffered saline pH 7.4 and five different solutions giving final concentrations of 0.75, 0.1, 0.125 and 0.15 mg/ml are prepared for use in the assay. PRP is prepared by centrifuging the test and control blood samples at 800 rpm for 10 minutes. The platelet count in the supernatant (PRP) is adjusted to about $250 \times 10^9/l$. 200 μl of patient or normal control (blank) is added to cuvettes containing a magnetic stir bar and placed in the 37 °C heating blocks of an aggregometer (Bio/Data 4-channel platelet aggregometer) for two minutes. Each cuvette is then inserted in one of the channels of the aggregometer and aggregation is started. 20 μl of ristocetin (starting with the weakest) is added to each of the specimens. Aggregation is allowed to occur for a minimum of three minutes. A trace of pattern of aggregation which is proportional to the light transmitted is printed out and a typical one is given in Fig. 29.4. Samples from type 2B vWD require less ristocetin than the normal samples to achieve a comparable aggregation pattern.

A series of missense mutations responsible for this type of vWD have now been identified and they are all grouped in the 2A domain of vWF, which contains the functional binding domain for glycoprotein Ib. With few exceptions, these are all confined to a short peptide ranging from amino acids 540 to 578.

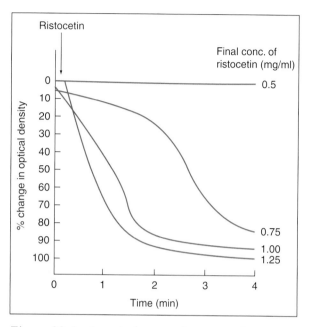

Figure 29.4: *A typical trace of pattern of aggregation for plasma from a normal individual with platelets in the presence of different final concentrations of ristocetin.*

vWF/FVIII binding assay

vWF and FVIII are closely associated and in plasma they form a noncovalent molecular complex. The integrity of the FVIII binding domain on the vWF molecule is an important factor for the formation of this and for the stability and transport of vWF/FVIII complex in plasma. In an investigation of several cases of vWD, it was noticed that the vWF had a defective binding capacity to FVIII, causing a reduction in the level of this factor, leading to a condition similar to mild haemophilia A. This condition was referred to initially as 'pseudo-haemophilia' but later it was recognized as a vWF abnormality and renamed 'Normandy' (after the area where the first defined patient came from) or type 2N vWD. The vWF:Ag multimers in this variant vWD are normal as the mutational defects present in these patients do not affect the mechanism of vWF multimerization. Recently, specific mutations within vWF, responsible for this condition, have been mapped to D' domain; most of the mutations are grouped in exon 18–20 between Arg 19 and Arg 91.

The method described here for determining the binding of FVIII to vWF is the Nesbit *et al.* modification of the original reported method. A suitable concentration of an anti-vWF monoclonal antibody, MAS 533p (Sera Lab) is bound to microtitre plates (Immulon 4, Dynatech Laboratories) overnight at 4°C. The plates are washed twice in 50 mM tris, 100 mM NaCl, pH 8.0 (TBS) containing 0.1% BSA. Serial dilution of patient plasma containing 1 U/dl, 0.5 U/dl, 0.25 U/dl and 0.125 U/dl of vWF:Ag are added in TBS containing 3% BSA and incubated again overnight at 4°C. The plates are washed as before and endogenous FVIII in the samples is removed by incubating with 0.35M $CaCl_2$ for one hour at room temperature. Recombinant FVIII (Bioclate, Baxter) at 0.05 U/ml diluted in TBS/1% BSA with 10 mM $CaCl_2$ and 0.002% Tween 20 is added and incubated for two hours at 37°C. After washing, the bound FVIII to vWF is determined using the Coamatic FVIII Chromogenic kit (Quadratech) and detected at 405 nm.

The results are plotted as vWF:Ag dilution (%) against absorbance at 405 nm for FVIII binding. In the example given here (Fig. 29.5),

the samples used are from a normal control, a homozygous and two heterozygous (P1 and P2) type 2N vWD patients with Thr28Met mutation as positive controls. For determination of any abnormal result, a range of normal control samples should be used.

Genotypic Tests for Mutation Identification

Screening for mutations

The mutations associated with all types of vWD have been identified since late 1980. However, because of the large size and complexity of the vWF gene and the presence of pseudogene on chromosome 22, with exclusion of large deletions, generally there is less information about molecular defects in type 1 and type 3 than in type 2 vWD. Searches for the mutations responsible for 2A and 2B subtypes have been more successful and these are as a result of the clues provided by the phenotype studies. A protease-sensitive region within the A2 domain near the Try842 to Met843 cleavage site was reported to induce structural changes similar to those seen in 2A vWD, and this domain has been targeted for mutation detection in 2A vWD. In 2B vWD where there is an increased affinity for platelet glycoprotein Ib, the mutation detection studies have been directed to the A1 domain of vWF which contains the functional binding domain for glycoprotein Ib. Indeed, almost all of the mutations responsible for these two subtypes of vWD have been found in exon 28 which maps to the A1 and A2 domain of vWF. A database of point mutations, insertions, and deletions identified in vWD, together with a large number of polymorphisms found in vWF, was published in 1993. This list is continuously increasing as more information becomes available. Some of the reported mutations have not been confirmed by functional studies where the recombinant vWF is expressed in a cell-line culture in which the mutations have been introduced by site-directed mutagenesis. In other reported mutations, not all of the vWF gene has been investigated to exclude the possibility of changes elsewhere.

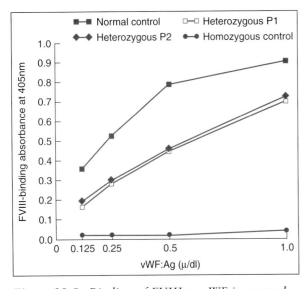

Figure 29.5: Binding of FVIII to vWF in normal control, two heterozygous patient P1 and P2 with Thr28Met mutation and a homozygous control with the same mutation.

Genotypic Tests for Mutation Identification
Mutation detection and authentication

As mutations responsible for type 2A and B are clustered in exon 28 of vWF, a screening of this exon will be useful for mutation detection. Chemical mismatch cleavage detection (CMCD), a method which can be used for mutation screening, has now been successfully utilized in this quest. Using this method, exon 28 from patients and normal subjects is amplified in two overlapping segments. Each amplified segment is initially purified by Gene Clean glass beads (Bio 101, Inc.) and denatured. Each of the patient's segments is annealed in a 10/1 ratio to homologous normal (probe) segment which is labelled at its 5′ end by phosphorylation with ^{32}P-ATP. Any mutation in the patient strands leads to mispaired or unstably paired cytosine (C) or thymine (T) residues of the heteroduplex formed by probe and patient DNA. Such a mismatched C or T residue is specifically modified by means of hydroxylamine (2.3 M, 37°C for 2 h) and osmium tetroxide (0.025%, 37°C for 2 h), respectively. The probes are cleaved by means of 1M piperidine (90°C for 30 min) at the site of the mismatch and any reduction in size is determined by electrophoresis of the denatured heterodimer in urea-acrylamide gels followed by autoradiography.

For mutation detection in the rest of the vWF gene, a methodology which has already been successfully used in haemophilia can be used. In this method the whole of the vWF gene is amplified in seven segments, one from the genomic DNA and from cDNA obtained by reverse transcription of the 'illegitimate' mRNA found in peripheral lymphocytes by means of a polymerase chain reaction (RT-PCR). These segments can then be similarly screened by CMCD for mutation not only in type 2 but also in type 1 and type 3 vWD.

Mutation detection and authentication
DNA sequencing
Screening methods such as chemical mismatched cleavage detection will identify the position of the mutation in a small area of the gene and is only an indication of where the mutation can be found. The actual nature of the mutation could, however, only be determined by DNA sequencing. It is now possible to directly sequence PCR products using the dideoxy chain termination method. Single-stranded DNA PCR product needed for this can be obtained either by using appropriate biotinylated primers and streptavidin-coated magnetic beads (Dynal) or by asymmetric PCR. These products can then be sequenced directly using dideoxy sequencing (Sequenase, USB) kit. Cycle sequencing is another alternative which relies on the synthesis of a new strand of DNA from a small amount of original double-stranded template in a further PCR process using a thermostable enzyme. Following mutation detection, it should be authenticated by one of the following two methods.

Allele-specific oligonucleotide (ASO) hybridization
For ASO-H or dot blot analysis, small (about 15 bp) oligonucleotides with wild type and mutant sequences are synthesized. Purified PCR products of the relevant exon are denatured in NaOH. Normal and patient's PCR products from the appropriate exon are applied to Hybond N$^+$ nylon (Amersham International) strips manually or using one of the commercially available apparatus. The nylon filter strips are then hybridized with the two different types of oligonucleotides labelled with ^{32}P-ATP using DNA Polymerase I Klenow Fragment (Pharmacia). After hybridization the filter strips are washed three times in differing concentrations of SSC with SDS for 10–20 minutes at an optimal temperature empirically determined for each ASO probe. Using autoradiography it is possible to visualize positive (annealed) and negative (not annealed) samples.

Restriction endonuclease analysis
A single base pair of substitutions can create or destroy a restriction endonuclease enzyme site. For confirmation of such a mutation, restriction products of relevant PCR products with one of the hundreds of suitable restriction enzymes can be analysed by electrophoresis on agarose or acrylamide gel and restricted DNA bands can be visualized by ethidium bromide staining. In type 2N vWD all the reported mutations can be detected in this way.

Further Reading

Enayat M S, Hill F G H. Analysis of the multimeric structure of factor VIII related antigen/von Willebrand protein using a modified electrophoresis technique. *Journal of Clinical Pathology* 1983; **36**, 915–919.

Evan Sadler J, Matsushita T, Dong Z, Tuley E A, Westfield L A. Molecular mechanism and classification of von Willebrand disease. *Thrombosis and Haemostasis* 1995; **74**, 161–166.

Ginsburg D, Bowie E J W. Molecular genetics of von Willebrand Disease. *Blood* 1992; **79**, 2507–2519.

Ginsburg D, Evan Sadler J. von Willebrand disease: A database of point mutations, insertions, and deletions. *Thrombosis and Haemostasis* 1993; **69**, 177–191.

Mancuso D J, Tuley E A, Westfield L A, Worrall N K, Shelton-lnoles B B, Sorace J M, Alevy Y G, Sadler, J E. Structure of the gene for human von Willebrand Factor. *J Biol Chem* 1989; **264**, 19514–19527.

Mazurier C. von Willebrand disease masquerading as haemophilia A. *Thrombosis and Haemostasis* 1992; **67**, 391–396.

Montandon A J, Green P M, Giannelli F, Bentley D R. Direct detection of point mutation by mismatch analysis: application to haemophilia B. *Nucl Acids Res* 1989; **17**, 3347–3358.

Nesbit I M, Goodeve A C, Guilatt A M, Makris M, Preston F E, Peake I R. Characterisation of type 2N von Willebrand disease using phenotype and molecular techniques. *Thrombosis and Haemostasis* 1996; **75**, 959–964.

Ruggeri Z M, Zimmerman T S. The complex multimeric composition of Factor VIII/von Willebrand Factor. *Blood* 1981; **57**, 1140–1143.

Ruggeri Z M, Zimmerman TS. von Willebrand factor and von Willebrand disease. *Blood* 1987; **70**, 895–904.

Ruggeri Z M, Ware J. The structure and function of von Willebrand factor. *Thrombosis and Haemostasis* 1992; **67**, 594–599.

30 PLATELET INVESTIGATIONS

Steven Walton

Introduction

Platelets are small fragments of megakaryocyte cytoplasm with a mean diameter of 1–2 μm and a mean volume of 5–8 fl, having an average life span in peripheral circulation of seven to ten days. Their function is to maintain the integrity of the vessel wall and to initiate haemostasis upon damage to the vasculature. Their functionality can be divided into three main areas: adhesion to the vascular endothelium; aggregation to each other; and release of chemicals into the plasma. This chapter will describe the principle behind the techniques used to investigate each of those areas.

In clinical situations loss of this functionality is expressed by patients showing increased bruising, petechial rashes or prolonged bleeding following minor traumas such as venepuncture or dental treatment. Patients who present with these problems should have a screen of platelet function, together with quantitation of the platelet count.

Structure and Function

Platelet function is closely related to the platelet structure. The platelet external membrane is a highly functional organelle containing at least nine different glycoproteins which transect the standard bilipid cellular membrane. Several of these glycoproteins are capable of activating various biochemical pathways within the platelet to induce any of the functions required in a normal platelet response. Abnormal platelet function has been shown to result from a lack of expression of one or more of these glycoproteins (see Table 30.1 and Fig. 30.1). Abnormal platelet adhesion is seen in Bernard Soulier syndrome, in which the platelet membrane glycoprotein Ib has been shown to be deficient. This glycoprotein has a specific binding capacity for the plasma protein von Willebrand's factor which coats subendothelial matrix upon exposure to plasma, thus adhering

platelets to the site of vascular injury via the glycoprotein Ib. Deficiency of complex glycoprotein IIb/IIIa causes an abnormality in the platelets' ability to aggregate (see Fig. 30.1). This condition is known as Glanzman's thrombasthenia. These and other glycoproteins act as a physiological receptor for various low and high molecular weight platelet agonists. Once one or more of these glycoprotein receptors have become activated there is a signal transduction into the internal organelles of the platelet. This is commonly via activation of the enzyme phospholipase C which is exposed on the internal ends of the glycoproteins upon activation by their respective ligands.

Within the platelet cytoplasm are many of the internal structures found in other secretory cells, however the platelet does not have a great capacity for synthesis of proteins. The platelet contains very little rough endoplasmic

Structure and Function

Table 30.1   Factors involved in a normal platelet response.

Glycoprotein	Ligands	Platelet function
GP IIb-IIIa	Vitronectin von Willebrand factor Fibrinectin Fibrinogen	Aggregation and adhesion at high shear rates
GP Ia-Iia	Vitronectin von Willebrand factor Fibrinectin Fibrinogen	Adhesion
GMP 140 (PADGEM)	Various glycoproteins and glycolipids	Platelet to leukocyte interaction

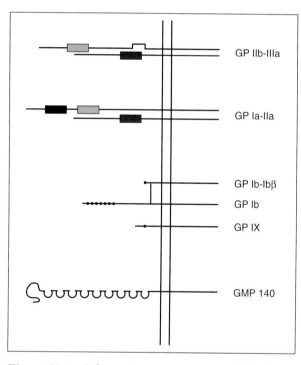

Figure 30.1: Schematic representation of platelet receptors.

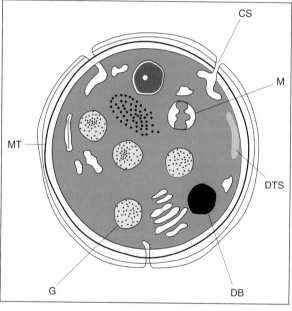

Figure 30.2: Schematic representation of platelet structure. The diagram illustrates the main internal structures of a discoid platelet. (CS) is the surface connected canalicular system. (M) is the platelet mitochondria. (DTS) is the dense tubular system. (DB) is a dense body. (G) represents one of the platelet granules. (MT) represents the circumferential band of microtubules.

reticulum and Golgi apparatus (see Fig. 30.2). It does contain extensive smooth endoplasmic reticulum which is often referred to as the dense tubular system. The cytoplasm also contains many alpha granules and dense granules. These granules contain a wide variety of chemicals which are involved in the inflammatory response and more importantly in accelerating the process of localized haemostasis.

The alpha granules contain coagulation factors such as factor V, VII and fibrinogen along with growth factors to aid vascular repair, notably platelet derived growth factor (PDGF) and endothelial growth factor (EGF). Another substance stored in the alpha gran-

314

ules is platelet factor IV and this is one of the main factors assayed to assess the platelet release response.

The dense granules contain a large proportion of the platelet's available nucleotides, mainly adenine and guanine diphosphate and triphosphate, along with calcium and magnesium ions, and 5-hydroxytryptamine (5HT). ADP is a major accelerant for platelet aggregation whilst ATP has an inhibitory effect on ADP and is therefore a part of the control mechanism to localize thrombus formation. 5HT is another powerful platelet aggregator, the platelet membrane containing numerous receptors for 5HT. These receptors are members of the super family of G proteins, a coupled neurotransmitter and hormone receptor, found both on nerve cells and in the gut endothelium in large numbers.

Platelet Counting

All aspects of platelet function are dependent upon the number of circulating platelets. It is therefore important to obtain an accurate platelet count before going on to more time-consuming and expensive techniques. Platelet numbers can be assessed by microscopy of a Romanowski stained blood film. This can only give an approximation of numbers, for instance low, normal or high. However it does give other valuable information on the platelets such as size and granularity, for example some platelet formation disorders such as Bernard Soulier syndrome are associated with giant platelets.

For many years manual counting of platelets has been the only way of obtaining a platelet count value. This involves dilution of a whole blood sample in a 1% (w/v) solution of ammonium oxalate; routinely as 1 in 100 dilution of blood to diluent. This is then placed in a previously cleaned or new modified Neubauer counting chamber, the chamber being left in a moist environment for at least 30 minutes to give time for the platelets to settle. By using phase contrast microscopy it is then possible to see the platelets as refractile particles and to count them using the graduated squares. The

number of platelets in one or more areas of one square mm is counted and a calculation used to multiply up to the whole blood figure. The calculation takes the average number of platelets per square mm and is multiplied by the dilution multiplied by 1,000. This gives the number $\times 10^9/l$, but is not suitable for platelet counts of less than $50 \times 10^9/l$. Due to the inaccuracy and the amount of time required to perform platelet counts this method is rarely used. Automated blood count machines capable of counting platelets are routine laboratory equipment, see Chapter 27. Greater accuracy than manual techniques enables counts as low as $5 \times 10^9/l$ and in excess of $1000 \times 10^9/l$.

Reduced platelet counts result either from a failure of marrow production (for example following cytotoxic chemotherapy) or from increased platelet consumption. The production of antibody to a platelet's membrane component or to a substance carried on the membrane of the platelet may result in increased sequestration in the spleen. The presence of platelet membrane-activated immunoglobulin is therefore an important investigation. The presence of platelet directed plasma immunoglobulins does not correlate with clinical severity of autoimmune thrombocytopenia, while the concentration of platelet-bound immunoglobulin is a better marker of disease activity.

The demonstration of platelet bound immunoglobulin is more difficult than red cell association immunoglobulin. Due to low platelet numbers and the difficulty visualizing platelets the method of choice is to use a flow cytometer and combine the antihuman globulin reagent with a fluorescent dye. A platelet-rich plasma is prepared by slow centrifugation. This plasma is then centrifuged hard in the presence of a buffer containing EDTA or some other platelet inhibitor to form a platelet button, which is then washed several times to remove any trapped plasma containing human globulins. Finally the platelets are resuspended in 5% bovine albumin. An aliquot of the platelets is then mixed with an antihuman globulin with either fluorescein isothiocyanate or another fluorochrome detectable by the flow cytometer. After incubation in the dark, platelets are given a final wash in a PBS EDTA buffer and resuspended in a sufficient quantity of buffer to allow easy flow through the flow cytometer. Patient's platelets without fluorescent dye tagged to them are used as a negative control. A positive reaction occurs when the fluorescent index is higher in the platelets tagged with the fluorochrome than those platelets without the dye.

Bleeding Time

One of the simplest platelet function tests is a bleeding time. An incision is made into the skin on the forearm using a bleeding device and the time taken for the bleeding to stop measured. In order to improve reproducibility of the method the technique is performed by using a dual incision using a spring loaded lancet of standard area. The spring is of a standard tension to give reproducible depth to the cut, while a sphygmomanometer cuff is inflated to a standard pressure of 40 mmHg. The time for bleeding to cease is measured by a stop-watch and detection is by mopping the excess blood from the arm with clean filter paper. Any major platelet defect will give a prolonged time, as will disorders of von Willebrand protein.

Platelet Adhesion

Physiologically the first stage of platelet activation is the adhesion of platelets to the subendothelial matrix. The measurement of platelet adhesion is difficult and seldom performed in routine laboratories. Several methods are reported which can be used to give a crude estimation of platelet adhesive function. The simplest is to take a citrated blood sample without venous occlusion and perform a platelet count on the sample. An aliquot of the sample is then passed at constant pressure over a tube containing standardized glass beads and a second platelet count performed on the emerging sample. A percentage of platelet adhesion can be calculated. A modification to this standard technique using a subcellular matrix such as collagen may give a better physiological picture. Problems with reproducibility of results have

restricted use to research laboratories including pharmaceutical companies evaluating the efficacy of drugs modifying platelet adhesion or activation. A more complex method involves a system to simulate normal venous pressure and requires the production of a loop of inert plastic with an area of subendothelial matrix. Blood is then passed into the system at normal physiological shear rates.

Investigations of Platelet Aggregation

A measurement of platelet aggregation is probably the most commonly used technique in the investigation of platelet disorders. Aggregation studies are based on a photometric technique. Aggregation is recorded as the change in absorbance of a mixture of platelet-rich plasma as aggregates form. The larger the clumps the heavier they are and as they fall out of the light

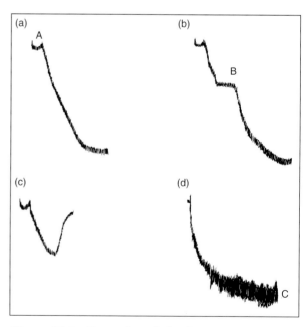

Figure 30.3: Examples of platelet aggregation traces. (a) ADP 5 μmol/l (note the indication of platelet shape change at A); (b) ADP 3 μmol/l (note the delay in secondary aggregation at B); (c) ADP 1 μmol/l (note the total reversion of primary aggregation); (d) Ristocetin 1.5 mg/ml (note the large aggregate formation at C).

path a higher transmission of the light is detected. There are several commonly used agonists including ADP, adrenalin, collagen and the antibiotic ristocetin. Ristocetin is an unusual agonist in that it has no direct effect on platelets but modifies part of the factor VIII complex known as von Willebrand factor. When modified this protein changes from a globular to a linear structure. The linear structure then binds to several platelets and gives a pseudo aggregation. An abnormal response to ristocetin is seen in patients with quantitative and qualitative changes in von Willebrand protein.

Investigations into Platelet Release

The techniques involved in studying platelet release can be divided into two, those that use radioisotopes and those that use the production of light using the enzyme luciferinase. Isotopic techniques can be performed in two ways. Platelets can be incubated with a radioisotope that can be incorporated into the molecule which is under investigation such as ^{14}C-labelled 5-hydroxytryptamine to look for release of 5-hydroxytryptamine. In these methods platelet-rich plasma is incubated for a time period with a relevant radioactive compound. The platelets are then separated from the plasma and the excess radioisotope. To do this the platelets are spun through an albumin density gradient leaving the platelet pellet at the bottom with the radioactive plasma on the top. The platelet pellet is then resuspended in a buffer, washed again and counted. After platelet aggregation with a potent agonist the platelet-poor plasma is also counted and the amount of radioactivity in the platelet-poor plasma expressed as a percentage of the activity in a full platelet sample.

A second technique using radio isotopes is to perform a radioimmune assay (RIA). With this methodology the compound under investigation is mixed with a portion of the same compound labelled with a radioactive tracer. To this mixture is added a specific antibody to the compound under investigation. After incuba-

tion antibody-bound compound is separated from unbound, usually by the addition of activated charcoal and then centrifuging. It is possible to count the radioactivity in either the pellet or in the free supernatant. Because the antibody binds radiolabelled and non-radiolabelled in equal quantity the proportion of radioactivity bound by the antibody is inversely proportional to the amount of compound in the plasma under investigation. The method is quantified by using known concentrations of control plasmas to construct a graph and then readings for samples are measured from the graph.

Chemiluminescence is another technique used in investigation of platelet release reaction. This is based on the same chemical reaction that takes place in the firefly where ATP and luciferinase reacts on luciferin to produce photons of light. The reaction is dependent upon the amount of ATP being produced. Within platelet reaction luciferinase and luciferin are added to a reaction vial along with platelet release compounds. The amount of ATP in the reaction vial determines the amount of light produced. A higher production of light results from a higher release of ATP from the platelets.

Flow Cytometry

Flow cytometry is used increasingly to investigate platelet function against specific antigens expressed on platelets. The methodology of flow cytometry is discussed in Chapter 32. For platelet investigations there are two main proteins that can be identified; those required for the binding of the platelet to the cell wall and those required for aggregating platelets to each other. Glycoprotein Ib is a surface antigen that is required for binding platelets to the subendothelial matrix via von Willebrand's factor. Glycoprotein IIb/IIIa is one of the main components required for the platelet aggregation reaction. A deficit of platelet function can therefore be identified using monoclonal antibodies raised against either of these proteins.

To investigate abnormalities in platelet membrane-bound glycoproteins, a platelet-rich

Flow Cytometry

Further Reading

plasma is prepared by slow centrifugation. The plasma is then diluted either in platelet-poor plasma or in albumin to give a platelet count of approximately $1 \times 10^9/1$. An aliquot of this is then mixed with a fluorescently tagged monoclonal antibody specific to the glycoprotein. After incubation the whole amount is again diluted to give about 0.5 ml. The sample is then analysed by a flow cytometer. For positivity the fluorescent index must be higher than a control sample of the same patient's platelets without the fluorochrome present. Platelets are the smallest cellular constituent of blood and it is not necessary to lyse red cells or to remove any debris from the sample as it is simple to gate around the platelets under investigation.

Platelet function disorders due to deficiency of glycoproteins are rare. There is, however, an increasing interest in the role of platelets in thrombotic disorders. This has led to the investigation of platelets to identify activated populations of platelets during thrombotic episodes e.g. after prosthetic heart valve replacements. Two major markers of activation have been identified. One is changes to the conformational shape of membrane glycoproteins, notably to IIb/IIIa. This change exposes sites to the external environment which in the resting platelet are hidden within coils on the molecules. Many antibodies have been produced to these activation epitopes. These activation antigens are only demonstrable on platelets that have been activated with weak thrombin solutions and negative on untreated platelets from the same volunteer. A second type of activation protein is when parts of the α-granules are actually expressed on the surface membrane of platelets. This happens when the granules have gone through the secretory process and the membrane of the granules has become incorporated into the platelet external membrane. The name for these has been given as PADGEM (Platelet Activation Derived Granular to External Membrane). By using antibodies to these markers either singly or in combination and using a flow cytometer with the technique briefly discussed above, it is possible to determine the proportion of activated platelets.

A more recent approach to this technique is to look for circulating activated platelet aggregates. In this technique an ordinary platelet marker CD41 to glycoprotein IIb/IIIa is used to identify populations of platelets. Using a second antibody CD62p with a different fluorochrome to the activation marker from α-granules, it is possible to identify three populations of platelets in patients suffering from TTP (thrombotic thrombocytopenic purpura). The first population is normal platelets which occur in singlets and only stain with CD41. The second population is activated platelets in singlets which stain with CD41 and CD62. The third population is small aggregates of platelets which show a larger volume on the flow cytometer and also stain positive with both CD41 and CD62. The latter population appear to identify activated aggregates of platelets in TTP.

Further Reading

Ahn Y S et al. Activated platelet aggregates in thrombotic thrombocytopenic purpura: Decrease with plasma infusions and normalisation in remission. *British Journal of Haematology* 1996; **95**, 408–415.

Chand I F, Keiffer N. A, Phillips B R. Platelet membrane glycoproteins. *Haemostasis and Thrombosis*, 3rd edn 1994: Lippincott, London.

Dacie J V, Lewis S M (eds). Basic Haematological Techniques. *Practical Haematology*, 7th edn 1991: Churchill Livingstone, London.

Rosenfield C S, Nicholls G, Bodensteiner D C. Flow cytometric measurement of antiplatelet antibodies. *American Journal of Clinical Pathology* 1987; **87**, 518–522.

White J G. Platelet ultrastructure. *Haemostasis and Thrombosis*, 2nd edn 1987: Churchill Livingstone, London.

31 A HOSPITAL TRANSFUSION SERVICE

Steven Walton and Peter E Rose

A hospital blood transfusion service undertakes three major serological investigations: (1) to identify a patient's blood group; (2) to detect and identify irregular antibodies including those inducing haemolytic anaemia; (3) to provide compatible blood components to patients.

Blood Group Identification

The laboratory methods applied to transfusion serology are rapidly changing to accommodate an increasing need to simplify and automate many aspects of the service. Long past are the days of blood grouping tests on glass slides or tiles. The principles of serology however remain the same. There are over a hundred recognized antigens on the red cell membrane, the presence of which can be identified by agglutination of the red cells on exposure to the corresponding antibody or antisera. Most blood group antigens are naturally occurring and exposure of the antigen may stimulate a primary antibody response in a person lacking the antigen. The resultant alloantibody is specific for that antigen and further exposure to the antigen may stimulate a rapid and prolonged antibody response with the potential to induce significant transfusion reaction. Rapid intravascular haemolysis may follow the binding of the antibody (usually IgM) to the antigen and complement activation. This results in ABO incompatibility when anti-A or anti-B naturally present in the recipient's sera is exposed to the appropriate antigen. Usually an individual produces naturally occurring antibodies against the AB antigens that are absent from their own red cells, due to stimulation from the same antigen found on other biological substances such as pollen or bacteria. An individual blood group can therefore be determined directly by adding specific antisera to the test red cells and indirectly by addition of red cells of known antigen specificity to the test sera. To determine a patient's blood group requires the characterization of red cell antigens. For routine blood grouping this requires identifying A, B and D antigens. People expressing the A antigen on the cells do not produce anti-A but can produce anti-B. People expressing B antigen do not normally produce anti-B but can produce anti-A, whilst group O do not express either A nor B antigen. Historically antigen identification was performed using purified antibodies from previously typed patients. Nowadays most typing antibodies are chemically modified monoclonal antibodies. For ease of use commercial antibodies have a specific coloured dye added to anti-A and anti-B antibodies.

Blood Group Identification

The rhesus system

Methods for Blood Grouping

An indirect method of checking a patient's blood group is to react a patient's serum which contains the antibodies with cells of known ABO specificity, which gives a reverse or back group. Thus a group A patient's serum will react with B cells, group B patients will react with A cells and group O patients will react with both A and B cells. The rare patients who possess both A and B antigens react with neither cell. A further check and part of the investigation for irregular antibodies is to put patient's serum with group O cells which should not react, irrespective of the patient's blood group.

It is important to include appropriate negative controls such as the patient's own cells or O cells. The control cells are necessary to identify reactions due to cold antibodies in the sample other than anti-A and anti-B.

The rhesus system

The rhesus system is the second most important blood group system to be identified. Unlike the ABO system, antibodies are not present naturally in the absence of the antigen, however antibodies can be readily formed following exposure of RhD-positive cells in a RhD-negative recipient. The antibodies formed are usually IgG, and can cross the placental barrier to result in second or subsequent pregnancies where the mother is RhD-negative and the fetus RhD-positive. It is therefore important that every effort is made to avoid sensitization of RhD-negative females of child-bearing age to the D antigen. Rhesus grouping should be performed in duplicate using an IgM monoclonal anti-D. Positive and negative controls must be included in each batch of

tests and the result read microscopically after centrifugation of tubes for one minute at a low speed. In Britain national guidelines recommend the use of two different anti-D reagents. The D antigen is a complex antigen made up of many different subantigens (epitopes). Monoclonal antibodies are highly specific and may react to single epitopes, therefore if the particular epitope to which the reagent reacts is missing there will be a false-negative result.

Using these eight reagents (anti-A, -B, -AB, -D1, -D2, A cells, B cells and O cells) it is possible to identify following common blood groups as shown in Table 31.1.

Methods for Blood Grouping

There are many methods using these basic reagents to group patients, which can broadly be divided into five categories: (1) Methods based on individual tubes with no enhancement, requiring approximately one hour's incubation with an optimum temperature of 16°C; (2) Methods in individual tubes with enhancement (rapid groups) usually requiring centrifugation and only performed on cell typing; (3) Methods using microtitre plates; (4) Methods using solid phase matrix; (5) Automated methods based on continuous flow principles. The method chosen depends on the volume of work to be undertaken and its urgency. Rapid methods usually only check the patient's antigens without a back check.

Visualization of results varies depending on the method employed, for tube and microtitre

Table 31.1:   Expected results for common blood groups.

Group	Anti-A	Anti-B	Anti-AB	A Cells	B Cells	O Cells	Anti-D1	Anti-D2
A RhD-positive	+	—	+	—	+	—	+	+
A RhD-negative	+	—	+	—	+	—	—	—
B RhD-positive	—	+	+	+	—	—	+	+
B RhD-negative	—	+	+	+	—	—	—	—
AB RhD-positive	+	+	+	—	—	—	+	+
AB RhD-negative	+	+	+	—	—	—	—	—
O RhD-positive	—	—	—	+	+	—	+	+
O RhD-negative	—	—	—	+	+	—	—	—

A HOSPITAL TRANSFUSION SERVICE

Methods for Blood Grouping
Microtitre methods
Gel systems
Automated systems
Antibody Screening

methods it is dependent upon agglutination of the red cells which can be interpreted either micro- or macroscopically. Microtitre and rapid group methodologies tend to use macroscopic visualization, while non-enhanced methods tend to be read microscopically.

Microtitre methods

Microtitre methodologies allow multiple groups to be performed easily in batches. A standard microplate consists of 96 wells in a solid plastic block, aligned in 12 rows of eight. Using eight reagents for a full group, 12 patients' blood can be grouped on a single plate. Visualization of all the groups on the plate can be rapid using a backlight to see positive and negative results. There are systems available using computers and micro-robotics to automate or semi-automate microtitre grouping systems. These systems incorporate micro-plate readers which can be programmed to identify blood groups by the reactivity pattern of the microtitre plate.

Gel systems

Gel phase systems rely on trapping the reacted cells in a solid or semi-solid matrix, with negative results falling through the gel. This occurs by having the monoclonal antibodies mentioned above chemically bonded to the matrix. Thus cells containing the corresponding antigen are stuck (trapped in the matrix) when they are pulled through the gel by centrifugation (see Fig. 31.1). This method is particularly useful for grouping patients with a high risk

from blood-borne microorganisms such as hepatitis or HIV. The high cost of manufacturing gels incorporating specific antibodies needs to be considered when implementing this methodology into routine laboratory practice.

Automated systems

Automated methods using equipment that can use positive sample identification are required in laboratories with high workloads. The benefits from using automated equipment are a reduction in sample handling time. While patients benefit from the removal of clerical errors as results can be reported directly from reading with no transcription, the large capital outlay required makes automated systems too expensive for laboratories with a low workload. Most laboratories will use two techniques, a rapid system for urgent analysis and a routine batch system for the bulk of the workload. Rapid grouping is performed to identify the patient's blood group in an emergency when blood is required for crossmatching, thus allowing a group-compatible blood to be selected with little delay.

Antibody Screening

Screening patient's sera for the presence of any irregular antibodies has now become a routine part of every hospital blood bank. It is now rare to undertake a blood group identification without antibody screening at the same time, with the possible exception of neonatal samples

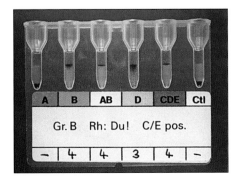
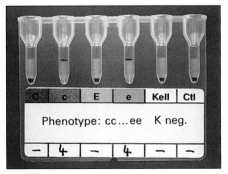

Figure 31.1: *ABO grouping of gel system. Showing a group B RhD Positive sample. (Reproduced with permission of Diamed U.K. Ltd.)*

Antibody Screening

The indirect antiglobulin test

where antibody production has not commenced and sample size is small.

For many patients undergoing elective and emergency surgical procedures, blood grouping and antibody screening is all that is recommended. This policy has dramatically reduced blood wastage, with cross-matched blood reserved for procedures with a greater than 30% likelihood of requiring cells. For patients in whom a clinically significant antibody is identified in the screening test procedure, a full cross-match is necessary.

There are a number of physiochemical properties displayed by different antibodies that are important in their identification. Firstly different blood group antibodies can be distinguished from each other on the basis that some antibodies agglutinate red cells better at low temperatures (cold antibodies), while others are active at 37°C. Cold antibodies are often IgM antibodies and may not be detectable or clinically significant at higher temperatures. Some naturally occurring antibodies such as anti-A and anti-B will still react at 37°C, however the titre will be much higher at 0–4 °C. Warm antibodies are usually IgG and agglutinate red cells more quickly at 37°C. Historically antibodies have also been classified as complete or incomplete depending on whether they agglutinate red cells suspended in normal saline. Incomplete antibodies do not agglutinate red cells under such circumstances and this has led to the search for other techniques to enhance the sensitivity of red cells suspended in 20–30% bovine albumin to identify many incomplete antibodies. Other methods employing polybrene or enzyme-treated cells have been routinely used. Enzymes such as trypsin, papain, bromelain or ficin have been used to remove neuraminic acid from the red cell surfaces and reduce the negative charge, causing the incomplete antibody to agglutinate the enzyme-treated cells. The saline tests at room temperature, albumin and enzyme methods have been superseded by the indirect antiglobulin test (IAT). The later test is superior in identifying clinically significant antibodies and does not have the disadvantage of identifying irrelevant antibodies which can result in a serious delay in the laboratory as further assessment and identification of the antibody is necessary.

Antibody screening is undertaken by reacting red cells containing the majority of common blood group antigens with the patient's sera. It is usual to have a set of three cells and the antigens known on each cell sample are given on an identification sheet (see Fig. 31.2).

The antibody screen can be performed using any of the techniques found in the laboratory, but commonly the indirect antiglobulin test is used as the initial screen. This is because the IAT test is the most sensitive test for most antibodies. Using the new gel systems it is being proposed that a negative IAT based antibody screen and selection of ABO RhD compatible blood are sufficient to issue blood for a patient and that cross-matching is no longer necessary. In the majority of cases this is true, but there is a risk that incompatible blood might be issued to a patient with antibodies to a rare antigen.

The indirect antiglobulin test

The IAT using red cells suspended in low-ionic strength saline (LISS) is the recommended method for antibody screening. In normal

	Rh-hr	Spender Donor Donneur		Rh-hr						Kell						Duffy		Kidd		Lewis		P	MNS				Luth.		Xg	
				D	C	E	c	e	Cʷ	K	k	Kpᵃ	Kpᵇ	Jsᵃ	Jsᵇ	Fyᵃ	Fyᵇ	Jkᵃ	Jkᵇ	Leᵃ	Leᵇ	P₁	M	N	S	s	Luᵃ	Luᵇ	Xgᵃ	
I	CʷCD.ee	R₁ʷR₁	21017730	+	+	0	0	+	+	0	+	0	+	0	+	+	0	+	+	0	+	+	+	+	+	+	0	+	+	F
II	ccD.EE	R₂R₂	21734192	+	0	+	+	0	0	0	+	0	+	0	+	+	+	+	0	+	0	+	+	+	0	+	0	+	+	M
III	ccddee	rr	41705967	0	0	0	+	+	0	+	+	0	+	0	+	0	+	0	+	0	+	0	+	+	+	0	0	+	+	F

Figure 31.2: Example of antibody screening cells. (Reproduced with permission of Diamed U.K. Ltd.)

322

saline the ionized groups on both antigen and antibody are partially neutralized by oppositely charged ions in the solution. The minimum incubation time for normal ionic strength techniques is 45 minutes and is no longer recommended.

If LISS is used as the medium, antigen and antibody reactions are more rapid. LISS is a solution of sodium glycine containing 0.03M sodium chloride. Rarely LISS dependent autoantibodies may be detected and in these circumstances normal ionic strength techniques may be helpful.

The screening cells used in antibody detection should have homozygous expression of appropriate antigens (RhD, Cc, Ee, Jk^a, Jk^b, Fy^a, Fy^b, Ss). It is expected that 99.9% of antibodies would be detected with only antibodies to red cell of very low frequency not detected. Following incubation of test serum with screening red cells, the cells are washed to remove any unbound antibody. Any contamination by free globulin will neutralize the antiglobulin component in the antiglobulin reagent, and must be avoided.

Monospecific anti-IgG may be used instead of a polyspecific antiglobulin reagent containing anti-complement sera using the LISS IAT method. This avoids the undesirable susceptibility to interference from low thermal optimum and LISS dependent antibodies that are complement binding. When an irregular antibody is identified further investigation to identify the specificity of the antibody is necessary.

Antibody identification

If a positive result is obtained in any of the antibody screening cells it is essential to identify the antibody specificity. This requires reacting the sera with a larger panel of typed cells. Commonly commercial panels contain 11 cells and are supplied with an antigram of the corresponding antigens (see Fig. 31.3). Antibody identification is produced by matching the antibody reactive pattern with the pattern of the antigens. If blood is required for transfusion, only units negative for the corresponding antigen can be selected. As with the antibody screen any method can be used, but it is best to start with the same technique as gave the

positive reaction in the antibody screen. Frequently this is the IAT. Inconclusive results from this panel can frequently be clarified by repeating the panel using an enzyme enhanced technique. If identification is still inconclusive a different panel of cells should be used. Inconclusive results may require a fresh sample to be taken to ensure the antibody is real and not a sample contaminant. If the identity of the antibody remains unknown it may be necessary to refer the sample to the reference centre, where a larger donor panel will be available to aid identification.

Cross-matching

Cross-matching is the procedure performed to ensure that potential donor blood is compatible with the recipient. Once the patient's ABO RhD group and a negative antibody screen has been obtained, cross-matching the blood should be straightforward. Donor units should be selected where possible of the same ABO and RhD group. The type of red cell product will need to be considered, for example, whole blood, concentrated red cells, cells with added supplement, leukocyte poor or depleted. This will depend on the condition requiring transfusion and on the age of the recipient. Furthermore it is necessary to ensure that women under 50 years old are given Kell-negative red cells. This is because antibodies produced to the Kell antigen are able to cross the placenta. Women stimulated to produce anti-Kell by transfusion who become pregnant may have an infant develop an intrauterine haemolytic anaemia.

Once the correct product has been selected the cross-match procedure is relatively straightforward, as cells from the donor bag are washed and reacted with recipient's sera. The choice of technique is the same as for antibody screening but must include an indirect antiglobulin method. Any units that give a positive reaction should not be transfused. Rarely there are instances where it is impossible to obtain compatible units, for example in patients with strong autoantibodies in the sera. In these patients an auto cross-match (recipient's cells

Cross-matching

	Rh-hr	Spender Donor Donneur		Rh-hr						Kell						Duffy		Kidd		Lewis		P	MNS				Luth		Xg		Spez. Antigene special types antigènes part.
				D	C	E	c	e	C^w	K	k	Kp^a	Kp^b	Js^a	Js^b	Fy^a	Fy^b	Jk^a	Jk^b	Le^a	Le^b	P	M	N	S	s	Lu^a	Lu^b	Xg^a	♀ ♂	
1	$C^wCD.ee$	$R_1{}^wR_1$	403/37728	+	+	0	0	+	+	0	+	0	+	0	+	+	+	+	+	0	0	+	+	0	0	+	+	+	0	M	
2	CCD.ee	R_1R_1	504/38187	+	+	0	0	+	0	+	+	0	+	0	+	0	+	+	+	0	+	v.w. +	+	0	+	0	0	+	+	M	
3	ccD.EE	R_2R_2	43/37566	+	0	+	+	0	0	0	+	0	+	0	+	+	+	0	+	0	+	+	+	0	+	+	+	+	nt	M	Co^b+, Co^a-
4	Ccddee	r′r	38016	0	+	0	+	+	0	0	+	0	+	0	+	+	+	0	+	0	0	+	+	+	+	+	+	+	0		Co^b+
5	ccddEe	r″r	36849	0	0	+	+	+	0	0	+	0	+	0	+	+	+	+	0	0	+	+	+	+	0	+	0	+	+		
6	ccddee	rr	112727	0	0	0	+	+	0	+	+	0	+	0	+	+	0	0	+	0	+	0	0	+	0	+	0	+	+	M	Co^b+
7	ccddee	rr	95/36818	0	0	0	+	+	0	0	+	0	+	0	+	+	+	+	0	+	0	w +	+	+	0	+	0	+	+	M	Bg^a+
8	ccD.ee	R_{0r}	818/38098	+	0	0	+	+	0	0	+	0	+	0	+	+	+	0	+	0	+	0	+	+	+	+	0	+	0	M	
9	ccD.EE	R_2R_2	71034080	+	0	+	+	0	0	+	+	0	+	0	+	0	+	+	0	0	+	0	+	+	0	+	0	+	+	M	Co^b+
10	ccddee	rr	01776470	0	0	0	+	+	0	0	+	0	+	0	+	+	0	0	+	0	+	+	+	0	+	0	0	+	0	M	
11	CCD.ee	R_1R_1	2573669	+	+	0	0	+	0	0	+	+	+	0	+	0	+	+	0	+	0	+	+	0	+	0	0	+	+		

Figure 31.3: *Example of an antigram showing a wide range of antigens. (Reproduced with permission of Diamed U.K. Ltd.)*

against recipient's sera) should be performed. Units that exhibit no greater strength of reactivity than in the auto autologous cross-match can be issued.

All autoantibodies should be further investigated to identify the specificity and thermal range of the antibody. This may require elution techniques.

Elution methods

It is possible to remove antibodies bound to red cell antigens without altering their antigenic specificity, by a process is termed elution. There are three main elution processes; temperature, low pH and organic solvents.

Temperature

The most commonly used temperature elution system is to heat washed red cells to 56°C for five minutes. After centrifugation the supernatant contains the antibodies. Freezing washed cells suspended in albumin elicits the same haemolysed supernatant which after centrifugation is ready for investigation. Both these methods are quick and easy to undertake in any laboratory.

Low pH

If washed red cells are suspended in buffers with a pH below 3.5 then IgG antibodies are

recovered from the cell membranes without lysis. Although low pH is the recommended elution technique, a pH above 10 appears to give better results for IgM antibodies.

Organic solvents

Although results of eluates using ether or xylene are very good for IgG antibodies, the hazards to works from exposure to these solvents restricts their use to laboratories with extraction hoods.

Once an eluate has been prepared the eluate is substituted for sera in an antibody identification method.

Autologous transfusions

With public awareness of the dangers of transmitting disease through transfusion of blood products and the continuing shortage of donors there has been an expansion of the procedure of donating and receiving one's own blood; namely autologous transfusion. There are two systems for autologous donations. One is a pre-deposit where patients attend a clinic prior to elective surgery, to donate blood for storage until the surgery. The second system is blood salvage using equipment in the operating theatre. If a patient loses blood during surgery it is collected, washed and given back to the patient.

Further Reading

Guidelines for Pretransfusion Compatibility Procedures in Blood Transfusion Laboratories. *Transfusion Medicine*, 1996; **6**: 273–283.

Issitt P D. *Applied Blood Group Serology*. 3rd edn 1985: Montgomery Scientific Publications, Miami, Florida, USA.

Knight R C, DeSilva M. New Technologies for Red Cell Serology. *Blood Reviews* 1996; **10**: 101–110.

Mollison P L, Engelfriet C P, Contreras M. *Blood Transfusion in Clinical Medicine*, 9th edn 1993: Blackwell Scientific Publications, Oxford.

32 FLOW CYTOMETRY AND MOLECULAR BIOLOGY IN HAEMATOLOGY

Ian Chant

Introduction

As technologies improve, the clinical and research applications of flow cytometry and molecular biology have expanded into diverse areas of haematological investigation. The ability of flow cytometers to measure multiple parameters on individual cells at high speed is ideal for the study of leukaemia and lymphoma cells. Immunophenotyping of cell surface antigens and intracellular components by flow cytometric analysis has become an essential tool for the diagnosis of leukaemia, providing information on lineage, stage of differentiation and clonality of malignant cells. Phenotypic and functional studies of platelets and red blood cells are similarly suited to the ability of the flow cytometer to analyse rapidly large numbers of cells in suspension.

The development of molecular biology techniques has led to a vast increase in our knowledge and understanding of the basis of human cancers and in particular haemopoietic neoplasms. In fact, more is known about the molecular basis of the malignant transformation of haemopoietic cells in leukaemias and lymphomas than for any other type of human malignancy. A variety of molecular biological techniques such as Southern blotting, Northern blotting, Western blotting, the polymerase chain reaction (PCR) and *in situ* hybridization (ISH) have provided information at the DNA, RNA and protein levels in terms of cancer-associated chromosomal breakpoints and gene rearrangements. As technologies become more 'user-friendly' we are now seeing a large transfer of this technology from research into the clinical diagnostic laboratory.

In particular, PCR has had a tremendous impact in molecular pathology, and PCR-based methods are now used widely for the identification of translocation-induced gene rearrangements in leukaemias and lymphomas

both as a diagnostic tool and for patient monitoring during treatment. Other haematological areas to which PCR is applicable are the

Introduction

Flow Cytometry and Immunophenotyping

demonstration of mutations within genes of the coagulation system such as factor X and identification of factor V Leiden. In the study of the haemoglobinopathies, the development of PCR-based methodologies for the demonstration of haemoglobinopathy-associated gene defects will have an increasing use in the clinical laboratory.

This chapter aims to demonstrate how the technologies of flow cytometry and molecular biology have complemented each other and together provide definitive information within the clinical haematology setting, particularly in terms of leukaemia and lymphoma diagnostics.

Flow Cytometry and Immunophenotyping

The most important application of the flow cytometer in the diagnostic haematology laboratory is the identification of cell lineage in leukaemias and lymphomas. The expression of surface antigens on leukocytes which are lineage and differentiation-dependent enables us to use fluorochrome-labelled monoclonal antibodies specific to these antigens in order to identify cell lineage. The various monoclonal antibodies which recognize specific epitopes of antigens are identified by a cluster of designa-

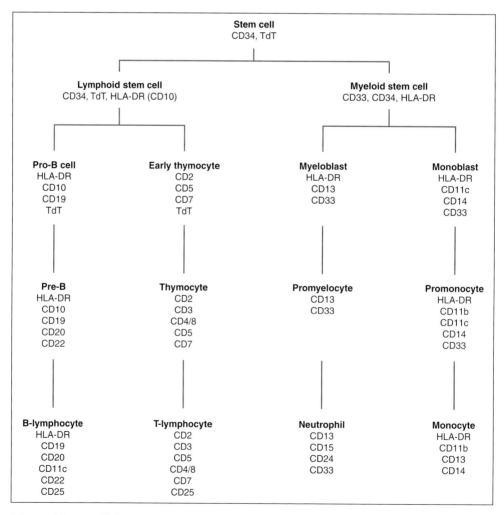

Figure 32.1: Cellular antigens expression of haematopoietic cells.

tion (CD) number. At the time of writing approximately 160 CD numbers have been assigned and a number of these are particularly important in the immunophenotyping of haematopoietic cells. Figure 32.1 illustrates some of the most important CD antigens which are lineage specific. These are especially useful in the differential diagnosis of myeloid and lymphoid leukaemias where immature blast cells may be morphologically similar, and in the differentiation of lymphoid and chronic myeloid leukaemia (CML) in blast crisis. An accurate classification of a newly diagnosed leukaemia is essential in terms of prognosis and subsequent treatment. Acute myeloid and lymphoid leukaemias are primarily classified according to morphological and cytochemical characteristics, as defined by the French–American–British (FAB) system. Flow cytometric analysis of leukocyte antigens is now an essential tool which complements morphological and cytochemical classification of the malignant cell.

Phenotypic analysis of the acute leukaemias

Immunophenotyping of a newly diagnosed acute leukaemia can in most cases be performed using a small battery of monoclonal antibodies which detect specific differentiation antigens expressed on early myeloid or lymphoid cells. A generalized first line antibody panel which will distinguish acute myeloid leukaemias (AML) and B- and T-cell lineage acute lymphoblastic leukaemias (ALL) is illustrated in Fig. 32.2. Expression of CD13 and CD33 will distinguish leukaemias of myeloid origin. All types of B-ALL will be CD19+, CD10+/– whilst T-ALL will be CD7+, CD3(cytoplasmic)+ and CD2+/–. Once the myeloid or lymphoid lineage of blast cells has been established, second line antibody panels can be used to further classify the various ALL and AML subtypes.

Acute myeloid leukaemias

In AML there are no specific markers which alone will distinguish the M1–M5 AML subtypes. However, some markers will be preferentially expressed within certain groups including CD14 in the M4 and M5 AML subtypes, and in the M2 subtype expression of the B-lymphoid marker CD19 is characteristic. The rarer M6 and M7 AML cases can be characterized by their expression of red cell and platelet markers respectively. Thus, M6 (erythroleukaemia) blast cells will express glycophorin A, and M7

Table 32.1: Classification of the acute myeloid and lymphoblastic leukaemias by the French–American–British (FAB) system based primarily on morphological and cytochemical criteria.

Category	Characteristic
Myeloid leukaemias	
M0	Morphologically and cytochemically undifferentiated
M1	Myeloblastic
M2	Myeloblastic with maturation
M3	Acute promyelocytic leukaemia
M4	Acute myelomonocytic leukaemia
M5	Acute monoblastic leukaemia
M6	Erythroleukaemia
M7	Megakaryoblastic leukaemia
Lymphoblastic leukaemias	
L1	Small, regular cells
L2	Large, irregular cells
L3	Large, uniform cells

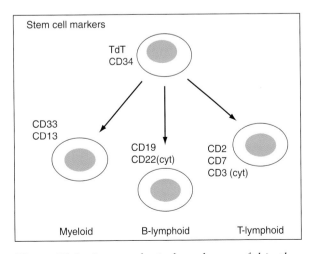

Figure 32.2: Immunological markers useful in the initial assessment of acute leukaemias.

Flow Cytometry and Immunophenotyping

Chronic lymphoproliferative disorders

(megakaryocytic) can be identified with CD41, CD42 and CD61, three monoclonal antibodies which recognize platelet glycoproteins.

Acute lymphocytic leukaemias

B- and T-cell ALL can be classified into various subgroups based upon the degree of lymphoid differentiation as determined by monoclonal antibody reactivity with differentiation-dependent antigens. B-ALL is the most common subtype of ALL (75–85%) comprising four distinct immunological groups. Early B-ALL (pro-B) is distinguished by CD10 negativity, common ALL expresses CD10, pre-B-ALL expresses characteristic cytoplasmic immunoglobulin and mature B-ALL is distinguished by surface immunoglobulin expression. The subtypes of T-ALL are generally classified according to levels of T-cell maturation, and immunophenotypic analysis defines three groups: early and pre-T-ALL (CD7+, cytoplasmic CD3+ and CD2+/−), cortical T-ALL (CD1a+) and mature T-ALL (membrane CD3+).

Chronic lymphoproliferative disorders

Flow cytometric analysis in chronic or mature lymphoproliferative disorders plays a diagnostic role by demonstrating the B- or T-cell nature of the malignant cell, by establishing monoclonality of kappa or lambda surface light chain expression in B-cell disorders, and by the distinction of lymphoblastic malignancies (TdT+) from mature lymphoid disorders (TdT−). There are also certain immunophenotypic characteristics which permit distinction of chronic lymphocytic leukaemia (CLL) from other B-cell malignancies. For example, hairy cell leukaemia (HCL) cells express most of the B-cell antigens, but not CD21, plus three markers which are HCL-specific, namely CD11c, CD25 and FMC7. In the T-cell disorders, expression of markers shows a great deal of overlap, but certain markers are characteristic, such as strong expression of CD25 (IL2 receptor) in adult T-cell leukaemia lymphoma (ATLL), strong reactivity with CD7 in T-prolymphocytic leukaemia, and CD56 (natural killer cell) expression in large granular lymphocyte (LGL) leukaemia.

Flow cytometric analysis of platelet function

The availability of monoclonal antibodies which recognize a variety of activation-dependent platelet antigens enables the analysis of the activation state of circulating platelets both in the absence and the presence of exogenous platelet agonists. One of the most widely used activation-dependent monoclonal antibodies is one specific for P-selectin (CD62P). This antigen is a component of the α granule membrane of resting platelets that is only exposed on the surface membrane following α granule secretion, so monoclonal anti-CD62 will bind only to degranulated platelets. Monoclonal antibodies are also available which recognize conformational changes in the glycoprotein IIb/IIIa complex (CD41/61), the platelet receptor for fibrinogen, von Willebrand factor and fibronectin.

At present, flow cytometric analysis has not replaced standard clinical tests of platelet function such as the bleeding time and platelet aggregometry. However, flow cytometry has several advantages over these traditional tests: the development of whole blood flow cytometric analysis involves minimal manipulation of samples thereby minimising artifactual platelet activation, and extremely small volumes of blood are required ($\sim$2 μl) making neonatal studies possible. The platelets of patients with profound thrombocytopenia can also be analysed accurately.

Enumeration of reticulocytes by flow cytometry

Standard techniques for reticulocyte enumeration are based on the presence of RNA in the cytoplasm of the reticulocyte and entail staining whole blood with supravital stains such as brilliant cresyl blue or new methylene blue. These methods are well established and simple, but are subject to significant variation depending upon unbiased visual counting of large numbers of cells.

Flow cytometric analysis of reticulocytes has been described utilizing a variety of fluorochromes, including acridine orange and propidium iodide, which bind to nucleic acids. One of the most useful fluorochromes is thiazole orange, a membrane-permeable basic dye which binds to RNA and can be excited by light at 488 nm, emitting fluorescence *within* the green region of the spectrum. Distinction of reticulocytes within the red cell population can then be performed on the basis of fluorescent intensity. Reticulocyte counting by flow cytometry can be precise, accurate and cost effective since a large number of cells can be analysed rapidly. In addition, further information regarding the age distribution of reticulocytes can be achieved using flow cytometry since young immature reticulocytes will contain more RNA and therefore have higher fluorescence intensity than older more mature reticulocytes.

Diagnosis of paroxysmal nocturnal haemoglobinuria (PNH) by flow cytometry

PNH is an acquired haematological disease characterized by intravascular complement-mediated haemolysis. The cause of the increased sensitivity to complement is a clonal stem cell disorder resulting in a deficiency of complement-regulatory proteins and other glycoproteins on the cell membranes of erythrocytes, platelets, granulocytes and monocytes. Proteins known to be deficient in PNH include CD14, CD16, CD24, CD55 and CD67. Quantitation of these five antigens by flow cytometry has been used to distinguish PNH patients from normal controls and, in addition, it has been reported to identify early PNH in patients where the Ham's test has been negative.

Molecular Biology

The greatest impact of molecular biology techniques in haematological investigations has been in the study of genetic abnormalities associated with leukaemias and lymphomas. The molecular analysis of translocation-induced gene rearrangements has been studied by a variety of techniques, including Southern blotting and Northern blotting, (see Table 32.2) at both the DNA and RNA levels. Whilst Southern blotting in particular remains the mainstay of many molecular diagnostic tests, this technique can be technically difficult and time-consuming and therefore not ideally suited for use in the clinical laboratory. However, two techniques which have had an enormous impact on molecular pathology diagnostics have been *in situ* hybridization and the polymerase chain reaction (PCR). Both *in situ* hybridization, especially fluorescence *in situ*

Table 32.2: Common molecular biology techniques which may have a place in clinical laboratories.

Method	Source material	Characteristics
Western blotting	Protein	Denatured proteins are size-fractionated on an agarose gel, transferred to nitrocellulose support and specific proteins detected using monoclonal antibodies coupled with variety of visualization procedures.
Northern blotting	RNA	Detects specific RNA sequences using antisense probes following size-fractionation and electrophoretic transfer.
Southern blotting	DNA	Detects specific DNA sequences using labelled antisense probe hybridized to nitrocellulose blot of electrophoresed sample.
Fluorescence *in situ* hybridization (FISH)	DNA or RNA	Hybridization of labelled probe to DNA or RNA in cellular or chromosomal preparations. Provides information on the localization of specific nucleic acid sequences.
Polymerase chain reaction (PCR)	DNA (or RNA by RT-PCR)	An *in vitro* amplification of nucleic acid sequence. Extremely sensitive and can be used quantitatively.

hybridization (FISH), and PCR have been used in the identification of chromosomal abnormalities and the detection of various genes or mRNA, e.g. oncogene expression, in haematological malignancies. These include: (1) abnormal translocation-induced gene rearrangements involving oncogene activation, which are consistently associated with lymphoid and myeloid malignancies; and (2) normal gene rearrangements involving immunoglobulin heavy and light chain genes and T-cell receptor genes which are used to demonstrate the monoclonality and cell lineage of lymphoproliferative lesions.

Examples of the first group include the detection of the t(9;22) (q34;q11) reciprocal translocation, which gives rise to the Philadelphia chromosome in chronic myeloid leukaemia (CML) and some acute lymphoblastic leukaemia (ALL) cases, and the t(14;18) (q32;q31) translocation which is the hallmark of follicular lymphomas and other lymphoid malignancies. Together with the second group where clonal gene rearrangement is a specific marker of neoplastic lymphocytes, these will be used as examples of how molecular biology is applied in the study of haematological cytogenetic abnormalities.

Detection of Philadelphia translocation by PCR

The Philadelphia chromosome results from a reciprocal translocation t(9;22) (q34;q11) causing gene rearrangement involving a cellular oncogene, c-abl (9q34), and the breakpoint cluster region or BCR (22q11) gene. This rearrangement is found in approximately 95% of chronic myeloid leukaemia (CML) patients and 25% of adult acute lymphoblastic leukaemias cases. Both in CML and ALL, the breakpoint in the c-abl gene is the same. However, in CML the breakpoints in the BCR gene occur at specific loci within the breakpoint cluster region (bcr) whilst in ALL the breakpoint within the BCR gene occurs further upstream, resulting in distinct chimaeric mRNA and fusion proteins. Since the breakpoints both in CML and acute leukaemias occur over relatively large stretches of DNA, detection of the fusion mRNA is the method of choice since mRNA sequences are much shorter, lacking the DNA intron sequences.

Figure 32.3 is a schematic representation of PCR detection of the BCR/abl gene rearrangement in CML and ALL. In both cases the starting material is mRNA extracted from peripheral blood or bone marrow leukocytes, which is first reverse transcribed to cDNA using a primer which is complementary to a common c-abl sequence. The selection of PCR primers in CML is aimed at amplifying sequences within the breakpoint cluster region to amplify specifically the fusion mRNA diagnostic of CML, whilst in ALL the primers are complementary to BCR exon 1 which covers the DNA region where breakpoints occur in de novo ALL. Both in ALL and CML the c-abl primer will be the same since the breakpoint within this gene occurs at the same point in both cases. Amplification of the cDNA sequence between the two primers will give rise to a characteristic amplification product and interpretation of the results is based on the examination of ethidium bromide-stained gels following agarose electrophoresis of the amplified products. Different types of fusion mRNA can be identified from the molecular weight of bands evident upon electrophoresis. The design of specific primers confers extreme specificity and sensitivity on PCR, to the level of being able to detect one Philadelphia-positive cell per 10^5 to 10^6 cells. The size of the fusion mRNA will vary for different CML and acute leukaemia breakpoints, but will be specific for that malignant clone and will remain constant throughout the clinical course of that patient's disease. This unique 'marker' can therefore be utilized for patient monitoring during treatment and can be used for the detection of minimal residual disease (MRD). The use of PCR to detect leukaemia-associated gene rearrangements as a means of monitoring MRD in patients in apparent clinical remission will be discussed later.

PCR detection of the t(14;18) translocation in lymphoid malignancies

The t(14; 18) (q32;q21) translocation is one of the hallmarks of follicular lymphoma, occurring in approximately 80% of cases, and is also seen in a significant number of patients with diffuse lymphomas (20%). This gene transloca-

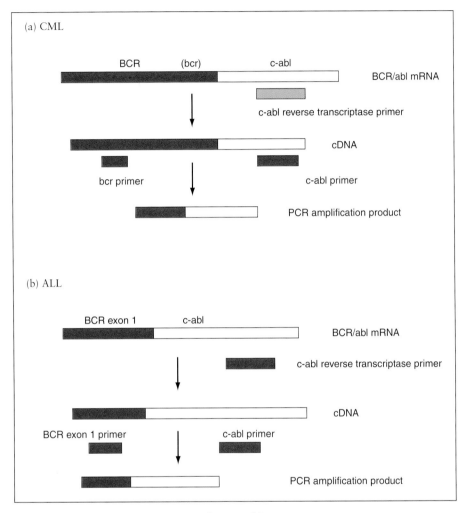

Figure 32.3: *RT-PCR detection of BCR/abl gene rearrangements in (a) CML and (b) ALL.*

tion involves the bcl-2 oncogene and the immunoglobulin heavy chain (IgH) locus, and results in upregulation of bcl-2 expression. Detection of this rearrangement is based upon the detection of the bcl-2/IgH fusion gene. Southern blotting, *in situ* hybridization and PCR have all been used successfully, but again PCR is most useful in clinical situations. Unlike detection of the Philadelphia (BCR/abl) chromosome, PCR detection of the bcl-2/IgH rearrangement is in this case possible at the DNA level because most breakpoints are clustered within short DNA sequences.

At present, detection of this translocation is of limited clinical value, and of course does not assist in the diagnosis of that small percentage of follicular lymphomas which do not have rearrangements of the bcl-2 gene. However, the rearrangement is a unique marker of malignancy which, when present, can be utilized in a variety of clinical situations where the detection of rare malignant cells within a larger normal population is desired.

Detection of rearranged immunoglobulin and T-cell receptor genes

The detection of clonal rearrangements of Ig and TCR genes is important in the identification of B- and T-cell malignancies. The result of a unique rearrangement is an alteration in the structure and size of the antigen receptor involved, which can be detected by Southern blotting or PCR. The chronic leukaemias including CLL, hairy cell leukaemia, prolymphocytic leukaemia and non-Hodgkin's lymphoma have clonal rearrangements both of heavy and light immunoglobulin chains whilst rearrangements of TCR genes are seen in leukaemias and lymphomas of T-cell lineage. Since such rearrangements are clonal and therefore unique for a particular cell and those derived from it, analysis of these gene rearrangements can be used to monitor disease.

Minimal Residual Disease

Minimal residual disease (MRD) can be defined as those leukaemic cells which survive following initial remission–induction chemotherapy. The ability to identify an extremely small population of malignant cells in bone marrow samples which are morphologically in complete remission may have important prognostic and therapeutic implications. Immunological and molecular biology techniques have been utilized to detect MRD in leukaemias and lymphomas, utilizing specific markers of malignancy which may be surface or cytoplasmic antigens or chromosomal rearrangements.

Immunological techniques suffer from the lack of availability of single antibodies which distinguish malignant from normal haemopoietic cells. However, some haemopoietic antigens are found on malignant cells in combinations not present in normal blood or bone marrow. For example, in most T-ALL cases, lymphoblasts will express nuclear terminal deoxyribonuclear transferase (TdT) as well as CD3, CD5 and CD1. This pattern of expression is not normally found in T-cells outside the thymus and can be used to detect lymphoblasts in blood or marrow. The same combination of markers may also be useful in ALL patients in order to demonstrate leukaemic meningeal infiltration. Other immunophenotypic combinations of analysis have been used in studies of MRD for B-lineage ALL and AML with varying degrees of success. A major problem with immunological techniques will always be sensitivity; under optimal conditions flow cytometry can realistically detect one target cell in 10^4 to 10^5. Most studies of residual disease have therefore taken advantage of the extreme sensitivity of PCR, and a large number of studies have used this technique to detect MRD by amplification of specific nucleic acid sequences such as breakpoints in chromosomal translocations, rearranged antigen receptor genes and sites of mutations in various oncogenes. Table 32.3 lists some of the genetic abnormalities which have been used as targets for the molecular detection of MRD.

At present the clinical significance of MRD detection is unproven. Systematic studies of serial samples from large numbers of individual patients will establish the clinical relevance of MRD detection and provide important insights into the kinetics and importance of MRD.

Table 32.3: Chromosomal translocations in leukaemias which have been used as the targets for PCR-based detection of minimal residual disease.

Disease	Genetic abnormality	Target	Frequency (%)
AML	t(8;21) (q22;q22)	AML1-ETO (RNA	5–10
	t(15;17) (q22;q11–22)	PML-RARA (RNA)	5–10
	t(9;22) (q34;q11)	BCR-ABL (RNA)	1–3
B-ALL	t(9;22) (q34;q11)	BCR-ABL (RNA)	25–40
	t(4;11) (q21;q23)	MLL-AF4 (RNA)	5
T-ALL	t(11;14) (p13;q11)	RHOM2-TCRδ (DNA)	5–10
	t(10;14) (q24;q11)	HOX11-TCRα (DNA)	1–3

Identification of Coagulation Factor Abnormalities

The genetic analysis of the genes encoding proteins involved in the coagulation system has led to a greater understanding of the molecular basis of many coagulopathies. Again, the technique of Southern blotting has been the mainstay of DNA analysis, but the transfer of PCR technology from research to clinical laboratory has meant that a variety of genetic screening tests can be performed.

One such test is the detection of the factor V Leiden mutation, in particular because of the high incidence of this mutation in the general population (it has been estimated that 2–6% of normal individuals carry this mutation). Individuals homozygous for this mutation have an estimated 80-fold increase in their thrombotic risk. A PCR-based method for the detection of the base substitutions which give rise to the FV Leiden gene utilizes sequence-specific primers (PCR-SSP). This technique involves PCR amplification using a sense primer complementary to both FV alleles plus an antisense primer which is complementary to either the normal FV allele or the FV Leiden allele. Identification of the FV genotype can then be determined from the analysis of the amplification products since either the normal or FV Leiden-specific primer will produce an amplified product.

Mutations in the gene encoding coagulation factor X have also been identified using PCR-based technologies. The demonstration of point mutations in genes coding coagulation factors has important clinical implications in the diagnosis of factor deficiencies and for the identification of individuals as carriers of these mutations.

Summary

Flow cytometry and molecular biology are powerful analytical techniques which have been used widely in research to investigate the molecular biology of human cancers. Breakthroughs in our understanding of carcinogenesis have been particularly significant in the study of leukaemias and lymphomas; in fact, the first chromosomal abnormality to be consistently associated with human malignancy was the Philadelphia chromosome in CML. The development of smaller, user-friendly benchtop flow cytometry analysers and PCR-based technologies has permitted the transfer of this technology to the clinical laboratory, and the clinical applications of these methodologies can only expand into more diverse areas.

Further Reading

Flow cytometry

General Haematology Task Force of BCSH. Immunophenotyping in the diagnosis of acute leukaemias. *Journal of Clinical Pathology*, 1994; **47**: 777–781.

Macey M G. Flow cytometric analysis of lymphocytes, leukaemias and lymphomas. *British Journal of Biomedical Science*, 1993; **50**: 334–349.

Matutes E. Contribution of immunophenotype in the diagnosis and classification of haematopoietic malignancies. *Journal of Clinical Pathology*, 1995; **48**: 194–197.

Michelson A D. Flow cytometry: A clinical test of platelet function. *Blood*, 1996; **87**: 4925–4936.

Riley R S, Mahin E J, Ross W. (eds.) *Clinical applications of flow cytometry*. 1993; Igaku-Shoin Medical Publishers, New York.

Further Reading

Molecular biology and haematological investigation

Campana D, Pui C-H. Detection of minimal residual disease in acute leukaemia: methodologic advances and clinical significance. *Blood*, 1995; **85**: 1416–1434.

Crisan D, Chen S-T, Weil S C. Polymerase chain reaction in the diagnosis of chromosomal breakpoints. *Haematology/Oncology Clinics of North America*, 1994; **8**(**4**): 725–749.

Kay N E. Clinical utility of molecular probes in lymphoproliferative disorders. *Blood Reviews*, 1996; **10**: 81–88.

33 HAEMATINIC INVESTIGATIONS

David I Fish

Anaemia may be caused by destruction of red cells, a failure in red cell production or by blood loss, which may in turn lead to a failure of production. A failure to produce cells is most often caused by a deficiency of vitamin B_{12}, folate, iron or a combination of two or more of these 'haematinics'.

The starting point for all investigations in the laboratory is the blood count. Macrocytosis and pancytopenia are the characteristic findings in the megaloblastic anaemias caused by vitamin B_{12} and folate deficiency, whilst microcytosis and hypochromia characterize deficiency of iron. Microscopical examination of blood and marrow also yields characteristic findings, but neither can quantify the absolute deficiency nor, in the case of megaloblastic anaemia, differentiate the specific deficiency.

The investigation of haematinic deficiency involves the demonstration of tissue deficiency, identification of specific deficiencies and establishment of the cause.

Vitamin B_{12} and Folate

A deficiency of vitamin B_{12} (cobalamin) and/or folate results in a disturbance in the production of DNA (megaloblastic anaemia). Deficiency is established directly by assay of these vitamins in the blood or indirectly by demonstration of the accumulation of intermediate products that accrue along the metabolic pathways that depend on the presence of these vitamin coenzymes (Fig. 33.1). Thus an increased level in serum or increased excretion in the urine of methylmalonic acid (MMA) indicates cobalamin deficiency, whilst increased excretion of formiminoglutamic acid (FIGLU) may indicate folate deficiency. The sensitivities of these tests are increased by giving the patient a 'loading' dose of valine and histidine respectively. FIGLU is measured by an electrophoretic technique and MMA by thin layer chromatography or gas chromatograph–mass spectrometry. Homocysteine is raised both in cobalamin and folate deficiencies and may be measured quantitatively in serum by HPLC. The findings in severe deficiency are shown in Table 33.1. FIGLU excretion is no longer used and in most laboratories the assay of serum cobalamin, serum folate and red cell folate are the methods of choice.

Deoxyuridine suppression test

This test is used to study a deficiency or the metabolic inactivation of cobalamin or folate. Thymidine is available from two sources: it may be 'salvaged' pre-formed from effete cells, or it may be synthesized. This requires both cobalamin and folate. The test utilizes these two alternative pathways. When deoxyuridine is added to bone marrow cells in culture thymidine is

Vitamin B$_{12}$ and Folate

Assay of vitamin B$_{12}$ and folate in blood

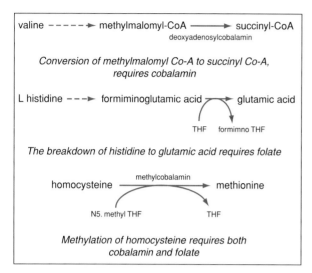

Figure 33.1: *Biochemical reactions dependent upon cobalamin and folate.*

Table 33.1: Laboratory test results in untreated cobalamin and folate deficiency.

Test	Result in severe B$_{12}$ deficiency	Result in severe folate deficiency
Serum B12	Low	Low in 30%
MMA excretion	Raised	Normal
Serum folate	Normal or raised	Low
Red Cell folate	Normal or low	Low
FIGLU excretion	Normal or raised	Raised
Homocysteine	Raised	Raised

produced along the synthesis pathway. Subsequent addition of ^{3}H thymidine provides the balance of the thymidine requirement of the cells. A normal marrow culture will typically take up less than 10% of the ^{3}H thymidine. However, a deficiency of the folate coenzyme, by whatever means, results in a greater uptake of the isotopically labelled thymidine. The addition of folate will correct the test regardless of the primary deficiency, whilst addition of cobalamin will only correct the test if the marrow culture cells are cobalamin deficient (see Fig. 33.2).

Assay of vitamin B$_{12}$ and folate in blood

Estimation of the amount of cobalamin in the serum yields direct evidence of cobalamin deficiency. The serum folate level, however, only reflects the recent folate dietary intake. Because of the cobalamin/folate metabolic interactions, serum folate may be increased in cobalamin deficiency. To measure folate 'status' an estimation of tissue folate is required and this may be obtained by assaying the folate within the red cells. Again, because of the inter-relationships between these two coenzymes, the level of 'red cell folate' is also influenced by cobalamin. It may be low when cobalamin is deficient (Fig. 33.1).

Microbiological assay

Microbiological methods were the first systems sensitive enough to measure the low level of B vitamin encountered in biological materials. These methods are 'functional' assays in that they estimate the vitamin quantity by measuring the ability of the serum under test to stimulate the growth of an organism, the amount of microbiological growth being directly proportional to the vitamin content of the serum under test. The essential factor in the microbiological assay is the organism, which should have a specific growth requirement for the vitamin being estimated. It should have a sufficiently high metabolism to ensure that growth is affected in the shortest time possible and it should not be pathogenic. The growth medium must contain all the necessary growth factors for the test organism except the vitamin under investigation. For cobalamin *Euglena gracilis* and *Lactobacillus leichmanii* are the most commonly used organisms, and a chloramphenicol-resistant *Lactobacillus casei* for folate. Generally such organisms cannot use protein-bound vitamins and some form of initial extraction procedure is necessary. The growth response is measured, usually the turbidity, and compared to the response of the organism to known amounts of vitamin standards.

Problems associated with these assays are those of contamination with organisms not having the specific growth requirement under test. In the clinical situation the presence of antibiotics or antagonists in the serum under investigation may also interfere with the growth.

Microbiological assays remain the yardstick against which alternative methods are compared, but they are technically demanding and time consuming.

Competitive protein bound assay: reagent limited (CPB)

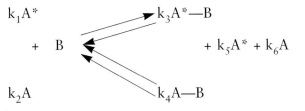

The general principle of CPB may be summarized by the following equation:
A* = Labelled analyte (usually radioactive)
A = Analyte under investigation
B = Specific binder
k$_{1-6}$ = Suitable constants

The system is dependent upon the labelled analyte having an equal affinity with the unlabelled analyte for the limited amount of specific binding agent being used. The binding agent must not exhibit significant cross-reactivity with interfering substances such as vitamin analogues.

Following the binding reaction the free analyte must be separated from the bound analyte. This is usually achieved by some physical means such as adsorption to dextran-coated activated charcoal. The ratio of bound labelled analyte to bound unlabelled analyte is the same as the ratio of the labelled analyte added to the total endogenous analyte in the test. This assumes the reaction has reached equilibrium and has followed simple mass action principles. These assumptions are seldom met and the amount of labelled analyte bound is measured and the response of the unknown sample is compared to the response of known standard preparations. The response is inversely related to the concentration of the analyte (see Fig. 33.3).

As in microbiological assay endogenous vitamin must be released from natural binders and those binders destroyed before the assay

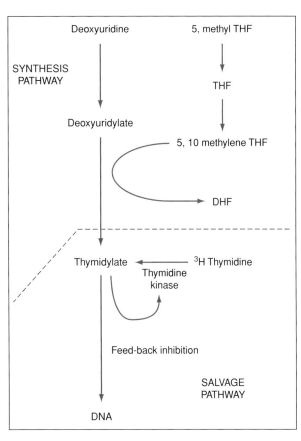

Figure 33.2: Mechanism of the deoxyuridine suppression test. THF: tetrahydrofolate; DHF: dihydrofolate.

can continue. This is usually achieved by boiling a dilution of the serum in a buffer of pH 9.3, however, boiling is not required if extraction solutions have a pH greater than 12.9. A reducing agent dithiothreitol (DTT) is included in the buffer systems. This has two uses; it protects the folate from oxidation and reduces the non-specific binding of the denatured proteins (NSB). This is important because the level of NSB influences the sensitivity and precision of the assay. For B$_{12}$ ^{57}Co is used as the label and the binding agent is intrinsic factor. ^{125}I is the label for folate and beta-lactoglobulin is the binding agent. ^{57}Co and ^{125}I isotopes have significantly different energy spectra enabling them to be counted on a gamma counter without interference from each other. Thus cobalamin and folate can be measured simultaneously in a single assay.

Vitamin B$_{12}$ and Folate

Investigation of the cause of cobalamin and folate deficiency

Iron

Demonstrable tissue iron

Serum iron and total iron binding capacity (TIBC)

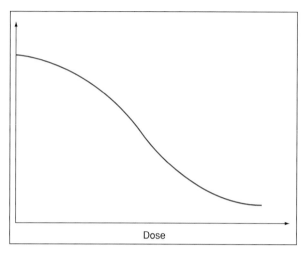

Figure 33.3: *Dose bound response curve.*

After dilution and pre-treatment to convert the red cell folate to a form suitable for the assay system, red cell folate may be measured in the same way as serum folate. The final result is expressed as the folate content of one litre of red cells. This is obtained by correcting the assay result for dilution, the level of interfering plasma folate and the percentage of blood occupied by red cells (haematocrit).

Investigation of the cause of cobalamin and folate deficiency

A clinical history is important and may indicate the cause of the deficiency. Dietary history is particularly important. Pernicious anaemia (PA) is the most important disease to exclude. The demonstration of serum intrinsic factor antibodies (IFAs) or malabsorption of free vitamin B$_{12}$, improved by the addition of intrinsic factor (IF), is required to make the diagnosis.

Folate absorption tests are rarely required.

Cobalamin absorption (Schilling test)

The patient is first 'saturated' with cobalamin, by giving intramuscular hydroxy-B$_{12}$. This ensures that any ^{57}CoB$_{12}$ absorbed is excreted through the kidneys into the urine. An oral dose of radioactively labelled cobalamin (1.0 μg) is then given and the urine is collected for 24 hours. Normal absorption is indicated by an excretion of >10% of the original oral dose. In patients with PA the excretion is improved if the test is repeated with the addition of IF to the oral dose. Failure to correct with IF indicates another cause of malabsorption such as ileal disease.

Iron

Iron is an important element and is to be found in all cells both in metabolically active and storage form. Excess iron within cells is stored as ferritin, which is a soluble protein. Iron within ferritin is mobilized easily, whereas that stored as insoluble haemosiderin is only mobilized slowly. The assessment of iron stores provides evidence in the diagnosis of iron deficiency or overload. In cases of overload the assessment of iron stores is important in the monitoring of treatment.

Demonstrable tissue iron

The assessment of iron may be achieved by liver biopsy or bone marrow aspiration. The iron present is detected by Perl's reaction and a qualitative assessment is made by microscopical examination. Potassium ferrocyanide combines with ferric ions to form potassium ferric ferrocyanide (Prussian blue). Prussian blue is not a dye, it is an insoluble, deeply coloured chemical product. Dilute HCl is included in the reagent to release ferric ions from protein.

$$Fe^{3+} + [Fe(CN)_6]^{4-} \rightarrow Fe_4[Fe(CN)_6]_3$$
$$\text{Prussian blue}$$

Serum iron and total iron binding capacity (TIBC)

Serum iron reflects the balance between input and output of iron and varies from hour to hour and day to day. Consequently, it is of little use as an indicator of iron stores. An abnormally high total iron binding capacity is, however, indicative of iron deficiency or overload.

Serum iron

A mixture of hydrochloric, thioglycolic and trichloracetic acids is used to release transferrin bound iron, reduce the ferric iron to ferrous and to precipitate protein. The ferrous iron in the supernatant gives an intense pink colour with 4,7-diphenyl-1,10-phenanthroline. This colour is measured at 535 nm. A standard and blank solution are treated similarly and the iron concentration is calculated.

TIBC

Sufficient ferric chloride solution is added to saturate the iron binding proteins and any excess iron is removed by adsorption to magnesium carbonate. After centrifugation the serum iron is measured.

Serum ferritin

There is a close relationship between the serum ferritin level and the total amount of storage iron in adults. Thus the assay of ferritin is useful for the assessment of iron stores in iron deficiency and iron overload. However, ferritin levels may be normal or elevated, even in iron deficiency, when infection, inflammatory disease or malignancy is present.

The two methods used are competitive radioimmunoassay (RIA) and a 'two site' immunoradiometric (IRMA) assay. If the label used is not an isotope but an enzyme, the assay is termed enzyme-linked immunosorbent assay (ELISA).

The principle of the competitive radioimmune assay is the same as that described for the assay of cobalamin and folate. In the immunoradiometric assay it is the binder (antibody) which is labelled.

Immunoradiometric assay (IRMA)

Proteins such as ferritin have many spatially separated antigen sites so that two antibodies may bind at the same time. Unlabelled 'capture' antibody is bound to a solid phase (e.g. plastic test-tube coated with ferritin antibody). Test sample or standard, suitably diluted, is added and ferritin within the sample is bound to the solid phase by the attached antibody in an amount proportional to its concentration in serum. The solid phase is then washed and ^{125}I-labelled 'detecting' antibody is added. The ferritin bound to the solid-phase antibody is then sandwiched between the solid-phase antibody and the labelled antibody. The excess labelled antibody is washed and the amount of labelled

antibody counted (see Fig. 33.4). It is worth noting that modern commercial assays have been designed to enable this two-site immunoradiometric assay to be carried out with a single incubation and single wash.

If the assay is of the ELISA type the enzyme label, usually horseradish peroxidase or alkaline phosphatase, is reacted with a suitable substrate to yield a coloured product that may be measured spectrophotometrically.

The amount of response signal (radioactive counts or colour intensity) is directly proportional to the concentration of ferritin in the original sample (Fig. 33.4). This is a method that is very sensitive and very low concentrations of analyte can be detected. However, one disadvantage is that very high concentrations of analyte saturate both capture and detecting antibodies. The response is lowered and in extreme cases a false low result may be reported. This phenomenon is called the 'high dose hook effect' (Fig. 33.5). It is recommended that when using such assays all samples that are suspected to have high values be assayed at two dilutions.

Competitive and immunoassays are widely used in pathology and with the advent of the non-isotopic label many have been automated to permit the routine assay of hundreds of samples daily.

Red cell zinc protoporphyrin

In the production of haem the final reaction is incorporation of ferrous iron into protoporphyrin. Zinc may also be chelated into the protoporphyrin ring and a reduction in the supply of iron results in an increased level of zinc protoporphyrin (ZPP). The ratio of ZPP to normal iron containing haem is therefore a functional measure of iron status.

A modified front-faced haematofluorimeter has been developed (Helena Laboratories, Gateshead, UK) to measure the ZPP/haem ratio. A beam of light at 420 nm is projected onto the sample of red cells. Both haem and ZPP absorb the light, but ZPP fluoresces and the amount of light emitted at 595 nm is measured. Results are expressed as the ZPP (μmol)/haem (mol) ratio. The finding of a normal ZPP/haem ratio is a clear indication

Iron

Red cell zinc protoporphyrin

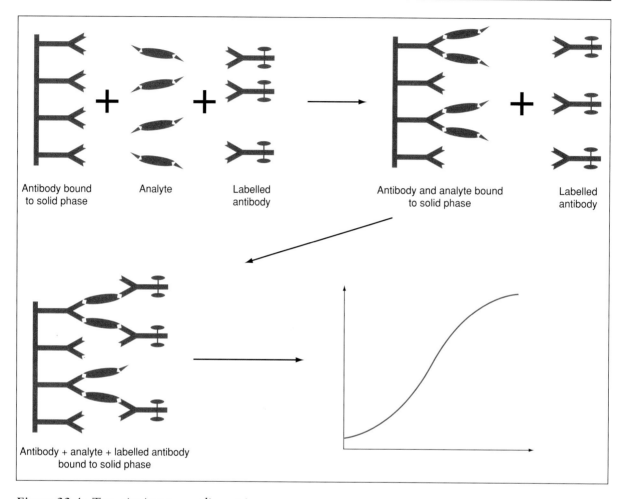

Figure 33.4: Two-site immunoradiometric assay.

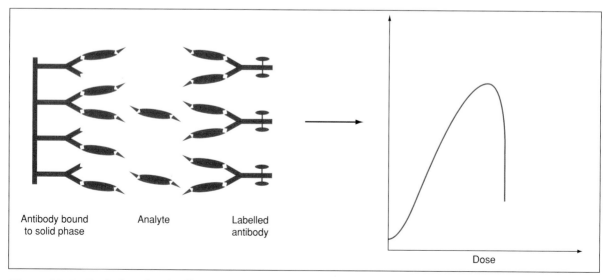

Figure 33.5: High dose hook effect.

of normal iron delivery; an abnormal ratio warrants further investigation.

The amount of fluorescence is influenced by a number of plasma constituents, notably bilirubin, but this is not generally a problem when screening for simple iron deficiency. For samples with significant amounts of bilirubin the problem may be overcome by washing the plasma from the cells with normal saline. The degree of oxygenation of haemoglobin also influences the level of fluorescence. To solve this problem all the haemoglobin present is converted to a cyanide derivative by adding Protofluor™.

Summary

The investigation of haematinic deficiencies, and of iron overload, always starts with the full blood count and blood film examination. The levels of cobalamin, serum and red cell folate, and serum ferritin are estimated to identify the specific deficiency. In cases of simple deficiency it is not necessary to employ invasive techniques such as bone marrow or liver biopsy. In the case of cobalamin deficiency PA must be excluded.

Haematinic assays give rise to numerical results that must be interpreted by comparison with a reference range derived from individuals deemed not to be deficient, the so-called normal range. These ranges should be determined by the laboratory. Typical reference ranges for the haematinic assays discussed are to be found in Table 33.2. Interpretation must always be made within the clinical context of the patient under investigation and with full knowledge of the assays and their limitations.

Table 33.2: Typical reference ranges for haematinic assays.

Haematinic assay	Typical reference range
Serum B_{12}	170–900 $\mu g/l$
Serum folate	3.0–20.0 $\mu g/l$
Red cell folate	160–600 $\mu g/l$
Serum ferritin	
Male & postmenopausal female	20–200 $\mu g/l$
Female	15–100 $\mu g/l$

Further Reading

British Committee for Standards in Haematology. Guidelines on the investigation and diagnosis of cobalamin deficiencies, *Clin Lab Haemat* 1994; **16**: 101–115

Chanarin I (ed) *Laboratory Haematology*, 1989: Churchill Livingstone, Edinburgh.

Dawson DW, Hoffbrand AV, Worwood M. In *Practical Haematology* 7th edn 1991: Churchill Livingstone, London.

Labbe RF, Rettmer RL. Zinc protoporphyrin: A product of iron-deficient erythroipoesis. *Semin Haematol* 1989; **26**: 40–46.

Wild D (ed). *The Immunoassay Handbook*, 1994: Stockton Press, New York.

34 LABORATORY INVESTIGATION OF HAEMOLYSIS

Paul Revell

Introduction

In normal life, red cells are recycled every 120 days. The haemolytic disorders are those in which there is accelerated red cell destruction accompanied by a compensatory increase in red cell production. If the marrow cannot 'keep up', anaemia will result. The accelerated destruction is usually because the red cell is abnormal. The associated abnormalities detected in the laboratory are shown in Fig. 34.1 and summarized in Table 34.1. Some of these are illustrated in Fig. 34.2.

Clinical Features

What happens to the patient is often rather non-specific and dependent on the *speed of onset* as much as the particular disease causing the haemolysis. The main clinical features which are seen in haemolytic anaemias are summarized in Table 34.2.

Table 34.1: **Laboratory abnormalities in haemolysis.**
They are not all found in every patient. The relative severity of each may depend on the stage in the illness that the patient has reached. Reduced red cell life span is rarely measured directly but see Fig. 34.5 for an example.
In general:
- Low haemoglobin if decompensated
- Increased reticulocyte count
- Increased (unconjugated) bilirubin
- Urobilinogen in urine
- Reduced red cell life span
- Abnormal red cells (depending on cause)

And if there is intravascular haemolysis:
- Haemoglobinaemia
- Methaemalbuminaemia
- Haemoglobinuria
- Haemosiderinuria
- Low serum haptoglobin

In very rapid onset conditions (e.g. incompatible blood transfusion) there will be prostration, fever, backache with haemoglobinuria and malaise, rather than the features in Table 34.2. The more chronic conditions reach a 'steady state' with destruction and production in balance though usually with some test results remaining abnormal. This can be punctuated by exacerbations of illness or 'crises'. There are four main types of crisis:

Clinical Features

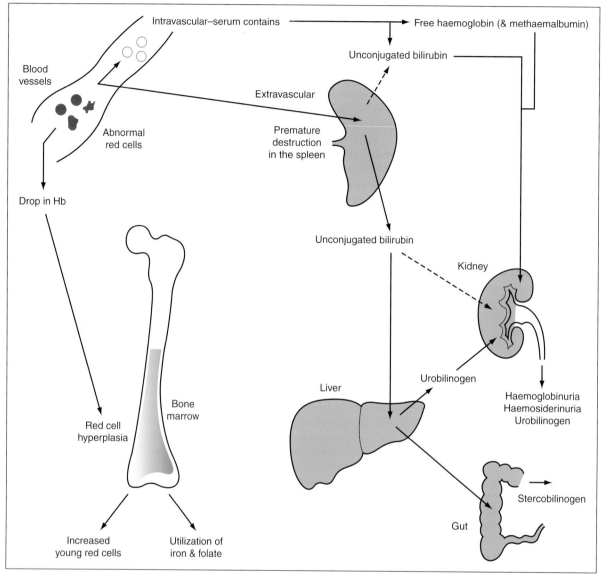

Figure 34.1: *The pathophysiological features of haemolysis.*
If destruction occurs within the blood vessels then free haemoglobin is liberated which will appear in the urine (see also Fig. 34.2). If the destruction is extravascular (spleen; sometimes liver) then this will be avoided but excessive unconjugated bilirubin will be liberated. This may result in the patient appearing jaundiced (yellow; pale yellow if also anaemic, first seen in the whites of the eyes) and the secondary product urobilinogen will be detected in the urine on testing (it does not discolour the urine). Increased production results in a shift of red cells to younger forms which creates polychromasia, a blue tinge, on the film, reflected in an increased reticulocyte count. Nucleated red cells, usually only seen in the marrow, can also be seen in the blood in active haemolysis.

A *haemolytic crisis* is the result of an increase in the accelerated haemolysis, often brought on by an intercurrent illness such as a viral infection. This causes an increase in jaundice and anaemia and a pouring out of reticulocytes (and sometimes nucleated red cells) from the marrow. This is one facet of a 'sickle crisis'.

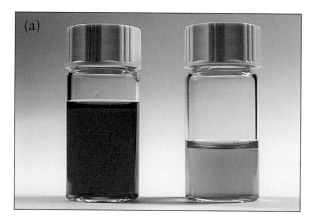

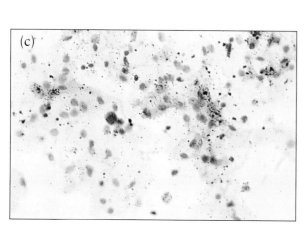

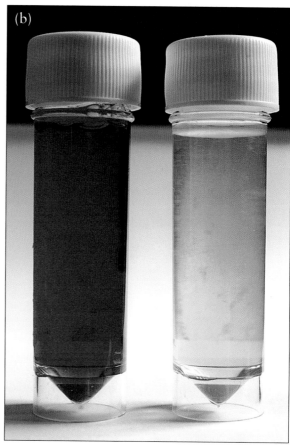

Figure 34.2: Some laboratory findings in intravascular haemolysis.
(a) Haemoglobin is released into the serum producing a 'muddy-brown' appearance. A normal serum is shown for comparison. (b) Some of this appears directly in the urine causing a similar discolouration. This should not be confused with the much commoner occurrence of haematuria where whole red cells appear in the urine. In haemoglobinuria, therefore, the stick test for blood will be positive but no red cells will be seen on microscopy of urine. (c) Some haemoglobin is taken up by kidney cells which are shed into the urine (red counterstain) and show up as small haemosiderin granules (blue).

An *aplastic crisis* is where the marrow stops working for a while, for example in parvovirus infection. In normal people this may have little effect but in a haemolytic condition, the patient can become very anaemic and ill quite quickly, since for most of the time they rely on a very active marrow to 'keep up'.

A *sequestration crisis* occurs in some conditions, like sickle cell disease in children, when the spleen suddenly enlarges and sequestrates the cells. The patient is either very ill or dead on arrival at hospital: fortunately this is rare.

A *megaloblastic crisis* occurs when the marrow runs out of folate (usually) from the excessive production of red cells required to 'keep up' and a frank megaloblastic anaemia results. 'Megaloblastic' refers to the bone marrow appearance where the nucleated red cells look abnormal, because the maturation of the nucleus and cytoplasm are out of step with each other.

General management of the patient
When the patient first presents, the diagnostic priorities are to establish that haemolysis is occurring (Fig. 34.1 and 34.2) and to try to

347

Table 34.2: Clinical features of haemolysis.
The clinical information provided by doctors can assist in the selection of primary as well as secondary investigations in suspected haemolysis.

- History of previous episodes
- Association of episodes with: infections
  - drugs
  - cold
  - foods
- Anaemia
- Jaundice
- Pigment gallstones
- Leg ulcers
- Growth retardation
- Family history of anaemia/jaundice
- Enlarged spleen
- Skeletal abnormalities

ascertain whether the process is slow or fast, intra- or extravascular. Tests to find the cause of the haemolysis then follow. Patients will generally need their vitamin B_{12} and folate levels checked and then be started on treatment doses of folic acid by mouth. Transfusion will be nec-essary in extreme clinical states. If the cause is found, then specific treatment will be started such as corticosteroids by mouth for immune haemolysis. Complications may need treatment such as the removal of symptomatic pigment gallstones in hereditary spherocytosis. Removal of the spleen (splenectomy, to reduce destruc-tion) will have to be considered in some cases.

Extra medical input is needed in times of stress (pregnancy, surgery, etc.) and support and education of the patient and family are always needed in chronic conditions. Genetic coun-selling and family studies may be appropriate in certain cases.

Haemolytic Disorders

There are hundreds of different conditions and many have had large tomes written about them! Table 34.3 gives a general outline of the broad groups seen and the common or impor-tant examples. A brief word about each of these is provided to illustrate where they fit into this general scheme; previous chapters

Table 34.3: The haemolytic disorders.
This way of dividing up the conditions enables a limited amount of clinical information to guide subsequent testing.

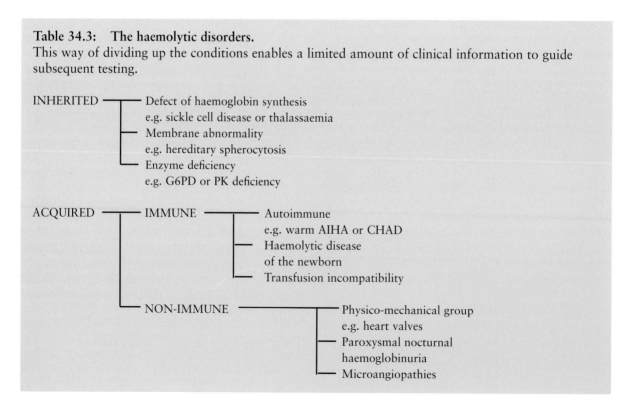

INHERITED ── Defect of haemoglobin synthesis
e.g. sickle cell disease or thalassaemia
── Membrane abnormality
e.g. hereditary spherocytosis
── Enzyme deficiency
e.g. G6PD or PK deficiency

ACQUIRED ── IMMUNE ── Autoimmune
e.g. warm AIHA or CHAD
── Haemolytic disease
of the newborn
── Transfusion incompatibility

── NON-IMMUNE ── Physico-mechanical group
e.g. heart valves
── Paroxysmal nocturnal
haemoglobinuria
── Microangiopathies

give greater detail about some of the individual conditions and the reading list at the end of the chapter provides further sources.

Sickle cell anaemias and other haemoglobin variants

These arise because the red cell contains haemoglobin made from abnormal globin chains. Haemoglobin A (Hb A) is normal. Hb F is a variant but would be normal in the fetus. The abnormal haemoglobin S arises from a genetic defect causing an amino acid substitution in the beta chain. In these conditions the red cell will contain various haemoglobins depending on the genes held. For example, in homozygous sickle disease with two S genes, the red cell will contain mostly Hb S and a little Hb F but no Hb A. In the trait (one S gene) they will contain 45% Hb S and the rest Hb A. It is worth bearing in mind that these are the percentages in every cell – in contrast, a homozygous sickle patient who has been transfused normal (Hb A only) blood may also have 45% Hb S and the rest Hb A but each cell will be *either* all Hb S *or* all Hb A.

Sickle cell anaemia (SS). The deoxygenated form of the abnormal Hb is less soluble than normal Hb A (this forms the basis of the screening test for Hb S). Hb S causes deformed red cells (sickle cells) due to 'tactoid' formation, and these cells are destroyed in the spleen and peripherally. The patients run a low haemoglobin (5–10 g/dl) and often have raised neutrophil and platelet counts. Sickle cells are visible on the blood film. Diagnosis is by Hb electrophoresis. The low Hb is sufficient to impair development in some children. Thrombotic phenomena occur due to sickling which can cause pain, classically in the limbs and also affect the chest, abdomen and brain. Infarction (localized destruction due to lack of oxygen) of the spleen causes hyposplenism with Howell–Jolly bodies in red cells on the blood film. Good medical care has a significant impact on the quality of life and mortality of patients with the condition.

In *Sickle cell trait (AS)* sickling does not occur (as there is less Hb S in each cell) except under very hypoxic conditions (unpressurized aircraft, general anaesthesia). There is little to see on the film.

Hb C Disease (CC) produces mild haemolysis and an enlarged spleen but extra problems arise in dehydration and pregnancy. The trait (AC) is of no significance to the individual except in genetic terms.

HbSC disease (S/C) produces mild haemolysis but patients can have sickling problems especially in pregnancy. Some are troubled by retinopathy (infarctions at the back of the eye) and bony destruction (e.g. of the head of the femur).

Sickle/thal disease (S/Thal). The severity depends upon the amount of normal Hb produced, which in turn depends on the precise thalassaemia gene. If none, then the disease is every bit as severe as the homozygous SS form.

Thalassaemias

In these conditions, there is abnormal production of globin chains (rather than production of abnormal types of chain). This ranges from β_0-thalassaemia (no beta chains) to the mild α- thalassaemias where there is a slight reduction in alpha chain synthesis and no clinical problems to speak of. Heterozygotes do not run into trouble but often have blood film abnormalities. Homozygous β_0-thalassaemia is a serious disorder requiring a lifetime of transfusions and is sometimes complicated by hypersplenism (the overactive spleen destroys all the blood cells). Target cells are characteristically seen on the film. The lack of production is of more importance than haemolysis of abnormal cells. Hyperplasia of the marrow leads to the characteristic childhood bony deformities. Children fail to thrive and die without transfusion. Survivors on transfusion suffer the effects of iron overload. If chelation, using desferrioxamine as a nightly subcutaneous infusion to increase iron excretion, fails then endocrine gland (pituitary, gonadal, pancreatic), liver and cardiac infiltration and damage occurs, with fatal result, often before the age of 25. Haemoglobin H disease is a form of α-thalassaemia (*not* an abnormal Hb

The Haemolytic Disorders
Hereditary spherocytosis

G6PD (Glucose-6-phosphate-dehydrogenase) deficiency

variant called H!) Here the absence of some alpha chains causes the excess beta chains to form tetramers (β_4), which condense as inclusion bodies (H bodies, seen on cresyl blue staining).

Hereditary spherocytosis
Hereditary spherocytosis is autosomally dominant (viz. with one gene, a person inherits the condition), and generally found in Caucasians. There is an abnormality of the red cell membrane contractile proteins which leads to reduced deformability. The abnormal cells are sequestered in the spleen and destroyed prematurely. Anaemia is usually mild and spherocytes are seen on the blood film (but they are easily missed!). The diagnosis is made by an increased 'osmotic fragility' (Fig. 34.3) and by electrophoretic analysis of the red cell membrane components.

G6PD (Glucose-6-phosphate-dehydrogenase) deficiency
The red cell has a reduced reductive energy from a lack of the first enzyme in the pentose phosphate shunt pathway of glucose metabolism. It is often a sex-linked recessive condition: the disease is expressed in males with one affected gene on the X chromosome but females need two affected genes. Females with one affected will show variable expression depending on which X chromosome is inactivated in which cells, according to the Lyon hypothesis. It is mostly seen in black and Mediterranean populations and affects 3% of the world's people. G6PD activity is present in reticulocytes but it falls off rapidly and prematurely in these individuals. Red cell integrity is therefore reduced on exposure to oxidant chemicals and drugs (e.g. sulphonamide antibiotics). Heinz bodies are seen on specially prepared blood films. Diagnosis is by assay of G6PD but only in the steady state (not when there is an excessive number of reticulocytes such as after haemolytic crises). Some episodes are caused by foods (classically, by fava beans – 'favism') as well as drugs.

Screening for 6GPD deficiency
Within the pentose phosphate pathway NADP is reduced by G6PD to NADPH. This product fluoresces under ultraviolet light. This forms

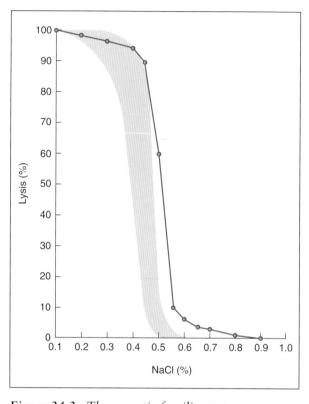

Figure 34.3: The osmotic fragility test.
Aliquots of well mix oxygenated blood are added to a series of buffered saline concentrations usually in the range 0.2–1.2% NaCl. The dilutions are incubated at room temperature for 30 minutes before the tubes are centrifuged and the amount of haemolysis in the supernatant read photometrically. Spherocytes are abnormally sensitive to hypotonic solutions and lyse in higher concentrations than normal red cells. Inconclusive osmotic fragility results can be repeated using the incubated osmotic fragility where the blood sample is incubated for 24 hours at 37°C prior to testing. This modification is much more sensitive in detecting mild spherocytosis than the original method. The graph for normal red cells will generally appear in the grey area. A representative graph for a patient with hereditary sperocytosis is shown.

the basis of the fluorescent spot test. Whole blood is mixed with:

- Glucose 6 phosphate
- NADP
- Lysing agent (usually saponon)
- Buffer

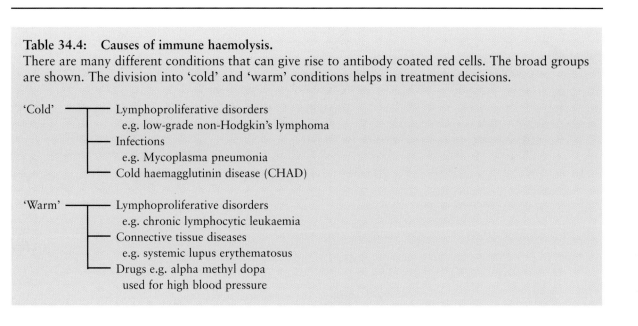

Table 34.4: Causes of immune haemolysis.
There are many different conditions that can give rise to antibody coated red cells. The broad groups are shown. The division into 'cold' and 'warm' conditions helps in treatment decisions.

'Cold'
— Lymphoproliferative disorders
  e.g. low-grade non-Hodgkin's lymphoma
— Infections
  e.g. Mycoplasma pneumonia
— Cold haemagglutinin disease (CHAD)

'Warm'
— Lymphoproliferative disorders
  e.g. chronic lymphocytic leukaemia
— Connective tissue diseases
  e.g. systemic lupus erythematosus
— Drugs e.g. alpha methyl dopa
  used for high blood pressure

It is then incubated for 5–10 minutes before being spotted onto filter paper, dried and examined under long wave UV light. Normal samples will fluorecense brightly, deficient samples will not fluorecense or only poorly. This screening test is the method recommended by the ICSH and as such is the only method to be discussed. Any abnormal screening test must be confirmed by a G6PD assay, here the production of NADPH by G6PD is measured spectrometrically with a change in optical density over time.

Pyruvate kinase deficiency
Pyruvate kinase deficiency is an autosomally recessive condition (with both genes abnormally, a person inherits the condition) and another enzyme problem — the commonest of the rarer non-G6PD diseases. The cells become deformed and vulnerable. The blood film shows poikilocytes (abnormally shaped red cells) and these are haemolysed spontaneously without a drug stimulus. Transfusions may be needed.

Screening for pyruvate kinase deficiency
Pyruvate kinase is the catalyst for the reaction:

ADP + Phosphoenolpyruvate PK ATP + Pyruvate

The product of this reaction, Pyruvate, then proceeds into the following reaction:

Pyruvate + NADH LDH Lactate + NAD

NADH will fluoresce under long wave UV light whereas NAD will not. Therefore when whole blood is incubated with ADP, Phosphoenolpyruvate and NADH in normal samples NADH is oxidised to NAD with a consequential loss of fluorescence. Deficient samples will fluoresce brightly. An abnormal PK screening test must be confirmed by a full assay of the enzyme where the oxidation of NADH to NAD is measured by a change in absorbance photometrically over time.

Immune haemolyses
Various conditions (such as those listed in Table 34.4) result in antibody-coated red cells, which have a shortened life span. Immune haemolysis is divided in the laboratory into 'warm' and 'cold' types depending on the thermal range of activity (and agglutination) in the laboratory, classically 37°C in warm and 4°C in cold, though there is sometimes a little overlap. As well as a broad screening direct Coombs (anti-globulin) test, which will be positive (DCT, Fig. 34.4), reagents giving a more specific profile (IgG, complement) can be used

The Haemolytic Disorders

Immune haemolyses

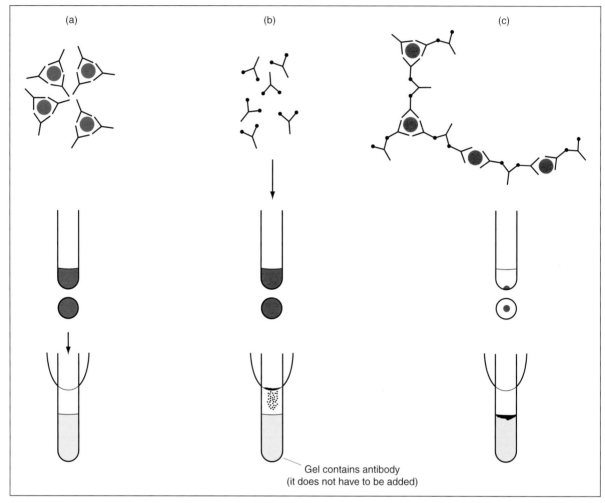

Figure 34.4: *The Direct Coombs (or Anti-Globulin) Test.*
The DCT (or DAGT) detects antibody-coated red cells. (a) To a suspension of the patient's red cells (already coated with antibody) is added (b) broad spectrum anti-globulin (e.g. rabbit antihuman). (c) Agglutination occurs. The result is shown in a traditional tube method (upper) or gel technology (lower).

in warm immune haemolysis. It is usual in suspected cold immune haemolysis to keep the specimen of blood warm until the serum is separated, then test against adult (containing I antigen) and umbilical cord (i antigen bearing) cells. The DCT is usually only positive with the complement reagent and the blood film shows agglutination, unless made warm. The distinction between warm and cold conditions is important for treatment. In the warm immune haemolyses, steroids and other immunosuppressive treatments aimed at switching off production of, or interfering with, the effect of

antibody production are often useful. Splenectomy often works. In cold immune haemolyses, however, cytotoxic chemotherapy (sometimes) and keeping the patient warm (nearly always) help but not steroids or splenectomy. Transfusion is generally avoided in immune haemolysis as the autoagglutination interferes with cross-matching. The clinical state of the patient occasionally demands transfusion and they should certainly not be allowed to succumb through lack of red cells, in which case the 'least incompatible' blood is issued.

Haemolytic disease of the newborn (HDN)

Rhesus positive cells from the Rh+ foetus pass into the circulation of an Rh– mother, for example in haemorrhage during pregnancy or threatened miscarriage. This causes the mother to produce anti-D (anti-rhesus) antibodies which later on in the same or subsequent pregnancies, will pass to the fetus and coat red cells, causing haemolysis if the baby is Rh+. ABO group incompatibilities can cause similar problems but of a lesser severity. High unconjugated bilirubin levels after birth (due to haemolysis) will cross the blood–brain barrier and cause 'kernicterus' with brain damage. Treatment, which may include exchange transfusion, will prevent this. Spherocytes may be seen on the blood film and the DCT will be positive. In severe cases the baby will be hydropic (anaemia/jaundice/swollen up with oedema). At times of potential feto-maternal haemorrhage, the production of antibody by the mother may be prevented by the passive administration of anti-D by intramuscular injection, which will prevent her producing her own response by mopping up Rh+ cells. Affected infants may be treated by intrauterine transfusion (a tricky manoeuvre!) or early induction of labour with exchange transfusion of the newborn.

Incompatible transfusion

Incompatible transfusion is an immune mediated haemolysis. In ABO incompatibility (a very rare occurrence it is hoped) the donor cells are destroyed intravascularly because of the patient's naturally occurring anti-A or anti-B antibodies (or both). The patient can become ill very rapidly, as previously described, and will pass haemoglobinuria. If the transfusion is not stopped or the patient is under anaesthesia the condition can be fatal. Incompatibility reactions due to other antigens will usually provoke extravascular haemolysis with anaemia and jaundice. Recovery is usual but there will be cross-matching problems thereafter on account of the allo-antibodies to red cell antigens.

Non-immune mechanisms

These can result in abnormal red cells (which therefore have a shortened life span). *Physico-mechanical* trauma to normal red cells, such as when passing through a leaking mechanical heart valve, can lead to fragmentation and either intravascular lysis or early recycling by the spleen.

Paroxysmal Noctural Haemoglobinuria (PNH) is a rare acquired haematological disease. The patient typically suffers intravascular complement mediated haemolysis resulting in haemoglobinuria, iron deficiency, aplastic crises and a predisposition to venous thrombosis. This is a stem cell disorder which produces cells deficient in complement regulatory proteins resulting in an increased sensitivity of the red cell membrane to lysis by complement. Traditional diagnosis was made using a variety of tests. The most sensitive being the acidified serum test (Hams' test) and the sucrose lysis test. These tests have now largely being replaced by the introduction of flow cytometry for the detection of surface molecules CD 55 (Decay-accelerating Factor-DAF) and CD 59 (Homozygous Restriction Factor-HRF/C8–binding protein (C8bp). These antigens are reduced or absent in PNH and is the most sensitive and specified-tool available for diagnosis at present.

Microangiopathies

The microangiopathies cause red cell shearing on fibrin strands in small vessels and are associated with a characteristic blood picture which contains lots of fragments, some helmet cells and a few microspherocytes. Thrombocytopenia and markers of haemolysis (anaemia, raised reticulocytes and bilirubin) are usually present. There are a number of causes of this which are summarized in Table 34.5. The diagnostic

Table 34.5: Causes of microangiopathy.
These three broad groups contain all the likely causes:

- Disseminated intravascular coagulation (DIC) (in obstetric problems, septicaemia, cancer, etc.)

- Systemic lupus erythematosus (SLE) and other renal and connective tissue disorders

- Thrombotic thrombocytopenic purpura (TTP) and haemolytic uraemic syndrome (HUS)

Endpiece

Table 34.6: Laboratory diagnosis of microangiopathic conditions.
The coagulation screen, renal biochemistry and clinical information will usually distinguish the cause.

Cause	Hb/Plats	Clotting	Renal failure	Clinical context
DIC	Low	Abnormal	+	++
SLE	Low	N	+	++++
TTP	Low	N	—	—
HUS	Low	N	+++	+++

pointers which distinguish between them are shown in Table 34.6. The diagnosis is well worth making because all of these conditions are serious and can kill otherwise young, fit patients, but are often treatable. The correct diagnosis between them is important because certain blood products are potentially dangerous in some but not in others and steroids are helpful in some but not in the rest.

Additional evidence of intravascular haemolysis can be obtained from the investigations shown in Table 34.7.

Endpiece

There will always be some cases which remain difficult to elucidate and direct measurement by isotope labelling of red cells may be needed (Fig. 34.5). There will, finally, be some patients who are clearly haemolysing but in whom no cause can be found. Most of these will have an as yet undefined disorder of red cell anatomy or physiology.

Table 34.7: Laboratory investigation of intravascular haemolysis.
During haemolysis, haemoglobin is released into the plasma. This binds rapidly to the plasma proteins haptoglobin and haemopexin before being cleared from the circulation by the liver. If haemolysis is severe haptoglobin and haemopexin concentrations are rapidly depleted and haemogolbinuria and methaemalbumin appear.

- Methaemalbumin gives plasma a 'muddy-brown' appearance which can be measured photometrically and has a characteristic absorbtion peak of 624 nm

- Serum haptoglobin and haemopexin levels can be measured in a number of ways that include gel filtration, and electrophoretic, photometric and immunological methods. The commonest in use today are the immunological methods utilising anti-haptoglobin or anti-haemopexin allowing demonstration by radial immunodiffusion or laurell rocket techniques

- Urinary haemosiderin demonstration is by the Perl's Prussion Blue iron stain method. A specimen of urine is centrifuged and the deposit spread onto a glass slide, dried in air before being fixed in methanol. Ferric iron present in the deposit reacts with acidified potassium ferrocyanide to produce ferric ferrocyanide which appears as blue stained granules

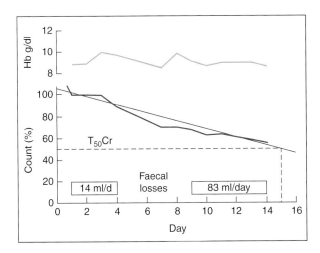

Figure 34.5: Red cell labelling.
Mrs ID, age 76, was suffering recurrent attacks of anaemia associated with palpitations, shortness of breath and exhaustion. She was known to have complex valvular heart disease including an aortic valve replacement, which had murmurs on listening to the heart which might indicate leakage. She was on warfarin and was known to have red cell allo-antibodies, making cross-matching difficult. An iron deficiency picture indicated loss of red cells but with a little fragmentation on the blood film, reduced haptoglobin but no haemosiderinuria it was unclear whether the intravascular destruction was significant. She had no bowel symptoms and full examination of the GI tract revealed no anatomical causes of blood loss. The patient's red cells were therefore labelled with ^{51}Cr and re-injected (day 0). Samples of blood were taken daily for isotopic activity (day 1 is taken as 100% to allow for early losses) and stools collected for activity as shown. It can be seen that the chromium half-life ($T_{50}Cr$) is reduced at 15 days (normal 25–33 days) although she maintained her Hb during the study. This modest reduction was accounted for by the considerable loss noted from the GI tract shown by the stool isotope counts. The loss is clearly variable and was assumed to be coming from an angiodysplasia in the large bowel (these are not demonstrable anatomically). She needed several elective and emergency transfusions during the first year but none in the second when it appeared that blood loss had ceased. The heart valve did not need replacing.

Further Reading

Chanarin I. (ed). *Laboratory Haematology. An account of laboratory techniques.* 1989. Churchill Livingstone, Edinburgh.

Dacie JV. *The Haemolytic Anaemias.* 3rd edn. Vols 1–4. 1988–95. Churchill Livingstone (Volume 5 in preparation), Edinburgh.

Dacie JV, Lewis SM. *Practical Haematology.* 7th Edn. 1991. Churchill Livingstone, Edinburgh.

Hall R and Malia RG. *Medical Laboratory Haematology.* 2nd Edn. 1991. Butterworth Heinemann, Oxford.

Lee GR et al. (eds). *Wintrobe's Clinical Haematology.* 9th Edn. 1993. Lea & Febiger, Philadelphia.

35 LABORATORY INVESTIGATION OF HAEMOSTASIS

Peter Rose and Catherine Caveen

Introduction

Blood flow within the vascular compartment is dependent upon the balance between procoagulant and anticoagulant activity. Under normal circumstances anticoagulant activity is dominant, however with damage to endothelial cells lining blood vessels, subendothelium may be exposed with local clot formation initiated. Initial platelet adhesion to the injured vessel and platelet aggregation form a platelet plug while local coagulation produces a firm fibrin clot. Subsequently a system of clot digestion (fibrinolysis), prevents clot extension and restores patency.

Laboratory investigation is routinely used to assess patients with increased thrombotic or haemorrhagic risk. In many acute medical conditions the normal balance of haemostasis is disturbed and requires correction. Furthermore, monitoring of therapeutic agents to promote anticoagulant activity or agents to restore normal haemostasis form part of routine investigations undertaken in the haematology laboratory. The separation of coagulation tests into investigation of the intrinsic and extrinsic activation pathways are convenient for *in vitro* testing. However *in vivo* there are numerous interactions between the pathways. Furthermore, different factors can act as both anticoagulant and procoagulant factors in different circumstances. *In vivo* clotting requires both calcium and phospholipid surfaces as an integral component for clot formation. *In vivo* coagulation factors circulate as inactive precursors which, under appropriate stimuli, are converted to active enzymes and cofactors, with generation of thrombin and subsequent convertion of fibrinogen to fibrin. With extrinsic pathway activity, tissue factor expressed on non-vascular cell membrane acts as a cofactor for activation of factor VII/VIIA with subsequent activation of factor X and eventual thrombin generation. Intrinsic pathway activation results upon contact to foreign surface of factor XII, high molecular weight kininogen and subsequent activation of the clotting cascade through factors XI, IX, X and prothrombin. *In vivo* small amounts of thrombin generation following activation of the extrinsic pathway result in an amplification of the haemostasis via activation of factor XI through the intrinsic pathway (see Fig. 35.1).

Prothrombin Time

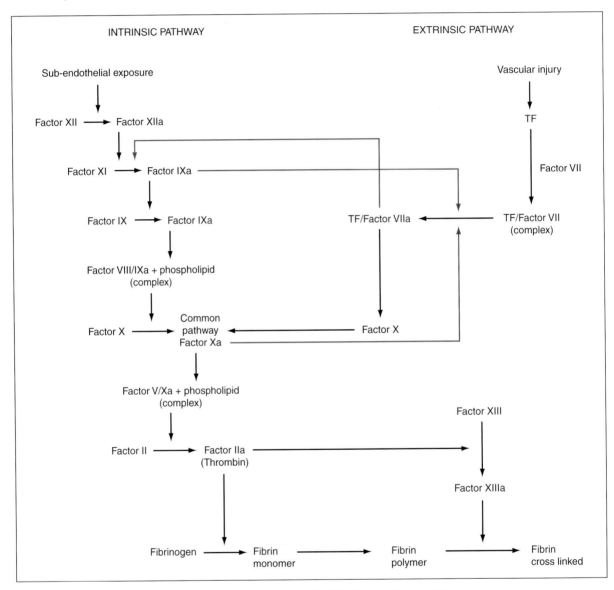

Figure 35.1: The coagulation cascade pathway Æ = feedback (accelerator) loops.

Prothrombin Time

The prothrombin time is used as a measure of extrinsic pathway activity, in which thrombo-plastin (tissue factor) and calcium are added to plasma and the time taken to clot formation is measured (see Fig. 35.2).

A prolonged prothrombin time may be due to: (a) oral anticoagulants; (b) deficiency of factor I, II, V, VII, or X, which may be inherited or acquired, for example in liver disease or disseminated intravascular coagulation; (c) high levels of heparin; (d) inhibitors to specific coagulation factors, including the lupus inhibitor. Further investigation of a prolonged prothrombin time may involve correction studies or assays of clotting factors.

A prolonged prothrombin time may correct in the presence of normal plasma. The pattern of correction may identify the factor or factors

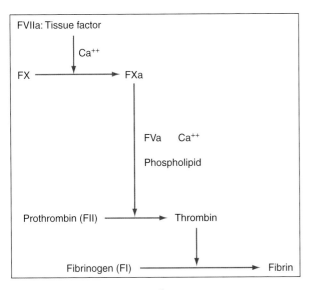

Figure 35.2: Extrinsic pathway.

which are deficient. Several reagents may be used in correction studies.

Normal citrate plasma This provides all the coagulation factors.

Aged serum Clotted blood is incubated for 24 hours at 37°C. The serum contains factor VII, IX, X, XI and XII.

Adsorbed plasma Normal plasma is treated with aluminium hydroxide which adsorbs

certain factors. The resultant plasma contains factors, I, V, VIII, XI and XII.

Oxalated plasma Normal plasma is added to sodium oxalate and incubated for 72 hours at 37°C. Contains all factors except V.

The results of correction studies are shown in Table 35.1.

Oral anticoagulant control

The international normalized ratio (INR) is the recommended method for reporting prothrombin time results for anticoagulant control. The INR system has been developed to compensate for the major source of discrepancy in prothrombin time assays, namely, variability in response of different thromboplastin reagents to changes in the vitamin K-dependent clotting factors induced by warfarin. With increasing numbers of patients requiring oral anticoagulant therapy, approximately 4 per 1000, this represents a major laboratory activity. The principle of oral anticoagulation is to provide a level of anticoagulation to prevent thrombotic problems but to avoid bleeding problems from over-anticoagulation. For most venous thrombotic problems an INR range of 2–3 is satisfactory. For patients with mechanical heart valves a high level of anticoagulation, INR range 3–4, is needed to prevent valve clot formation. See Table 35.2.

Table 35.1: Correction studies of a prolonged prothrombin time.

Normal plasma	Aged serum	Adsorbed plasma	Oxalated plasma	Factor deficiency	Further tests
+	—	+	+	I	Fibrinogen assay
+	—	—	+	II	Factor assay
+	—	+	—	V	Factor assay
+	+	—	+	VII	Factor assay
+	+	—	+	X	RVV time
—	—	—	—	Inhibitor	Reptilase time
					Protamine neutralization

+ = corrected
— = not corrected
RVV = Russell's Viper Venom Test

Prothrombin Time

Prothrombin errors

Table 35.2:   Oral anticoagulants for various clinical conditions.

Condition	INR Range	Recommended duration
Venous thromboembolism		
• Postoperative calf vein thrombosis without any risk factors	2–3	6 weeks
• Calf vein thrombosis in non-surgical patients without any risk factors	2–3	3 months
• Calf vein thrombosis in non-surgical patients with risk factors	2–3	indefinite (while risk factors persist)
• Pulmonary embolus and proximal vein thrombosis	2–3	6 months
• Recurrent DVT and/or PE	2–3	indefinite
• Recurrent DVT and/or PE while on warfarin (INR range 2–3)	3–4	indefinite
Atrial fibrillation		
• Atrial fibrillation or other high risk arrhythmias	2–3	indefinite
Heart valve prostheses & other cardiac indications		
• Mechanical prosthetic valves	3–4	indefinite
• Bioprosthetic heart valves (not aortic)	2–3	3 months*
• Cardiomyopathy, mural thrombus or akinetic segment	2–3	indefinite

Aspirin is first-line therapy for the following conditions; if aspirin is contraindicated, the following INR ranges for warfarin therapy are recommended:

Condition	INR Range	Recommended duration
• TIA / Ischaemic stroke	3–4	indefinite
• Peripheral arterial thrombosis and grafts	3–4	indefinite
• Coronary artery thrombosis	3–4	indefinite
• Coronary artery graft thrombosis	3–4	indefinite
• Coronary angioplasty and coronary stents	3–4	indefinite

*discontinue warfarin if there is no AF, intracardiac thrombus or history of systemic embolism. Patients not requiring warfarin should be considered for anti-platelet therapy (e.g. aspirin)

The INR is expressed as:

$$INR = \frac{PT \cdot ISI}{GMNPT} \qquad INR = \frac{PT \cdot ISI}{GMNPT}$$

where the ISI in the International Sensitivity index of the thromboplastin reagent and the GMNPT is the geometric mean normal prothrombin time.

Important sources of error remain in INR measurement and may result from problems in measurement of the prothrombin time, ISI or GMNPT.

Prothrombin errors

Errors with estimation of the prothrombin time can arise from problems with sample collection, the concentration of anticoagulant and the type of collection tube used. Furthermore, differences between manual and automated methods are recognized, with the latter producing shorter prothrombin times. While manufacturers are required to produce an ISI value for each batch of thromboplastin reagent, incorrect calibration of thromboplastin reagents by local laboratory or manufacturers is a problem. For calibration of a thromboplastin a pool of plasma samples from 20 normal adults and 60 patients on warfarin is recommended. In addition, different international reference preparations from different species may result in ISI differences. The geometric mean normal prothrombin time should be derived from a pool of 20 normal adults' plasma samples and the geometric mean calculated from this.

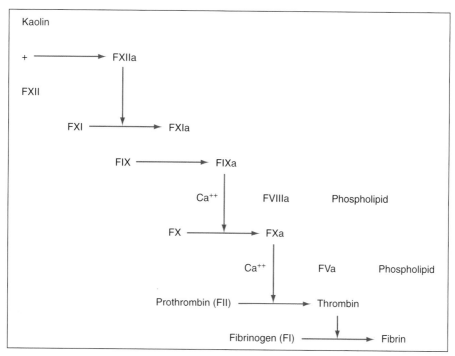

Figure 35.3: Intrinsic pathway.

Activated Partial Thromboplastin Time (APTT)

This test measures the intrinsic pathway of coagulation. An activator, such as kaolin, triggers the pathway by activating the contact factors (see Fig. 35.3). In the presence of calcium ions and phospholipid, this culminates in the generation of thrombin and ultimately fibrin clot formation. The APTT is also used in the monitoring of heparin therapy. A prolonged APTT in a patient with history of a bleeding diathesis would require further investigation, particularly to exclude haemophilia A or B.

A prolonged APTT may be caused by deficiency of factors I, II, V, VIII, IX, X, XI or XII which can be inherited or acquired due to liver disease or consumption as in disseminated intravascular coagulation. Heparin therapy, inhibitors to specific coagulation factors, the presence of lupus anticoagulant or high levels of FDPs (fibrinogen degradation products) may also produce a prolonged APTT. Correction studies may also be used to investigate further the cause of a prolonged APTT. If mixing studies show correction of the APTT then specific factor assays are performed to determine the deficient factor. The failure to correct would require further investigation to exclude a further specific inhibitor or lupus anticoagulant (see Fig. 35.4).

The most frequent use of the APTT is to monitor heparin treatment and to adjust the infusion schedule as illustrated in Table 35.3.

Thrombin Time

The thrombin time is used as a rapid screen for abnormalities of fibrinogen and to assess whether heparin is the cause of a prolonged APTT. Thrombin is added to citrated plasma and the time taken for fibrin formation is

Thrombin Time

Reptilase time

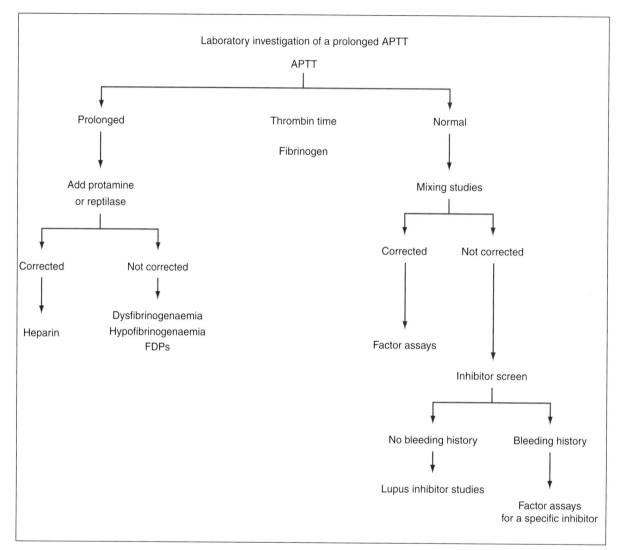

Figure 35.4: Laboratory investigation of a prolonged APTT.

measured (see Fig. 35.5). A prolonged thrombin time may be due to: (1) dysfibrinogens can be inherited or acquired, with a structurally abnormal fibrinogen molecule with altered functional properties; (2) low fibrinogen level lg/l; (3) raised FDP levels; (4) heparin therapy. The presence of heparin in a sample is confirmed by correction of the thrombin time with protamine sulphate which neutralizes the anticoagulant activity.

Reptilase time

Reptilase is an enzyme from the venom of *Bothrops atrox*, which clots human fibrino-

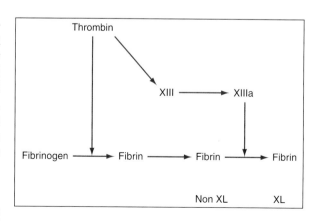

Figure 35.5: Thrombin time.

Table 35.3: This shows a heparin infusion regime, with laboratory monitoring of treatment using the APTT. The therapeutic range should be determined from the APTT range equivalent to a plasma heparin concentration of 0.2 iu/ml to 0.4 iu/ml.

Heparin infusion schedule

I.V. bolus	5000 units		
I.V. infusion	15000 units/12 hours		
Check APTT after **2–6** hours			
• acceptable range	1.5–2.5		
• in pregnancy	1.5–2.0		
Adjust heparin as follows:-			
>5.0	stop for 1 hour		
	decrease by 6000 units/12 hours	recheck APTT	in **2–6** hours
4.1–5.0	decrease by 3600 units/12 hours	recheck APTT	in **2–6** hours
3.1–4.0	decrease by 1200 units/12 hours	recheck APTT	in **2–6** hours
2.6–3.0	decrease by 600 units/12 hours	recheck APTT	in **2–12** hours
1.5–2.5	no change	recheck APTT	within **24** hours
1.2–1.4	increase by 2400 units/12 hours	recheck APTT	in **2–12** hours
<1.2	increase by 4800 units/12 hours	recheck APTT	in **2–6** hours

Check APTT 2–6 hours after starting heparin
Do not re-prescribe heparin for more than 24 hours
Checking APTT on a daily basis is the mandatory minimum for all patients receiving intravenous heparin
Monitor platelets after four days heparin treatment

gen by cleaving fibrinopeptide A from fibrinogen. Reptilase is not inhibited by heparin or antithrombin III. A prolonged thrombin time and normal reptilase time is also in keeping with the presence of heparin in the sample. The reptilase time is prolonged in dysfibrinogenaemia and hypofibrinogenaemia.

Fibrinogen

While inherited disorders of fibrinogen are rare, acquired disorders are common in patients with consumptive coagulopathies, liver disease and following major surgery including cardiopulmonary bypass. Furthermore the association of high fibrinogen levels and increased risk for ischaemic heart and peripheral vascular disease is well recognized. Fibrinogen is also an acute phase reactant with increased levels commonly seen in inflammatory diseases. The interpretation of results is therefore difficult, and the most appropriate method is dependent on the reason for the investigation. Confirmation of low

fibrinogen levels with a manual Clauss method is advisable. There are numerous methods used to measure fibrinogen, with clotting methods used most commonly to measure functional fibrinogen, based on fibrin formation. In the thrombin time method (Clauss) the thrombin time is proportional to the concentration of fibrinogen in the test sample. A calibration curve is prepared from known fibrinogen concentrations and used to convert the thrombin time to a fibrinogen concentration. There is little interference from FDPs or heparin, unless they are present in high concentration.

A fibrinogen titre may be obtained using a series of dilutions of plasma followed by the addition of thrombin. The dilution at which the fibrinogen is diluted out is a measure of the concentration of fibrinogen present. The test is usually run in parallel with protamine sulphate and EACA as indicators of FDPs and fibrinolysis respectively. Physicochemical methods used less commonly measure the total fibrinogen and may not reflect the functional activity, while immunological methods measure factor-related antigen present both in fibrinogen and FDPs. The increased use of automated coagulometers has led to the automation of fibrinogen assays as a derived parameter from the prothrombin time, based on a turbidometric analysis using a spectrophotometer.

Fibrinogen Degradation Products

FDPs increase following plasmin degradation of fibrinogen and non cross-linked fibrin and result in a prolonged thrombin time or reptilase clotting time. The most commonly performed FDP assay, however, uses a latex agglutination technique in which an antibody that recognizes FDPs is coated on the surface of latex particles. The particles agglutinate in the presence of FDPs and the concentration is determined by their dilution that sustains agglutination. As antibodies used in the assay may cross-react with fibrinogen, the latter must be removed from the patient's sample. This is accomplished by clotting the sample with thrombin or a snake venom in the presence of a plasmin inhibitor to prevent *in vitro* generation of split products. These reagents are incorporated in special collection tubes.

The D-Dimer assay is similar to the FDP assay except that the antibody is specific for cross-link fragments derived from fibrin and there is no cross-activity with fibrinogen. This can therefore be performed on a plasma sample. A common method involves a card covered by a membrane carrying D-Dimer-specific monoclonal antibodies. A conjugated solution carrying D-Dimer-specific monoclonal antibodies is conjugated with gold particles which bind the D-Dimer in a sandwich-type reaction. In the presence of increased levels of D-Dimer in the sample the membrane produces a colour intensity proportional to the D-Dimer concentration. Raised levels of FDPs and D-Dimers are seen in disseminated intravascular coagulation, deep vein thrombosis, pulmonary embolism, pregnancy and postoperatively. As the D-Dimer assay is more specific and distinguishes between fibrinogenolysis and fibrinoly-

sis, this is particularly helpful in monitoring disease progress in disseminated intravascular coagulation following *in vivo* plasmin activation. The assay may also be used to assess whether a fibrinolytic response to a therapeutic fibrinolytic agent, such as streptokinase or urokinase, has been achieved.

Factor Assays

Specific coagulation factor assays are based on either the prothrombin time or APTT. A range of dilutions of a plasma standard are added to a specific factor-deficient plasma. The clotting times obtained show a linear relationship to the factor concentration when plotted on log paper. The activity of the factor in the test plasma can then be determined from the graph. These assays are particularly important in identification of patients with inherited bleeding disorders and also in the monitoring of factor concentrate replacement therapy. Factors II, V, VII and X are commonly assayed using a one-stage prothrombin time, while factors VIII, IX, XI and XII are based on an APTT method. Factor XIII deficiency is not detected by any of the routine coagulation tests as it does not participate in the reaction leading up to the formation of fibrin. A urea solubility test is a commonly used method to screen for factor XIII deficiency. A fibrin clot is formed and either acetone or urea added to the plasma sample incubated at 37°C. Fibrin cross-linked by the action of factor XIII is insoluble in these solutions, but in the absence of factor XIII activity a fibrin clot will dissolve within an hour.

Natural anticoagulants
In vivo there is continuous low-grade activation of coagulation and there are natural inhibitors of activated coagulation factors. A deficiency of such factors may be associated with a prothrombotic tendency.

Antithrombin III
Antithrombin III is a major regulator of thrombin *in vitro*. Functional assays are preferred as a variety of molecular forms are recognized

which produce normal quantitation as measured by immunological techniques. Most functional assays measure neutralization of thrombin or factor Xa in the presence of added heparin.

Protein C and Protein S

Protein C is activated following thrombin generation. Thrombin binds to thrombomodulin on the surface of endothelial cells and binds and activates protein C. Thrombin in this situation loses its procoagulant activity and is no longer able to convert fibrinogen to fibrin. Activated protein C acts as a natural anticoagulant by activating factors Va and VIIIa, limiting further thrombin generation. Protein S serves as a cofactor for activated protein C. A further recent important finding is that activated protein C resistance may occur due to a defect of the factor V molecule, the factor V Leiden mutation. This is associated with an increased risk of venous thrombosis and is the most prevalent inherited prothrombotic risk factor known. PCR screening is recommended for patients with a prothrombotic history, to exclude this defect.

Fibrinolysis

Fibrinolysis results in the breakdown of the fibrin clot and is initiated by the release from vascular endothelium of tissue type plasminogen activator (tPA) and urokinase type plasminogen activator (uPA). These activators convert plasminogen into the active enzyme plasmin, which degrades fibrin. There is also a natural inhibitor to plasmin, αII anti- plasmin and plasminogen activator inhibitor type 1 (PAI–1) released by endothelium, which binds to and inactivates free tPA and uPA.

Markers of Activated Coagulation

Over the last few years there has been increasing interest in hypercoagulability and tests available for its detection. Assays for markers of coagulation activation have several potential uses, including characterizing patients with clinical conditions predisposing to thrombosis, aiding the diagnosis of acute thrombotic events and monitoring anticoagulant therapy. This may be achieved by measuring the enzymatic forms of coagulation zymogens generated during coagulation activation, or indirectly by measuring activation peptides generated when zymogens are activated. In addition, by measuring complexes that result from enzyme inactivation by naturally occurring plasma inhibitors, a further approach is available. A number of immunoassays are available to measure fragments generated from the activation of clotting factors such as factor IX and X activation peptides. Prothrombin fragment 1 + 2 which results from thrombin-mediated activation of prothrombin, and fibrinopeptide A cleaved from the alpha chain of fibrinogen by thrombin, are indices of thrombin generation and activity respectively. Immunoassays for quantifying protein C activation peptide or activated protein C can be regarded as indices of thrombin and thrombomodulin function. Immunoassays are also available for the measurement of enzyme inhibited complexes such as thrombin, antithrombin and other complexes which result from the inhibition of activated protein C by protein C inhibitor and antitrypsin. Currently the usefulness of markers of coagulation activation is better for assessing hypercoagulability than in the diagnosis of acute thrombotic events. For the latter purpose it is more effective to measure markers of fibrinolysis activation such as D-Dimer.

Automated Coagulation

Recent advances in technology have heralded the introduction of automated instruments for coagulation screening. An increase in workload, the demand for greater specificity and the reduction in manual labour have ensured that most laboratories now have semi- or full automation. Most manual methods can be modified for instrumentation, although results vary greatly between instruments. All routine coagulation screening tests, including factor assays, can be analysed on automated instruments. More advanced instruments allow chromogenic assays for specialized coagulation tests. The early instruments involved detection of the fibrin clot through electrodes. An electrode moves in and out of the reagent/plasma. Calcium is added and as soon as the first fibrin clot is formed, the electrical circuit is completed and the timer stopped. The majority of modern-day instruments involve photo-optical endpoint detection. As the clotting process takes place, the light scattered from a fixed beam increases. The clotting time is obtained from the coagulation curve as the time required for the sample to reach the preset percentage of the scattered light intensity. Full instrumentation includes robotic sampling, barcode reading of samples, automatic reagent dispenser and a data management system. However, as clotting times vary between different instruments, depending on the method of endpoint detection, results from automation are not strictly comparable. Therefore, manual techniques are still used as reference methods.

Further Reading

British Society for Haematology. Guidelines on oral anticoagulation: second edition. *Journal of Clinical Pathology* 1990; **43**: 177–183.

British Society for Haematology. Guidelines on the use and monitoring of heparin: second edition. *Journal of Clinical Pathology* 1993; **46**: 97–103.

Ludlam C, Bennett K A, Fox A, Lowe G, Reid A. Guidelines for the use of fibrinolytic therapy. *Blood Coagulation and Fibrinolysis* 1996; **6**: 273–285.

Poller L, Hirsh J. *Oral anticoagulants*. 1996: Arnold, Hodder Headline, London.

SECTION 5
CYTOGENETICS

36 CHROMOSOME BANDING AND ANALYSIS

Mervyn Humphreys

Chromosome Banding

Since the first banded chromosome preparations were described in the early 1970s, there has been a rapid proliferation of chromosome staining techniques which has enabled the very precise characterization of the normal human karyotype. The Giemsa banding (G-banding) method developed in the mid 1970s is the most widely used technique for routine chromosome analysis. The numerous other banding methods are generally only utilized to aid the identification of specific chromosome abnormalities whose exact nature is uncertain with G-banding. Clinical cytogenetics is now established as a vital medical speciality enabling the clinical diagnosis of many genetic conditions.

Although the biochemical basis of chromosome banding is poorly understood, the various patterns obtained appear to reflect the highly organized fashion by which the enormous stretch of human DNA is packaged into the chromosomes.

This chapter will describe and explain the underlying principles of the main chromosome banding techniques which are available, and highlight their main applications in the laboratory.

Giemsa Banding

G-banding is produced by digesting chromosomes with the proteolytic enzyme trypsin, followed by Giemsa staining. The chromosomes exhibit a consistent pattern of dark and light bands along their length [Fig. 36.1(a)]. It is essential that slides are aged either at room temperature for three to four days or at 60°C overnight before banding. Trypsin digestion of freshly made chromosome spreads is too severe and yields very poor banding quality. The ageing of chromosome preparations strengthens the integrity of chromosomes, making them less vulnerable to over-digestion by trypsin.

Giemsa Banding

Quinacrine Banding (Q-Banding)

Mechanism

Although the G-banding method presumably involves the selective removal of proteins from different chromosome regions, the mechanism by which the pattern of G-bands is revealed is still not completely understood and many explanations have been proposed. Chromosomes are believed to contain a basic structure which is enhanced by the G-banding procedure. Each length of about 146 base pairs of human DNA is wound around a core consisting of eight histone protein molecules to produce repeating units called nucleosomes or chromomeres. Successive nucleosomes are arrayed like beads on a string. The elementary fibre of linked nucleosomes is coiled further to form the chromatin fibre. Chromatin fibres are further looped and coiled into the final chromosome packages. It is believed that the dark G-bands may simply correlate with the bead-like chromomeres and the G-banding pattern therefore reflects the structural organization of chromatin along the chromosome length.

It has been suggested alternatively that the dark and light G-bands correlate with the differing functional content of the DNA in these chromosome regions. Replication studies have shown that regions of DNA with similar replication times are clustered together with the DNA in dark G-bands, replicating late in S phase compared to light G-band DNA. *In situ* hybridization studies have shown a correlation between the G-banding pattern and the location of repetitive DNA sequences. Dark G-bands have been shown to be rich in L1 type repetitive DNA sequences which are relatively AT-rich and encode very few expressed genes. Light G-bands have similarly been shown to be rich in Alu type repetitive DNA sequences which are relatively GC-rich and encode many expressed genes.

Applications

G-banding is by far the most widely used chromosome banding method for routine cytogenetic analysis in clinical investigations. This method enables the majority of numerical and structural chromosomal abnormalities to be detected and identified. Laboratories that do not routinely use G-banding generally use R-banding. Other chromosome banding methods are generally only used when an initial G-banding analysis detects a chromosome defect which requires further investigation for accurate characterization. The G-banding pattern is generally similar to the Q-banding pattern.

Quinacrine Banding (Q-Banding)

Q-banding was the first chromosome banding pattern to be reported, in 1970. Q-banding is produced by treating chromosomes with quinacrine dihydrochloride. A series of bright and dull fluorescing regions is revealed along the chromosomes when viewed with fluorescence microscopy (450–500 nm) (Fig. 36.1 (b)) The Q-banding pattern strongly resembles the G-banding pattern with brightly fluorescing Q-bands corresponding to dark staining G-bands. Notable exceptions include the distal long arm of the Y chromosome which shows extremely bright fluorescence. Also, the heterochromatic regions of chromosomes 1, 9 and 16, as well as the satellite regions of the acrocentric chromosomes, show characteristic Q-banding patterns.

Mechanism

Because Q-banding and G-banding patterns show such similarities, the mechanisms are influenced by the same parameters of chromosome composition (see G-banding). DNA rich in AT sequences has been shown to enhance the fluorescence of quinacrine whereas GC-rich DNA tends to quench quinacrine fluorescence. Therefore Q-bands, which are rich in AT base pairs, fluoresce brightly, providing further evidence that the varying DNA content of chromosome bands explains differences in staining intensity.

Applications

Q-banding is a non-permanent staining method and is therefore not suitable for routine cytogenetic investigations. It is very useful, however, for the specific examination of the heteromorphisms associated with the Y chromosome and the satellite regions of the acrocentric chromosomes and for the characterization of structural abnormalities involving Y chromosome mater-

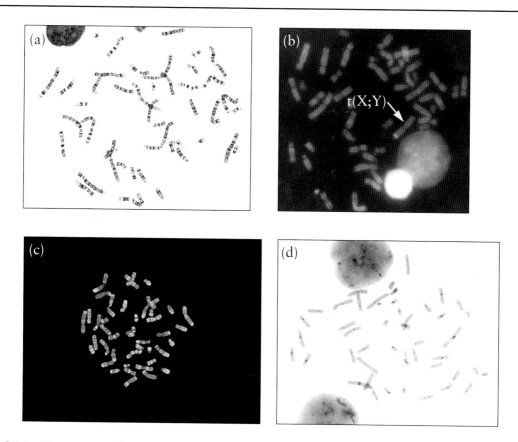

Figure 36.1: *Human metaphase spreads stained by: (a) G-banding, (b) Q-banding (arrow indicates the X, Y translocation in this patient), (c) R-banding, (d) C-banding. [a], (c) and (d) courtesy of Applied Imaging International Ltd.]*

ial. Q-banding patterns of *p* arm and satellite heteromorphisms can sometimes be used to determine the parental origin and stage of meiotic non-disjunction in trisomies of the acrocentric chromosomes.

Reverse Banding (R-Banding)

Reverse banding of chromosomes (R-banding), using phosphate buffer (pH 6.5) at high temperature followed by Giemsa or acridine orange staining, yields a banding pattern which is the reverse of G- or Q-banding. Chromosome regions which are G-dark or Q-bright are stained lightly (weakly fluorescing) when R-banded [Fig. 36.1(c)]. R-banding is most successful when slides have been aged at room temperature for several days or at 60°C overnight. Freshly made slides require shorter incubation times in buffer.

Mechanism

As for G- and Q-banding, the R-banding pattern appears to reflect the structural and functional makeup of chromosomes. The chemical basis of the pattern of bands is still not understood fully. Chromosomal proteins and AT-rich DNA sequences of the G-bands are denatured preferentially by the heat treatment, leaving behind the GC-rich DNA of the R-bands. The fact that aged slides require shorter incubation times and yield better R-banding again suggests that as slides are aged their general structure becomes more stable and less vulnerable to degradation by various agents (see G-banding).

Constitutive Heterochromatin Banding (C-Banding)

Nucleolar Organizer Region Staining (NOR-staining)

DA–DAPI Banding

Applications

Although most cytogenetic laboratories use G-banding for routine investigations, the remainder use R-banding. This banding pattern reveals no new information on chromosome preparations which have already been analysed by G-banding.

Constitutive Heterochromatin Banding (C-Banding)

The C-banding procedure involves treating chromosomes with acid (HCl), alkali ($Ba(OH)_2$) and hot salt solution (2XSSC). C-banded chromosome preparations show dark staining of the regions of constitutive heterochromatin, which are located at the centromeres of all the chromosomes except the Y chromosome where it is located on the distal long arm [Fig. 36.1(d)].

Mechanism

The harsh C-banding treatments are thought to facilitate preferential loss of DNA and protein from the non-C-band chromosome regions. Successive depurination and denaturation of the chromosomal DNA occurs during the acid and alkali treatments. Further small DNA fragments are lost during the salt treatment, leaving only the tightly compacted centromeric heterochromatin. Non-histone proteins bound to the C-band regions may prevent the same DNA denaturation occurring at these loci.

Applications

The C bands of all chromosomes, especially chromosomes 1, 9, 16 and Y, vary in size between homologues within an individual as well as between individuals. Where it is unclear whether an extra band, or an abnormal chromosome segment, represents a normal variation of a heterochromatic region or a euchromatic chromosomal abnormality of possible clinical significance, C-banded analysis enables conclusive interpretation. C-banding is also invaluable for the accurate identification of structural abnormalities involving breakpoints at or near centromeres.

Nucleolar Organizer Region Staining (NOR-Staining)

The ribosomal RNA genes that form and maintain the nucleolus in interphase nuclei are located on the short arms of the acrocentric chromosomes (13–15 and 21–22). When chromosome preparations are treated overnight with silver nitrate solution these nucleolar organizer regions (NORs) stain darkly [Fig. 36.2(a)].

Mechanism

NOR staining involves the extraction of DNA, RNA and histones. It is actually the residual non-histone proteins adjacent to the NORs rather than the NORs themselves which are stained selectively by this method. Studies have shown that this method only stains the active NORs which participated in the formation of the nucleolus in the preceding interphase of the cell cycle.

Applications

The number of NORs detected per metaphase spread varies between individuals because only active NORs which participated in the formation of the nucleolus during the preceding interphase stage are stained. The NOR pattern of acrocentric chromosomes is consistent within an individual and is heritable. The NOR patterns and Q-banding appearance of acrocentric satellites are therefore useful for determining parental origin and/or the stage of meiotic non-disjunction involved in trisomies involving these chromosomes.

DA–DAPI Banding

When chromosomes are stained with the fluorescent dye 4,6-diamino-2-phenyl-indole (DAPI) and treated with the non-fluorescent counterstain diastamycin (DA), the heterochromatic regions of chromosomes 1, 9, 16, the distal long arm of the Y chromosome and the proximal short arm of chromosome 15 are brightly fluorescing (Fig. 36.2(b)).

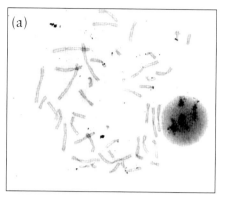
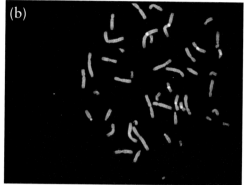
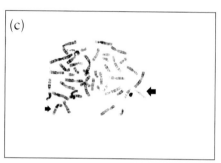
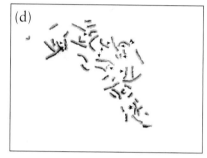

Figure 36.2: *Human metaphase spreads stained by:* (a) *NOR staining showing the active NORs (arrows) and a derivative chromosome 14, with chromosome 7 material translocated to the end short arm (large arrow), in this patient, (b) DAPI banding, (c) Replication banding using late pulse BrdU showing the early replicating, normal X chromosome (small arrow) and the late replicating, structurally abnormal X chromosome (large arrow) in this patient, (d) SCE (SCEs arrowed).* [*Figure (b) courtesy of Applied Imaging International Ltd.*]

Mechanism

DAPI binds to DNA and has an affinity for AT base pairs. DAPI binding alone yields a weak Q-banding pattern. Although DAPI fluorescence is enhanced both by AT and GC base pairs, there is a significant enhancement of fluorescence in regions of AT-rich DNA. DA also shows AT-specific DNA binding affinity. Although the two dyes used have similar base-pairing preference they have non-identical binding affinities and dissimilar structures. The differential fluorescence obtained may be due to competitive binding between the two dyes which bind at similar but not identical sites. Alternatively DA may block DAPI binding in euchromatic regions, whereas DAPI binding sites remain available in heterochromatic regions.

Applications

DA–DAPI banding is used predominantly for the interpretation of certain chromosome abnormalities detected using more routine banding methods (G- or R-banding). For example, DA–DAPI banding may be of use where a structurally rearranged chromosome has a breakpoint close to a region selectively stained with DA–DAPI banding. DA–DAPI banding is particularly useful for studying small satellited marker chromosomes. This technique can identify those marker chromosomes involving the proximal end of chromosome 15. DAPI staining is also commonly used as the counterstain for fluorescence *in situ* hybridization of chromosome preparations.

Replication Banding

A G- or R-banding pattern can be produced on chromosome preparations if they are grown in the presence of the thymidine analogue 5-bromodeoxyuridine (BrdU) and stained with the

373

Replication Banding

fluorescent dye Hoechst 33258. This method utilizes the fact that different regions of the chromosome complement replicate at different stages during S phase. The type of banding pattern obtained depends when the pulse of BrdU is administered relative to the harvest time. If BrdU is added at culture initiation, but removed about six hours before harvest at 48 hours, a G-banding pattern is obtained. If BrdU is added only about six hours before cultures are harvested, R-banding results [Fig. 36.2(c)].

If cells undergo two complete cycles of replication in the presence of BrdU the sister chromatids of each chromosome are stained differentially. The harlequinization pattern obtained enables the detection of sister chromatid exchanges which are points along the length of chromosomes where the chromatid material is swapped between sister chromatids (Fig. 36.2(d)). Preparations are either viewed by fluorescence microscopy (360–400 nm) or, if they are exposed to UV light and stained with Giemsa stain, permanent preparations are obtained (fluorescence plus Giemsa (FPG) technique).

Mechanism

BrdU is a thymidine analogue which is readily incorporated into chromosomes. When chromosomes are stained with the fluorochrome Hoechst 33258 (which binds to AT-rich base pairs) chromosome regions which replicate in the presence of BrdU contain BrdU-substituted DNA and are weakly fluorescing (lighter with Giemsa). When BrdU is present at culture initiation it is present for the early part of one cycle and therefore chromosome regions which replicate early in S phase (R-bands) become BrdU-substituted and are therefore weakly fluorescing or light-staining with Giemsa. The G-bands replicate late in S phase, after the BrdU has been removed from the cultures, and therefore incorporate thymidine and are brightly fluorescing, or dark-staining with Giemsa (G-banding).

Alternatively if BrdU is only added to cultures about six hours before harvesting it is only present for the late part of one replication cycle and early replicating regions (R-bands) have already been replicated, incorporating thymidine, and fluoresce brightly or stain darkly with Giemsa. Only the late replicating regions (G-bands) become BrdU-substituted and therefore fluoresce weakly or stain lightly with Giemsa (R-banding). The harlequinized staining pattern obtained when BrdU is present in cell cultures for two cycles of replication reflects the asymmetric incorporation of BrdU into chromosomal DNA. By semi-conservative replication each new strand of DNA consists of one original DNA strand and one newly constructed strand. After two cycles of replication in the presence of BrdU one chromatid contains DNA with BrdU substituted into one nucleotide strand while its sister chromatid contains two BrdU substituted DNA strands. This chemical difference between the sister chromatids explains the difference in staining intensity obtained. The staining intensity is proportional to the amount of DNA present in each chromatid. When chromosome preparations are stained more DNA is lost from the bifiliarly BrdU-substituted chromatid than its counterpart, thereby producing the characteristic harlequinized staining pattern.

Applications

Apart from providing alternative methods for G- and R-banding, the staining patterns obtained after a pulse of BrdU is administered early or late in the cell cycle is useful for replication studies. Although homologous chromosomes show similar replication patterns, in normal females one X chromosome is inactivated in each cell by a random process (Lyonization). The inactivated X is always the last chromosome to complete its replication in each cell cycle and therefore the early and late replicating X chromosomes can be distinguished using replication banding. The late replicating X chromosome is darker staining with early pulse BrdU replication banding and lighter staining with late pulse BrdU replication banding. In females carrying structural abnormalities involving the X chromosome the pattern of X-inactivation can generally be shown to be a non-random event by replication banding [Fig. 36.2(c)].

The production of harlequinized chromosome staining patterns enables the detection of sister chromatid exchanges (SCEs). These are points along the length of chromosomes where there is exchange of material between the two sister chromatids of individual chromosomes producing a checker-board appearance [Fig. 36.2(d)]. Normal human cells show a mean frequency of five to eight SCEs per cell but SCE levels have been demonstrated to increase with exposure to most mutagens. The main application of this technique is therefore as a method for monitoring mutagen-induced chromosome damage. In many cases SCE has proved more sensitive for the detection of chromosome damage compared to measurement of chromosomal aberrations. However not all test mutagens show a positive correlation between induced chromosomal aberrations and induced SCEs, thereby indicating that these two parameters reflect different and independent expressions of mutagen-induced damage.

This method is also used as a diagnostic test for the chromosome instability syndrome, Bloom's syndrome, in which cells show a significant increase from the normal baseline level of spontaneous SCE. SCE can also be used to demonstrate the increased level of chromosome damage induced by specific types of mutagens in other chromosome instability syndromes, e.g. by cross-linking agents in Fanconi's anaemia or by X-irradiation in ataxia telangiectasia. SCE can also be used to study cell kinetics by indicating the duration of the various stages of the cell cycle.

Chromosome Analysis

The majority of routine cytogenetic analyses are carried out by the examination of banded metaphase preparations (G- or R-banded). Cytogenetic analysis is a highly skilled laboratory discipline and several years' training are required before a cytogeneticist becomes competent in recognizing the normal karyotype and detecting karyotypic abnormalities.

Classification of banded chromosomes and nomenclature
Chromosomes are identified, karyotyped and described using the guidelines proposed in the International System of Chromosome Nomenclature (ISCN). This is the report pub-

lished by the Standing Committee on Human Cytogenetic Nomenclature. The basic terminology for describing human karyotypes was put forward by this group in 1971 (Paris nomenclature). The main features used to distinguish chromosomes are length, centromere position, presence of secondary constrictions (satellites) and banding pattern. The autosomes are numbered in pairs by decreasing size from 1 to 22, leaving the sex chromosomes (X and Y). Based on length, centromere position and satellites alone the chromosomes of the human karyotype can be sorted into seven groups, A–G (X chromosome included in C group and Y chromosome included in G group). Based on centromere position there are three types of chromosome: metacentric (centromere in the middle), acrocentric (centromere at one end) and sub-metacentric (centromere off-centre). Individual chromosome pairs can, however, only be identified accurately and sorted into the karyotype from banding patterns (Fig. 36.3). ISCN provides a standardized numbering system for describing the bands visualized in chromosome preparations. These are illustrated in diagrammatic chromosome maps (ideograms) which show, and label, the exact layout of bands associated with each normal chromosome pair. This permits an accurate description of breakpoints in chromosome rearrangements. Each chromosome is divided into a number of chromosome regions using the telomeres,

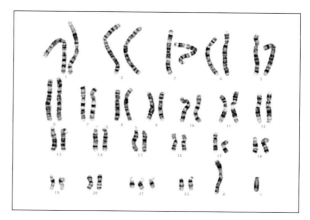

Figure 36.3: G-banded karyotype from a male patient with Down's syndrome showing trisomy 21. [Courtesy of Applied Imaging International Ltd.]

Chromosome Analysis

Chromosome variation

Chromosome analysis

Chromosome analysis for acquired chromosome abnormalities

---

centromeres and most prominent bands as landmarks. The centromere divides each chromosome into a short (p) arm and a long (q) arm. Most arms are divided into two or more regions of prominent bands and each region may be subdivided further depending on the number of visible bands. Therefore band 1p34.2 is to be found on the short arm of chromosome 1 in region 3, band 4, sub-band 2. As improving techniques have enabled increased resolution of chromosome preparations (more elongated) the ISCN has been updated accordingly with new ideograms. The most recent update was in 1995. When using ISCN to describe karyotypic abnormalities the cytogeneticist must utilize the most appropriate ideogram showing equivalent banding resolution.

Chromosome variation

In order to recognize any chromosome abnormality present in any human chromosome preparation the cytogeneticist must be very familiar with the appearance of the normal human karyotype. This is complicated by the occurrence of considerable variation in certain heterochromatic regions including centromeric and satellite polymorphisms. It is important that these regions of normal chromosome variation are recognized and distinguished from other clinically significant chromosome abnormalities. This often requires the use of specific banding techniques such as C-banding.

Chromosome analysis

The majority of routine chromosome analysis is performed by microscopically examining G- or R-banded metaphase preparations. Suitable metaphases are first located by screening prepared slides using low-power microscopy ($\times 100$ magnification). Suitable metaphases are then examined using higher magnification (usually $\times 1000$). For constitutional karyotype analysis only five to six metaphases of suitable quality need be examined, except where a possible chromosome mosaicism may be expected (mixture of normal and abnormal cells), when more cells should be analysed. The quality of metaphases analysed depends largely on the reason for carrying out the cytogenetic investi-

gation. If checking for an obvious numerical abnormality (e.g. trisomy 21) then high quality metaphases are not required. However, if a subtle abnormality may be present (small deletion or rearrangement involving small segments) then more elongated chromosome spreads must be examined.

If the cytogeneticist is satisfied that all chromosome pairs show the recognized normal banding pattern, a normal karyotype can be reported. Karyotypes are described using ISCN nomenclature. In general this has the order: total number of chromosomes; sex chromosome constitution; description of abnormality. Thus the normal female karyotype is described as 46, XX and the normal male karyotype as 46, XY. Where a chromosome abnormality is recognized then the appropriate karyotype nomenclature is assigned. Each type of structural abnormality has an associated ISCN abbreviation (e.g. 't' for translocation; 'i' for inversion, etc.). If the abnormality is indistinct or breakpoints are unclear by microscopic examination, the preparation of karyotypes may help characterize the exact nature of the abnormality. The final karyotype formula assigned should indicate the exact nature of any numerical and/or structural abnormalities identified from cytogenetic analysis.

Chromosome analysis for acquired chromosome abnormalities

The cytogenetic analysis of cancer (leukaemias and solid tumours) is routinely carried out to detect any associated acquired chromosome abnormalities. Detection of such abnormalities provides vital information in relation to disease diagnosis, patient prognosis and for monitoring the response to therapy. A cytogenetic analysis for acquired chromosome abnormalities bears a few important differences from the constitutional chromosome analysis procedure. Acquired chromosome abnormalities are clonal, being confined only to the malignant cells. In addition metaphases obtained from malignant cells typically show inferior morphology (short and poor bands) compared to non-malignant cells. It is important that the cytogeneticist analyses firstly a larger number of cells to enable detection of small clonal abnormalities, and secondly examines a repre- sentative selection of all metaphases to avoid the inadvertent selection of the better quality but non-malignant cells.

Further Reading

Benn P A, Perle M A. (1992) Chromosome staining and banding techniques. In Rooney DE, Czepulkowski (eds). *Human Cytogenetics: A Practical Approach: Vol I* 1992: Oxford University Press New York pp. 91–118.

Bickmore A, Summer A T. Mammalian chromosome banding – an expression of genome organization. *TIG* 1989; 5(5): 144–148.

Comings D E. Mechanisms of chromosome banding and implications for chromosome structure. *Ann Rev Genet* 1978; **12**: 25–46.

Goldman M A, Holmquist G P, Gray, M C, Caston L A, Nag A. Replication timing of genes and middle repetitive sequences. *Science*. 1984; **224**: 686–692.

Holmquist G, Gray M, Porter T, Jordan J. Characterization of Giemsa dark and light band DNA. *Cell* 1982; **31**: 121.

ISCN. *An International System for Human Cytogenetic Nomenclature*. Mitelman F (ed). 1995; S Karger, Basel.

Summer A T. The nature and mechanisms of chromosome banding. *Cancer Genet Cytogenet* 1982; **6**: 59–87.

Verma RS, Babu A (eds). *Human Chromosomes: Manual of Basic Techniques* 1989: Pergamon Press, New York.

37 FLUORESCENCE *IN SITU* HYBRIDIZATION

Ivor Hickey

Fluorescence *in situ* hybridization (FISH) is a powerful technique that plays a significant part in several current areas of genetical research. It refers to a series of related procedures in which single-stranded nucleic acid molecules (probes) tagged with chemicals which are either themselves fluorescent, or can be detected by immunofluorescence microscopy, are used to identify specific target sequences in cytological preparations.

The technique derives directly from the original nucleic acid hybridization experiments first pioneered by Speigleman in the 1960s, which were adapted by several groups using radio-labelled probes to identify nucleic acid sequences in fixed material on microscope slides. Early examples included the identification of ribosomal RNA genes in the nucleoli of *Xenopus* oocytes and centromeric satellite DNA in metaphase mouse chromosomes. Although protocols have developed greatly since then, the basic steps have remained largely unaltered. All variations of the technique include a nucleic acid probe, a cytological preparation and a detection system. The principal steps in the system will be described at this point before variations and applications of the technique are encountered.

Choice of Probe

In most cases a genomic clone of DNA can be used although, as will be seen later, other sources of DNA can also be utilized for chromosome painting. In some applications RNA molecules may be used, although this is rarely done today. The probe must be labelled prior to use in order to detect the hybridized material at the end of the procedure. It is important to realize that a limiting factor in probe detection is the length of a probe. Under the same labelling and detection systems a smaller probe will always give a weaker signal than a longer probe. Although probes as small as 500 base pairs can be detected in certain circumstances, cosmids, vectors

derived from bacteriophage λ which contain approximately 40 kb of cloned DNA, are the most popular sources of probe. DNA cloned in vectors carrying larger inserts, such as bacterial artificial chromosomes (BACs), P1 artificial chromosomes (PACs) or yeast artificial chromosomes (YACs) will work well in all instances.

Labelling of Probes

The most frequently used labels for probes in FISH experiments are modified deoxyuridine triphosphates. The modifications involve addition of haptens, immunoreactive groups such as digoxigenin or biotin, which are linked to the 5 position of the pyrimidine ring by a long spacer arm. These may be detected by indirect immunofluorescence techniques. Alternatively probes may be labelled with nucleoside triphosphates containing a fluorochrome such as fluorescein which can be detected directly by its own fluorescence. Probes can be labelled using any of the systems frequently employed elsewhere in molecular biology. These include polymerase chain reaction (PCR), nick translation and random primer labelling. Of these nick translation is probably the most popular, since it will produce labelled DNA fragments of small size. The size of probe is important as large probe molecules have difficulty in diffusing through cytological material to reach their target DNA, and their use often results in high background fluorescence. The optimal size of probe is between 200 and 500 bases. Probes produced by PCR are increasingly important in the techniques of chromosome painting and fibre FISH which will be described in detail later.

Hybridization

Here the procedures broadly follow those of other molecular nucleic acid hybridization protocols. Differences relate to attempts to maintain the morphology of the cytological preparation in good condition, and to prevent binding of the probe to repeated sequences distributed throughout the genome. To maintain the integrity of the cytological preparation, hybridization is usually carried out at reduced temperatures, typically 35–42°C in 50% formamide. Most eukaryote genomes contain large amounts of dispersed repeated DNA sequences. For this reason if genomic material is used as probe, it is likely to contain DNA sequences which are repeated elsewhere in the genome. This will result in a level of fluorescence across all regions of the chromosomes which will reduce the specificity of the probe. To prevent this and thus to improve the quality and sensitivity of the final image, unlabelled DNA from the repetitive fraction of the genome (Cot1 DNA) is usually added to the probe during hybridization.

Detection of Hybridized Probe

When probes are labelled directly with fluorescent nucleotides detection simply requires observation of the material using a fluorescence microscope with appropriate filters. Since the signal is not amplified this method will result in less intense fluorescence, but the level of background is low. The use of coupled charge device (CCD) cameras to detect low level fluorescence can make this method sensitive enough for use with small DNA targets. When probes are labelled with haptens their presence is detected with antibodies conjugated to fluorochromes. Digoxigenin and biotin labelled probes may both be detected in this way, but biotin has the added advantage that it has an extremely high affinity for the egg-white protein avidin. This allows the use of avidin conjugated with fluorochromes to be used in detection. The only shortcoming of this technique is where the target tissue contains enough biotin to give rise to background fluorescence. In the case of cytogenetics this is not a major problem. Frequently the fluorescent signal from a target is amplified by using more than one layer of antibody in the detection process.

One of the major advantages of FISH technology is the fact that different fluorochromes can be used simultaneously in conjunction with a series of probes labelled with different haptens. The result is a two-colour FISH image. For example two probes may be hybridized to the same chromosome preparation. If one is labelled with biotin and detected with fluorescein conjugated antibodies and the other is labelled with digoxigenin and detected using Texas red, then both loci will be detected simultaneously as areas of green or red fluorescence. This approach can be extended by also using directly labelled probes in the same experiment, or when probes labelled with a mixture of two haptens are used. If such probes are detected by antibodies conjugated to two different fluorochromes, the result is a signal of intermediate colour; red fluorescence by Texas red and green fluorescence from fluorescein will give an orange signal. A series of probes can be labelled with different ratios of the same two haptens. The resulting fluorescence can be converted to a digital signal in a CCD camera and dedicated software will recognize subtle differences in fluorescence. These will then be allocated new false colours. The ultimate development of such an approach is the recently described multiplex

FISH where each homologous chromosome pair in humans or mice can be detected as a different colour.

After detection of the probes it is necessary to detect the remaining areas of the chromosomes or nuclei to which probe has not hybridized. This is done using the fluorochromes 4,6-diamino-2-phenyl-indole (DAPI), Hoechst 33258, or propidium iodide. Combinations of DAPI and propidium iodide will produce a banding pattern which can be helpful in chromosome identification. However, due to the fact that it is excited by more than one wavelength and fluoresces at several different wavelengths, propidium iodide may cause problems where images are captured using monochrome CCD cameras.

Applications in Basic Research

Although this technology can potentially be used with all species of eukaryote, this author will concentrate on uses in human genetics. FISH can be used to detect genes or other DNA sequences from specific chromosomal regions. The precision required by the experiment determines the approach to be used. At the simplest level the process can be used to identify whole chromosomes, a technique known as chromosome painting. In this case it is necessary to isolate DNA from a single human chromosome in order to make a probe. This is carried out in one of two ways. Originally the human chromosome of interest was separated from other human chromosomes by use of an inter-specific cell hybrid. Somatic cell fusion of a diploid human cell and a mouse or hamster cell line results in the formation of hybrid cells which lose human chromosomes in a random manner. A rapid initial loss of human chromosomes is observed in these hybrids. Eventually, when most cells have lost all but a small number of human chromosomes, the cells become karyotypically stable. Sub-clones of these hybrids can be isolated which contain only a single human chromosome. This is particularly easy where the human chromosome contains a selectable gene such as thymidine kinase on

chromosome 17. Total DNA extracted from such hybrids is labelled and used as a probe for the specific human chromosome. This is, however, an inefficient use of resources since most of the label will be wasted as it will be incorporated into rodent DNA. A better approach is to label only human specific regions of DNA. Human DNA contains a common interspersed repeat sequence known as *alu*. This is absent from rodent gnomes. By carrying out PCR using specially designed primers complementary to *alu* repeats, a probe is produced containing only human sequences specific to the single chromosome present.

It is now possible to isolate specific human metaphase chromosomes directly using fluorescence activated cell sorting (FACS). DNA from the pellet of purified chromosomes is amplified by PCR using degenerate primers. This is now the method of choice for commercial suppliers of chromosome paints. Chromosome painting is particularly useful for the study of translocations. Figure 37.1 shows a tumour cell in which chromosome 17 has undergone complex rearrangements. The particular strength of chromosome painting lies in the ability to identify

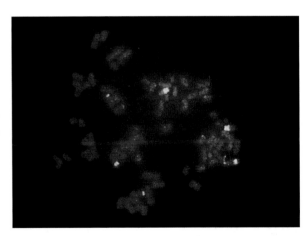

Figure 37.1: *Chromosomes of an ovarian cancer cell line painted with biotin-labelled chromosome 17 paint. The paint is detected with fluorescein isothiocyanate (FITC) and the chromosomes stained with propidium iodide. The chromosomes fluoresce brick red, the FITC green; the yellow coloration is due to a mixture of green and red fluorescence. This shows the presence of chromosome 17 translocations.*

Applications in Basic Research

small translocations which cannot easily be picked up by conventional G-banding. In this example the two large translocations could be identified by banding carried out by a trained cytogeneticist, but the two small interstitial translocations can only be detected by painting. To confirm which chromosomes are involved in any translocation it is possible to carry out two-colour painting with paints specific for different chromosomes.

A more sophisticated use of FISH is required to map the chromosomal location of a specific gene sequence. For this task DNA cloned in YACs or cosmids is normally used as probe. This provides sufficient fluorescence to be easily detectable. The procedures involved are similar to those employed for chromosome painting, but a greater amplification of the signal may be required. FISH is much more successful for this task than the previously used radio-labelled probes, because of the reduced background and the short time required to complete the experiment (two days as compared to several weeks needed for exposure of autoradiographs). As described earlier, more than one probe may be used simultaneously. This approach can be used in different ways. When attempting to localize a probe on a chromosome it is often necessary to identify unambiguously the chromosome at the same time. This is done by using a probe for a centromeric DNA repeat sequence specific to the chromosome in question. To determine the order of closely linked genes along the chromosome, dual or triple colour FISH can be used. Because of the colours used this process is often referred as 'traffic lighting'. The position of probe on a chromosome can sometimes be identified by the banding pattern but is often expressed simply as F/pter units. These represent the fractional distance from the telomere of the p arm of the chromosome as compared to the length of the entire chromosome.

A serious limitation to the mapping of genes by FISH is caused by the relatively condensed state of mitotic metaphase chromosomes. This means that signals from genes lying within approximately 1–2 Mb of each other will overlap and it is not possible to distinguish the two separate signals. A number of approaches

have been used to overcome this problem. Chromatin is much less condensed during interphase and sequences which could not be separated on metaphase chromosomes are often resolvable by hybridization of probes to the nuclei of non-dividing cells. A drawback in this system is that it is not possible to orient genes in relation to the centromere. An alternative process which allows this is the use of meiotic chromosome preparations. These are considerably more elongated than mitotic chromosome preparations. However they are not so convenient to prepare. One approach which has been used successfully to produce elongated mitotic chromosomes has been to use cytospin preparations of unfixed metaphases. A cytospin is a device frequently used in haematology to prepare slides of blood cells. It consists of a modified centrifuge in which cells are spun directly onto slides. When unfixed metaphases that have been swollen in hypotonic saline are treated in this way, the shear forces produced during centrifugation stretch the chromosomes up to twenty times their normal length. Even though this causes many of the metaphases to be disrupted and chromosomes to be deformed, it has an advantage over interphase analysis in that individual chromosomes can be identified and the orientation of FISH signals to centromeres and telomeres can be observed. The ultimate degree of resolution that can be obtained with FISH analysis is found in the technique of fibre FISH. Here the probe is hybridized to DNA which has been spread on a slide after removal of most or all of its chromatin packaging. No information at all can be obtained on the orientation of the signal to the chromosome but the technique is extremely powerful for fine scale analysis of small regions of the genome. Spreading of DNA can be achieved in a number of ways.

Extended chromatin fibres can be obtained from nuclei of unfixed interphase cells treated on microscope slides with detergent and high salt to remove histones. This causes the looped structure of chromatin to untangle and the DNA extends to a length comparable with that of pure DNA. Such techniques are known as halo production or DIRVISH (direct visual hybridization). These allow ordering of probes to a lower resolution limit of 3–5 kb. Purified DNA can also be spread on microscope slides for use in fine structure analysis. The DNA may be entrapped in agarose plugs, such as those used for pulsed field gel electrophoresis which are melted and gently spread on the slide, or DNA in solution can be allowed to spread on silanated slides. In this case the end of the molecule binds to the glass and the rest of the DNA is combed out into a pattern that is more or less linear by the meniscus as the solution evaporates.

Both of these protocols facilitate extremely fine-scale study. Typical examples include ordering of probes produced by PCR along DNA cloned in Yacs or cosmids. This can be very useful in circumstances where a contig (a group of ordered overlapping cloned DNA fragments) is incomplete and the size of gaps need to be estimated.

Applications in Medical Genetics

As noted above, chromosome painting is particularly useful for detecting translocations that would be too small to be resolved unambiguously by conventional G-banding. Other uses that can be made of FISH include detection of aneuploidy, particularly in amniocentesis. Here analysis of interphase nuclei can again be undertaken. Rather than using whole chromosome paints to detect numbers of homologues, probes specific to repeated DNA sequences found at the centromeres of different chromosomes are used. This can detect the presence of extra copies of the chromosomes involved in the common aneuploid syndromes such as Down's, Edward's and Pateau's. The sex of an embryo can also be determined in amniotic cells using two-colour probes for X and Y chromosomes. In these procedures FISH allows for a result to be obtained in a much shorter time than conventional chromosome analysis where cells must be cultured, and has the added advantage that as only interphase cells are necessary the number of cells scored can be very high. However it is more expensive and does not give as much information on the nature of

any cytogenetic abnormality as G-banding does. For instance, it will not distinguish between the presence of an intact extra chromosome and a fragment of the chromosome containing the centromere.

Applications in Cancer Diagnosis and Research

It is in the study and accurate diagnosis of cancers and leukaemia that FISH currently makes its major contribution to medicine. In the vast majority of cases malignant tissue shows at least some cytogenetic aberrations. Conventional cytogenetics can be applied only with some difficulty to these situations but FISH, particularly on interphase nuclei, can produce results accurately and in a short period of time, two criteria that are of obvious importance in patient management.

Although random translocations are common in tumour cells many cancers, particularly leukaemias and lymphomas, carry specific translocations that can be used to make an accurate diagnosis. These often result in fusion between copies of two different genes, creating a novel gene. An example of this is the Philadelphia chromosome which is detected in chronic myeloid leukaemia. Here, highly specific translocations between chromosomes 9 and 22 bring about fusion of the *abl* and *BCR* oncogenes to produce a novel tyrosine kinase. Here conventional G-banding is problematical. This is because the malignant cells may not provide significant numbers of metaphases *in vitro* and the quality of chromosome spreads is usually well below that obtained from normal lymphocytes. Chromosome painting can be applied even where the quality of chromosome preparations is poor, as the target chromosomes will be identifiable due to fluorescence even though they may not be clearly detected by G-banding. The main advantage of FISH technology in this instance is again the ability to obtain cytogenetic information from non-dividing cells. The use of fluorescent probes, often cosmids, for regions on either side of the tumour-specific translocation will allow an

Applications in Cancer Diagnosis and Research

accurate diagnosis. The two probes are labelled with different haptens so that they can be detected as two different colours, usually red and green. In normal cells, where no translocation is present, two red and two green fluorescent spots will appear on the nucleus. The dots will be distributed randomly across the nucleus. In the presence of a translocation one red and one green dot will be found in close proximity to each other in every tumour cell. Overlap will often occur and a yellow region of mixed signal will be observed. This approach allows a clear-cut detection of translocation in a large number of cells and can differentiate between normal cells and leukaemic cells in the sample. In addition to diagnostic work this system can also be used to look for the presence of residual leukaemic cells in patients after therapy. Specific aneuploidies can be detected in leukaemic tissue by the same methods as described above for amniotic cells.

Cytogenetic analysis of solid tumours has always lagged behind that of blood cancers. This is in part a consequence of the greater difficulty of obtaining usable chromosome preparations. Despite this, many solid tumours have been found to carry specific chromosomal aberrations. These can be looked for by interphase FISH either in touch preparations, where excised tumour material is 'touched' onto microscope slides to leave behind a film of cells, or by the use of cytological smears of small numbers of cells obtained in fine needle aspirates.

In addition to translocations and changes in chromosome number, tumours often contain multiple copies of the oncogenes or genes conferring resistance to chemotherapeutic drugs. These arise either as elongate regions of chromosomes where the gene has ampified *in situ*, known as homogenously staining regions (HSRs), or in small extrachromosomal elements referred to as double minutes (DMs). Oncogene amplification is an important factor in prognosis. FISH allows for the detection of amplification in interphase nuclei of tumour samples. An example of this is screening of breast cancer biopsies for amplification of the oncogene *erbB-2* on chromosome 17. Normal cells in the biopsy will provide a control showing two small fluorescent spots corre-

sponding to the two unamplified copies of the gene present, whereas the area of fluorescence is much greater where amplification has taken place. Examples of this are seen in Figure 37.2.

A somewhat different application of FISH both in cancer research and treatment has been the development of a novel technique that will provide an overall estimate of specific gains and losses of chromosomes, or chromosome regions from a particular tumour. This is known as Comparative Genome Hybridization. Here DNA is extracted from the tumour after removal from the patient. This DNA is labelled with a fluorochrome (green). It is mixed with DNA extracted from normal cells, which has been labelled red and the mixture hybridized onto normal metaphase chromosomes. The differently labelled probes compete for sites on the chromosomes. If the tumour shows no gains or losses of chromosomal material the resulting *in situ* hybridization will contain 46 chromosomes, all of which will fluoresce an even yellow. However regions of the tumour which have undergone amplification will be over-represented in the extracted DNA and will out-compete the red fluorescing normal DNA. Such regions will therefore appear green. Conversely, regions lost from the tumour, which are likely to contain tumour suppressor genes, will fluoresce red. Analysis of this two-colour competitive hybridization requires sophisticated computer software, but it may become a major tool for providing a broad spectrum molecular analysis of individual tumours.

FISH appears to have established a central role in molecular biology. How the technique evolves in future will depend on the increased understanding of the role of genetic processes in disease. In some of the applications to which it is put it may be replaced by non-cytological techniques such as PCR. Areas where this may happen include the detection of cancer-specific translocations, or the determination of sex in amniotic cells. However one of the most important advantages of FISH is that it does not destroy the cells on which it is carried out. In many areas this ability to obtain molecular genetic information whilst still being able to identify cellular and tissue structure is essential,

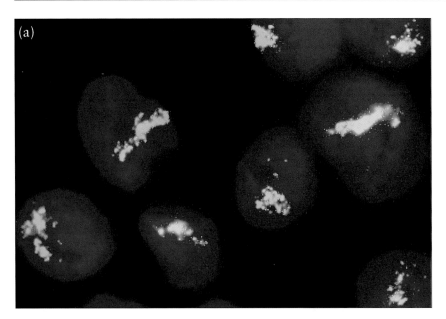
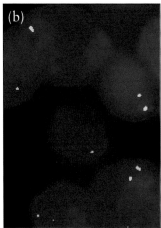

Figure 37.2: *(a) Interphase cells from a fine needle aspirate of a breast tumour which have been hybridized with a probe for the oncogene erbB-2. In this case the cells show amplification of the oncogene, while in (b) the aspirate contains cell in which the oncogene has not been amplified, and each cell shows one or two spots corresponding to the normal genes. In smear preparations made from fine needle aspirates the cells are not flattened which explains why the erbB-2 signal is not in the same focal plane in each cell. In these examples the probe was directly labelled with FITC and the nuclei counterstained with DAPl. [Courtesy of Dr Damien McManus, Royal Victoria Hospital, Belfast.]*

for instance in the molecular pathology of cancer. In addition the coupling of molecular and cytological techniques provides a valuable control against erroneous results arising from contamination of samples. For these reasons the technique is likely to remain of importance both in research and in the applied biosciences for some time.

Further Reading

Haaf T, Ward D C. Structural analysis of α-satellite DNA and centromere proteins using extended chromatin and chromosomes. *Human Molecular Genetics*, 1994; **3**: 697–709.

Heiskanen M, Hellsten E, Kallioniemi O-P, Makela T P, Alitalo K, Peltonen L, Palotie A. Visual mapping by fibre – FISH. *Genomics* 1995; **30**, 31–36.

Kallioniemi A, Kallioniemi O-P, Sudar D, Rurovitz D, Gray J W, Waldman F, Pinkel D. Comparative genomic hybridization for molecular cytogenetic analysis of solid tumours. *Science*, 1992; **258**: 818–821.

Pardue M L, Gall J G. Chromosomal localisation of mouse satellite DNA. *Science*, 1970; **168**: 1356–1358.

Speicher M R, Ballard S G, Ward D C. Karyotyping human chromosomes by combinatorial multi-fluor FISH. *Nature Genetics*, 1996; **12**: 368–375.

SECTION 6
CLINICAL CHEMISTRY

38 THE ACQUISITION, USES AND INTERPRETATION OF CLINICAL BIOCHEMICAL DATA

William J Marshall

Introduction

Clinical biochemical tests are used extensively in medicine, for a variety of purposes (see Table 38.1). The majority of the more familiar tests involve the measurement of a substance in a body fluid, usually serum (or plasma) or urine. Tests may also be made on spinal fluid, fluid obtained by paracentesis, intestinal secretions and faeces, and on biopsy samples of body tissues.

The results of most clinical biochemical tests are expressed quantitatively as a concentration or, in the case of enzyme measurements, as an activity. Molecular genetic analysis, though increasingly part of the repertoire of clinical biochemistry laboratories, is not discussed in this chapter or this section of this book. The fact that results are expressed numerically means that biochemical data appear easy to assess and to compare with normal rangesor with results obtained previously in the same patient(s). Whereas for example a subtle sign on a radiograph might be open to a variety of interpretations (or might be missed by an inexperienced observer), a serum sodium concentration of 143 mmol/l appears unequivocally 'normal' (the normal range is usually given as 135–145) and is clearly different from a value

of 147 mmol/l which, in turn, is by definition 'abnormal'.

But let us examine these statements. A serum sodium concentration may be within the normal range, but that does not mean that an abnormality of sodium or water homeostasis cannot be present, nor that the individual is necessarily healthy; conversely, finding a

Table 38.1: The Uses of biochemical tests in medicine.
- Diagnosis
- Assessment of severity
- Prognosis
- Monitoring disease/treatment
- Long-term follow up
- Screening
- Detecting drug toxicity
- Stratification for clinical trials

sodium concentration of 147 mmol/l does not necessarily mean that a disorder of sodium or water homeostasis is present and indeed the individual may be perfectly healthy. When a measurement is repeated, the result can be compared with the previous result. To decide whether a concentration of 147 mmol/l is clinically significantly different from a previous value in the same individual of 143 mmol/l requires a knowledge of the reliability of the data, not only in terms of analytical quality but also in relation to extent of any natural, biological variation which affects the concentration of sodium *in vivo*. Finally, any interpretation will be unreliable if the sample to be analysed has not been collected and handled prior to analysis in a way that does not affect sodium concentration.

Lest readers be concerned about whether any conclusions at all can be drawn from clinical biochemical data (or, and worse, be dismissive that these matters are trivial and of no consequence) it should be emphasized that laboratories go to considerable efforts to ensure that the data that they provide are reliable. Particularly with less familiar tests, they may provide helpful information on the significance of results. But it is still important to be aware of potential sources of error and of pitfalls in the interpretation of results if the maximum information is to be obtained from clinical biochemical tests. The bulk of this chapter is divided into two sections: the first deals with sample collection and analysis; the second with the uses and interpretation of biochemical data.

Sample Collection and Analysis

Laboratory personnel distinguish between factors affecting the quality of results which arise before a sample is analysed (pre-analytical phase); those directly relating to the analysis (analytical phase), and those arising after the results have been generated (post-analytical phase).

Pre-analytical factors

Biochemical variables can be affected by many physiological factors (Table 38.2). In addition, however, biochemical variables all show intrinsic random biological variation. For some analytes, particularly those whose concentrations are subject to tight feedback control, this variation may be small but for others it may be a significant factor to take into account when interpreting results.

Biochemical variables can also be affected by artefact, including drugs that may interfere physiologically with the analyte or interfere

Table 38.2:   Examples of physiological factors affecting biochemical tests.

Factor	Test
Age	Cholesterol, urate, alkaline phosphatase
Sex	Gonadotrophins, gonadal steroids
Body mass	Triglycerides
Time	Cortisol (diurnal variation)
	Gonadotrophins (in women, catamenial variation)
	25-hydroxycholecalciferol (seasonal variation)
Stress	Cortisol, prolactin, growth hormone, catecholamines, glucose
Posture	Renin, aldosterone, plasma proteins
Food intake	Glucose, triglycerides, phosphate

From: *Clinical Biochemistry*. Marshall W J, Bangert S K O Churchill Livingstone, 1995. (Reproduced with permission of Churchill Livingstone)

THE ACQUISITION, USES AND INTERPRETATION OF CLINICAL BIOCHEMICAL DATA

Analytical factors
Post-analytical factors
The Interpretation of Laboratory Data
Normal ranges and reference intervals

with the analysis itself. Drug interference is a potentially huge problem, though practically the number of important examples is relatively small. Finally, errors can occur pre-analytically because of poor sample collection technique (for example into the wrong container) or careless sample handling (for example, causing haemolysis or allowing evaporation of water). Exceptionally, errors can arise because of misidentification of samples. Extreme vigilance is necessary to prevent this. Request forms must be properly completed and matched to the patient, and the sample(s) obtained positively identified at all stages of handling (for example, if serum must be transferred from the initial (primary) container to a secondary container for analysis). In many hospitals and clinics, blood and other samples are collected by trained nurses or phlebotomists. Many laboratories find that errors of identification are more likely to occur when samples have been collected by doctors. In laboratory medicine, as in other activities, it is a good principle to take as much care with apparently simple procedures as with complicated ones.

Analytical factors

Laboratory personnel take considerable care to ensure the accuracy (correctness) and precision (reproducibility) of the results that they produce, whether they are generated by manual analysis or by automated equipment. It is a condition of accreditation by Clinical Pathology Accreditation (UK) Ltd (CPA) that laboratories use acceptable internal quality control and external quality assessment procedures to this end. Problems affecting the quality of results are discussed in the chapters on individual techniques.

Post-analytical factors

Once results have been generated, errors can still arise during any transcription of results. With the increasing use of on-line computing and electronic transmission, the risk of such errors has decreased considerably, but it can never be entirely eliminated.

The Interpretation of Laboratory Data

Although biochemical data are extensively used in the investigation and management of patients, they rarely provide a complete diagnosis. Biochemical changes usually reflect pathological processes rather than distinct diseases, and may not even be specific for one process, although in a particular clinical situation or in the light of the results of other investigations one may be more likely than any other. For example, a low serum albumin concentration can occur as a result of decreased synthesis, increased volume of distribution or increased catabolism or excretion of the protein, and each of these has several potential causes. In a patient known to have chronic liver disease, for example, decreased synthesis would be the most likely cause. According to the reasons for performing biochemical tests, their results can be assessed in relation to one of several criteria: the normal ranges (for a group of comparable healthy individuals); the values known to be characteristic of a particular condition; cutoff points or action limits, or results obtained previously in the same individual.

Normal ranges and reference intervals

The term 'normal' has many meanings. A normal distribution describes a symmetrical distribution of data around a mean that can be described by a specific mathematical function. Statistically, the normal range is the range of values for such data extending from the mean minus two standard deviations to the mean plus two standard deviations, and encompasses approximately 95% of values. For many people, however, normal means 'conforming to type' or 'expected', or by implication 'healthy' since normal ranges for human biological variables are usually based on measurements made on a sample of individuals from a 'normal' (that is, healthy) population.

There are many pitfalls in the use of normal ranges. Within the disciplines of laboratory medicine, it has been argued extensively that the term should not be used. Instead of 'normal population', the term 'reference population' is

The Interpretation of Laboratory Data

Normal ranges and reference intervals

preferred, since this does not imply that such a population is necessarily healthy. (Indeed, there is no reason why one should not attempt to define the ranges of test results seen in patients with specific diseases.) The upper and lower ends of the distribution are termed 'reference limits' and the range between them, the 'reference interval'. Worthy though this endeavour is to direct more objective analysis of data, the terms described are not used widely outside laboratories and, indeed, many laboratory personnel continue to refer to 'normal ranges'. Furthermore, reference intervals are often based on the same data as were used to calculate normal ranges.

By definition, since the normal range encompasses only 95% of values from the sample studied, 5% of values fall outside its limits – 2.5% above and 2.5% below. Thus some values falling outside the normal range would be expected to occur in healthy individuals, although common sense tells us that the further away a result is from that range, the more likely it is to be 'abnormal', that is, potentially characteristic of disease. The more tests that are performed in an individual, the greater the probability that the result of at least one will fall outside its normal range even if the person is healthy by every possible criterion. If twenty independent analytes were to be measured, the probability that the result of at least one would be 'abnormal' is 0.64 (better than evens!). Many autoanalysers routinely measure this number of analytes and falsely 'abnormal' results are an inevitable occurrence.

Another problem in interpretation stems from the fact that the range of variation of a test result in an individual is likely to be less than the range observed in a population, since the population, even when healthy and comparable in terms, for example, of age, sex, ethnic origin, etc., is composed of individuals whose characteristics will differ due to genetic and environmental influences. For example, although the normal range for serum creatinine concentration in adult males is approximately 60–120 μmol/L, the range of values that would be found with repeated measurements on a single individual with normal renal function would be much less than this. An individual

might have a value for an analyte within the normal range as conventionally defined which was actually abnormal for him.

Normal ranges can be misleading, and are not always appropriate as standards against which to judge patients' results, as the following examples illustrate.

Example 1. A result within the normal range may falsely suggest normal function. Creatinine is measured in serum as an index of renal function, specifically of the glomerular filtration rate (GFR). Because it is inversely related to the GFR, a considerable fall in GFR (approximately half) must occur before mean serum creatinine concentration increases sufficiently to exceed the 'upper limit of normal' (Fig. 38.1).

Example 2. A result within the normal range may falsely suggest no risk of disease. There is a relationship between increasing serum cholesterol concentration and the risk of coronary heart disease even within the normal range as conventionally derived (Fig. 38.2). For cholesterol, it is better to define ideal concentrations (which themselves depend on the presence or absence of other risk factors for coronary disease) and target concentrations for treatment.

Example 3. Any concentration is abnormal. Since drugs are not physiological constituents

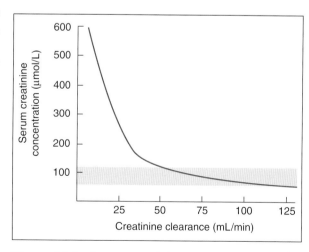

Figure 38.1: *Serum creatinine concentration and creatinine clearance. Clearance may fall to half its normal value (approx. 120 mL/min) before serum creatinine concentration becomes abnormal. (The shaded area shows the reference range for serum creatinine concentration.)*

of the body, drug concentrations in patients cannot be compared with normal ranges. For therapeutic drug monitoring, 'therapeutic' and 'toxic' ranges are more appropriate (although even these terms must be used with caution); in cases of poisoning, 'action levels' are used to help determine appropriate management.

Critical differences

The preceding discussion relates to the comparison of measured data with expected values based on observations of other people. When a measurement has been repeated, it is more relevant to consider it in relation to the previous value. The relevant question is then whether the two measurements differ significantly.

This will depend on two factors, the innate variability of the measurement even when sampling conditions are identical (biological variation), and the unavoidable (although it is to be hoped small) analytical imprecision. Both of these can be determined from the results of repeated measurements of the same and a series of samples, and a function known as the critical difference (CD) calculated from the equation: $CD = 2.8 \times (SD_A^2 + SD_B^2)^{\frac{1}{2}}$, where SD_A and SD_B are respectively the analytical and biological standard deviations. The CD indicates the difference between two values that is unlikely to have occurred as a result of analytical and biological variation alone at a level of $p = 0.05$, i.e. if two values differ by the CD, the probability that this is a true difference is 0.95. Whether any change is clinically significant is a different matter, but clearly a change cannot be considered to be of potential clinical significance if it is less than the CD.

The concept of critical difference appears not to be widely known outside the laboratory but is fundamental to the use of laboratory data in monitoring the responses of patients to treatment, or the natural history of a disease. Values for some CDs should be obtainable from the local laboratory. Critical differences are independent of normal ranges. Indeed, two results may be critically different yet both be within the normal range, for example an increase in serum creatinine concentration from 80 to 100 μmol/L (the CD for creatinine at this order of concentration is approximately 15 μmol/L).

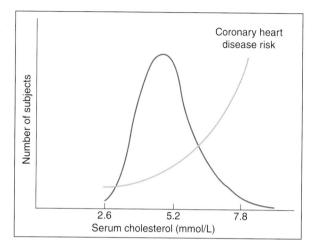

Figure 38.2: *The distribution of serum cholesterol concentrations in healthy adult subjects and risk of coronary heart disease. Approximately one third of values exceed the recommended ideal maximum concentration (5.2 mmol/L) and are associated with significantly increased risk. Note also that the distribution is non-Gaussian, being skewed to the right.*

Action limits, cutoff points and predictive values

For some laboratory tests, it may be appropriate to consider the results against *action limits*, that is, values used to determine whether specific action should be taken. Obvious examples include action limits for the concentrations of poisons to direct therapy, for example, serum paracetamol concentration to indicate whether treatment with N-acetylcysteine should be initiated (or continued) to prevent hepatic damage. Many laboratories have action limits for telephoning the requesting clinician with results outside a certain range which may require that appropriate action is taken urgently, for example to treat dangerous hyperkalaemia, or for instigating further tests themselves (e.g. thyroid function tests in a patient with hypercholesterolaemia).

Because for most laboratory data there is an overlap between the range of values that are usually seen in healthy people and those that occur in disease, the selection of action points is particularly critical when tests are used for screening (detecting subclinical disease). Setting the action limit (more frequently called a *cutoff*

The Interpretation of Laboratory Data
Likelihood ratios

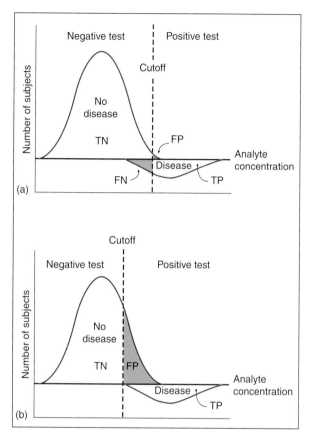

Figure 38.3: *The effect of moving the cutoff point that determines positivity/negativity of a test result. Hypothetical distributions for the concentrations of an analyte with and without disease are shown. Because these overlap, if the cutoff is selected to decrease the numbers of false positive results (and hence increase specificity) (a) there are a significant number of false negative results (decreasing the sensitivity). If the cutoff is set lower (b), false negatives are eliminated (maximizing sensitivity) but at the expense of increasing the number of false positives (and decreasing specificity). The distributions for individuals with disease have been shown below the horizontal axis for clarity.*

value in this context) too low will mean that everyone with a condition will be detected by the test, but at the expense of miscategorizing a significant number of healthy individuals (false positives). Setting the cutoff too high will exclude all healthy individuals, but some with disease will be missed (false negatives) (Fig. 38.3). The performance of screening tests can

be measured by calculating the functions known (in this context) as sensitivity (a measure of the ability of the test to detect people with disease) and specificity (a measure of the ability to identify people who do not have the disease) (Table 38.3). Such calculations require identification of false and true positives and negatives which in turn requires a 'gold standard' test that uniquely identifies the presence or absence of disease. Histological or molecular genetic tests may provide the gold standard, but sometimes true positivity or negativity can only be determined in retrospect, by observing outcome.

The numbers of true and false positive and negative results can also be used to calculate the predictive value (PV) of a positive or negative result, that is, the probability that a result of either type will correctly classify a patient.

The concepts of sensitivity, specificity and predictive value can also be used to describe the performance of tests done for diagnostic purposes, but both in this case and in screening it is important to appreciate that they can only be applied reliably to similar groups of patients to those on whom the data were derived. A test for, say, rheumatoid arthritis may appear to have a very high sensitivity if most of the people from whom the data are derived have rheumatoid disease. The sensitivity might be much lower in a group of people in whom the disease had a very low prevalence. This is a major drawback to (and frequent source of error in) the use of these concepts.

Likelihood ratios
These functions express the odds that a given finding (e.g. a certain test result) would occur in a person with, as opposed to without, a particular condition. The likelihood ratio (LR) for a positive result is given by: LR_{pos} = sensitivity/ (1 − specificity). The odds that a negative test result would occur in a person with, as opposed to without, a particular condition (LR_{neg}) is given by: LR_{neg} = (1 − sensitivity)/specificity. Likelihood ratios can be used to convert pre-test probability (e.g., in a screening test, the prevalence of the condition being tested for in the population from whom a patient is drawn) into the post-test probability of the condition being

Table 38.3: Sensitivity, specificity and predictive values of test results.

		Test Result	
		Positive	Negative
Disease status	Positive	True positive (TP)	False negative (FN)
	Negative	False positive (FP)	True negative (TN)

Sensitivity = TP/(TP + FN) Specificity = TN/(TN + FP)
Positive predictive value (PV+) = TP/(TP + FP)
Negative predictive value (PV–) = TN/(TN + FN)

present. Such data can be used to direct management and are potentially of great value in clinical audit.

Evidence-based Clinical Biochemistry

It will have been seen that biochemical and other laboratory test results must be interpreted with care. Many currently available tests provide less reliable information than is often appreciated, not usually because of analytical problems, but rather because of poor sensitivity and specificity. New diagnostic tests are being introduced all the time, often enthusiastically promoted by the manufacturers of test kits, and supported by clinicians who are looking for improved diagnostic performance. Their evaluation, however, is often poor. Ideally, all diagnostic tests should be evaluated with a similar rigour to that used for the introduction of new treatments, so that they can be used rationally, on the basis of scientifically sound evidence.

Conclusion

Biochemical tests have become an essential part of modern medicine. They have many potential uses but, for many tests, the ease with which they can be requested and performed belies their complexity. They should all be performed with care and interpreted through an appreciation of the underlying physiological and pathological principles, whatever the purpose for which they are to be used.

Further Reading

Fraser C G. *Interpretation of clinical chemistry laboratory data.* 1986: Blackwell Scientific Publications, Oxford.

Fraser C G, Fogarty Y. Interpreting laboratory results. *British Medical Journal* 1989; **298**: 1659–1660.

Jones R, Payne B. *Clinical Investigation and Statistics in Laboratory Medicine* 1997: ACB Venture Publications, London.

Marshall W J. The uses of biochemical data in clinical medicine. The acquistion of biochemical data. The interpretation of biochemical data. In: Marshall W J, Bangert S K (eds). *Clinical Biochemistry* 1995: Churchill Livingstone, New York, pp 1–24.

Moore R A. Evidence-based clinical biochemistry: a personal view. *Annals of Clinical Biochemistry* 1997; **34**: 1–7.

Read M C, Lachs M S, Feinstein A R. Use of methodological standards in diagnostic test research: getting better but still not good. *Journal of the American Medical Association* 1995; **274**: 645–651.

39 IMMUNOASSAY IN CLINICAL BIOCHEMISTRY

Joan Butler

Introduction

Immunoassay uses the antigen–antibody reaction as a means of quantitating either the antigen or the antibody. Most applications in clinical biochemistry have used the technique to quantitate the antigen, whereas in immunology and microbiology it is also used to quantitate (or detect) circulating antibody. For clinical biochemistry, the antigen is the analyte of interest. Antibodies can be raised against a wide variety of substances. Small molecules can be made immunogenic by chemical coupling to a large molecule such as albumin or polylysine, and are then referred to as haptens.

Assay Design

Despite the apparent complexity of published methods, there are two basic assay designs, competitive or limited antibody methods using antigen labelled with a tracer or reporter molecule and having the generic title immunoassay, and noncompetitive or excess antibody methods using labelled antibody and having the generic title immunometric assay. In a *competitive assay*, the analyte in the sample (or calibrant) competes with labelled analyte for the binding sites on a limited amount of antibody. It is essential that the amount of antibody is insufficient to bind all the labelled analyte, so that competition for binding sites must occur. At equilibrium the amount of labelled analyte bound to the antibody will be inversely related to the amount of unlabelled analyte in the sample or calibrant. Determination of the label in the bound fraction will provide a measure of the amount of analyte, by comparison with a calibration curve.

$$Ag + Ag^* + Ab \rightarrow AgAb + Ag^*Ab + Ag^*$$
$$\textit{initial state} \qquad \textit{final state}$$

In order to determine the amount of labelled analyte in the bound (or free) fraction, these fractions must be separated, except in the rare cases where the signal from the label is modified by binding of the labelled analyte to the antibody.

In a *noncompetitive or immunometric assay*, the analyte is reacted with an excess of labelled antibody. The unreacted antibody is then separated, and the amount of labelled antibody bound to analyte is measured.

$$Ag + Ab^* \rightarrow AgAb^* + Ab^*$$
$$\textit{initial state} \qquad \textit{final state}$$

Assay Design

Labels

This simple design is the basis for a number of more complex formats. Analytes which are large molecules may be reacted with another antibody, termed the capture antibody, directed against a different and spatially distinct epitope on the analyte molecule, and usually linked to a solid phase.

$$Ab_1 + Ag + Ab_2^* \rightarrow Ab_1AgAb_2^* + Ab_1 + Ab_2^*$$
initial state   *final state*

where Ab_1 = capture antibody
       Ab_2^* = labelled antibody

This assay design is the so-called sandwich or two-site immunometric assay, and is the design presently most used for assay of polypeptides. The analyte must be large enough for simultaneous binding by two antibodies. Antibody addition to the sample may be simultaneous (a one-step format), or sequential with removal of the sample before addition of the labelled antibody (a two-step format). More than one capture or labelled antibody may be used, giving a multisite assay.

In requiring two distinct but connected epitopes, the two-site assay design offers considerably greater specificity than a competitive single antibody design. Although polyclonal antisera can be used in sandwich assays, this design came into general use only when monoclonal antibodies became available.

In immunometric assays for small analytes, the unreacted labelled antibody is usually removed by the addition of analyte coupled to a solid phase. Attachment to a solid phase impairs reactivity and the coupled analyte will therefore not compete with free analyte from the sample. Alternatively, antibody specific for the complex of hapten and anti-analyte antibody and not reactive to either of these components separately (anti-immune complex or anti-metatype antibody) can be used.

$$Ag + Ab_1 \rightarrow AgAb_1 + Ab_1 \rightarrow + Ab_2^* \rightarrow$$
initial state

$$\qquad AgAb_1Ab_2^* + Ab_1 + Ab_2^*$$
           final state

where Ab_1 = anti-Ag
       Ab_2 = anti-$(AgAb_1)$

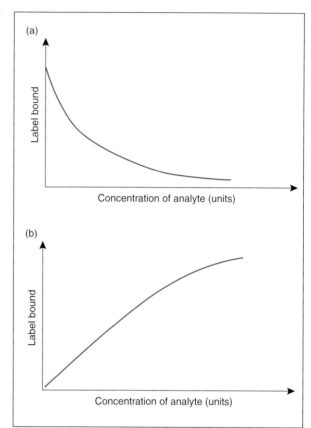

Figure 39.1: *Typical standard curves for*
a) a competitive immunoassay
b) a two-site immunometric assay.

This format demonstrates the fundamental difference between competitive and antibody excess immunoassays, namely that the former measures signal from antibody not bound to analyte and the latter measures signal from antibody bound to analyte or antibody occupancy. The latter is inherently more sensitive, since it is easier to distinguish a small number from zero than to distinguish a large number from a slightly larger number. Moreover, antibody excess methods are more rapid and affected less by variations in reagent quality and quantity, and may have a wider working range. Figure 39.1 shows typical calibration curves for a competitive immunoassay and a two-site immunometric assay.

Labels

Many different types of label or reporter molecule are in use. Labelling procedures are designed

Table 39.1:   Types of label in common use.
- radioisotopes
- chemiluminescence
    enhanced chemiluminescence
    electrochemiluminescence
- fluorescence
    time-resolved fluorescence
- enzymes
    colorimetry, rate colorimetry
    fluorescence
    chemiluminescence
    amplification (cascades)

not to impair the binding of the labelled substance to its appropriate antibody or analyte. Measurement (detection) of the label may require further reagents and/or highly specialized equipment. Types of label in common use are given in Table 39.1.

Homogeneous assays

The term homogeneous is used for immunoassays in which separation of bound and free label is not required. In such systems the signal is modified by antibody binding such that bound and free label can be distinguished in the reaction mixture. For example, binding of enzyme-labelled analyte to the antibody may sterically inhibit binding of substrate to the enzyme. Another example is the turbidimetric assay for small molecules in which crosslinking of analyte-coated latex particles by antibody is inhibited by free analyte from the sample, causing a decrease in turbidity. If the analyte is a large molecule and in sufficiently high concentration, the formation of antigen–antibody complexes can be measured by nephelometry, and no label is needed. Some types of homogeneous assay available are given in Table 39.2.

Table 39.2:   Homogeneous immunoassays.
- enzyme inhibition or de-inhibition
- fluorescence polarization
- cloned enzyme donor assay
- nephelometry
- turbidimetry

However, these techniques are not generally applicable, and most immunoassays are of the heterogeneous type, in which separation of bound and free label is required.

Separation methods

Any technique used to separate bound from free analyte or antibody must not disturb the primary reaction.

The difference in molecular size between free and antibody-bound analyte was exploited in early systems such as protein precipitation with ammonium sulphate or polyethylene glycol and adsorption of free analyte with charcoal. Immunological separation through the use of an anti-species antibody proved much more reliable. For example, since antibodies are bi- or multivalent, if the primary antibody was raised in a rabbit, antibodies to rabbit immunoglobulins raised in a donkey will produce complexes with the rabbit immunoglobulins that are sufficiently large and insoluble to form a precipitate. Usually some serum or immunoglobulin from a non-immunized rabbit (carrier serum) is added to ensure precipitation. Such reagents are of general applicability. This separation system (in the example donkey anti-rabbit) is called a second antibody, and assays using it are called double antibody methods, although this name is occasionally also used to mean a two-site assay. The formation of the second antibody precipitate is slow, assays usually being left overnight, but this stage can be shortened considerably by the addition of polyethylene glycol. After centrifugation, the supernatant is removed by aspiration or decantation, procedures requiring skill and experience with the very small precipitates produced.

Solid phase separation methods

These techniques, which have largely superseded all other methods, involve attaching reagents to solid phases by covalent bonding or by absorption. The solid phase can be the wall of a plastic tube, the well of a microtitre plate or the surface of large beads or small particles. Particles with a magnetizable core offer exceptionally rapid and efficient separation. Separation is by simple and convenient decantation or aspiration of the liquid phase, usually followed by washing of the solid phase with buffer to ensure completeness of separation and to reduce the non-specific binding (the apparent binding in the absence of antibody).

The solid phase can be a multipurpose reagent made by coating with second antibody or with streptavidin, one specific reagent being coupled with biotin which has a very high affinity for streptavidin. Other pairs include fluorescein with anti-fluorescein. This technique has the additional advantage that the specific reactions occur in the liquid phase. Coupling to a solid phase diminishes the affinity of an antibody and the speed of reaction, and may alter other characteristics. Solid phase techniques also permit variations of assay protocol from the basic form of simultaneous addition of all reagents to the sample. Such variations may result in increased specificity and other improvements. Reagents immobilized onto strips of paper form the basis of dipstick tests, for example for pregnancy testing.

Assay conditions and calibrators

Many factors must be controlled within- and between-batch in the optimization of an assay. Rate of reaction and position of equilibrium are dependent on temperature, pH and ionic strength. Cross-reactivity of structurally related molecules will be affected by changes in these variables. As far as possible these factors especially the sample matrix, must be kept constant. If a reaction is not permitted to reach equilibrium, then lack of constancy of timing can lead to drift, systematic error in the result according to the position of the sample in the batch.

Calibrants or standards can pose a special difficulty in immunoassay, since for many substances there is no alternative assay system. If the analyte is a heterogeneous protein, the assignment of concentration may depend on the set of antibodies and the preparation of analyte used. For this reason, International Standards have been set up for many proteins, with unitage assigned by collaborative studies involving different assay systems in a number of laboratories. Use of such Standards tends to minimize but does not eliminate differences between assays.

Calculation of Results

Since the calibration curve (a plot of label bound vs. concentration of analyte) is not a straight line, fitting a curve to the data, with its attendant imprecision, is a matter of judgement. Various empirical manipulations have been employed to make some or all of the graph linear. Bound label (or percentage bound if the total amount of label added is known) vs. concentration or log concentration, log bound label vs. log concentration, and logit-log plots are commonly used (logit = $\log (B/B_0/(1 - B/B_0))$ where B_0 = bound label in the zero calibrator). Lin-log, log-log and logit-log graph papers are available. Modern instruments designed for immunoassay have computer programs for curve fitting, including complex methods like cubic spline or 4-parameter log-logistic curve fits.

Accuracy and Precision

The accuracy of the result of an assay is the closeness to the true concentration of the analyte, for many substances still the subject of research and debate. Precision is the variability of the result obtained, and imprecision can be minimized by the use of appropriate reagents, for example a label with superior detectability, by reduction of the number of steps and by close control of technique. Internal quality control gives information only about imprecision. Manual assays are usually performed in duplicate. Imprecision varies with the concentration of analyte. A typical example is shown in Fig. 39.2.

The concentration range of low imprecision should ideally match the range over which clinical results will be obtained, and the imprecision be appropriate for clinical utility of the results. Some workers define the working range of an assay as that over which the coefficient of variation (CV) is less than 10%.

The sensitivity or minimum detectable concentration can be defined in several ways, for example as the concentration corresponding to 2, 2.5 or 3 standard deviations (SDs) of the signal of the zero calibrator above (for immunometric assays) or below (for competitive assays)

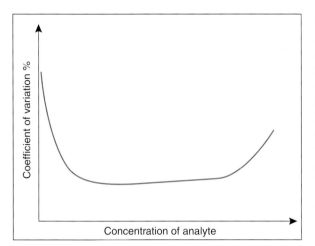

Figure 39.2: A typical precision profile.

the mean value for the zero calibrator, the SD being obtained from, say, 20 replicates of the zero calibrator in a single batch. This is sometimes termed the analytical sensitivity. More realistic may be the use of between-batch SDs, and analyte-free serum, giving the 'biological detection limit'. Others use the concentration at which between-batch CV is 20% on biological samples to give a value termed 'functional sensitivity'. Note that 'sensitivity' has alternative meanings; it is also the slope of the standard curve at any given concentration, and clinical sensitivity is a measure of the ability of a test to detect the presence of disease.

Quality Control

Internal quality control (IQC) provides information about precision within- and between-assay and about variability of reagent quality, but not about accuracy or validity, nor about errors with individual samples. IQC requires materials of similar composition to clinical samples, in sufficient quantity for repeated use both within and between batches of an assay. Liquid materials are usually stored frozen. Commercial QC materials are supplied lyophilized. During lyophilization (and subsequent storage) some components may be damaged, e.g. unstable analytes or binding proteins for steroids. The concentrations of the

analyte chosen for the QC materials (usually low, middle and high values) should correspond to significant points of the assay, for example clinical decision points, but should avoid areas of high imprecision, which might make interpretation difficult. Commercial QC materials achieve the required values by the use of stripped serum and the addition of analyte, which may limit the similarity to clinical samples. Materials of human origin must be used.

Results are generally plotted (Shewhart or Levey–Jennings plots) with the batch number or date on the x-axis and the result on the y-axis, either as a value or in terms of the SD from the mean value for that material. The latter implies that data must be accumulated to determine the mean and SD before the chart can be used. The usual rules are that the batch should be rejected if the values of all three controls are outside 1 SD on the same side of the mean, if two are outside 2 SDs or if one is outside 3 SDs. Interpretation of QC rules is often somewhat subjective but should be explicit. More complex acceptance rules have been formulated (Westgard analysis). Plots of other assay parameters can also be useful.

External quality assurance schemes (EQAS) seek to provide information about the comparability of methods and to investigate validity via recovery of added standard, linearity on dilution, specificity, performance with low-analyte serum, interference and other factors. Such schemes are available only for established assays.

Specificity, Cross-reactivity and Interference

The high specificity of the binding site of an antibody for its antigen is a major advantage of immunoassays. A single epitope on a complex molecule may involve amino acids spatially close only in the tertiary or quaternary structure of the molecule, and an antibody to such an epitope will therefore not react with denatured forms or fragments. However, a polyclonal antiserum will contain antibodies of differing affinities and specificities. If the antigen preparation used for immunization was impure, then the antiserum will contain antibodies to the impurities, and the resulting lack of specificity may compromise the validity of the assay, especially if the calibrant and label are also impure. Selection of monoclonal antibodies may minimize cross-reactivity, but closely related molecules may still be recognized by the antibody. Cross-reactivity in a competitive assay is arbitrarily defined as that concentration of cross-reactant giving 50% of the signal found in the absence of analyte, expressed as a percentage of the concentration of analyte giving the same signal. The measured cross-reactivity will vary at different points on the dose–response curve, and will also vary with the presence or absence of analyte and with assay format and reaction conditions such as temperature and time of incubation.

In two-site immunometric assay, it is important to test potential cross-reactants in the absence and in the presence of analyte, since the cross-reactant may react with either or both antibodies. Reaction with both antibodies will give an increase in signal, whereas reaction with one antibody may produce a decrease in signal at high cross-reactant concentrations, which can be detected only in the presence of analyte.

Hyperspecificity of an assay may occur if a monoclonal antibody is directed to an epitope occurring in some but not all biologically active forms of a heterogeneous analyte.

Interference from unrelated substances in clinical samples is an occasional but difficult problem. Complement binding may lead to destruction of the immune complex. Heterophilic antibodies and rheumatoid factor can bind to a single antibody, reducing its affinity for its antigen, or crosslink two antibodies thereby mimicking antigen. These effects can be blocked by the addition of immunoglobulins from the same animal species as the primary antibodies. Antibodies specific for the analyte may occur, for example anti-triiodothyronine and anti-thyroxine. Their effect in an assay will depend on the assay design.

A simple test for the presence of an interferant is examination of linearity on dilution with a diluent of similar matrix. Lack of linearity suggests a problem, though good linearity does not exclude one.

High Dose Hook Effect

In a two-site immunometric assay with simultaneous addition of the two antibodies to the sample (a one-step assay), when the concentration of analyte is very high and the antibodies are no longer in excess there will be sufficient analyte present for some binding sites on the antibodies to be occupied by separate molecules of analyte. Crosslinking of capture and signal antibodies will be diminished, and the signal will be reduced. At extremely high concentrations the signal may fall below that of the top calibrator and a falsely low result will be read off (Figure 39.3). This phenomenon is known as the high dose hook effect, and will be important only for those analytes which occur clinically in a concentration range of several orders of magnitude, as seen for tumour markers such as human chorionic gonadotrophin, alphafetoprotein and prolactin. The

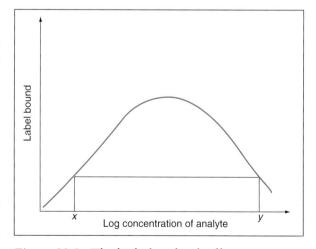

Figure 39.3: The high dose hook effect.
x = concentration of highest calibrator,
y = concentration above which falsely low
values will be obtained on undiluted samples.

position of the hook is dependent on the concentrations of the antibodies. The hook effect can be avoided by using a two-step format, in which the sample is incubated with solid phase capture antibody, and the labelled antibody added after separation and washing.

Further Reading

Bangham D R, Cotes P M. Standardisation and standards, *British Medical Bulletin* 1974; **30**: 12–17.

Brown E N, McDermott, T J, Bloch, K J, McCollom A D. Defining the smallest analyte concentration an immunoassay can measure, *Clinical Chemistry* 1996; **42**: 893–903.

Chan D W, Perlstein M T, eds. *Immunoassay: a practical guide*. 1987: San Diego. Academic Press,

Ekins R P. The precision profile: its use in assay design, assessment and quality control. In Hunter W M, Corrie J E T (eds) *Immunoassays for clinical chemistry*, 2nd edn 1983: Churchill Livingstone, Edinburgh. 76–105.

Price C P, Newman D J, eds. *Principles and practice of immunoassay*. 1991: Stockton Press, New York.

Self C H, Dessi J L, Winger L A. High-performance assays of small molecules: enhanced sensitivity, rapidity, and convenience demonstrated with a noncompetitive immunometric anti-immune complex assay system for digoxin. *Clinical Chemistry* 1994; **40**: 2035–2041.

Wild D G, ed. *The immunoassay handbook*. 1994: Stockton Press, New York.

40 ION SELECTIVE ELECTRODES

Alan D Hirst

Introduction

Production of a colour – a coloured compound – is the basis of most conventional forms of chemical measurement. Electrochemistry is different in that the measurement is based on the production of a voltage (potential) or current, and the measuring system is a voltmeter or ammeter rather than a photometer.

Ion-selective electrode (ISE) is a term given to an electrochemical detector which responds specifically to a given analyte. The early electrodes responded to ions, hence the name, but more recently electrodes have been developed which respond to metabolites such as glucose and urea, but these are usually included in the same category because they share a common technology. Glucose sensors in common use in clinical areas are often ISE devices, and all blood gas analysers are based on ISE technology.

The basis of ISEs is that they produce a potentiometric (voltage change) or amperometric (current change) response to changes in the analyte, i.e. there are two type of primary electrode. Secondary electrodes use other features such as enzymes to achieve specificity and release a product which can be detected by an ISE.

Electrodes with Clinical Applications

Ions: hydrogen (pH), sodium, potassium, chloride, fluoride, calcium, magnesium, lithium, ammonium (NH_4^+)

Gases: oxygen, carbon dioxide, ammonia (NH_3)

Secondary or complex electrodes: glucose, urea, lactate

Advantages and limitations

There are a number of good reasons for using ion-selective electrodes but in looking at these

Electrodes with Clinical Applications

A Potentiometric Cell

Measurement and reference half cells

---

for a solution to an analytical problem it must be recognized that there are also many limitations.

Advantages of ISEs

(1) Non-photometric, which means that an optically clear solution is not needed, i.e. whole blood can be used; (2) Rapid; (3) Direct, allowing measurement of (a) true concentration or (b) biological activity; (4) Usable by non-technical staff; (5) Portable; (6) Size (hence low sample volume); (7) Direct control (e.g. an insulin infusion pump can be directly controlled by a glucose electrode); (8) Possible invasive applications.

Potential limitations

(1) Suitable for a limited number of analytes (ionic or capable of an electrochemical reaction); (2) Properties of membrane, e.g. electrical conductivity; (3) Properties of selective agents (e.g. pH dependence of enzyme membranes such as urease for urea electrode); (4) Limited selectivity, e.g. for lithium over sodium; (5) Limited electrode life, e.g. if selective agents are leached out of the membrane; (6) Electrode maintenance such as removal of protein deposits; (7) Temperature stability – the potential of electrodes vary with temperature and may take time to stabilize; (8) Stability after maintenance. New electrodes can take up to 1 h to stabilize; (9) Properties of reference electrode, e.g. a calomel electrode with a concentrated KCl internal solution could contaminate a chloride or a potassium electrode; (10) Requirements for sample preparation: a calcium electrode requires 'balanced heparin' which is presaturated with calcium and will not bind the calcium in the sample; (11) Variation in sample: ionic strength, viscosity and sedimentation can all affect electrode potentials; (12) Response times vary with electrode and concentration and some electrodes such as fluoride can take minutes to reach a steady state; (13) Sensitivity is related to the range of concentration (small in plasma sodium) and to the selectivity of the electrode; (14) Linearizing the signal: potentiometric electrodes have an inverse logarithmic response which is not easily converted to a linear form; (15) Capital and running costs: electrodes need regular checking

for drift and recalibration. This requires an instrument with ancillary reagent pumps, valves and control processors; (16) Safeguards are needed to monitor the performance of the instrument.

While this may seem to be a daunting list of limitations, most of them have been overcome for a number of clinically useful applications, as the following accounts indicate.

A Potentiometric Cell

To make a measurement with a potentiometric ISE four elements are required: (1) a measuring half cell; (2) a reference half cell; (3) a salt bridge (or equivalent electrical connection; (4) a measuring device.

A functional electrode (cell) is made up of two half cells – a measuring electrode and a reference electrode. Each half cell produces a potential and it is the potential difference (i.e. voltage) between the two half cells which produces a measurable signal. The reference half cell should be designed to have a constant potential while the measuring electrode has a potential which varies with the concentration of the substance being measured, and so the potential difference or voltage will vary in a reproducible way with the concentration of the substance. A schematic view of this arrangement is shown in Fig. 40.1.

Measurement and reference half cells (giving rise to electrode potentials)

The potential of each half cell arises from a charge separation as follows: At the electrode surface, or at any junction, liquid or solid, there will be a tendency for ions to pass from one phase into the other. If this is at the electrode surface, for example, ions will go from the electrode into solution. If these ions are hydrogen ions, for a pH electrode, and they go into the solution without a corresponding negatively charged ion, a charge separation will be created with the solution becoming more positively charged with hydrogen ions and the electrode becoming more negatively charged (with elec-

<u>A Potentiometric Cell</u>

Measurement and reference half cells

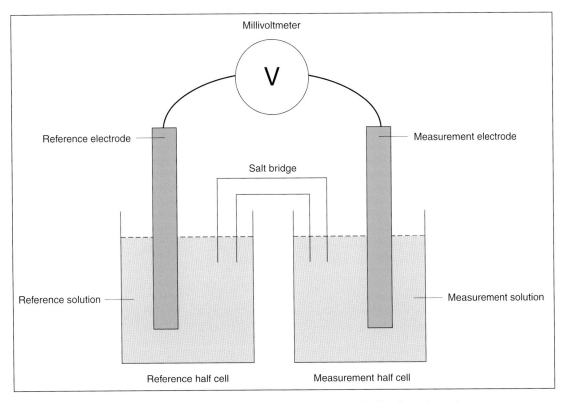

Figure 40.1: *A simple electrode consisting of a measurement half cell and a reference half cell connected by a salt bridge.*

trons). As this process continues the increasing charge separation produces an increasing potential between the electrode and the solution which will oppose further ionic migration, until an equilibrium is reached at which there is no further net movement of ions. This process is illustrated with a zinc electrode in Fig. 40.2.

If the electrode is in contact with a solution with a low concentration of ions, there will be a relatively large outflow of ions from the electrode before equilibrium is reached, and a relatively large potential will be established. Conversely, a concentrated solution will tend to oppose migration of ions from the electrode and will produce a lower potential. In other words the potential produced will vary inversely with the concentration of ions in the solution. The reference electrode works in exactly the same way as the measuring electrode, but is in contact with a solution of constant concentration and should have a constant potential.

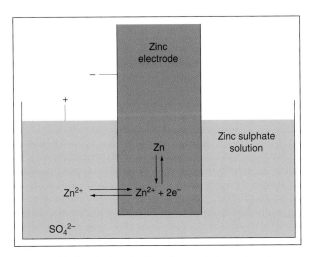

Figure 40.2: *A zinc half cell consisting of a zinc metal electrode in contact with a zinc sulphate solution. Zinc ions will migrate from the electrode into the solution, leaving a small negative charge on the electrode and making the solution more positively charged.*

A Potentiometric Cell

Salt bridge (giving rise to a junction potential)

Measuring system

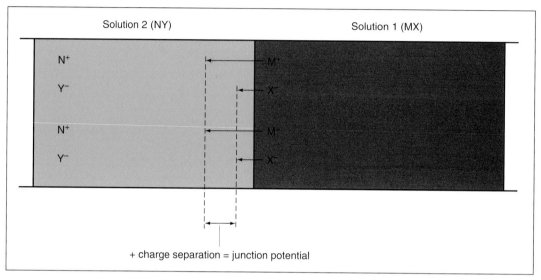

Figure 40.3: *Illustration of junction potential. Solution 1 is a salt consisting of a relatively small metal ion (M) and large anion (X). At the liquid junction, the smaller metal ion will diffuse into the other solution (NY) at a greater rate than the anion, causing a charge separation which is the junction potential.*

Salt bridge (giving rise to a junction potential)
To be able to measure the potential difference between the two half cells there must be an electrical circuit, and to do this there must be electrical contact between the reference electrode solution and the measuring electrode solution. This is usually by direct contact or by a 'salt bridge' as shown in Fig. 40.1.

Just as there is ion migration between electrodes and solutions, there is also ion migration between solutions in contact. If the anions and cations in one of the solutions are a different size they will migrate at different rates, as shown in Fig. 40.3, and this will result in a charge separation, just as with the electrodes above, which will produce a potential which will oppose further charge separation. All electrode systems have liquid junctions and therefore junction potentials. One of the main features of the design of a reference electrode is to minimize the size and variability of the junction potential. For this reason, the most common reference electrode is the 'calomel' (mercuric chloride) electrode. This is a chloride electrode which uses saturated potassium chloride as the reference electrode solution because potassium ions and chloride ions have a similar

ionic size and migrate at a similar rate. However this does not eliminate entirely the junction potential because the unknown solution it is in contact with has a variable composition.

Measuring system
The potential difference is measured with a millivoltmeter, as shown in Fig. 40.4. Typical measuring voltages are 59 mV for each decade (tenfold) change in concentration for a monovalent ion such as hydrogen and sodium, and 29.5 mV for a divalent ion such as calcium. A measurement error of 1 mV from any source (e.g. junction potential) would result in a readout error of 4% for a monovalent ion and 8% for a divalent ion. This means that sensitive, stable millivoltmeters are required for the measurement.

Another requirement for measurement is that the circuit must allow minimal current, because to allow a large current would disturb the ion equilibrium at the electrode surfaces. Electrode membranes must be theoretically capable of electrical conductance, but in practice they have a very high resistance, of the order of 10^9 ohms. Similarly, the millivoltmeter must draw a minimal current from the circuit

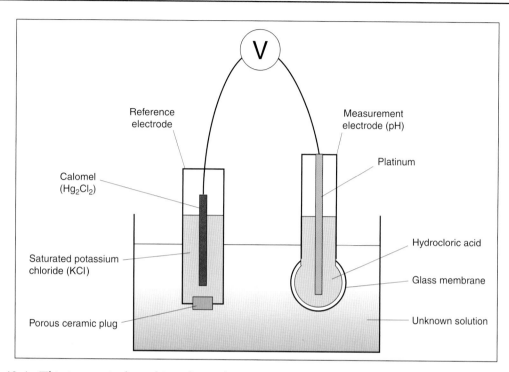

Figure 40.4: *This is a typical working electrode system consisting of a glass pH electrode and a calomel (mercuric chloride) reference electrode, both immersed in a solution whose pH is being measured. The porous ceramic plug forms the salt bridge and controls loss of the internal solution from the reference electrode.*

by having a very high input resistance. This requires special voltmeter design, and a standard voltmeter would not be adequate. Needless to say, in a system which requires high electrical resistance and negligible current to operate, cleanliness is very important, and systems need to be carefully sealed and insulated to give reproducible results.

The electrodes described so far are simple systems with no element of selectivity, and low resistance, and are the basis of the common battery. For measurement purposes a selective membrane is needed and a typical working system is shown in Fig. 40.4.

Calibration

To make useful measurements with a working electrode system, as shown in Fig. 40.4, the system must first be calibrated.

The response of an electrode system is an inverse logarithmic response defined by Nernst equation:

$$\text{EMF (voltage)} = E_{reference} - E_{unknown}$$

$$= \frac{RT}{nF} \ \log_e \ \frac{(A_{references})}{(A_{unknown})}$$

where
R = the gas constant
T = absolute temperature
n = valency charge
F = Faraday constant

It can be seen by this that there is a complex inverse logarithmic relationship between the concentration (or rather the 'activity') of an ion and the voltage produced by an electrode. This means that calibration of the system, and producing a readout, is not a simple matter, as it would be, say, for a colorimetric blood glucose system.

The usual approach is to measure the logarithmic 'slope' of the electrode, by measuring the voltage at two concentrations. Ideally this should be 59 mV for a tenfold change in con-

A Potentiometric Cell

Ways of achieving specificity

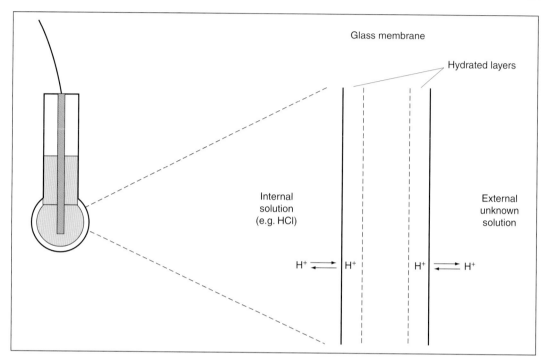

Figure 40.5: *A pH electrode operates on the principle of hydrogen ion exchange on both sides of the membrane. There is no transfer of hydrogen ions through the membrane – an equilibrium is established – although theoretically there must be electronic conduction for the electrode to form part of a measuring circuit. In practice the membrane will have a resistance of 10^9 ohms and there will be a negligible current.*

centration. However electrodes are rarely ideal, and the signal deteriorates with time, so the slope needs to be checked regularly.

Ways of achieving specificity (How do you measure what you need?)

In simple electrodes, specificity for a particular ion is determined by the electrode membrane, which acts by selective ion exchange, e.g. the pH electrode has a glass membrane which acts as a hydrogen ion exchanger. Glass is a complex silicate crystal lattice which contains charged ions (sodium for soda glass). At the surface there is a very thin hydrated layer where these ions can exchange with ions in the liquid in contact (Fig. 40.5). Exchange of ions between the membrane and liquid will take place provided that the physical size of the ion and its electrostatic charge are compatible with the crystal lattice structure, but as membranes become more complex other factors play a more important part.

With standard sodium silicate glass, hydrogen ion exchange is favoured, but an 'alkaline error' occurs due to interference from sodium ions at alkaline pH. At alkaline pH conditions, as the hydrogen ion concentration becomes very low, the relative contribution to the electrode response from sodium ions becomes more significant until it exceeds the hydrogen ion response. In practice, no electrode is absolutely specific for a single ion, and the preference it shows for a particular ion is called the 'selectivity'. In this example, at neutral or acid pH the glass electrode is a hydrogen ion electrode with a high selectivity for hydrogen ions over sodium, but at alkaline pH it has the reverse characteristics. The prime objective of membrane design is to maximize selectivity to avoid interference from other similar ions. In the case of halides, e.g. chloride, this can easily be achieved by using a silver chloride crystal membrane, in which only a chloride ion can fit easily into the crystal lattice. More difficult problems arise when trying to measure calcium in the presence of magnesium and vice versa (both present in similar concentrations in blood), because the ions are similar in size. Even more difficult is the design of an electrode to detect lithium in blood at a concentration of 1 mmol/l against a background of 140 mmol/l of sodium.

By altering the glass composition, electrodes can be produced which respond to sodium and potassium. The best sodium electrode has a selectivity for sodium over potassium of 100:1 and this is clinically useful for biological fluids with high sodium concentration and low potassium. However the best glass potassium electrode has a selectivity for potassium over sodium of 20:1, which is not ideal for blood applications where the sodium concentration is normally about 30 times the potassium concentration. For these applications more selective membranes are needed.

Ion selective membranes

The paradox in developing ion selective membranes is that the membrane must be impermeable to water, so that there is no electrical conduction which would short-circuit the electrode, but ions by their nature have a preference for solution in water. The membrane needs to have a component for which the ion has an equivalent preference either by electrostatic attraction, as in the case of ion exchange, or by substitution of the hydration shell (provided by the water solvent), as in the case of neutral carriers. Living cells often use such carriers for transporting ions and water-borne nutrients across cell membranes which are usually hydrophobic barriers, and this has provided models for the design of ISE membranes.

To have a functional membrane which uses an ion exchanger or neutral carrier, the membrane needs an inert support which must be able to contain and retain the ion carrier, and this usually means it traps the solvent in which the carrier is dissolved.

In the case of calcium sensors, ion-exchange materials have been found which bind calcium with a high selectivity. The electrode consists of a calcium salt of an alkyl phosphate dissolved in di-*n*-octophenyl phosphonate – a solvent

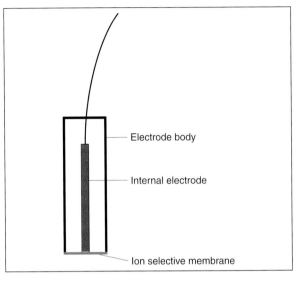

Figure 40.6: A solid-state ion-selective electrode. Because there is electronic conduction across the membrane rather than transfer of ions, there is no necessity for an internal solution, provided that the internal electrode has good electrical contact with the membrane.

which is not volatile and not soluble in water. This is mixed with polyvinyl chloride (PVC) dissolved in a volatile solvent and the mixture is poured onto a flat surface and the volatile solvent allowed to evaporate away. This leaves a thin PVC layer with the calcium exchanger trapped within it. Fig. 40.6 shows a typical example of a solid-state calcium electrode.

In an ideal electrode the carrier would be completely insoluble in water, but in practice it is gradually leached away, leading to a gradual loss of the response of the electrode, which is why electrode membranes usually have to be changed regularly.

Neutral carriers are an alternative to ion exchange, and the most widely used is valinomycin for potassium electrodes. Valinomycin is a large complex ring compound containing six oxygen atoms within the ring structure. It is believed to be able to complex potassium by acting as an alternative to the hydration shell which the ion has when dissolved in water, i.e. the ion will exchange its aqueous hydration shell for valinomycin and migrate from an aqueous solution into a hydrophobic

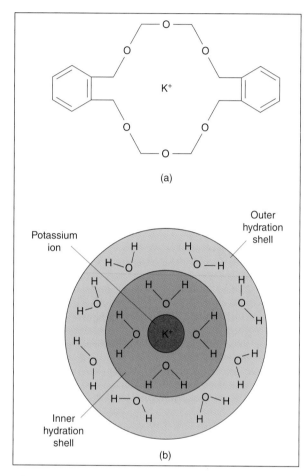

Figure 40.7: *(a) An example of a 'crown ether' compound (dicyclohexyl-18-crown 6) which acts as a substitute hydration shell for an ion such as potassium and is able to transport the ion through a hydrophobic membrane. (b) A potassium ion in solution surrounded by an inner hydration shell and an outer hydration shell of water molecules.*

membrane. The oxygen atoms in the ring structure play an important part in this function, and synthetic analogues of valinomycin have been produced with very similar selectivity. An example of such a compound and a metal ion surrounded by a hydration shell is shown in Fig. 40.7. One of the advantages of neutral carriers is that they tend to be less water-soluble than ion exchangers, which must of necessity have slight solubility. They make membranes which have a longer life. Neutral carriers have been developed for a number of

ions, including sodium, potassium, chloride, lithium and ammonia.

The narrative above is all related to potentiometric electrodes, which have been used for illustration because they include all the problems related to electrochemistry.

Electrochemical Reactions

The description of electrode potential given above is a simplification of the real situation to help illustrate how the electrode works. In fact what is really happening at the electrode surface is that an electrochemical reaction is taking place to produce a charged species prior to the charge separation.

$$Zn \rightarrow Zn^{++} + 2e^-$$

In a conducting material such as a metal electrode, the electron structure is similar to a 'sea' in which the electrons are free to move throughout the solid. The energy of the electrons are filled to a level called the Fermi level. In the solution there is a different situation. The ions are surrounded by a hydration shell (see Fig. 40.7) which effectively separates them from the other ions and the electrons are restricted to different (lower) energy bands. At the instant the electrode comes into contact with the solution the difference in energy levels favours a flow of electrons to equalize the energy and an equilibrium is quickly reached at the state of lowest free energy (known as the Gibbs free energy level). This is the basis of the electrode potential.

This electrochemical reaction takes place spontaneously because of the property of the electrode material to lose an electron and form an ion, and so the main application of these (potentiometric) electrodes is measurement of ions. The concept of electrochemical reactions can be expanded to include reactions which do not occur spontaneously but are promoted by an applied potential. This opens up the possibility of analysis of substances, which do not necessarily exist as ions in solution but which will give rise to an electrochemical reaction in suitable circumstances.

412

Amperometric Electrodes

There is another class of electrodes called amperometric electrodes, because they produce a current rather than a voltage. These electrodes are designed to measure an electrochemical reaction – a chemical reaction which produces or consumes electrons – by measuring an electrical current instead of measuring the voltage produced by a charge separation. The most common of these in clinical use is the oxygen (pO_2) electrode. In the case of the oxygen electrode the reactions are:

oxygen electrode:

$$O_2 + 2H_2O + 2e^- \xrightarrow{-0.7V} H_2O_2 + 2\ OH^-$$

peroxide electrode:

$$H_2O_2 \xrightarrow{+0.7V} 2H^+ + O_2 + 2e^-$$

The first reaction is used in the standard oxygen (pO_2) electrode, known as the Clarke electrode while the second is used in some glucose electrodes, as described later, to measure peroxide produced by the enzyme glucose oxidase.

It can be seen from these electrochemical reactions that the reactions are facilitated by an applied voltage (0.7 V) and this voltage can add to the specificity of the electrode response. The main feature of these electrodes is that a constant voltage is applied to the measurement electrodes and the resulting current (in microamps) is proportional to the rate of the reaction. This is a direct linear relationship, in contrast to the complex inverse logarithmic response of potentiometric electrodes. Because current is being measured, these electrodes (e.g. a pO_2 electrode) do not need a reference electrode. However, the reaction and current will also be related to the surface area of the electrode.

Polarography

This application of electrochemistry is also known as polarography. The voltage applied is a polarizing voltage, and the electrochemical cell is called a polarographic cell.

To get a measurement of the analyte concerned, or pO_2 (the partial pressure of oxygen is not strictly speaking 'concentration' but is equivalent in gaseous terms), the rate of reaction should be constant, so the pO_2 concentration should be constant. A key requirement of this type of system is that the electrode should not consume the oxygen at the electrode surface at a faster rate than oxygen can diffuse through the electrode solution to the electrode surface, otherwise the current will fall as the pO_2 in contact with it falls. To maintain a steady state to allow measurement, measuring cells must be designed so that the electrode at which the reaction takes place is very small (e.g. a needle point), so that a minimal amount of the analyte is consumed in the measurement. This means that a typical system will only produce a current of microamp proportions, which will require a specifically designed ammeter for measurement.

Oxygen electrode

To have a functional electrode, the electrodes at which the electrochemical reaction takes place must be in contact with a constant solution – one with a constant resistance so that there will be no variation in resistance which would affect the applied voltage, and hence the current produced. The Clarke oxygen electrode consists of electrodes in contact with an electrolyte solution which is contained by a silicone rubber membrane. Gaseous oxygen can pass freely through the membrane, but the membrane is hydrophobic, not allowing water or dissolved electrolytes to pass through and change the composition, and resistance, of the electrolyte solution. This is shown in Fig. 40.8.

Glucose electrodes

Glucose electrodes use a combination of a specific enzyme and a specific polarization voltage to provide a response which is specific for glucose. At the present time there are two different enzymes and three different electron transfer reactions in common use. The simplest form of glucose electrode is to use the enzyme glucose oxidase in conjunction with an oxygen electrode. Glucose oxidase catalyses the reaction:

glucose + O_2 + $2H_2O$ → gluconic acid + H_2O_2

413

Amperometric Electrodes

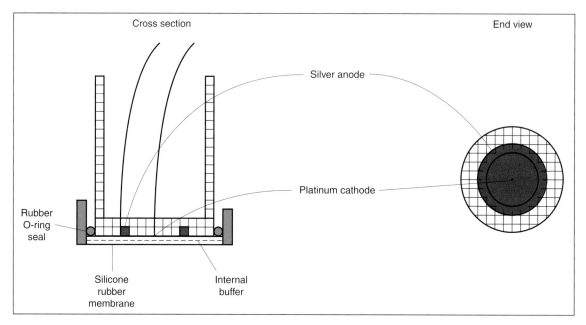

Figure 40.8: *A Clarke oxygen electrode. This consists of a very small area platinum cathode surrounded by an annular silver anode. Both are in contact with an internal buffer enclosed within a hydrophobic silicone rubber membrane. Oxygen can diffuse freely through the membrane and dissolve in the internal buffer. The resulting electrochemical reaction at the platinum cathode is measured.*

The oxygen electrode can measure the fall in pO_2 as a measurement of glucose consumed in the reaction. Unfortunately, if the cell is open to the atmosphere, oxygen will be replenished from atmospheric oxygen, and there will also be problems if whole blood is used from the oxygen binding effects of haemoglobin. Because of these problems better applications have been developed.

The glucose oxidase/peroxide electrode. This is used to detect the peroxide produced by the reaction, with an applied potential of + 0.7 V.

The glucose oxidase/ferrocene electrode. This electrode uses ferrocene as an electron transfer agent in the following electrochemical reaction.

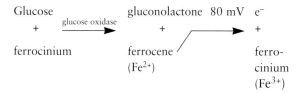

This is the basis of the 'Medisense®' glucose stick assay, and is illustrated in Fig. 40.9.

The glucose dehydrogenase/ferricyanide electrode. This electrode works in a similar way, but with a different enzyme and electron transfer agent.

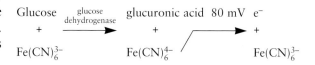

This is the basis of the Boehringer Mannheim Corporation (BMC) 'Advantage®' glucose stick assay.

Drug interference

The three types of glucose electrode described here are in common use and are in general good measuring devices, but it is known that a number of substances including common drugs such as paracetamol can interfere and give a signal with these systems. This is because many compounds, including most drugs, can produce an electrochemical reaction, given a large enough polarizing voltage. It is on this basis that therapeutic drugs and many other biological compounds can be measured by chro-

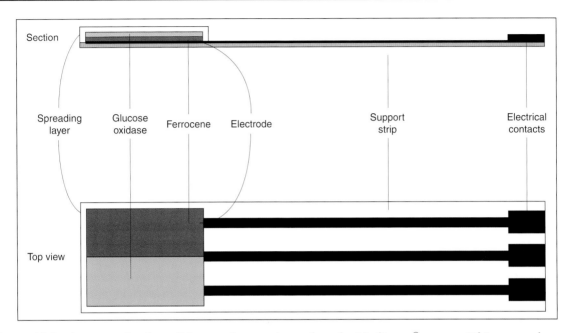

Figure 40.9: *An example of a solid-state glucose electrode – the Medisense® system. This system has three contacts – a central common electrode, one in contact with the ferrocene alone (for non-specific reactions) and one in contact with glucose oxidase plus ferrocene. The difference in the two signals is the measurement of glucose.*

matography using a polarographic cell as an electrochemical detector.

Electrochemical detectors

These detectors are a development of the polarographic electrode for use as a detector in high performance liquid chromatography (HPLC). A typical laboratory application for this would be measurement of catecholamines (adrenaline, noradrenaline) for the detection of phaeochromocytoma.

The electrodes described so far operate in stable conditions, e.g. they are in contact with a constant solution. In a chromatographic system, selectivity is provided by chromatographic separation of similar compounds, e.g. adrenaline and noradrenaline (as opposed to having a selective membrane), but the solvent systems used for the separation are variable, so the resistance of the solution in the measuring cell will vary, and that would affect the applied voltage. To overcome this problem a third electrode is used in the HPLC measurement cell which has the function of monitoring the

applied voltage and holding it at a steady value through a feedback circuit.

Complex Electrodes

These consist of an electrode within an electrode, and the most common example is the pCO_2 (carbon dioxide) electrode found in all blood gas analysers.

This electrode consists of a standard pH electrode in contact with a weak bicarbonate buffer and encased in a PVC membrane. This is shown in Fig. 40.10. The PVC membrane is permeable to gases, e.g. carbon dioxide, but impermeable to water. Carbon dioxide diffuses across the membrane and dissolves in the buffer and changes the equilibrium of the bicarbonate buffer.

$$CO_2 + H_2O \rightarrow H_2CO_3 \rightarrow HCO_3^- + H^+$$

In doing so the pH of the buffer will change, and this change is measured by the pH electrode.

Safeguards

Policy

Software

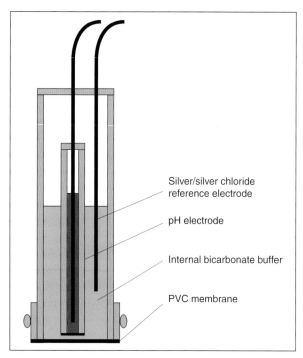

Silver/silver chloride
reference electrode

pH electrode

Internal bicarbonate buffer

PVC membrane

Figure 40.10: *A pCO$_2$ electrode consisting of a pH electrode and an internal silver/silver chloride reference electrode. The CO$_2$ diffuses through the PVC and changes the pH of the internal buffer.*

Ammonia electrodes are made in a similar way, with a pH electrode immersed in a buffer. The differences are that the buffer is different; and the membrane contains the neutral carrier nonactin to assist the transfer of the ammonia.

$$NH_3 + H_2O \rightarrow NH_4^+ + OH^-$$

Safeguards

Policy
One of the main applications of ISEs is Point of Care Testing (POCT) where the tests will be done by nurses and clinicians without formal laboratory training. As there are numerous problems which can occur with ISE measurements, there must be safeguards built into the whole process (not just the measurement system) for this application to be acceptable, and they should be made clear in a hospital

policy on POCT. Without this safeguard patients are placed at risk and the institution has a risk control issue.

The main input of the laboratory is the production of the specification which the instrument must meet (i.e. instrument performance). The specification will (should) address issues such as selectivity of the electrodes. Fortunately modern technology allows us to build in suitable safeguards, as outlined below.

Software
Instrument checks
Clearly modern instruments will be operated by computers which will check the performance of functions such as electrode signal (e.g. slope, mV/decade) and response time, and other checks such as temperature, air bubbles, membrane leaks, etc. For a laboratory-based instrument, where the staff should understand the electrode characteristics, it is acceptable to have a high level override facility to produce measurements in an emergency situation. For POCT applications, if an electrode response falls outside specified limits the test must be disabled until the problem is resolved.

There are other useful functions which are enabled with a computer-controlled instrument.

Identification
Training is an important feature of POCT, and an operator function can be used so that only those trained to operate the instrument are allowed to use it.

Remote lockout
This is facility where the instrument is connected to the laboratory computer, which monitors the quality control performance of the instrument, and locks the instrument if the quality control falls outside predefined limits. The laboratory computer then alerts laboratory staff of the problem.

Quality control and assurance
Quality control is real-time checking of the instrument. This involves analysing material of known composition and checking that the results obtained are within clinically significant

limits, as defined by the professional bodies (such as the national quality assurance bodies). Quality control should be performed regularly by the operators (e.g. nurses and clinicians) doing the tests, and an essential part of their training is the significance of doing quality control, recording results and what action to take should the QC check fail. This training should be given by experienced laboratory professionals.

Quality assurance is a retrospective examination of instrument performance, usually done as part of an external EQA scheme. The UK laboratory accreditation agency, CPA (UK) Ltd, require that laboratories participate in a recognized EQA scheme and maintain an adequate performance. If POCT instruments are under the control of the main laboratory, the laboratory accreditation is applied to the POCT service provided that it is operated to an acceptable standard. This approach is recommended as the best way of providing quality patient care at minimal risk.

External quality assessment is best supervised by trained laboratory staff, although the tests can and probably should be done by the actual users. A large-scale audit showed no evidence of the operator being a source of error.

Maintenance checks
Maintenance checks are usually planned preventative maintenance such as replacing tubing, seals, electrodes, etc. These tests are best done by experienced laboratory professionals, but if they are done by non-laboratory staff, rigorous training on the significance of the checks is vital.

Training
Training of all users is an essential feature of a hospital POCT policy. For modern instruments the training need not be in great depth or time consuming, provided that adequate safeguards have been built into the instrument.

Training should include not only operation of the instrument, but an understanding of all error signals, the significance of results, and the importance of recording results and QC procedures.

Economics

While low capital cost is often coupled with high revenue costs, it does not necessarily follow that the expensive instruments are cheap to run. In practice POCT is not cheap, and an outline of the possible costs involved are as follows:

- Capital cost £0 to £30 000
- Revenue consumables, calibration, quality control, syringes, etc.
  * cost of each request £0.10 – £5
  * cost of calibration £1000 – £5000 p.a.
  * consumables £0.20
- Internal QC Typically £3 per QC or £250 per year.
- Operator time Time taken by doctors/ nurses to do the tests
- Electrodes/spares up to £150/electrode. An instrument with five replaceable electrodes may cost up to £2000 per year in electrodes
- Maintenance contract 10%–20% of the purchase price.
- In-house support Ten major POCT analysers would require one WTE
- External QA External QA schemes currently cost typically £40 per instrument per year.

Summary of costs
For a hospital with five blood gas instruments of varying complexity, the summary of costs for one year was as follows:

Reagents & consumables	£20 900
Internal QC material	£1 250
External QA scheme	£200
Maintenance contracts	£13 000
Staff (laboratory)	£8 240
Total	£43 590

This cost should be assessed against the cost of vacuum tube systems, particularly when a survey showed that POCT did not have a significant impact on patient waiting times.

Further reading

Crompton R G, Sanders G H W. *Electrode Potentials*. 1996: Oxford University Press.

Hirst A D, Stevens J F. Electrodes in Clinical Chemistry. *Annals of Clinical Biochemistry*, 1985; **22**: 460–488.

Van Ysek P (ed). *Modern Techniques in Electroanalysis*. 1996: John Wiley & Sons, Chichester.

41 ULTRAVIOLET AND VISIBLE SPECTROPHOTOMETRY, FLUORIMETRY, NEPHELOMETRY AND TURBIDIMETRY

Bernard F Rocks

Few of the chemical constituents of blood, plasma or urine can be determined directly. Clinical biochemists have, however, developed indirect means of measuring quantitatively many of the constituents of clinical interest. Frequently the method involves adding to the diluted sample a substance (the reagent) that reacts specifically with the particular component to be quantitated (the analyte) to form a product that is measured relatively easily. Whenever possible the assay conditions are such as to produce a product, the quantity of which is directly proportional to the original concentration of the analyte.

When light strikes matter of any kind, the interaction may change the intensity, direction, wavelength or phase of the incident light. Absorption, fluorescence, and scatter are three of the many optical effects that have been exploited for analytical purposes. The majority of quantitative measurements made in clinical biochemistry laboratories are based on the production of coloured reaction products, so that most frequently photoelectric absorbance devices such as colorimeters or spectrophotometers are used. Other common light measurement based methods include fluorimetry, nephelometry and turbidimetry. The essential features of these techniques are discussed in this chapter.

Ultraviolet and Visible Spectrophotometry

Absorption photometry forms the basis for most of the quantitative analyses carried out in clinical biochemistry laboratories. The primary reasons for this are ease of measurement, satisfactory accuracy and precision, and that the instrumentation is stable, reliable and relatively inexpensive.

Spectrophotometers
Single-beam instruments
Spectrophotometers may be divided into two basic types, the single-beam and the double-beam instrument. In each type, although the light paths are different, many of the basic

Ultraviolet and Visible Spectrophotometry

Spectrophotometers

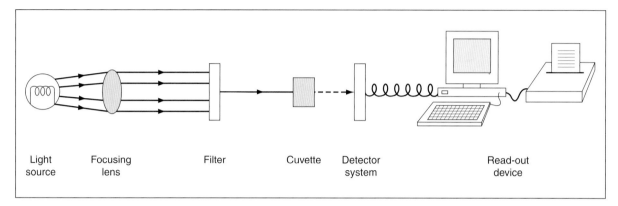

| Light source | Focusing lens | Filter | Cuvette | Detector system | Read-out device |

Figure 41.1: Basic components of a simple photometer.

components are the same. A simple single-beam photometer is illustrated in Fig. 41.1. Clinical biochemists often refer to this type of photometer as a colorimeter.

The light source provides radiant energy over the wavelengths of interest. For work in the visible range it is now common to use tungsten–quartz–halogen lamps (340–800 nm). These lamps may also be used for near infrared and near ultraviolet measurements. For work at shorter UV wavelengths a deuterium discharge lamp is normally used. Below 360 nm these sources provide a strong continuum which, together with fused silica lenses and cuvettes, fulfils most needs in the UV region. The power supply to the lamp must be of high stability.

The wavelength appropriate for the particular assay is usually selected by using narrow-bandwidth high-transmittance interference filters. Interference filters are expensive and some inexpensive colorimeters use filters of coloured glass or dyed gelatin (sandwiched between layers of glass). Spectrophotometers generate monochromatic light by means of a prism or grating monochromator rather than by using filters.

The cuvette is a transparent vessel which holds the solution being measured. The design of the cuvette and the means of admitting the sample to it and subsequently removing it vary with instrument and analyser type. The sample solution, held in the cuvette, absorbs a proportion of the incident radiation; the remainder is transmitted to a detector where it generates an electrical signal.

Many different types of photodetectors are in use. Various solid-state photodiodes and diode arrays are now frequently used in visible and near infrared instruments. These detectors are sturdy, inexpensive and have a linear response over several decades of light intensity. However, they give a low response to UV light. Where high sensitivity is required, and for UV work, vacuum photomultiplier tubes are used. The output from the detector may need amplifying and will need to be expressed as its logarithm in order for it to be linearly related to concentration. Both of these operations are conveniently carried out by means of a logarithmic amplifier. The signal, after any necessary transformations, may be displayed by a meter, printed or stored for future use.

In single-beam instruments a blank (for example a cuvette containing water) is used to set zero, then the standards and samples are read. Interferences from variations in sample turbidity and source intensity changes and other instrument fluctuations are not automatically compensated for. In some modern designs a second detector is used to monitor the intensity of the light source and to electronically compensate for lamp drift. Single-beam instruments are well suited for quantitative absorption measurements at a single wavelength. Easy maintenance and low cost are distinct advantages of this type.

Double-beam spectrophotometers

A double-beam instrument has two light paths, both originating from the same source. One beam passes through the sample cuvette and the other through the blank or reference cuvette. This is usually achieved by directing the light beam from the monochromator towards a rotating mirror or chopper that alternately directs light through the reference cuvette and the sample cuvette. Light emerging from each cuvette is then reflected towards the detector. The detector output is consequently an alternating signal with an amplitude proportional to the ratio of the intensities of the sample and reference beams. The resulting electrical signals are processed electronically to give the absorbance on a readout device. Double-beam systems correct automatically for changes in light intensity from the light source, fluctuations in instrument electronics, and absorption by the blank. An instrument of this kind is often provided with a motor-driven monochromator so that automatic scanning and recording of an entire spectrum is possible.

Beer's law

The mathematical basis for quantitative measurements is based on the experimentally derived Beer–Lambert relationship. Lambert's law states that the proportion of radiant energy absorbed by a substance is independent of the intensity of the incident radiation. Beer's law states that the absorption of radiant energy is proportional to the total number of molecules in the light path. It is not possible to measure directly the amount of radiation absorbed by a substance and it is usually determined by measuring the ratio of incident radiation falling on the sample, I_0, and the transmitted radiation which finally emerges from the sample, I. Using these measurements, the Beer–Lambert law can be expressed as

$$log_{10} (I_0/I) = \varepsilon c l$$

where c is concentration of the substance in moles per litre, l is the optical path length in centimetres and ε is the molar absorption coefficient for the substance expressed as litres per mole per centimetre. The values for I and I_0 cannot be measured in absolute terms and measurements are most conveniently made by expressing I as a percentage of I_0. This value is known as the percentage transmittance, T, and gives a linear relationship with concentration if the logarithm of its reciprocal is used. This reciprocal logarithmic function of I and I_0, is known as absorbance, A.

$$\%T = ((I/I_0) \times 100 \text{ and}$$
$$A = log_{10} (100/T) = -log_{10}(I_0/I).$$

Absorbance is a most convenient parameter since, from Beer's Law, it is directly proportional to the concentration of the absorbing species.

Spectrophotometers are usually linear over the range 0–2 A and chromophores can be measured at concentrations as low as 10^{-6} mol/l. Test values are usually calculated by comparing the absorbance readings of the test samples with readings obtained from assaying a series of standards or calibrators of known value.

Applications

Some of the many substances determined by UV and visible spectrophotometry include the following: albumin, bilirubin, calcium, chloride, cholesterol, creatinine, glucose, iron, phosphate, proteins, urea, uric acid, and the enzymes acid phosphatase, alkaline phosphatase, aspartate transaminase, creatine phosphokinase and lactate dehydrogenase. Information on analytical methodologies can be found in Burtis & Ashwood and a more detailed account of UV/visible spectrophotometry has been given by Skoog, West & Holler.

Fluorimetry

When light impinges on a molecular substance, enough energy may be absorbed to cause the substance to alter its electron configuration and place some of the electrons in an excited state. This state is short-lived and the excited electrons quickly return to the ground state. If the substance is of a certain chemical structure, the transition may be a multi-step process with the major step resulting in release of emitted light of lower energy than the excitation light. The other steps in

Fluorimetry

Fluorimeters

the transition to the ground state are mostly vibrational energy loss due to electron collisions. Emitted light that is produced as the substance passes from an excited state to the ground state is called fluorescence. Many molecules demonstrate fluorescence and this property provides the basis of a sensitive method of quantitation. In general most compounds which exhibit fluorescence are those which contain multiple conjugated bond systems with the associated delocalized π electrons. Most molecules that fluoresce intensely have rigid planar structures and electron-donating groups. For dilute solutions, the intensity of fluorescence is directly proportional to the concentration of the fluorophore. The wavelength maxima of absorption and emission are also useful in the identification of substances. Analysis of blood and urine for porphyrins is a good example of the qualitative and quantitative use of fluorimetry.

Fluorimeters

When a substance displays the property of fluorescence it will, if irradiated at a specific wavelength, absorb some of that radiant energy and emit it, with varying degrees of loss, at a longer wavelength. The basic components of a fluorimeter are essentially similar to those of a photometer. Figure 41.2 indicates the optical arrangement in most fluorimeters. The appropriate excitation wavelength is filtered from the source and is directed into the solution held in the cuvette. The resulting fluorescent light is emitted in all directions but it is usual to select that part emerging at right angles to the incident beam, the unabsorbed part of which passes through the cuvette and enters a light trap. The emission wavelength is selected from the emitted or secondary light and the beam is directed onto the detector, usually a photomultiplier. The output from this is amplified and displayed. If the amplifier gain and the excita-

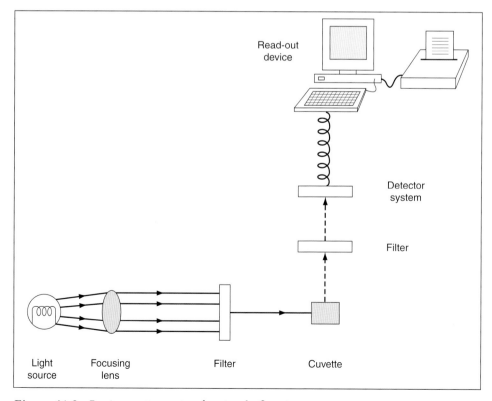

Figure 41.2: *Basic components of a simple fluorimeter.*

tion source are constant the fluorescent output reading is linearly related to the concentration. Linearity is maintained over a 100-fold concentration range: this is a range much wider than is feasible with light absorption measurements, which are prone to considerable error at low or high absorbances. A spectrofluorimeter employs monochromators instead of filters for wavelength selection.

In fluorimetry, measurements are not based on difference, as in absorption, therefore increasing the intensity of the light source will correspondingly increase the fluoresence signal. Fluorescence measurements are generally 10 to 1000 times more sensitive than absorption measurements. A typical commercially available fluorimeter should be able to measure high quantum yield fluorophores at concentrations as low as 10^{-9} mol/l. Many older fluorimeters use mercury vapour lamps. These lamps have their output concentrated into a relatively small number of sharply defined bands which limit the choice of excitation wavelength. A high-intensity source with a nearly continuous spectrum is the xenon arc. However, this source generates ozone and runs very hot. Most fluorimeters aimed specifically at the clinical market use either a tungsten halogen bulb or a rapidly firing xenon flash tube.

Ratio mode fluorimeters
To compensate for lamp instability, single-beam instruments are often operated in ratio mode. Light from the source is reflected alternatively between the sample cuvette and a second reference photomultiplier tube. The ratio of the signals from the detectors is used to compensate for changes in intensity caused by an unstable source.

Double-beam spectrofluorimeters
Typically the beam of light from the source is chopped and split between the sample cuvette and a reference cuvette. The fluorescence produced by each cuvette is monitored by a single photomultiplier tube electrically phased with the chopper. The difference signal allows subtraction of the fluorescence produced in the reference cuvette and also compensates for lamp drift and flicker.

Fluorescence polarization analysers
These instruments are basically filter fluorimeters to which a set of excitation and emission polarizers have been fitted. Fluorescence intensity is measured both parallel and perpendicular to the plane of the excitation beam. The degree of fluorescence depolarization depends on molecular rotation, which depends on molecular size. This technique has been applied to homogeneous (non-separation) immunoassays. In these applications, typically, a competitive binding immunoassay is performed in which an antigen and a fluorescent labelled antigen compete for binding sites on an antibody. The binding of the fluorescent label to the large antibody, which rotates slowly, will cause the fluorescent light to remain highly polarized. Conversely, the unbound fluorescent labelled antigen is free to rotate more rapidly and will produce depolarized fluorescence.

Some fluorimeters of this type are dedicated to the measurement of only one fluorescent species. For example the Abbott TDx® analyser system uses fluorescein labelled immunoassay reagents exclusively. Because fluorescein absorbs in the visible region a tungsten halogen light source can be used. Compared with other fluorimetric techniques sensitivity is low and is applicable only to the assay of small molecules. The TDx polarization fluorimeter is relatively simple and reliable and is widely used for therapeutic drug monitoring.

Time-resolved fluorimeters
A problem often encountered with fluorescence based immunoassays (particularly homogeneous assays) is the high background fluorescence associated with biological samples. The use of time-resolved measurements and labels with long fluorescence decay times have circumvented this limitation. Using this technique the fluorescence from the analyte is monitored only after the background fluorescence has decayed. Automated systems using highly fluorescent lanthanide chelates are commercially available for a wide range of immunoassays. In the Wallac DELFIA® system measurement is with a time-resolved fluorimeter which, for europium chelates, supplies 1000 pulses of light per second. The detector

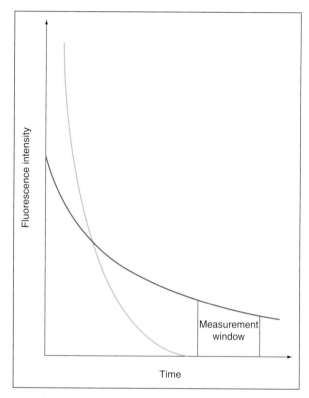

Figure 41.3: Principle of time-resolved fluorimetry. The long decay-time emission is measured in a time window after the background fluorescence has become insignificant.

switches on 400 microseconds after each excitation pulse and collects emitted light, at 613 nm, for 400 microseconds (see Fig. 41.3). Detection limits as low as 10^{-14} mol/l of lanthanide chelates are possible. For a comprehensive account of fluorescence measurement see the textbook by Skoog, West & Holler.

Turbidimetry and Nephelometry

These related techniques are commonly employed in clinical laboratories. Both are based on the measurement of particle-induced light scatter. When light is directed through a solution containing suspended particles some of the light will be scattered, some will be absorbed and the remainder will be transmitted through the liquid. This interaction can be used to measure the concentration of particles in suspension by measurement of light transmitted (turbidimetry) or of the light scattered (nephelometry).

Light scatter involves a direct interaction between light and the particle it strikes. When a light beam strikes a particle, its electric field moves the particle's electrons in one direction relative to the nucleus. The electrons move back and forth in phase with the frequency of the incident light wave. This produces an oscillating dipole the size of which depends on the electric field strength (related to frequency) and polarizability of the particle's electrons. The oscillating dipole becomes a source of electromagnetic radiation radiating light, of the same frequency as the incident light, but in all directions. The amount and distribution of scattered light also depends on particle concentration and size, and on the polarization of the light beam.

For particles smaller than one-tenth the wavelength of the incident light, the re-radiated light waves are in phase and reinforce each other resulting in a symmetrical, though not spherical, pattern of scattered light. This is termed Rayleigh scattering. Larger particles (immunoglobulin–antigen complexes, for example) act as a number of randomly spaced point sources, and destructive interference between light arising from different sites within the particle will occur, resulting in a maximum and minimum pattern of re-radiated light. This is known as Rayleigh–Debye scattering and together with Rayleigh scattering is illustrated in Fig. 41.4. More light is scattered forward as the particle size increases and measurement of this asymmetric scatter can be used to measure particle size. Short wavelength light (blue) is scattered much more than longer wavelength light (red). The principles of light-scattering immunoassays have been reviewed.

Applications

Immunoassays involving nephelometry and turbidimetry as detection systems are widely used to measure the concentrations of specific proteins. The protein solution and the appropriate antibody are mixed together and allowed to react to form large complexes that scatter

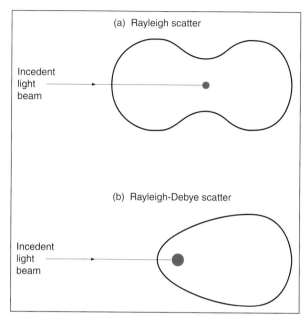

Figure 41.4: Two-dimensional angular distribution patterns for: (a) Rayleigh light scatter from a small particle, (b) Rayleigh–Debye scatter from a large particle (diameter similar to or less than the wavelength of the incident light).

more light than the antibody or protein alone. The turbidity produced by precipitation of proteins with sulphosalicylic acid has been used for many years as a non-specific method for determining the total amount of protein in urine and CSF. The large light scatter produced when cetylpyridinium chloride is added to urine containing mucopolysaccharides is another well-established use of turbidimetry.

Turbidimeters
In theory turbidity can be measured in any standard photometer or spectrophotometer. Because a small change in transmitted light is measured in the presence of a large background signal, instruments with a low signal to noise ratio are desirable. A simple dedicated turbidimeter would consist of a quartz halogen light source, an narrow band interference filter, sample cuvette holder and a photodiode or photomultiplier (Fig. 41.5). Use of short wavelength light offers the advantage of increased scatter and thus a larger signal, but in biological solutions

absorption of the light will also increase. Consequently antigen–antibody complex formation is usually measured in the range 340–400 nm. For good precision timed reagent addition, mixing and reading are necessary. When particle size increases slowly with time the rate of decrease in transmitted light is best calculated from multipoint measurements. Many automated discretionary photometric analysers are commonly used for turbidimetric assays.

Nephelometers
Nephelometers usually comprise a light source, incident light filter, sample holder and a detector set at an angle so as to avoid direct transmitted light. Provided the filters (or monochromators) for incident and emitted light are set to the same wavelength fluorimeters, in which the scattered light is measured at 90°, can be used, though with limited sensitivity. (Dedicated nephelometers do not require an emission monochromator but cutoff filters may be used to prevent fluorescent light from reaching the detector.) Light scatter measured at 90° is weaker than forward light scatter. Theoretically the best sensitivity is attained by placing the detector angle as close to 180° as possible. This requires a tightly focused incident light beam and excellent optics. In practice clinical nephelometers use detector angles between 90° and 170° to the axis of incident light (see Fig. 41.5). Nephelometric measurements made at angles other than 90° to the incident light are best made from round rather than square faced cuvettes. At these detector angles, round cuvettes minimize reflection of the measured light by the cuvette walls.

A tungsten or quartz halogen bulb is frequently used. Alternative sources include xenon lamps, mercury-arc lamps, light-emitting diodes and lasers. The helium neon laser is especially useful for nephelometry because it has a high intensity, narrow beam that does not require focusing or collimating optics. Unfortunately the long wavelength, red light (632.8 nm), is not scattered as much as short wavelength light. The detector must be well shielded to minimize interference from stray light. Low noise photomultiplier tubes are the most commonly used.

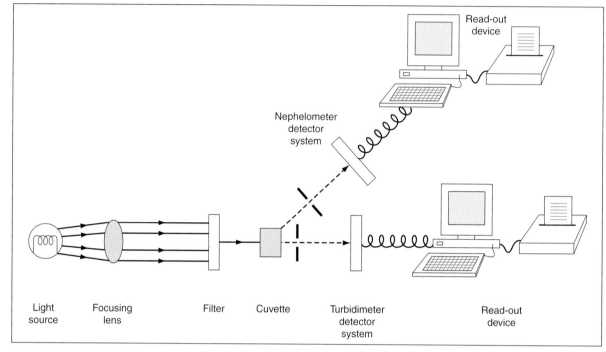

Figure 41.5: Basic components of a turbidimeter, which measures transmitted light, and a nephelometer, which measures scattered light.

The wavelength for optimum scatter by fully formed antibody–antigen complexes is about 460 nm. However, in kinetic immunoassays it has been shown that the optimum wavelength changes as the immune complexes grow. For these widely used assays monochromatic light is undesirable and incident light over a broad band (typically 450–550 nm) provides more reproducible peak rates.

The Beckman Array® is a well-established example of a clinical laboratory nephelometer. Automated sample dilution, antiserum addition and antigen excess checking are some of the features of this type of dedicated analyser. Electronic differentiation of the light signal is used to identify and record the maximum rate of reaction and through a stored calibration curve relate it to concentration.

Nephelometry or turbidimetry?

In general nephelometry has the potential to be more sensitive and give faster results than turbidimetry. Turbidimetry, on the other hand, does not require specialized instruments and can be carried out on many of the currently available automated clinical analysers.

Maintenance and Quality Assurance

The manufacturers of most analytical instruments and automated analysers publish operating manuals that describe routine maintenance and specific detailed performance checks. These procedures should be carried out, and documented, at the intervals specified by the manufacturer.

The accuracy of monochromators needs particular attention to ensure reliable instrument performance. Monochromator drive mechanisms wear and fail periodically. The use of a light source that emits narrow bands at known wavelength (often the instrument's own source) can be used for wavelength checking and calibration. For example, xenon and mercury lamp lines are suitable. Didymium glass filters, and standard solutions of known absorbance, are available for checking wavelength calibration and linearity of absorbance readings. Manufacturers of fluorimeters and nephelometers may supply special cuvettes (containing a fluorescent substance or a stable colloid) that are designed to be used for checking and adjusting their instruments.

Further Reading

Burtis C A, Ashwood E R. *Tietz Fundamentals of Clinical Chemistry*. 4th edn, 1995: WB Saunders Company, Philadelphia.

Chen A K. Nephelometry. In: Sheehan C. *Clinical Immunology: Principles and Laboratory Diagnosis*. 1990: JB Lippincott Company, Philadelphia: 179–189.

Skoog D A, West D M, Holler F J. *Fundamentals of Analytical Chemistry*. 2nd edn 1992: Saunders College, Fort Worth.

42 ATOMIC ABSORPTION AND EMISSION SPECTROMETRY

Andrew Taylor

Introduction

Atomic absorption and emission spectrometry are techniques that can be used to measure the concentrations of individual elements in body fluids and tissues. The major applications are to the measurement of essential minerals and trace elements e.g. sodium, magnesium, zinc and copper, and toxic substances such as aluminium and lead. These techniques allow for accurate measurements at very low concentrations in complex biological samples.

Principles

Spectroscopy is the study of interactions between matter and electromagnetic radiation, and when applied to quantitative analysis, the term spectrometry is used. Different types of spectroscopy are concerned with various regions of the electromagnetic spectrum (e.g. X-rays, UV light, infrared radiation), properties of the matter with which the interactions occur (e.g. molecular vibration, electron transitions) and the physical interactions involved (i.e. scattering, absorption or emission of radiation). Analytical atomic absorption and atomic emission spectrometry are quantitative techniques which exploit interactions between UV and visible light and the outer shell electrons of free, gaseous, uncharged atoms.

Every element has a characteristic atomic structure with a positively charged nucleus surrounded by the number of electrons necessary to provide neutrality. These electrons occupy discrete energy levels but it is possible for an electron to be moved from one level to another within the atom by the introduction of energy (Figure 42.1). This energy may be supplied by collisions with other atoms or with free electrons, or as photons from light. Such transitions will occur only if the available energy is equal to

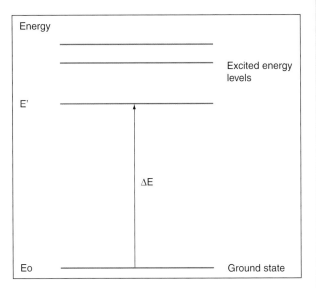

Figure 42.1: Partial energy level diagram showing absorption of energy to raise the atom from the ground state to an excited level.

Principles

the difference between two levels (ΔE). Uncharged atoms may exist at the lowest energy level or ground state, or at any one of a series of excited states depending on how many electrons have been moved to higher energy levels, although it is usual to consider just the first transition. Energy levels and the ΔEs associated with electron transitions are unique for each element.

The ΔE for movements of outer shell electrons in most elements correspond to the energy equivalent to UV–visible radiation and it is these transitions which are used for atomic spectrometry. The energy of a photon is characterized by

$$E = h\upsilon \qquad (1)$$

where h = the Planck constant and υ = the frequency of the waveform corresponding to that photon (the dual concept of light as waveform and discrete particles is not considered further here). Furthermore, frequency and wavelength are related as

$$\upsilon = c/\lambda \qquad (2)$$

where c = the velocity of light and λ = the wavelength. Therefore,

$$E = hc/\lambda \qquad (3)$$

and it follows that a specific transition, ΔE, is associated with a unique wavelength.

When light (radiant energy) of a characteristic wavelength enters an analytical system, outer shell electrons of the corresponding atoms will be excited as energy is absorbed (Fig. 42.1). Consequently the amount of light transmitted from the system to the detector will be reduced. This is understood as *atomic absorption spectrometry* (AAS). Under appropriate conditions outer shell electrons may also be excited by thermal energy (i.e. collisions with other atoms). As these electrons return to the more stable ground state energy is lost, some of which will be in the form of emitted light, which can be measured with a detector (Fig. 42.2). This is *atomic emission spectrometry* (AES).

It follows from equations (1) and (2) that the wavelengths of the absorbed and emitted light are the same and are unique to a given element. It is this which makes AAS and AES *specific*, so

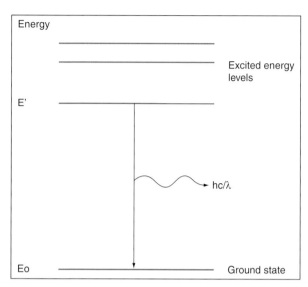

Figure 42.2: *Partial energy level diagram showing emission of energy as light as atom drops from the excited level to the ground state.*

that one element can be measured even in the presence of an enormous excess of chemically similar element.

The Boltzmann equation relates the energies associated with different states to the atomic structure and, from the equation, the proportion of an atom population present as excited atoms compared with ground state atoms can be calculated. The proportion is influenced by two features, temperature and the element. At the typical operating temperatures of around 2000°C, the ratio is at least 10^{-6}:1 for most elements and AAS affords superior sensitivity to AES. With systems that provide higher temperatures (see below) the proportion changes and AES may be favoured. The atomic structures of the alkali metals (e.g. sodium, potassium, lithium) are such that the ΔEs are relatively small, corresponding to longer wavelengths and although at about 2000°C the proportion of excited atoms is not high (10^{-4}–10^{-6}:1), the concentrations of sodium and potassium in biological specimens are such that flame AES (also called flame photometry) is a well established technique for measuring these metals in clinical laboratories.

Atomic absorption spectrometry can be used for the determination of more than 60 elements with instrumentation that is comparatively cheap and simple to operate and it affords sufficient sensitivity to measure many of these elements at the concentrations present in clinical specimens. A similar range of elements can be measured by atomic emission spectrometry. Flame photometry is convenient for the alkali metals at high concentrations but AES is most useful with high temperature energy sources (see below) when multi-element analysis can be undertaken.

Instrumentation

An atomic absorption spectrometer consists of the following modules: light, source, atomizer, monochromator, detector, readout/display, where the monochromator, detector and display are similar to those of other spectrometers. The essential feature of a good light source for AAS is to provide high intensity monochromatic output, which is achieved with hollow cathode lamps. The lamps are constructed with the element to be measured as a major component of the cathode, so that the emitted light is of the same wavelength as is required for atomic absorption by the sample. Consequently a different lamp is required for each element to be measured and because of the costs involved a comprehensive range of lamps is generally maintained at only a few specialist laboratories.

The atomizer is any device which will generate ground state atoms as a vapour within the instrumental light path. If we consider calcium in a specimen of serum, the element is present in solution, bound to protein, complexed with phosphate and with some as the inorganic Ca^{2+}. Formation of the atomic vapour (atomization) requires the following steps:

removal of solvent (drying)
$\downarrow$
separation from anion or other components of the matrix $\rightarrow Ca^{2+}$
$\downarrow$
reduction: $Ca^{2+} + 2e^- \rightarrow Ca^\circ$
$\downarrow$
$\rightarrow$ absorption of light $\rightarrow$

The energy necessary to accomplish the first three of these steps is supplied as heat, either from a flame or an electrically heated furnace.

Flame atomizers

The typical arrangement involves a *pneumatic nebulizer*, premix chamber and an air-acetylene laminar flame with a 10 cm pathlength (Fig. 42.3). The high speed auxiliary air flow causes sample solution to be drawn continuously through the capillary due to the venturi effect. The sample emerges from the nebulizer as an aerosol with a wide range of droplet sizes and is mixed with the flame gases and transported to the flame for atomization. However, only droplets less than 10 μm actually enter the flame because those of larger size fall to the sides of the premix chamber and run to waste. Consequently, no more than about 15% of the sample enters the flame. Thus, with the pneumatic nebulizer, the original sample undergoes dilution with the flame gases, losses in the premix chamber and considerable thermal expansion (i.e. further dilution) within the flame. In addition to dispersion of sample through the flame there are losses of atoms due to the formation of oxides or other species in the margins of the flame. The nebulizer sample uptake rate is usually about 5 ml/min and aspiration for several seconds is necessary to achieve a steady-state signal.

The advantages and disadvantages of the pneumatic nebulizer–flame atomization system are shown in Table 42.1. Because of its simplicity, speed and freedom from interferences, this approach is preferred wherever the analyte concentration is suitable. The lowest concentrations which can typically be determined are approximately 1 μg/ml. Air–acetylene burns at about 2000°C while the hotter nitrous oxide–acetylene flame is approximately 3000°C and is used for elements which form refractory oxides and have no effective atomization in an air–acetylene flame.

Improved sensitivity is obtained with devices which overcome the limitations of pneumatic nebulizers listed above. These (i) trap atoms to give a greater density within the lightpath, (ii) bypass the nebulizer so that 100% of the sample is atomized and (iii) introduce the

Instrumentation

Hydride generation

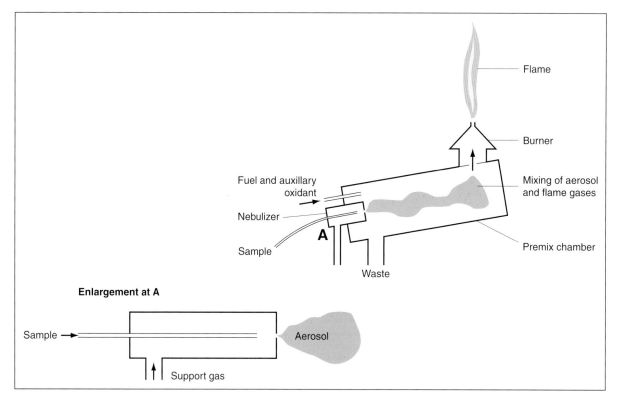

Figure 42.3: Diagram of pneumatic nebulizer, premix chamber and burner; the lower image shows the nebulizer in greater detail.

Table 42.1: Features of pneumatic nebulization with flame atomization.	
Rapid	Only about 15% of sample enters the flame
Reproducible	Wide range of droplet sizes
Few interferences	Low atomic density of sample in the flame
Steady-state signal	Burner conditions impose limitations on nebulizer

sample as a single, rapid pulse rather than as a continuous flow. Some employ a combination of these features. Devices used in a flame, e.g. the slotted quartz tube and Delves' cup, are most effective with more volatile elements such as zinc, cadmium and lead. These three approaches to improved sensitivity also feature in other atomizers used in AAS and AES.

Hydride generation

Certain elements such as arsenic, selenium and bismuth readily form gaseous hydrides, e.g. arsine (AsH_3). Using simple additional instrumentation, a reductant such as sodium borohy-dride is added to the reaction flask containing acidified sample. Hydrogen is formed which reacts with the analyte, the gaseous hydride is evolved and is transferred by a flow of inert gas to a heated silica tube positioned in the light path. The tube is heated by the air–acetylene flame or by an electric current and the temperature is sufficient to cause dissociation of the hydride and atomization of the analyte (Fig. 42.4). Thus there is no loss of specimen, all the atoms enter the light path within a few seconds and they are trapped within the silica tube which retards their dispersion. Hydride generation AAS allows the detection of a few ng of

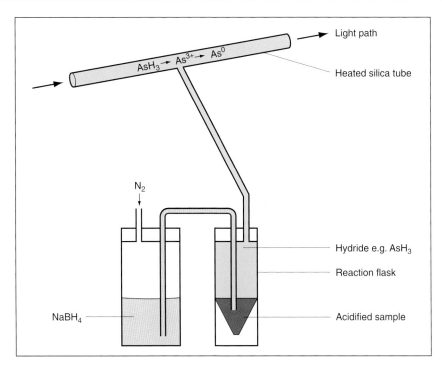

Figure 42.4: *Diagram of system for hydride generation and atomization.*

analyte from whatever sample volume is placed into the reaction flask. Variations to the instrumentation are possible to give a continuous flow arrangement which is simpler to automate.

Mercury vapour generation

Mercury forms a vapour at ambient temperatures and this property is the basis for cold vapour generation. A reducing agent is added to the sample solution to convert Hg^{2+} to the elemental mercury. Agitation or bubbling of gas through the solution causes rapid vaporization of the atomic mercury which is then transferred to a flow-through cell placed in the light path (Fig. 42.5). As with hydride generation, the detection limit is a few ng and common instrumentation to accomplish both procedures have been developed by some manufacturers.

Electrothermal atomization

Most systems use an electrically heated graphite tube and this technique is often called *graphite furnace atomization* although different materials are sometimes employed. Electrical contact

is made with the furnace and a voltage is applied. Resistance to the flow of current causes the temperature of the furnace to increase (as with the element of an electric fire). A programmed temperature sequence (Fig. 42.6) can be set up so that solution placed inside the furnace is carefully dried, organic material is then destroyed and the analyte ions dissociated from anions. With a rapid increase in temperature, ions are reduced to ground state atoms for absorption of light, and a small further temperature increase ensures the graphite tube is clean for the next sample.

The atomization temperatures achieved by this technique can be up to 3000°C so that refractory elements such as aluminium and chromium can be measured. Typically only 10–50 μl of sample is injected into the furnace so very small specimens can be accommodated and, because all the sample is atomized within a small volume, a dense atom population is produced. The technique is, therefore, very sensitive allowing measurement of μg/l concentrations. Although slow compared with flame AAS the analysis can be automated and modern

Instrumentation

Electrothermal atomization

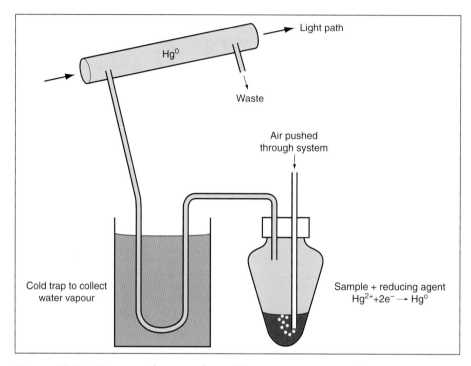

Figure 42.5: *Diagram of system for cold vapour generation (mercury).*

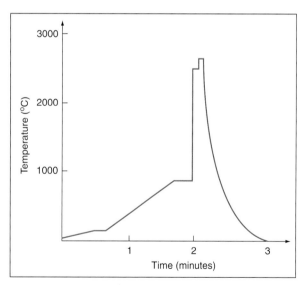

Figure 42.6: *An example of a simple heating programme for electrothermal atomization.*

instruments will shut down at the end of a run so that unattended overnight operation is possible. Electrothermal atomization AAS is subject to greater interferences than flame AAS and various procedures to eliminate or compensate for these are necessary. Optimization of methodological detail and careful attention when the instrument is set up each day are necessary to obtain accurate and precise results. Surveys of laboratory performance demonstrate that such expertise is usually found in centres where trace element analysis is a major activity.

Instrumentation for *atomic emission* includes: atomizer/excitation source, monochromator, detector, readout/display. As indicated above, the heat source for atomization and excitation to a higher energy level can be a flame. Historical alternatives include arcs and sparks but modern instruments use argon or some other gas in an ionized state, which is called a *plasma*. The plasma is initiated by seeding from a high voltage spark to ionize the atoms (Ar + e^- ↔ Ar^+ + $2e^-$) and is sustained with energy from an induction coil connected to a radio-frequency generator. This is known as an *inductively coupled plasma* (ICP).

Plasmas exist at temperatures of up to 10 000°C and in the instrument have the

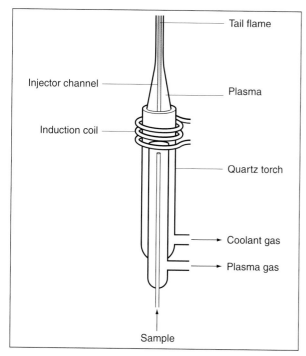

Figure 42.7: *Torch unit for the inductively coupled plasma.*

appearance of a torch (Figure 42.7). Samples can be introduced via a nebulizer or, as for AAS, by hydride generation, cold vapour generation, by electrothermal vaporization from a graphite atomizer or by laser ablation of solid specimens. The main feature of AES is that it permits multi-element analysis. Optical systems direct the emitted light either via a monochromator to a single detector or to an array of monochromators and detectors positioned around the plasma. With the first arrangement a sequential series of readings can be made with the monochromator driven to give each of the wavelengths of interest, in turn. Simultaneous readings can be made with the second arrangement as each of the monochromators is set to transmit light of predetermined wavelengths. A sequential reading instrument is less expensive than a simultaneous reading instrument, but more sample is required to take a series of readings. For most elements the analytical sensitivity for ICP–AES is similar to that obtained with flame AAS.

Applications

Measurements of minerals and trace elements are required for many different clinical investigations. Certain groups may have poor nutritional intakes of essential elements, e.g. elderly, deprived children, women during pregnancy, and deficiencies of iron, zinc and selenium are well recognized in these groups. Essential trace element deficiency also can occur during total parenteral feeding and protocols for regular monitoring of patients are generally recommended. In other situations iatrogenic poisoning can occur. Serum aluminium concentrations are regularly measured in patients with chronic renal failure because of the use of oral aluminium-containing phosphate-binding agents and, also, from possible contamination of dialysis fluids. Dialysis fluids can become contaminated with other elements and toxic events associated with copper and zinc have been reported. The diagnosis and monitoring of inborn errors of trace element metabolism usually require measurements of the element involved.

Increased exposure to minerals and trace elements can cause morbidity and some are carcinogenic. While the function of many organs may be perturbed by accumulation of metals, the kidney, liver, nervous, intestinal and haemopoietic systems are more likely to be involved. Accidental (or even deliberate suicidal or homicidal) exposures to trace elements feature in the differential diagnosis when considering signs and symptoms involving these sites. Undue exposure may be consequent on sources within the environment or in the home, associated with hobbies or from unusual cosmetics and remedies.

In an occupational setting there may be increased exposure to materials with recognized toxic potential. Determination of concentrations in appropriate specimens is a statutory requirement for lead and biological monitoring is also important in the implementation of the Control of Substances Hazardous to Health (COSHH) regulations.

The usual specimens for analysis are body fluids (blood, serum and urine). Hair and nails are occasionally taken to investigate situations of over-exposure. The clinical conditions in which *tissues* are most likely to be analysed are Wilson's disease and haemochromatosis; the concentrations of copper and iron in liver are such that even biopsy specimens can be investigated. Larger specimens of tissues removed during surgery or post-mortem may be analysed for special investigations. It is unusual for a multi-element analysis to be required in all except a few clinical situations.

Quality Assurance

Apart from the actual analysis, adventitious contamination is the factor which has the greatest impact on the quality of results. Contamination can occur during collection and storage of specimens, the preparative procedure and the spectrometric measurement. Scrupulous attention to cleanliness and to methodological detail are essential for obtaining meaningful results. Data from external quality assessment schemes indicate that while some general hospital laboratories obtain good results it is the specialist trace element centres that tend to maintain the highest standards of performance. This observation reflects the continuing application of practices which minimize contamination and their expertise and experi-ence in ensuring optimal functioning of equipment. Such centres also accumulate experience with unusual clinical cases and are well placed to provide advice and interpretation.

Because of the stability of inorganic analytes and the purity with which standard materials can be prepared there are reasonable numbers of reference materials available for use to validate methods and for internal and external quality control. Unlike many other clinical laboratory procedures, and partly as a consequence of the wide use of certified reference materials, accuracy is a straightforward concept and is not defined in the context of particular methodologies.

Conclusions

With recent improvements in reliability of equipment and developments to reduce interferences associated with electrothermal atomization, AAS remains the most suitable technique for the measurement of minerals and trace elements in clinical samples. The importance of flame photometry is decreasing with the introduction of sodium and potassium ion-selective electrodes while other approaches for AES currently fail to match the sensitivity of AAS.

Further Reading

Haswell S (ed). *Atomic Absorption Spectrometry. Theory, Design and Applications*. 1991: Elsevier, Amsterdam.

Taylor A (ed). Trace Elements in Human Disease. *Clinics in Endocrinology and Metabolism* 1985; **14**: 513–764.

Taylor A. Detection and monitoring of disorders of essential trace elements. *Annals of Clinical Biochemistry* 1996; **33**: 486–510.

Walker A W (ed). SAS Trace Element Laboratories. *Clinical And Analytical Handbook*, 3rd edn 1997; Royal Surrey County Hospital, Guildford, UK.

43 DRY REAGENT CHEMISTRY TECHNIQUES

Jacqueline C Osypiw and Gordon S Challand

Introduction

Dry reagent chemistry, thin film chemistry, reagent strip chemistry, and solid support analytical chemistry are all synonyms. They describe the incorporation of one or more chemical reagents into a convenient portable unit, which can then be used to carry out chemical analyses without the necessity to make up and transport reagents in liquid form. Probably the earliest and most familiar example is litmus paper, still used in school chemistry departments, analytical laboratories, and for in-the-field use testing soil pH. Made by incorporating the vegetable pigment derived from moss (described in English in 1502) into the interstices between cellulose fibres of paper, it was used by Peacham to colour paper blue in 1606, and is likely to have been in use as an indicator for at least 300 years.

A profound stimulus to the development of thin film chemistry techniques was the development of photography. The property of silver halides to change colour on exposure to light was first noted by Fabricius in 1556, and the first photographic image may have been produced by Schultze in 1727. The first practical photographic films and papers were development in the nineteenth century, and today a modern instant colour print film may have as many as fifteen discrete layers, each involving a chemical reaction or physical function, all integrated into a single stable portable unit.

The first application of these techniques for clinical biochemistry appeared in the mid-1950s, with the development of reagent strips for the measurement of glucose in urine. A comparatively untrained analyst, nurse, or patient could dip the reagent strip into a urine sample, and within a couple of minutes could obtain a semi-quantitative measurement of the amount of glucose by comparing the colour developed to a preprinted colour chart. This, together with the subsequent application of similar technology to blood glucose analysis, revolutionized the monitoring of diabetic patients.

Accurate quantitation was improved with the development of simple photometers to measure reflected light for reading glucose reagent strips (so-called glucose meters) and further major developments occurred in the 1970s when the technology of photographic film manufacture was applied to clinical chemistry analyses. Today, many hundreds of analyses are available in thin film format, and machines have been produced that are capable of measuring colours (or other signals) developed on a wide range of reagent strips, and producing an accurate and precise result every few seconds.

The technology has the potential to revolutionize clinical chemistry practice, both in reducing the requirement for analytical skills needed for common analyses, and in the capacity for analyses to be simply and rapidly performed outside an analytical laboratory: in wards or clinics; in family practitioner offices, and in the patient's own home. Walter & Boguslaski have reviewed the field and described the range, and technology, of available assays.

Principles of Methodology

Structure of reagent strips

In their simplest form, thin film chemistry analyses consist of a pigment or other reagent trapped between the cellulose fibres of a strip of paper. These produce a visible reaction when an analyte diffuses into the matrix, either in liquid form (e.g. litmus and other indicator papers for the estimation of the pH of a liquid) or gaseous form (e.g. ferrous hydroxide paper for the detection of hydrogen cyanide; mercuric bromide paper for the detection of arsine).

More complex systems consist of a series of layers each of which has one or more functions. From the bottom up, these are as follows.

(1) A support layer. This is the foundation for the dry reagent elements. It usually is thin plastic, which may either transmit or reflect light.

(2) A reflective layer. Its purpose is to reflect back to the eye or mechanical detector as much as possible of the light emitted by the chemistry of the reagent layer(s). This may be included with the support layer, by using a reflective plastic. Alternatively it may be a layer of a pigment such as titanium dioxide, or a reflective material such as a metal foil.

(3) One or more analytical layers. These commonly consist of thin porous gelatin films in which one or more reagents have been included during manufacture of the film. The reagents are stable once the gelatin layer has dried. A single layer is adequate when the incorporated reagents do not interact with each other in the absence of an analyte. Multiple layers (each one of which is dried before the next is applied) are necessary to separate reagents which react with each other in the absence of analyte. As well as gelatin, fibrous materials such as cellulose can be used. These may function as filters (for example, to separate red blood cells from plasma). Alternatively, reagents can be introduced by immersing the fibrous matrix in the appropriate solution(s), and then drying. Instead of containing reagents, individual analytical layers may carry out other functions such as molecular sieving to separate one reaction product from another.

(4) A spreading layer. This usually consists of a fibrous material or a membrane. When a drop of sample is applied, it rapidly spreads the sample out laterally and enables a uniform diffusion into the analytical layers.

Complex reagent strips require very accurate manufacture in which, particularly for the analytical layers, the concentration of reagents in the gelatin, the pore size of the gelatin, the thickness of each layer, and the extent of drying of each layer must be carefully controlled. However, once manufactured, each strip contains all of the analytical steps required to carry out an assay. No prior reconstitution of reagents is needed, the strip is portable and can be stable for many weeks or months, and the analyst need only apply the sample to initiate the analysis.

Semiquantitative results can be obtained by matching the colour developed after a fixed time to pre-printed colour charts. In daylight or good artificial light, an experienced analyst with normal colour vision can usually obtain a result within ±25% of the true value. However, for reactions monitored by UV or fluorescence detection, and where more accurate quantitation is needed, a meter to measure the colour or other signal is required. Most dry reagent chemistries are monitored by diffuse reflectance photometry; front-face fluorescence can also be used.

Monitoring of reactions

It is not obvious that the properties of reflected light are different to those of transmitted and absorbed light familiar to analysts. But the primary colours of paints and other pigments (red, yellow, blue) are not the same as transmitted light (red, yellow, green). In an art gallery, we usually look at paintings from the front, with the painting being illuminated from above. If a painting is illuminated directly from the front, colouring and detail are lost to the observer because of non-coloured reflected light from its surface. We are dealing with the laws of reflectance photometry.

Some light falling on a reagent strip will simply be reflected by the surface (specular reflection). Since this does not interact with chromophores within the analytical layers, it will have the same properties as light from the origin, and cannot be used to monitor a reaction. Some light, however, enters the analytical layers and can interact with chromophores before being returned by the reflectance layer. Light scattering and reflection without chromophore interaction can also take place within the analytical layers. The light returned after transmission through the analytical layers (diffuse reflection), which contains a mixture of interacted light and scattered light, is used to monitor a reaction. It is detected by measuring the light returned at an angle away from the main specular reflection beam.

After reaction, the concentration of analyte in a sample can be calculated by comparing the amount of diffuse reflected light with that of a standard. The relationship is governed by the equation $R_u = R_s . I_u/I_s$ where R_u is the percentage reflectivity of the sample, R_s is the percentage reflectivity of the standard, I_u is the intensity of reflected light from the sample, and I_s is the intensity of the reflected light from the standard. Like transmittance, percentage reflectivity measurements are not linear with respect to concentration, and in practice, linearizing algorithms are used to convert a measurement of percentage reflectivity to concentration, such as that of Williams & Clapper.

Fluorescent products of a reaction can be monitored using front-face fluorimetry. Mono-chromators are used to separate fluorescent light emitted by the analytical layers from reflected light. If quenching within the reagent strip is negligible, the measured fluorescence is linear with respect to fluorophore concentration.

Specific Examples

Dry reagent chemistries can be used to measure many hundreds of urine analytes and blood metabolites and proteins. Some can be carried out using a single analytical layer; others require multiple layers or the incorporation of physical structures into the analytical layers. Even trace quantities of analytes such as hormones and drugs can be measured by utilizing immunoassay techniques within the analytical layers. Specific examples are given below.

Glucose

Glucose was the first biological analyte to be measured using dry reagent techniques. Modern glucose methods rely on enzymatic assays which generally utilize glucose oxidase. A typical example is the Dextrostix reagent strip, illustrated in Fig. 43.1. A blood sample is applied to the surface layer, which both acts as a spreading layer and is a semipermeable membrane which separates blood cells from plasma. Plasma diffuses into the paper analytical layer which contains the buffered enzyme reaction system. Within this, glucose and atmospheric oxygen are acted on by glucose oxidase producing hydrogen peroxide and gluconic acid. In the presence of peroxidase, also incorporated into the analytical layer, hydrogen peroxide oxidizes a redox indicator to produce a visible colour change. The plastic support layer is reflective, and after blood cells have been wiped from the surface layer, the colour developed can be read from the top, either visually (by comparing with a pre-printed colour chart) or by using a glucose meter.

Many alternatives to this simple reagent strip for glucose have been developed. For example, the Fuji Strip incorporates a masking and reflective layer containing titanium dioxide between the spreading layer and the analytical layer. The support layer is transparent rather

<u>Specific Examples</u>

Alanine aminotransferase

Creatinine

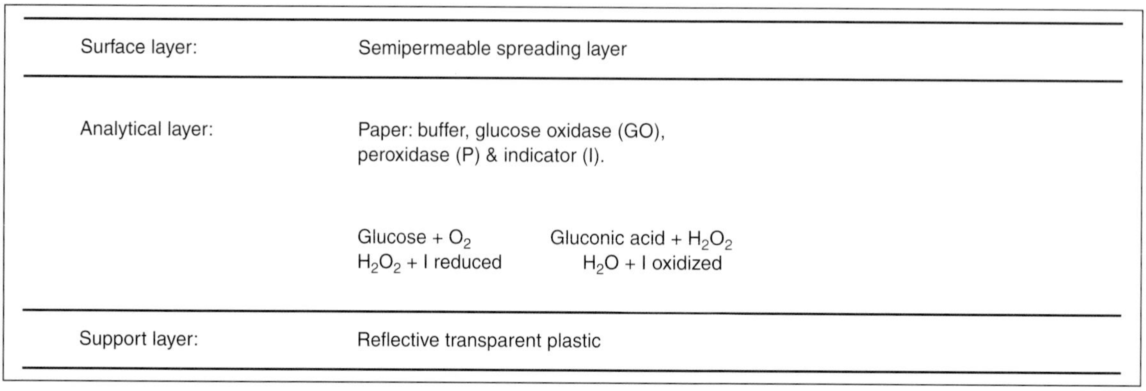

Surface layer:	Semipermeable spreading layer
Analytical layer:	Paper: buffer, glucose oxidase (GO), peroxidase (P) & indicator (I).
	Glucose + O_2 Gluconic acid + H_2O_2
	H_2O_2 + I reduced H_2O + I oxidized
Support layer:	Reflective transparent plastic

Figure 43.1: *The structure of a Dextrostix glucose reagent strip (adapted from Walter & Boguslaski.)*

than reflective plastic and the reaction is monitored from below. This removes the need for wiping blood cells from the strip.

Alanine aminotransferase

Serum enzymes can also be measured using dry chemistry techniques, although analytical systems are more sophisticated as enzymes are large molecules which do not readily diffuse through matrices. Also, the measurement of enzymes relies frequently on multi-step reactions which are themselves enzymatic. Careful manufacturing control both of the enzyme reagents and other participating reagents such as cofactors are therefore necessary. Some dry reagent systems for enzyme analysis have open lattices which allow serum enzymes to enter the reagent layers of a slide, whilst others have closed lattices which retain the serum enzyme on the surface layer of the slide.

A typical example of a closed lattice system is the Vitros (formerly Ektachem) method for alanine aminotransferase (ALT) assay. The spreading layer, which is semipermeable and retains the serum enzyme, also contains the ALT substrates L-alanine and sodium α-oxoglutarate. ALT catalyses the transfer of an amino group from L-alanine to α-oxoglutarate producing pyruvate and glutamate. Unchanged substrates and reaction products diffuse into the analytical layer, which contains lactate dehydrogenase (LDH) and NADH. Pyruvate produced by ALT is acted on by LDH to produce lactate, while NADH is converted to NAD^+. The rate of change in absorbance at 340 nm is monitored from below using reflectance photometry.

In this system, the spreading layer is also used to initiate the reaction, and the activity of ALT can be measured without the enzyme itself entering the traditional analytical layer. Although pyruvate in the sample can itself participate in the reaction, the concentration in serum is usually too low to cause significant interference.

Creatinine

Serum and plasma creatinine can be measured using a multi-layered slide which has an internal separation layer. The structure of a typical slide is shown in Fig. 43.2.

For this slide, the spreading layer contains titanium oxide, so that it also serves as the reflectance layer. When serum is applied, creatinine enters the first analytical layer. Here, ammonia is produced from creatinine by a specific enzyme (creatinine iminohydrolase) incorporated within the layer. The gas-permeable membrane between the first and second analytical layers allows ammonia to diffuse into the second analytical layer. However, constituents such as buffers and hydroxyl ions which interfere with the subsequent reaction cannot traverse the membrane and are trapped in the first analytical layer. The second analytical layer contains an indicator, bromophenol blue, which changes colour in response to ammonia. Viewed from below, the colour change in bromophenol blue can be related to creatinine concentration. Ammonia can inter-

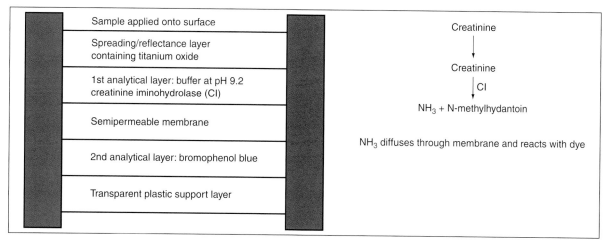

Figure 43.2: The structure of a Vitros creatinine reagent strip.

fere, but the concentration in serum is usually too low to give erroneous results.

Potassium

Electrolytes can be measured using ion-selective electrodes constructed as a reagent strip. In a typical ion-selective electrode, an electrically conducting membrane separates the sample from an internal solution of constant composition. A difference in concentration produces an electrochemical gradient across the membrane, which gives rise to a potentiometric difference. An internal reference electrode, usually silver/silver chloride, is also immersed in the filling solution. The change in potential at the internal reference electrode is measured by comparison with an external reference electrode.

Figure 43.3 shows the structure of a Vitros ion-selective electrode reagent strip. Like a conventional ion-selective electrode, the concentration of an ion is measured from the potentiometric difference generated between two electrodes: the bridge forms a stable liquid junction connecting the two electrodes. Unlike a conventional ion-selective electrode, a solution of known composition is applied to the

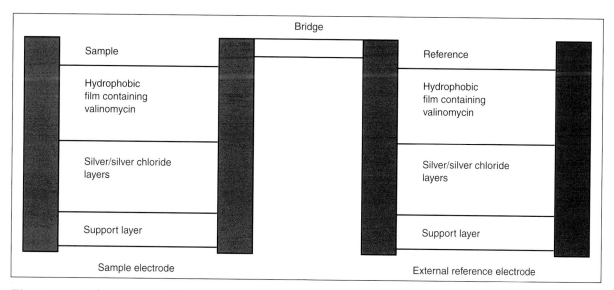

Figure 43.3: The structure of a Vitros potassium ion-selective electrode.

Specific Examples

Human chorionic gonadotropin

---

second (external reference) electrode, so the sample is referenced directly to a standard solution. Different ions can be measured using different ion-selective membranes. For potassium measurement, each electrode includes a hydrophobic film containing a high concentration of valinomycin. This permits the passage of potassium ions, but excludes anions and other cations. A potentiometric difference then solely reflects any difference in concentration between the sample and the standard solution.

Ions such as potassium can also be measured using more conventional dry reagent chemistry. The analytical layer typically contains a hydrophobic organic phase, which excludes all ions except those whose passage is mediated by an ionophore such as valinomycin for potassium. The ionophore mediates a cation–H^+ interchange between the aqueous (sample) and organic phases. The resulting change in pH within the organic phase causes a change in colour of a redox dye incorporated within the analytical layer. A similar approach is also used for the measurement of 'specific gravity' – actually a measurement of total ionic activity – in reagent strips for urine analysis.

Human chorionic gonadotropin

Probably the most widely used dry reagent chemistry strips are those for the measurement of human chorionic gonadotropin (HCG). Designed for visual reading and available over-the-counter, they can be sensitive enough to permit the diagnosis of pregnancy within a few days of conception.

Classical techniques for the measurement of trace quantities of hormones such as HCG relied upon the immunoassay techniques developed in the 1960s. Such techniques relying on limited quantities of an antibody and subsequent differentiation between bound and free antigens have been adapted for thin film methodology. The structure of a typical format, for the measurement of serum thyroxine, is shown in Fig. 43.4. The second analytical layer consists of an antibody to thyroxine covalently bound to the matrix. Diffusion of the sample through this layer gives partition between thyroxine in the sample and peroxidase-labelled thyroxine incorporated into the

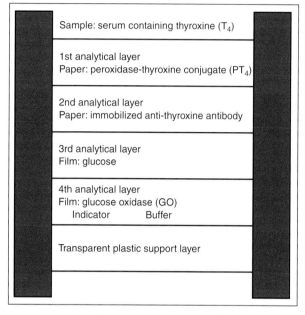

Figure 43.4: The structure of a Fuji thyroxine reagent strip.

first analytical layer. The third analytical layer incorporates glucose, and the fourth layer utilizes glucose oxidase to generate hydrogen peroxide from glucose. Peroxidase from free labelled thyroxine diffusing through the layers then catalyses the oxidation of a redox dye, which results in a colour change proportional to the amount of free label, which is in turn inversely related to the amount of thyroxine in the original sample.

Such reagent strips are complex to manufacture, and because classical immunoassay techniques require long incubation times, the sensitivity of these methods in dry reagent formats is inadequate to detect trace quantities of hormones such as HCG in early pregnancy. Most modern pregnancy test kits utilize immunometric techniques, in which an excess of antibody is present and for which short incubation times are possible. Early versions used a mixture of wet and dry reagent techniques. A monoclonal antibody to the α-subunit of HCG was covalently bound to a matrix. The sample was added first, any HCG present binding to the antibody. A solution containing an enzyme-labelled antibody to the β-subunit of HCG was added and incubated for a short time, allowing the reaction to proceed in which intact HCG was sandwiched between matrix-bound antibody and labelled antibody. After adding buffer to wash surplus sample and enzyme-labelled antibody from the strip, a third solution containing an dye substrate for the enzyme label was added, which generated a coloured product. In the absence of HCG from the sample to form the sandwich, no colour was developed on the matrix. A convenient positive control for the reaction could be incorporated by binding in one area of the strip the first antibody which had already been allowed to react with intact HCG. This area of the strip then should then have given a positive reaction even in the absence of HCG in the urine sample.

Later versions of immunometric assay technology have included all the components of a monoclonal antibody reaction in a dry reagent format. Some have used particle agglutination techniques, relying on the ability of particles such as those containing a gold sol to change colour when bound together in the presence of HCG. Others have relied on a region of immobilized HCG antibody covalently bound to a reagent strip. Urine travelling along the strip rather than through it mobilizes coloured particles linked to a different HCG antibody. In the presence of HCG in the urine sample, these form a sandwich, and produce a discrete coloured line over the immobilized antibody. Again, a positive control can be incorporated within the strip by including a region of immobilized antibody already bound to HCG.

Quality Control of Dry Reagent Chemistry

Controlling the quality of results given by reagent strips poses different problems to those of traditional wet chemistry analyses. For the latter, new reagents can be made up, and the concentrations of reagents used in the assay can be modified by the analyst. It is therefore comparatively easy to change assay ingredients in response to unacceptable performance. But dry reagent strips cannot be modified by the analyst, and it is seldom obvious from exam-

ination or inspection of the strip itself that analytical performance is unacceptable. A major quality control problem is therefore identifying unacceptable performance and determining its cause. In practice, the cause is seldom the reagent strip itself.

For the manufacturer and the analyst, dry reagent chemistries pose a further problem, because the long-term stability of each batch of strips can only be predicted from the stability of previous batches. In practice, there is always some batch-to-batch variation in stability, even when reagent strips are stored in ideal conditions. As part of a quality control programme, it is therefore necessary to monitor long-term trends in performance, so that appropriate action can be taken before quality becomes unacceptable.

Identification of unacceptable performance – extra-laboratory semiquantitative assays

At present, the main area of clinical use for semiquantitative dry reagent assays is in urine testing. A wide range of reagent strips is available, which may include just one analyte (e.g. for glucose or for protein), or a range of analytes, the colours of each reagent pad having to be matched visually in strict time sequence to a preprinted colour chart (see Fig. 43.5). Although semiquantitative assays for blood glucose have been largely superseded by the use of reagent strips read in blood glucose meters, these assays pose similar quality control problems. In addition, many new extra-laboratory reagent test strips have recently been introduced, which range from the measurement of whole blood lipid fractions to the detection of drugs of abuse in urine. These semiquantitative assays are carried out in a wide range of settings – wards, clinics, GP practices, and by patients. Little attention has been paid to performance, because there is a widespread belief that such assays are foolproof; and in a hospital setting they are often delegated to the most junior member of ward staff, who has no experience of analytical chemistry and who frequently receives no training.

The first survey of the performance of urine analyses on hospital wards showed that the correct result (i.e. matching to the right colour

Quality Control of Dry Reagent Chemistry

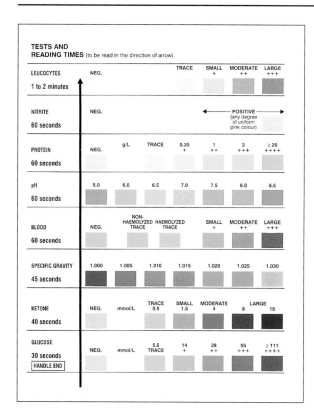

Figure 43.5: The pre-printed colour chart for a Bayer Multistix 8SG urine analysis reagent strip.

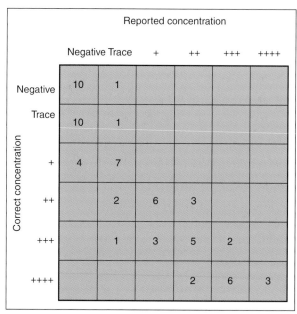

Figure 43.6: Bias in urine protein assays.
Six pre-prepared urine samples with protein concentrations corresponding to a different colour block, were distributed 'blind' to 11 nurse analysts. The Figure compares the known protein concentrations with the numbers of analysts reporting each colour block. As well as the expected scatter of results, a systematic bias exists, analysts tending to underestimate the true protein concentration by one colour block.

pad) was only obtained in only about 50% of analyses. Around 5% of all measurements gave grossly aberrant values. Similar finding have since been obtained in studies from many different locations.

With quantitative assays, it is comparatively easy to define acceptable performance numerically, either in terms of analytical achievability (the approach of most external Quality Assurance (QA) schemes) or in terms of clinical utility. Semiquantitative assays do not lend themselves to an easy numerical approach. One cannot use the mean value obtained from QA distributions as the best estimate of the true value, since this often has a bias, introduced either by approximation to the nearest colour match, or through deficiencies in technique (e.g. Fig. 43.6). Samples distributed as part of a survey or a QA programme are therefore usually synthetic, with weighed-in constituents defining the true value (although this is difficult for some analytes, such as bilirubin). When the weighed-in value corresponds to the concentration required to match exactly one pre-printed colour block for each analyte, in practice only about half of the people carrying out the test achieve the correct match; approximately 95% achieve a result within one colour block of the correct figure. Results outside this range can be taken to be unacceptable performance. An alternative approach is to weigh in amounts of constituents which produce a colour halfway between two colour blocks. Results corresponding to either of the two adjacent colour blocks are taken to be acceptable; in ward surveys, 10–20% of returns are unacceptable by this rather tighter criterion [Tighe P, personal communication]. When unacceptable performance is identified, a cause needs to be identified; some of the possible causes are listed in Table 43.1. Almost all of these are due to deficiencies in understanding, in training, and

Table 43.1:   Some causes of poor performance in carrying out manual reagent strip analyses.

- Use of out-of-date reagent strips
- Keeping reagent strips in conditions which shorten shelf-life
- Leaving the top off the strip container, or removing the desiccant
- Cutting the strip in half to save money
- Using an unsuitable sample container (e.g. a bleach container for a urine sample)
- Failure to dip a urine reagent strip completely into the sample
- Insufficient sample applied to a blood reagent strip
- Carrying out the test at the wrong temperature
- Reading the colour pad too soon, or too late
- Reading the wrong colour pad on a multi-analyte reagent strip
- Poor lighting conditions
- Poor colour vision
- Wrongly transcribing a result on to a report form
- Using the wrong units when reporting

in technique (all of which can be remedied locally). The cause is seldom attributable to manufacturing deficiencies in the reagent strip.

Assessment of long-term trends – quantitative assays

Automated instruments using dry reagent chemistries have been available for several years. These can carry out many different analyses on small quantities of serum, with throughput and precision of analysis matching more traditional wet chemistry analysers. Reagent slides are typically bought in single batches sufficient to last six months. If stored in ideal conditions, each batch may need just a single calibration before use, the stability being good enough to maintain quality for the six-month lifetime of the batch. However, in practice storage conditions may not be ideal (temperature differences between the floor and ceiling of a cold room have been sufficient to change stability!), and the very slow deterioration of reagent strips is not identical from batch to batch. Quality control is therefore aimed at ensuring that the initial calibration is adequate, and then monitoring slow drift to identify the point at which either a second calibration is required or unused slides should be discarded.

Conventional quality control sera can be used for both purposes, but suffer from disadvantages. They are expensive; matrix effects particularly relating to viscosity and subsequent diffusion through the layers of a slide may make their behaviour different to patient samples; and the results for some analytes may change markedly in the first few hours after reconstitution. The authors find that the results obtained from patient samples give more reliable QC information. Although patient results are obviously more scattered than the results of a conventional QC serum, many more patient results are available for statistical analysis. For most analytes, parameters such as the mean patient result (after exclusion of extreme values) and the number of results falling outside a preset limit (such as an 'automatic telephone' limit for serum sodium) are sensitive and provide almost all of the necessary QC information. Initial calibration can be judged by the comparability of a patient daily mean following previous calibrations. A drift in daily mean can be used to judge the point at which recalibration or new slides are necessary. Figure 43.7 shows a daily patient mean plot for serum sodium analyses, showing the period before and after recalibration.

Quality control statistics based on patient samples can be used to ensure long-term comparability of results within a laboratory, but do not of course ensure that results are comparable to those produced by other laboratories. Participation in external quality assurance

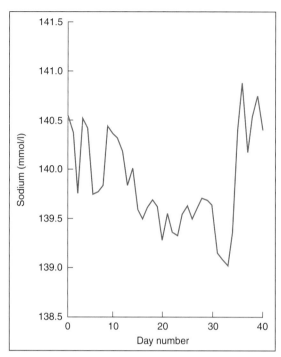

Figure 43.7: *Daily patient means, sodium analyses. The plot shows successive daily mean values for serum sodium analyses carried out using a Vitros analyser over the period from late August 1996. A fall in results is apparent, which averaged approx. 0.04 mmol/l each day. Recalibration was carried out after day 34.*

but aberrant results. The incidence of these is likely to be less than 0.2%. Short of analysing all samples in duplicate, such errors are not detectable by standard quality control procedures.

Summary

The technology of dry reagent chemistry has now advanced to the point at which almost all conventional wet clinical chemistry analyses can be reproduced in dry reagent format. Although reagent costs are usually higher, sample volumes are usually low, sensitivities are comparable to conventional techniques, and precision can be at least as good. These assays offer major advantages to the analyst in speed, convenience and reliability, and carrying them out requires little specific analytical skill. They are therefore appropriate in a clinical chemistry laboratory, where they free scarce technical and scientific resources for development and application of new assays and new techniques. They are also easily adopted to a near-patient environment, e.g. on wards, in clinics, in general practice, and for use by patients themselves.

Despite its apparent simplicity, this technology is not foolproof. Without careful attention to detail in ensuring the identity of the patient, the appropriateness of the sample, the correct procedure of the analysis, including timing, temperature, and quality control, and the accurate and appropriate recording of the reaction, analyses can give dangerously misleading results. With an increasingly wide utilization of the technology there are major benefits to the patient and to the clinician in the speed with which results can be obtained. The challenge to the manufacturer is continual development, not only in introducing new assays but also in simplifying current assays and ensuring that they are as accurate and as free from interference as possible. The challenge to the analytical laboratory is ensuring that, wherever this technology is used, the analyst is trained in the appropriate analytical procedures and educated to be aware of not only the strengths but also the limitations of the technique.

schemes can provide this information, and gives more reliable information than, for example, the results obtained by analysing a quality control sample of known composition.

The temperature of the dry reagent strip, and of the sample, affect both the speed of diffusion of sample, and the rate of reaction within the strip; good temperature control is essential. The overall performance, as judged by external QA data, of two reagent strip analysers over a two-year period is shown in Fig. 43.8. Temperature control in the laboratory in which they were situated was less than ideal; the deterioration in performance over the hot months of summer is obvious.

Automated analysers using dry reagent chemistry, and those using wet chemistry, on occasion produce 'fliers' – apparently correct

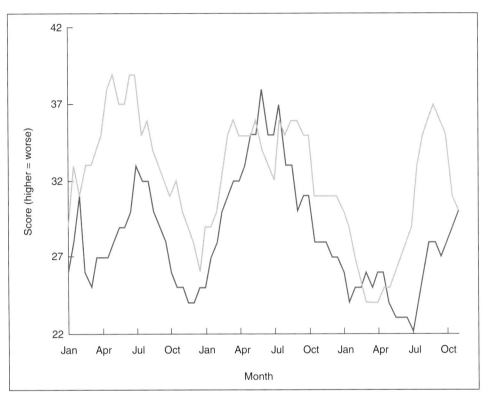

Figure 43.8: *Overall external QA results – seasonal trends. The overall mean running variance index score (OMRVIS, an index of imprecision) is shown for two identical Vitros analysers housed in the same laboratory between January 1995 and December 1997. The precision in summer months is worse than in winter months, probably due to inadequate temperature control in the laboratory.*

Further Reading

Adams E C Jr, Burkhardt C E, Free, A H. Specificity of glucose oxidase test for urine glucose. *Science* 1957; **125**: 1082–1083.

Bevan D. Case study. Better comparability means better business for Kodak. *VAM Bulletin* 1996; **15**, 10–12. (Laboratory of the Government Chemist, Teddington, Middlesex, UK).

Challand G S. Is ward biochemical testing cheap and easy? *Intensive Care World* 1987; 4, 9–11.

Charlton S C, Zipp A, Fleming R I. Solid-phase colorimetric determination of potassium. *Clin Chem* 1982; **28**, 1857.

Curry A S. *Poison detection in human organs*. 4th edn 1988: Charles C Thomas, Springfield, Illinois, p. 79, p. 103.

Fraser C G, Hyltoft Petersen P. Desirable standards for laboratory tests if they are to fulfill medical needs. *Clin Chem* 1993; 39, 1447–55.

Fraser C G, Hyltoft Petersen P, Libeer J-C, Ricos, C. Proposals for setting generally applicable goals solely based on biology. *Ann Clin Biochem* 1997; **34**, 8–12.

Kobyashi N, Tuhata M, Akui T, Okuda K. Evaluation of multilayer film analytical elements in plasma and in serum by Fuji dry chem slide GLU-P. *Clin Rep* 1982; **16**, 484–7.

Further Reading

Kortum G. *Reflectance Spectroscopy: Principles, Methods, Applications* 1969: Springer, New York.

Marks V, Dawson A. Rapid stick method for determining blood-glucose concentration. *Br Med J* 1965; **1**, 293–4.

Mazzaferri E L, Lanese R R, Skillman T G, Keller M P. Use of test strips with colour meter to measure blood-glucose. *Lancet* 1970; i: 331–3.

Nagatoma S, Yasuda Y, Masuda N, Makiuchi H, Okazzaki M. *Multilayer analysis component utilizing specific binding reaction.* Eur Pat Application No 81108365.8, October 15, 1981.

Pesce A J, Rosen C H, Pasby T L. *Fluorescence Spectroscopy* 1971: Dekker, New York.

Russell L J, Buckley B M. Ion-selective electrodes. In *Principles of Clinical Biochemistry: Scientific Foundations*. Williams D L, Marks V (eds). 2nd edn 1988: Heinemann Medical Books, Oxford, pp. 201–214.

Stenger E. *The History of Photography*, 1939: Mack Printing Co, Easton, Pa, p. 1.

Sunberg M W, Becker R W, Esders T W, Figueras J, Goohue C T. An enzymatic creatinine assay and a direct ammonia assay in coated thin films. *Clin Chem* 1983; **29**, 1267.

Test Methodology, Kodak Ektachem Clinical Chemistry Slides (ALT). Publication No. MP2-36 4/92, 1992: Eastman Kodak Co, Rochester, New York.

The Oxford English Dictionary, 2nd edn 1989: Clarendon Press, Oxford. Entries under *litmus*, and *litmus paper*.

Walter B, Co R, Makowski E. A solid-phase reagent strip for the colorimetric determination of serum alanine aminotransferase (ALT) on the Seralyser. *Clin Chem* 1983; **29**.

Walter B, Boguslaski R. Solid-phase Analytical Elements for Clinical Analysis, in *Principles of Clinical Biochemistry: Scientific Foundations*, Williams D L, Marks V (ed) 2nd edn 1988: Heinemann Medical Books, pp. 250–265.

Williams F C, Clapper F R. Multiple internal reflections in photographic colour prints. *J Optical Soc Am* 1953; **43**, 595–9.

44 SEPARATION TECHNIQUES IN LABORATORY MEDICINE

Roy A Sherwood

Why Separate?

Most of the analyses carried out in clinical laboratories involve the detection and quantitation of individual compounds in body fluids, usually blood or urine. For this purpose, specific chemical or immunological methods are used for the compound of interest. Whilst such assays account for the bulk of analyses in the clinical laboratory, in some instances a family of closely related compounds may need to be measured. Although specific assays could be developed for each compound of the family group, this approach is often economically or practically less viable than using a technique which can separate and quantitate all the compounds simultaneously. A wide variety of separation techniques are used in clinical laboratories, but the vast majority are based on the principles of chromatographic or electrophoretic separation. Chromatography in its various guises, e.g. thin layer chromatography (TLC), high performance liquid chromatography (HPLC) or gas chromatography (GC), can be used to separate many different types of compounds from small molecules such as amino acids and drugs to proteins such as glycated haemoglobin. Electrophoresis, on the other hand, is typically used for the separation of proteins, either coarsely (e.g. serum proteins), or specifically to identify variants of a particular protein (e.g. inherited variants of haemoglobin).

Chromatography

The principle of all the different types of chromatography is the interaction of molecules of interest between a mobile phase (liquid or gas) and a stationary phase (solid). Those molecules which interact with the stationary phase will move more slowly across a plate or through a column than those which do not interact, therefore resulting in separation of molecules from within a mixture. Control of these interactions, and hence separation, is achieved by exploiting

Thin Layer Chromatography (TLC)

Principles

Applications

Table 44.1: Molecular properties which govern separation in various forms of chromatography.

Property	Type of chromatography
Adsorptive properties	TLC, HPLC
Partition	GC, HPLC
Antigen–antibody or enzyme–substrate interactions	Affinity
Molecular size and shape	Gel filtration
Ionic charge	Ion exchange

subtle differences in certain physical properties of the different molecules in samples, e.g. their solubility in either water or organic solvents, net charge and size. Table 44.1 details the molecular properties that govern separation in the various forms of chromatography.

Thin Layer Chromatography (TLC)

Principles

TLC superseded paper chromatography in the 1960s and is itself now largely being superseded by HPLC. In TLC the stationary phase (commonly alumina, silica gel or cellulose) is coated onto a glass, plastic or metal plate. A solvent mixture (mobile phase) applied to one end of the plate travels along the plate by capillary attraction and results in chromatographic separation of solutes in a sample applied to the plate. Unless they are fluorescent, most compounds will require derivatisation (chemical modification) to enable then to be visualized, which is achieved typically by spraying with or dipping the plate into chromogenic reagents. Qualitative information can be gained simply by viewing the plate and identification of individual spots can be achieved by measurement of the retention factor (Rf, distance travelled by the spot divided by total distance travelled by the solvent front). Greater resolution can be obtained by running the plate again with the solvent direction at 90° to the first run (two-

dimensional TLC). The disadvantage of 2-D TLC is that only one sample can be applied to each plate. Quantitation either requires the use of a densitometer which can scan the plate, or elution of the spot from the stationary phase followed by colorimetric measurement.

Applications

TLC is predominantly used now as a screening technique as it is relatively quick, cheap and easy in comparison to other chromatographic methods. The applications for TLC in a clinical laboratory include assay of amino acids, drugs and carbohydrates.

Amino acids

Neonatal screening programmes exist in many countries for the early detection of children with phenylketonuria. Although specific spectrophotometric or HPLC methods exist for phenylalanine, many screening laboratories prefer to use a 1-D TLC method which separates the basic, neutral and acidic amino acids, because this has the potential for identification of other amino acid disorders, e.g. tyrosinaemia, maple syrup urine disease, etc. Confirmation of the identity of an abnormally raised amino acid can then be achieved by 2-D TLC or HPLC, e.g. the characteristic pattern of abnormally raised branched chain amino acids (leucine, isoleucine and valine) in maple syrup urine disease.

Drugs

Urine drug screening is complicated by the diversity of drugs available for 'recreational' use or taken in deliberate or accidental overdose, which include basic, neutral and acidic compounds. In the unconscious or non-cooperative patient little information may be available about the consumption of specific drugs. TLC is often the technique of choice for initial screening, and commercial systems e.g. Toxilab^R are available. These tend to have separate plates and solvent systems for acidic and basic drugs with the neutral drugs included in either one of the systems. Sequential spraying of different chromogenic reagents results in different drugs staining different colours, thus permitting easier identification.

SEPARATION TECHNIQUES IN LABORATORY MEDICINE

High Performance Liquid Chromatography (HPLC)
Principles
Equipment for HPLC
Sample preparation for biological samples
Applications

Carbohydrates

TLC is the technique of choice for initial screening of urine or faecal samples from symptomatic infants for disorders of carbohydrate metabolism, e.g. fructosuria, etc. Only qualitative results are required for this application but the development of tests for gastrointestinal tract function and integrity using orally administered sugars has resulted in the need for quantitative TLC of sugars.

High Performance Liquid Chromatography (HPLC)

Principles

HPLC is the commonest form of chromatography used in the clinical laboratory. Enhanced performance is achieved by containing the solid phase in narrow columns (typically 150 mm × 5 mm) and pumping the mobile phase through the column under pressure (typically $1.5–2.0 \times$ atmospheric pressure). Although ion-exchange or size exclusion mechanisms of separation are occasionally used in HPLC, most methods are based on the adsorption of molecules to the solid phase. In *normal phase* HPLC hydrophilic binding groups on the surface of a silica packing material attract hydrophilic but not hydrophobic molecules, the opposite being true for *reverse phase* HPLC. Thus in normal phase HPLC a mobile phase of increasing polarity will more effectively remove polar molecules from the solid phase, while in reverse phase HPLC increasingly hydrophobic (organic) mobile phases will more readily remove non-polar molecules from the solid phase. Reverse phase HPLC is, therefore, particularly suited to the separation of uncharged molecules which predominate in biological fluids.

Equipment for HPLC

The components of an HPLC system comprise: a pump(s), sample introduction system (syringe injector or autosampler), column, detector and data collection system (chart recorder or computer). For most applications a single liquid phase can be used throughout at a constant flow rate (typically 1–2 ml/min) i.e. isocratic

elution. However, in some complex applications where the compounds being separated are very similar in structure it may be necessary to vary the composition of the liquid phase during the analysis, i.e. gradient elution. An example of gradient elution is the separation of amino acids in blood or urine.

The choice of the method of detection for HPLC is dependent on the type of analyte, with ultraviolet (UV), fluorescent and electrochemical (EC) detection being routinely used. UV detection predominates in reverse phase HPLC but is seldom used in normal phase methods as the high concentration of organic solvent in the mobile phase results in a large background absorption between 190 and 230 nm. Fluorescence detection has high sensitivity but requires compounds either to have native fluorescence or to be chemically modified to induce fluorescence. Electrochemical detection is based on the oxidation of compounds at a carbon or metal electrode and can offer excellent sensitivity and specificity for particular compounds.

Sample preparation for biological samples

A complication of analysing biological samples using HPLC is the high protein content present in many body fluids (approximately 70 g/l in plasma and serum). This can produce background interference and can lead to column clogging, so some form of sample preparation is usually required prior to analysis. The exact form of sample preparation will vary with the specific application, but usually deproteinization and/or extraction of the compounds of interest is carried out. Both liquid–liquid and solid-phase extractions are used for HPLC methods involving blood samples. When urine is used, interference in UV or fluorescent detection methods can occur if coloured or fluorescent pigments are present and some form of extraction will often be necessary.

Applications

The majority of applications of HPLC in laboratory medicine fall in the field of clinical biochemistry although haematologists also use the technique. Groups of compounds that are regularly analysed by HPLC in the clinical

High Performance Liquid Chromatography (HPLC)

laboratory include biogenic amines, amino acids, porphyrins, drugs, vitamins, haemoglobin including glycated haemoglobin, and carbohydrates. Many other specific applications have been described for research purposes including nucleosides, collagen degradation products and steroids, but these have not often become part of the routine repertoire of tests.

Biogenic amines

The catecholamines, adrenaline, noradrenaline and dopamine and their metabolites are measured in plasma and urine samples for the detection of tumours of neural crest origin – phaeochromocytoma and neuroblastoma. Phaeochromocytomas secrete large amounts of adrenaline and/or noradrenaline which is further metabolized to 4-hydroxy-3-methylmandelic acid (HMMA). Increased concentrations of both the catecholamines and HMMA can be detected in urine from patients with phaeochromocytoma using reverse phase HPLC with electrochemical detection. This technique can also be used to detect the abnormally high amounts of dopamine and its metabolite homovanillic acid (HVA) produced by neuroblastomas.

Serotonin (5-hydroxytryptamine, 5-HT) is synthesized from tryptophan and metabolized to 5-hydroxyindole acetic acid (5-HIAA) by monoamine oxidases. Carcinoid tumours secrete abnormal amounts of 5-HT and measurement of blood/urine serotonin concentrations or urinary 5-HIAA excretion is useful in detecting tumours and in monitoring therapy. Methods for the simultaneous determination of HMMA, HVA and 5-HIAA by reverse phase HPLC are in routine use in clinical laboratories.

Amino acids

The use of TLC for qualitative identification of abnormalities of amino acid metabolism has been described previously. Quantitation of specific amino acids is often necessary, particularly for monitoring therapy in disorders such as phenylketonuria or maple syrup urine disease. The first specialist HPLC system was the amino acid analyser which is based on the separation of amino acids by cation exchange chromatography with spectrophotometric detection

following post-column reaction with ninhydrin to produce coloured derivatives. Many alternative derivatization methods have now been described to separate amino acids by reverse phase HPLC with UV, fluorescent or electrochemical detection (see 'Further reading').

Porphyrins

The porphyrins are cyclic tetrapyroles which are formed by oxidation of the porphyrinogens, the intermediates of the haem biosynthetic pathway. A class of inherited disorders exists (the porphyrias) in which specific enzyme deficiencies lead to accumulation of the precursors. The clinical presentation of the porphyrias is diverse, ranging from chronic photosensitivity to acute abdominal pain and, although some idea of the exact diagnosis can be gained from the symptoms, characterization of the type of porphyria requires the identification of the pattern of

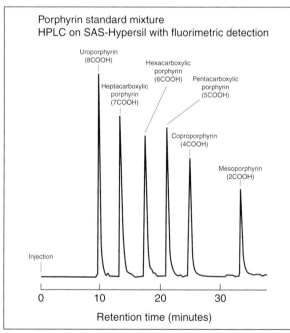

Figure 44.1: HPLC of standard mixture used for urinary porphyrin analysis. Peaks correspond to uroporphyrin (8 COOH), heptaporphyrin (7 COOH), hexaporphyrin (6 COOH), pentaporphyrin (5 COOH), coproporphyrin (4 COOH) and mesoporphyrin (2 COOH). Column–0.8 ×15 cm SAS-Hypersil (5 μm). Gradient elution and UV detection (400 nm).

porphyrins in blood, urine and faeces. This can be achieved by liquid–liquid extraction of the porphyrins followed by reverse phase HPLC with either UV or fluorescent detection since the porphyrins have native fluorescence. An example of porphyrin separation by HPLC is shown in Fig. 44.1.

Drugs

Immunoassay techniques have now replaced HPLC as the routine method for many of the established anticonvulsants e.g. phenytoin, phenobarbitone and carbamazepine. However, the newer generation of anticonvulsants including lamotrigine, vigabatrin and oxcarbazepine are measured by reverse phase HPLC with UV detection.

The methylxanthines, caffeine and theophylline, are used for the prevention of neonatal apnoea; theophylline is also used as prophylactic treatment for asthma. Specific immunoassays exist for these compounds but two assays are required for each sample. Reverse phase HPLC with UV detection can measure both simultaneously and can also provide information on the other metabolites in the xanthine pathways.

Other drugs

Assays for many thousands of other drugs in biological fluids have been developed. Readers seeking further information should consult the 'Further reading' at the end of this chapter.

Vitamins

The vitamins are a diverse group of compounds, but virtually all have been measured in blood or urine by HPLC (see 'Further reading' for details).

Haemoglobins including glycated haemoglobin

Over 400 structural variants of haemoglobin are known, most of which have no clinical sequelae for the individual. However, some variants are associated with disease, for example Hb S (the haemoglobin of sickle cell disease). A definitive diagnosis requires the identification of the variant present. Until relatively recently, separation of haemoglobins was achieved by electrophoresis but several commercial dedicated HPLC systems have now appeared based on ion-exchange chromatography. These have a faster sample throughput and are useful in population screening for the haemoglobinopathies. Modifications to these systems enables them to be used to quantitate the glycated fraction of haemoglobin, HbAlc, with an analytical cycle time of four to eight minutes. A HPLC version of the boronate gel affinity chromatography method is also available, which has the benefit of being unaffected by the presence of haemoglobin variants.

Carbohydrates

Screening for inherited disorders of carbohydrate metabolism is usually carried out by TLC as previously described. Quantitation of specific carbohydrates is often not necessary but the development of intestinal sugar absorption/permeability studies has necessitated accurate measurement of specific sugars in urine, e.g. lactulose, rhamnose and xylose, when quantitation is required. Separation can be achieved using ion exchange chromatography but detection has been difficult as carbohydrates have neither usable UV or fluorescent properties. The advent of pulsed amperometric electrochemical detection has improved the situation vastly.

Gas Chromatography (GC)

Principles

In GC the compounds of interest are separated by partition between the solute in an inert carrier gas stream (nitrogen, argon or helium) and a liquid of low volatility held on an inert support (hence its former name, gas–liquid chromatography or GLC). The inert support is usually glass microbeads or synthetic halogenated polymers and a derivatized polyalcohol or silicone. Conventional GC columns are typically 1–3 m long with a 2–6 mm internal diameter, but the majority of clinical applications use capillary columns which can be up to 40 m in length with an internal diameter of 0.2–0.5 mm. The benefits of capillary GC are generally improved resolution and shorter run

Gas Chromatography (GC)

Applications

times. The detection systems available for GC are: flame ionization (FID), electron capture (ECD) and mass spectrometry (GC–MS). A comparison of normal versus capillary GC and details of the mode of action of the types of detectors is given in a review by Lewis & Sampson.

Applications

Compounds that can be separated by GC must be volatile or capable of being converted to a volatile state by derivatization. These include alcohols, steroids, drugs, organic acids and bile acids.

Alcohols

Ethanol and methanol are volatile compounds readily measurable by GC with FID. A normal GC column can be used as the extra resolution of capillary GC is unnecessary. Ethylene glycol measurements in suspected toxicity are also feasible.

Steroids

Urine steroid profiling provides information on the production and metabolism of steroids from the adrenal gland, testes and ovaries. It is particularly important in assessing children of uncertain gender or with precocious sexual development. Using capillary GC with FID following derivatization of the steroids, up to 25 steroids and metabolites can be detected and quantitated in one run (Fig. 44.2).

Drugs

Drugs which are not easily measured by HPLC e.g. valproate, the tricyclic anti-depressants, etc. are often assayed by GC, either for therapeutic drug monitoring or for toxicological purposes. Most systems use normal GC columns with FID, but GC–MS has a particular role in confirming positive drugs of abuse screens obtained using TLC, EMIT or other immunoassays. Specific methods for many drugs can be found in the book by Ghosh.

Organic acids

Inherited diseases which produce changes in organic acid excretion include specific diseases

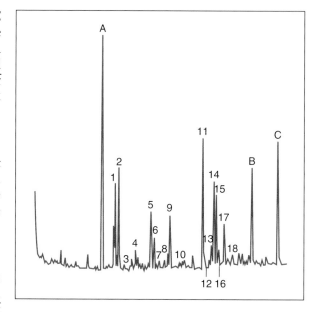

Figure 44.2: Typical chromatogram from the capillary GC analysis of methyl oxime-trimethylsilyl ether (MO-TMS) derivatives of steroids in urine from a normal adult female. The peak identities are as follows: A, B, C, internal standards; 1. androsterone, 2. aetiocholanolone, 3. dehydroepiandrosterone, 4. 11-oxo-aetio-cholanolone, 5. 11β-OH androsterone, 6. 11β-OH aetiocholanolone, 7. 16α-OH dehydroepiandrosterone, 8. pregnanediol, 9. pregnanetriol, 10. androstenetriol, 11. tetrahydrocortisone, 12. tetrahydro-11-dehydrocorticosterone, 13. allo-tetrahydrocorticosterone, 14. tetrahydrocortisol, 15. allo-tetrahydrocortisol, 16. α-cortolone, 17.β-cortolone, 18. α-cortol.

e.g. propionic acidaemia, and families of diseases associated with abnormalities of the urea cycle. Urinary organic acid measurements are usually carried out using capillary GC–MS. The added benefit of mass spectrometry as the detector is the positive identification of any unusual compounds.

Bile acids

Disorders of bile acid synthesis are rare but can be confirmed by bile acid analysis in blood or urine. Like organic acid analysis, bile acids require capillary GC–MS for optimal separation and identification.

Electrophoresis

Principles

Electrophoretic separation is based on the differential migration of charged molecules under the influence of an applied electric potential. Molecules that can be separated by electrophoresis must either carry a net positive or negative charge in their native state (e.g. many proteins and amino acids) or must be able to accept a charge (e.g. carbohydrates complexed with borate ions). The chemical environment around the molecule, the electrolyte solution, must be capable of conducting an electric current, but also has a critical role in determining the state of ionization and hence the charge on any molecule in contact with it. The choice of electrolyte and its pH is critical to achieving optimal mobility and separation. Movement of the charged particle is brought about by the action of the electrical force. The migration velocity is dependent on the relationship between the applied potential and the distance between the electrodes – greater migration can be obtained by increasing the voltage applied or by decreasing the distance between electrodes. The passage of an electric current will inevitably generate heat and optimal conditions will need to balance this with maximizing separation. A retarding force, which is a function of the size of the molecule and the viscosity of the solution, counteracts the forward migration induced by the electric field. The rate of migration is therefore directly proportional to the field strength and to the net charge of the molecule and inversely proportional to the size of the particle and the viscosity of the solution. Electrophoretic separation can be achieved in free solution but usually some form of solid support medium is used such as paper, cellulose acetate, agar gel or polyacrylamide gel. In the past ten years much interest has focused on carrying out electrophoresis in narrow capillaries at high voltage, capillary electrophoresis.

Applications

Electrophoresis was first used in the clinical laboratory in the 1950s for the separation of serum proteins. Since then applications have been developed to separate serum proteins, isoenzymes (e.g. creatine kinase, alkaline phosphatase etc), haemoglobin variants and DNA fragments following the polymerase chain reaction (PCR). As for chromatography, many other applications exist such as separation of lipoproteins, but these have tended to remain in the research domain and have not become routine tests.

Serum protein electrophoresis

The principal use of electrophoretic separation of serum proteins is the identification of monoclonal gammopathies, although it continues to be used to demonstrate the (non-specific) changes associated with a variety of conditions e.g. nephrotic syndrome. The early methods for serum protein electrophoresis used cellulose acetate as a support medium which produces limited resolution of serum proteins into the main bands: albumin, α_1-globulins, α_2-globulins, β-globulins and γ-globulins. If plasma is used rather than serum then an additional band from fibrinogen occurs, usually between the β- and γ-globulin regions. Visualization following staining with Ponceau red or Coomassie brilliant blue stains is usually adequate to detect gross abnormalities but densitometric scanning can be used if quantitative data on the individual fractions are required. Whilst the resolution using cellulose acetate is adequate for most purposes, considerably improved resolution can be obtained by using agar gel as the support medium. Additional bands are seen with agar gel electrophoresis including prealbumin, C-reactive protein and differentiation of the β_1- and β_2-globulins (Fig. 44.3). Even greater resolution can be obtained using polyacrylamide gels but this is seldom of value in routine clinical use.

Isoenzymes

Many of the enzymes which are routinely measured in serum exist as a mixture of isoenzymes, each of which may be produced in a different organ system in the body. For example, creatine kinase (CK) in serum is a mixture of CK-MM (from skeletal muscle), CK-MB (predominantly from the heart) and CK-BB (from brain). Electrophoresis can differentiate whether the cause of a raised total CK is

Electrophoresis

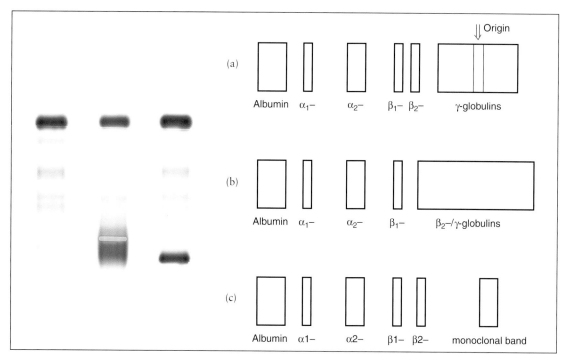

Figure 44.3: *Agar gel serum protein electrophoresis: (a) Normal pattern, (b) Polyclonal increase in γ-globulins due to cirrhosis of the liver, (c) Monoclonal gammopathy (IgG) with immune paresis.*

damage to cardiac or skeletal muscle. Separation is achieved using agar gels and these are overlaid with a synthetic substrate to the enzyme which produces a fluorescent compound visible under UV light when acted on by CK. Although immunological methods for CK-MB are now replacing electrophoretic methods for CK in many laboratories, electrophoresis remains the only method capable of detecting the presence of macro-CK complexes. Electrophoresis is also used to separate alkaline phosphatase into its liver, bone, placental and intestinal forms or to determine the pattern of isoenzymes of lactate dehydrogenase.

Haemoglobin
Until the recent introduction of HPLC, methods for the identification of haemoglobin variants, electrophoretic methods were in common use, based on the different overall charge on the haemoglobin molecule caused by the amino acid substitutions. Cellulose acetate was normally the support medium for screen-

ing methods with citrate agar gel electrophoresis used for positive identification of any abnormal variants seen on screening. The separation of haemoglobin variants by citrate gel electrophoresis relies on the interactions of the substituted amino acids with agaropectin. Those variant haemoglobins with substitutions near the surface, e.g. Hb S and Hb C, are retained whilst those with deeper substitutions such as Hb D and Hb G are not. Complex combinations of electrophoresis or isoelectric focusing are required to identify rare haemoglobinopathies.

DNA fragments following PCR
Whilst outside the scope of this section it is worth remembering that many of the molecular techniques now being introduced into the clinical laboratory include the electrophoretic separation of the restriction fragments of DNA following PCR and treatment with restriction enzymes. Agar gel is the support medium used in the vast majority of applications in molecu-

lar biology with visualization either by radio-labelling or by staining with ethidium bromide.

Capillary Electrophoresis (CE)

Although electrophoresis in a narrow capillary was first described in 1937, it has only been since 1985 that the technique has come into its own. Capillaries between 20 and 100 μm in diameter and 25 to 100 cm in length are used, the ends of which are placed in buffer vials which also contain the electrodes. Very high voltages (10–30 kV) are applied to produce the electroendosmotic flow within the capillary. The type, pH and ionic strength of the buffer filling the capillary are critical to achieving the desired separation.

There are four major modes of separation by capillary electrophoresis: capillary zone electrophoresis (CZE) or free solution separation; micellar electrokinetic capillary chromatography (MECC); capillary isoelectric focusing (CIEF); capillary isotachophoresis.

The principles of these different modes of separation and potential applications in laboratory medicine have been reviewed recently. Although still in its infancy as a routine technique, CE is likely to replace conventional electrophoresis for serum proteins and possibly haemoglobin variants over the next five years. CE is also being used in conjunction with DNA amplification techniques in molecular biology.

Further Reading

Ghosh M K. *HPLC Methods in Drug Analysis*. 1992: Springer Verlag, Berlin.

Jenkins M A. Capillary electrophoresis – an overview. *Clinical Biochemist Reviews*. 1995; **16**: 98–103.

Lewis J, Sampson D. Chromatography for the Clinical Biochemist. *Clinical Biochemist Reviews*. 1994; **15**: 56–63.

Sherwood R A. Amino acid measurement by HPLC with electrochemical detection. *Journal of Neuroscience Methods*. 1990; **34**: 17–22.

Sherwood R A, Rocks B F. Liquid chromatography: Applications in clinical analysis. *Encyclopaedia of Analytical Science*. 1995: Academic Press, London. Vol 5, 2677–2685.

SECTION 7
IMMUNOLOGY

45   PROTEIN ASSAYS

David Burnett

Introduction

Qualitative and quantitative techniques for protein analysis are essential tools in the routine immunology laboratory, whose remit includes the analysis of some proteins in blood and other body fluids. Specifically, the proteins of major interest to the immunologist include the immunoglobulins (antibodies), the proteins of the complement system and, most recently, cytokines which have a role in the immune system. The purpose of this chapter is to describe briefly the principles of the methods used for routine protein analysis. Although some of the methods described are used for the study of proteins of the complement system, the nature of that system demands special considerations for accurate interpretation. Assays for complement proteins are therefore described in detail in Chapter 46. Similarly, assays for autoimmune antibodies are addressed in the chapter on immune complex disease and cryoglobulins (Chapter 48).

The main purpose of the routine laboratory is to detect, characterize and measure the quantity of (1) deficiencies of specific proteins as in immunoglobulin deficiency, and (2) abnormal or inappropriate expression of proteins, for instance in monoclonal gammopathies, autoimmune disease or atopy.

Methods for the analysis of proteins rely on a variety of principles. For most routine assays such as those which are described in this chapter there are, however, really only two basic properties utilized: (1) Individual proteins have a characteristic electrical charge which means that different specific proteins can be separated by electrophoresis. (2) Each specific human protein has a unique structure and this can be used to produce antibodies to that protein, either polyclonal antibodies by immunizing animals with that human protein or monoclonal antibodies by hybridoma technology. Antibodies specific for a protein are the basis of immune assays.

The selection of an appropriate assay method will depend upon whether a qualitative or quantitative result is required. Furthermore, the concentration of the protein of interest will be crucial to the choice of test. The detection or measurement of oligoclonal and monoclonal immunoglobulins in CSF and urine, for instance, may require sample concentration or the choice of a method more sensitive than that required for serum specimens.

Historical Perspective

The study of human plasma proteins began essentially with the work of Liebig and Mulder in the 1830s. At the time blood proteins were regarded simply as the 'albuminoid' component of tissues. By 1864, however, it was discovered that blood serum could be fractionated into 'albumin' and a second component that was called globulin. By the early 1900s the 'globulin' fraction was still thought to consist only of two components, named pseudoglobulins and euglobulins. The principles of electrophoresis, the method of separating molecules in an electric charge, had been known for some time when the Swede, Arne Tiselius, in 1930, suspecting the complex nature of blood proteins, began experimenting with the electrophoresis of serum in a liquid buffer medium. In 1937 he identified several discrete protein zones which could be seen after the electrophoresis of serum; these he designated albumin, α-globulin, β-globulin, and γ-globulin, albumin having the fastest mobility towards the anode and γ-globulin the slowest. This basic nomenclature is still employed today (see below). The use of a liquid buffer as the support medium for electrophoresis limited the definition of the protein bands which were separated. In the 1950s paper began to be used as a support medium, followed in later years by cellulose acetate and gels such as agar, agarose and polyacrylamide.

As early as 1905 Bechhold showed that a protein *antigen* and an antibody to that antigen could form a precipitate. It was 1946, however, before Oudin described a useful development of this principle and in 1948 'double diffusion' in a gel was introduced independently by Elek and Ouchterlony. This simple method, which is still used (described below) continues to be referred to as the 'Ouchterlony method'. Grabar and Williams in 1953 combined electrophoretic separation of serum proteins with immunoprecipitation (qualitative immunoelectrophoresis) using polyclonal antibodies to whole serum and the true nature of the heterogeneity of serum proteins was recognized. As specific proteins began to be purified and antibodies to them raised in animals, specific quantitative immune assays became possible. Radial immunodiffusion (the Mancini technique) was introduced in 1965 and this too is still used routinely (see below). The sensitivity of quantitative protein assays has since been improved, with radioimmunoassays and enzyme-immunoassays allowing realistic measurements down to the order of several ng/ml.

Qualitative Techniques

Electrophoresis

Serum protein electrophoresis, although giving limited resolution, is a fundamental method for analyzing samples for gross protein abnormalities. The support medium is usually a cellulose acetate membrane or agarose gel. Buffers vary but usually are based on barbitone with a pH of about 8.5. Gels or membranes for routine electrophoresis are available commercially and these are frequently used to minimize preparation time and to ensure consistent results. The support membrane is placed on an electrophoresis tank, connected at each end to buffer solution. The sample to be analysed is loaded at the cathode end and an electric current applied for 30 minutes to one hour. The proteins in the sample migrate in the current at rates proportional to their charge. After completion of electrophoretic separation, the gel or membrane is removed and the proteins insolubilized by fixation, usually in acetic acid solution, and visualized by staining with an appropriate protein dye (Fig. 45.1a). The gel can be semi-quantitated by densitometry, that is, the gel is scanned using a densitometer which measures the density of staining. (Fig. 45.1b)

Only proteins with a concentration of 0.1–0.5 g/l or greater will contribute to the serum protein bands seen, of which usually six are represented. These are designated, in order of electrophoretic mobility, as:

1. The albumin band (represented by serum albumin)
2. The α_1 band (represented usually by α_1 antitrypsin, orosomucoid and α lipoprotein)
3. The α_2 band (represented by haptoglobin and α_2 macroglobulin)

462

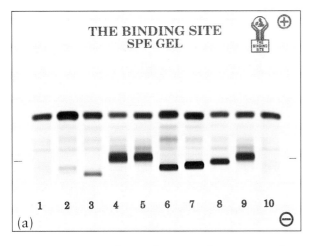
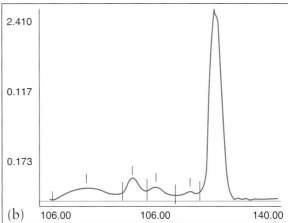

Figure 45.1: *(a) Electrophoresis of serum samples in agarose. Samples were loaded at the cathode (bottom). The dark band at the top represents albumin. Dark-staining bands in the γ-protein area (nearest the cathode) represent paraproteins. (b) Densitometry scan of agarose gel electrophoresis of serum from a healthy subject. The tall peak on the right represents albumin.*

4. The β_1 band (represented by transferrin)
5. The β_2 band (represented by complement proteins and β lipoprotein)
6. The γ band (represented by the immuno-globulins IgG, IgM and IgA)

Although most serum proteins, being present in blood at concentrations below the threshold for this method, do not contribute to the bands seen, much valuable information can be obtained using this technique. For instance, a reduced α_1 band usually indicates a deficiency of α_1 antitrypsin (also known as α_1 proteinase inhibitor). Since inherited α_1 antitrypsin deficiency may be associated with an increased risk of pulmonary emphysema, the absence of an α_1 band is an indication for further quanti-tative estimations of α_1 antitrypsin in the patient's serum and possible haplotyping of the protein by isoelectric focussing of the serum or gene analysis using leukocytes as the source of genetic material.

For the immunologist perhaps the most rel-evant information obtained from electrophore-sis is the detection of immunoglobulin deficiency or monoclonal gammopathy. Because immunoglobulins usually represent many different antibody molecules they are by nature heterogeneous and are not represented by a discrete γ band. Rather, this band is seen as a broad smear *unless* there is a monoclonal (or M band). In cases of monoclonal gam-mopathy there is production predominantly, by a single expanded clone of immunoglobu-lin-producing cells, of immunoglobulin of one isotype (IgG, IgM or IgA) with discrete specificity. These immunoglobulin molecules are thus essentially identical and produce a dis-crete γ band, or M band (Fig. 45.1). The identification of the nature of the monoclonal M protein in serum and free light chains (Bence Jones proteins) in urine can be carried out using immunofixation by precipitating the protein in the support medium, after elec-trophoresis, with a specific antibody to each isotype. Non-precipitated proteins are washed out and the remaining precipitate visualized by staining with a protein dye (Fig. 45.2). The M protein can also be characterized by immuno-diffusion or immunoelectrophoresis and the concentration measured by quantitative immunoassay (these methods are described below). By contrast, a reduced γ band suggests an immunoglobulin deficiency and this should be investigated further by quantitative assay (see below).

Ouchterlony immunodiffusion

Immunodiffusion is carried out usually in agar or agarose gels. Classically, a rosette of wells is

<u>Qualitative Techniques</u>

Countercurrent immunoelectrophoresis

Immunoelectrophoresis

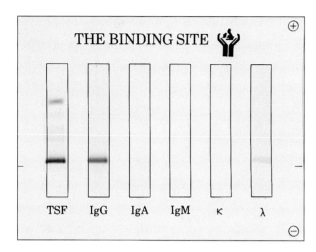

Figure 45.2: *Immunofixation and staining of proteins following electrophoresis of serum in agarose gel (from cathode at bottom towards top). The separation on the left (TSF) shows the pattern for total serum proteins. Note the paraprotein band in the γ fraction near the cathode. Immunofixation with anti-IgG, anti-IgA and anti-IgM reveals the paraprotein to be of the IgG heavy chain. Fixation with antibodies to κ-light chain and λ-light chain show this paraprotein was IgGλ.*

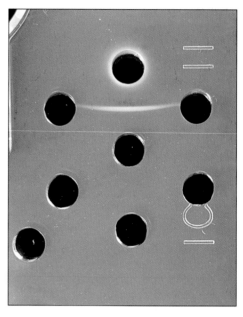

Figure 45.3: *Ouchterlony immunodiffusion showing the classic rosette pattern of wells cut in agarose gel. An antibody was placed in the central well and serum samples into each of the six satellite wells. The serum in the well at the bottom contained the protein to which the antiserum is directed, as revealed by a visible immunoprecipitate line.*

cut into the gel with a well also cut at the centre of the rosette (Fig. 45.3). The central well is filled with test specimen and each surrounding well in the rosette with an antiserum of different specificity. The gel is incubated in a humid atmosphere for several hours. The proteins in the central well and those from the rosette diffuse into the gel. If the specimen contains a protein to which one of the antisera is raised, a precipitate begins to form which is insoluble at concentrations of 'equivalence' and is visualized easily in the gel. The gels can be washed, dried and stained for archiving. Using this method the presence of several proteins can be detected simultaneously in the test specimen. Alternatively, several test samples can be analysed for the presence of a specific protein by putting a specific antiserum in the central well and a different test sample in each of the surrounding wells. Commercially supplied Ouchterlony plates are now available, to identify, for example, the isotype and subclass representing a paraprotein in a serum sample.

Countercurrent immunoelectrophoresis

Countercurrent electrophoresis is similar in principle to immunodiffusion but the antigen and antibody are electrophoresed towards each other in the gel (Fig. 45.4). The use of electrophoresis rather than diffusion means that results are obtained more quickly. It has been recommended that countercurrent immunoelectrophoresis should be used as a rapid initial screening method (for example for detecting antibodies to extractable nuclear antigens) and positive results confirmed by other methods such as Ouchterlony immunodiffusion.

Immunoelectrophoresis

Qualitative immunoelectrophoresis (described originally by Grabar & Williams) begins with electrophoresis in cellulose acetate, agar or agarose. A trough is cut in the membrane or gel, adjacent to the electrophoresis track. Following electrophoresis, antiserum is placed in the trough and the membrane or gel is incubated in a moist atmosphere for several hours.

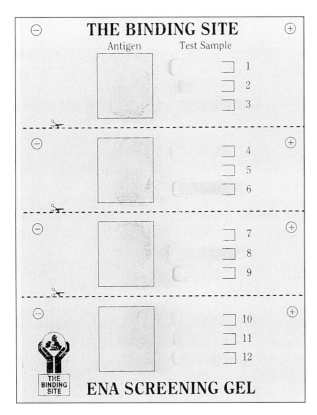

Figure 45.4: Countercurrent electrophoresis. This example is of a commercial kit designed to detect autoantibodies. The target antigen is in the square section at the left (cathode side) and patient's sera applied at the anode side (right). Under the influence of electrophoresis, the antigen at the cathode and the antibodies in the patient's sera move towards each other. An immunoprecipitate (stained with protein dye in this example) indicates the presence of autoantibody in a sample.

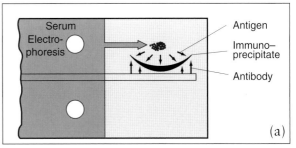

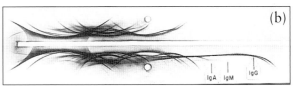

Figure 45.5: (a) Diagram showing the principle of qualitative immunoelectrophoresis. Sample is placed in a trough cut into agarose gel on a glass plate and the proteins separated by electrophoresis (from cathode, left to anode, right). After electrophoresis a well is cut in the agarose parallel to the electrophoretic separation. Antiserum is put into the trough and the plate incubated to allow antibodies and sample proteins to diffuse into each other. The presence of proteins to which antibodies are present in the antiserum results in an immunoprecipitate arc. (b) Immunoelectrophoresis of two serum samples. The two sample application wells are at the centre of the picture, separated by a trough which contained antiserum raised against whole human serum. Electrophoresis was carried out with the cathode towards the right. The immunoprecipitate arcs in the serum at bottom show a normal pattern; those for IgG, IgA and IgM are labelled. Note the absence of these immunoprecipitates in the upper serum sample, indicating that this subject was deficient in all three immunoglobulins.

During this time, the electrophoretically separated proteins and the antibody molecules from the trough diffuse through the support medium. If antibodies to the separated proteins are present, an immunoprecipitate forms in the gel, which is insoluble at a point of 'equivalent' concentrations. These precipitates are often visible in the unstained 'wet' gel but sensitivity can be increased after the gel is washed, fixed and stained (Fig. 45.5). An antiserum raised to whole serum reveals precipitate arcs representing all the proteins present to which there are antibodies in the antiserum. The absence of a precipitin arc (when compared to a reference specimen) indicates a protein deficiency. Monoclonal paraproteins will also be evident because of abnormally shaped or pronounced precipitates. The presence or identity of a specific protein, such as a paraprotein, can be confirmed by putting a specific antiserum (for instance antiserum specific for human IgG, IgA or IgM heavy chains or κ or λ light chains) into the trough.

Qualitative Methods

Radial immunodiffusion

Rocket immunoelectrophoresis

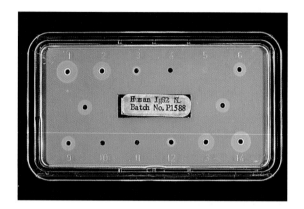

Figure 45.6: Single radial immunodiffusion. An example of this method shows an agarose gel into which is dissolved antiserum to human IgG subclass 2. Human serum samples were aliquoted into the sample wells and, after incubation, immunoprecipitate rings were formed, the areas of which are proportional to IgG2 concentration. Note the absence of immunoprecipitate in three samples, showing IgG2 deficiency.

Quantitative Methods

Radial immunodiffusion (Fig. 45.6)
This method is also known as single radial immunodiffusion or the Mancini method. Agar or agarose, melted in a suitable buffer, is cooled to about 55°C and precipitating antiserum specific for the protein to be measured is added at the appropriate concentration. The antiserum-containing gel is poured onto a glass or plastic plate or tray and allowed to cool, whereupon the gel solidifies. Wells are cut into the gel and each of these is filled with several μl of test serum. A series of wells is each filled with reference serum (or reference solution) containing known concentrations of the protein to be assayed. The plate is left in a humid atmosphere to allow the proteins within the samples and reference solutions to diffuse into the surrounding antiserum-containing gel. As the protein molecules being assayed diffuse into the gel they form precipitates with the antiserum molecules. These precipitates are partially soluble as long as the antigen (protein) concentration remains in excess of that of the antiserum. Thus some protein molecules continue to diffuse radially from the sample well

until the antigen concentration is 'equivalent' to that of the antibodies. At this point an insoluble precipitate ring is formed around the sample well.

The area (and therefore the diameter) of the ring is directly proportional to the concentration of the protein in the test sample. Indeed, provided the antiserum concentration in the gel, and the sample protein concentrations, are within appropriate limits and the diffusion process has been allowed to run to completion, the immunoprecipitate ring area is linearly proportional to protein concentration. This requires that the test system be titrated by experimentation. It also means that the plates may have to be left for a considerable time (perhaps several days) for diffusion and precipitate formation to run to completion. These constraints may be inconvenient and too slow for some routine laboratories but commercial radial immunodiffusion plates are now available for the measurement of clinically relevant proteins, including the immunoglobulin isotypes, subclasses and light chains. These commercial plates are produced to within such fine tolerances that accurate and precise results are obtained before the diffusion has run to completion (the Fahey & McKelvey method), giving results in only a few hours. Indeed, the antiserum concentrations are incorporated so accurately that, with a small and usually irrelevant loss of accuracy, protein concentrations can be interpolated from the ring diameters to standard reference curves supplied with the kit, without using standard reference solutions. The limit of sensitivity of a radial diffusion assay will depend largely upon the quality of the antiserum but is usually in the order of about 5 mg/l. Some commercially developed plates can measure proteins down to as low as 0.5 mg/l.

Rocket immunoelectrophoresis
Rocket immunoelectrophoresis or electroimmunodiffusion involves the electrophoresis of proteins in a sample into agarose gel containing a specific precipitating antiserum. Protein-antibody precipitates are formed by a principle similar to that of radial immunodiffusion, but have a characteristic flame-like (or rocket-like) shape (Fig. 45.7). The area of the precipitate is

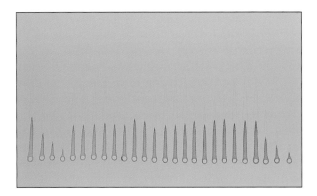

Figure 45.7: *Rocket immunoelectrophoresis. This figure shows the simultaneous assay of two proteins in serum samples. Agarose gel incorporating one antisera specific to human α-1-antitrypsin and a second antiserum, specific to human α-2-macroglobulin, was poured onto a glass plate and allowed to solidify (thickness 1mm). Wells were punched in the gel (bottom of picture) and serum samples put into the wells. Electrophoresis was performed with the cathode at bottom. Immunoprecipitate peaks (rockets) were formed as the two target proteins migrated through the gel. The taller, lighter-staining peaks represent α-1-antitrypsin. The four samples at each end of the plate were standard solutions of known concentrations, used to calibrate the plate. Peak area is proportional to protein concentration, but peak height is a convenient and good approximation.*

proportional to protein concentration but, if conditions are right, peak height is a fair approximation to area.

The method relies on the antibody molecules in the gel remaining immobile. In fact this is not really possible, but antibody electrophoresis is kept to a minimum in two ways. Firstly, agarose gel, rather than agar, is used. Agar is charged and causes a bulk flow of water molecules (endosmosis) in the gel towards the cathode. This carries the antibody with it and depletes antibody at the anodal end, resulting in disproportional precipitation of protein in the gel, with loss of accuracy. Agarose has less charge than agar and therefore endosmosis is not effectively a problem. Secondly, the pH of the buffer used is about 8.6, which is the average isoelectric point of immunoglobulin

molecules and results in minimal electrophoresis of the antibody molecules during the assay procedure. Clearly, however, this means that immunoglobulins and other proteins with a basic charge cannot be measured by this technique since they will not electrophorese into the antibody-containing gel. In theory, this method is faster than radial immunodiffusion and some claim that the measurement of peak height is easier and more precise than that of the diameter of a precipitate ring.

There are some adaptations of this method which have applications for specific investigations, mostly in a research setting. Nevertheless, despite the visually aesthetic nature of this method, in practical terms radial immunodiffusion (especially in the form of commercial kits) is more convenient than rocket immunoelectrophoresis and offers equal accuracy and precision.

Turbidimetry and nephelometry

The quantitative methods described above rely upon the formation of insoluble protein-antibody complexes in supporting gel media which can be visualized by eye. If the precipitate is formed by a protein and antibody at low concentrations in a liquid medium a finer precipitate is formed in suspension. This property can be used to measure the protein concentration. The amount of suspension, at a constant antibody concentration, will be proportional to protein concentration and will impede the passage of a light beam passed through the suspension (turbidimetry). Alternatively, the light scattered by the suspension can be detected at an angle to the incident light (Fig. 45.8). This method is called nephelometry. Clearly this approach, unlike even more 'low-tech' methods such as radial immunodiffusion, requires dedicated apparatus but does offer a degree of automation and large through-put of specimens. Some laboratories use centrifugal analysers in which reagents are mixed during centrifugation and this reduces assay time. The limit of sensitivity of this method, as with most immunoassays, will depend upon the specific system and, especially, the quality of antiserum. In a good system, the limit is about 100 mg/l but this can be improved several-fold

Qualitative Methods

Enzyme-linked immunosorbent assays

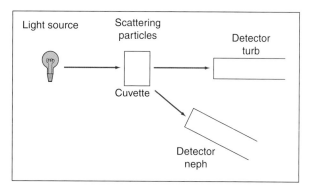

Figure 45.8: *A simplified schema showing the difference between the principles of turbidimetry and nephelometry (see text for explanation).*

if the antibodies are bound to tiny polystyrene beads. Reagents for turbidimetry and nephelometry of clinically important proteins such as immunoglobulin isotypes and subclasses are available commercially.

Enzyme-linked immunosorbent assays

Enzyme-linked immunosorbent assays (ELISA), also called enzyme-immuno assays (EIA), represent a versatile and sensitive principle for protein measurement which has largely replaced radioimmunoassays. These assays can measure proteins down to a concentration of about 1 μg/l, and are therefore convenient if the protein of interest is present at low concentrations. The assays are performed in 96-well plastic plates and reagent handling is usually done by means of multi-channel pipettes or even automated pipetting stations. The ELISA is eminently suited to automation or semi-automation and, therefore, even if the protein being measured is at high concentration, necessitating sample dilution, if large numbers of samples are being processed this technique may be more convenient than other simpler methods such as radial immunodiffusion. Many laboratories construct their own in-house ELISA systems but commercially available kits are available for a wide range of applications including assays to measure clinically important serum proteins, cytokines, microbial antigens (e.g. Chlamydia, HIV, hepatitis B virus), IgE antibodies to allergens and antibodies to pathogens.

Different assay systems vary in detail but the essential principle remains the same (Fig. 45.9). The wells of 96-well microplates (also obtainable as 8-well strips) are coated with an antibody to the protein being measured. This need not be a precipitating antibody, and monoclonal antibodies are often used. Each well is filled with a test sample (100–200 μl) or one of a range of reference solutions of known concentrations. The wells are incubated for an appropriate time (at least one hour) after which the wells are washed to remove material which has not been captured by the antibody on the well surface. The wells are then filled with a solution of another antibody to the protein being measured. Clearly, if the primary antibody was a monoclonal, the same monoclonal antibody might not be effective in this step because the target protein might have only one antigenic determinant (epitope) recognized by that antibody. This is where some experimentation is needed, to identify a second antibody that will recognize the protein after it has been captured by the primary one immobilized on the plate wells. This second antibody is conjugated with an enzyme, usually horseradish peroxidase (HRP) or alkaline phosphatase. The plate is incubated again to allow the second, enzyme-conjugated antibody to bind to captured protein. The plate is washed further and the substrate to the conjugated enzyme is added to the wells. The substrate produces a soluble, coloured reaction product. Since the amount of enzyme-conjugated antibody that binds will be proportional to the amount of protein captured by the primary antibody, it follows that the amount of enzyme reaction product will be proportional to the protein concentration in the original sample. The amount of reaction product is measured using an ELISA plate reader which passes light through each well at a wavelength that is absorbed by the reaction product (450 nm for HRP, 492 nm for alkaline phosphatase) and, for quantitation, results are interpolated from those obtained with the reference solutions.

If the ELISA is to be used to detect specific antibodies in a body fluid the plate wells are coated with proteins of the relevant target (protein from a pathogen, for example). The

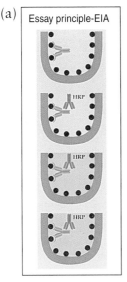

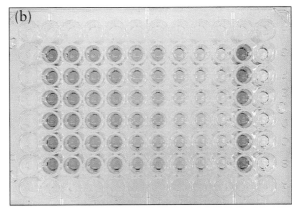

Figure 45.9: (a) Diagram showing a simple scheme for an ELISA to detect antibodies in samples directed against a specific protein. Microtitre wells are coated with the protein (red). The sample is added to the well. If an antibody to the protein is present, it will bind (green antibody molecule). After washing, an antiserum to the human protein raised in an animal and labelled with horseradish peroxidase (HRP) is added (blue antibody molecule). If the sample contained the antibody of interest and was captured by the well-coating protein, the anti-human antibodies (blue) will also bind. After washing the plate again, a substrate for HRP is added and any bound antibody-conjugated HRP will react with the substrate giving a yellow product. The amount of product is measured by absorbance of light of the appropriate wavelength and is proportional to the amount of peroxidase-conjugated antibody (blue) bound, and hence proportional to the concentration of the antibody of interest (green) in the original sample. (b) A completed ELISA plate showing the resulting colour development, resulting from a peroxidase-labelled antibody.

samples being tested are applied to the wells, followed by an enzyme-conjugated antibody to human immunoglobulin. The choice of the anti-human immunoglobulin will allow the detection of all isotypes (by using antiserum raised against human immunoglobulins IgG, IgA & IgM), or of a specific isotype (IgE antibodies to allergens, for example) or subclass.

Conclusion

Routine immunology laboratories have at their disposal a range of methods for protein analysis from which to choose. The methods employed will be dictated by considerations including the nature of the specimens, the identities of the proteins being measured and their concentrations in the specimens. Also, the numbers of specimens routinely processed will dictate whether automated systems need to be used. Many of the methods used today have changed only in detail since specific proteins began to be identified and measured and some of these will probably continue to be employed for decades to come. Others, such as ELISA, represent newer technologies and will displace those with technical or practical disadvantages, such as radioimmunoassay. Who knows what new methods wait around the metaphorical corner?

Acknowledgements

I should like to thank Mr. Roger Drew, ISRL, University of Birmingham Medical School and Mrs. Suzanne Fahy, The Binding Site, Birmingham for providing some of the figures.

Further Reading

Chapel H, Haeney M. *Essentials of Clinical Immunology*. 3rd Ed 1993: Blackwell Scientific, Oxford. A good textbook on clinical immunology, with discussion of appropriate tests to use and their interpretation.

Sheehan C. *Clinical Immunology. Principles & Laboratory Diagnosis*. 2nd Ed 1997: Lippincott, Philadelphia & New York. [About half of this textbook is devoted to immunological techniques and their interpretation.]

Two useful little booklets by A R Bradwell are *IgG & IgA Subclasses in disease* (1995) and *The Binding Site Guide to paraprotein testing* (1994). [These can be obtained from The Binding Site Ltd, P.O. Box 4073, Birmingham, B29 6AT, UK.]

46 COMPLEMENT ASSAYS

Keith Whaley and Jonathan North

Introduction

Complement is a system of serum proteins and cell receptors that has several functions, most of which help the host prevent or fight infection. Originally described as a heat-sensitive substance that could, together with specific antibody, lyse certain bacteria, we now know that complement proteins act through two main pathways. Activation of these pathways leads to the deposition of a potent opsonin on the surface of microorganisms as well as producing an inflammatory response by releasing vasoactive and chemotactic factors. Further components can damage the surfaces of cells and yet another group of components controls the spontaneous and potentially harmful activation of these pathways.

Complement protein levels can be assayed by several methods and it is also possible to determine the functional activity of the majority of components. To appreciate fully the conditions required for these assays it is important to understand the process which is occurring. Accordingly a brief overview of complement is given in the following section with more detailed descriptions to be found in the individual assay sections.

The classical pathway

The first pathway to be described is termed the classical pathway (Fig. 46.1). The components in this system are prefixed with 'C' and comprise C1q, C1r, C1s, C4 and C2 (the numbers being ascribed at the time of the components' definition, not sequence of activation). The classical pathway can be activated by IgG or IgM which has bound antigen. C1q binds to such antibody and, once attached, activates C1r which in turn activates C1s. Activated C1s is a protease whose substrate is C4 which becomes cleaved. Cleaved C4 (C4b) will bind C2 and C1s will then activate C2 (to form C2a) by limited proteolysis. The active C4b2a complex (classical pathway C3 convertase) activates C3, again by limited proteolysis.

Calcium and magnesium ions are both required for activation of the classical pathway. Activated C3 (C3b) will bind covalently to surfaces and act as a high affinity ligand for C3b receptors on phagocytes.

This pathway can also be activated by C1q binding to C-reactive protein which is an acute phase protein, similar in shape to IgM, that binds to the carbohydrate on some bacteria. Mannan binding lectin (MBL) is a functionally similar protein which resembles C1q itself and MBL forms a macromolecular complex with MBL associated serine protease (MASP) which has much the same properties as C1s. The MBL/MASP complex can therefore activate the classical pathway through C4 when it binds to a suitable carbohydrate.

Introduction
The alternative pathway

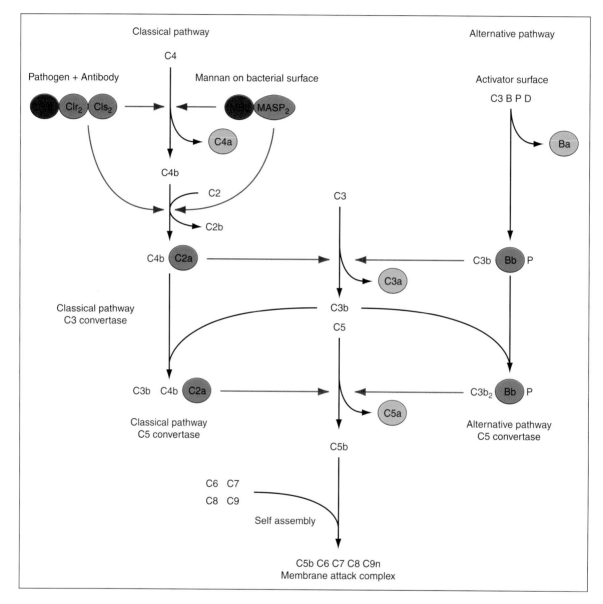

Figure 46.1: *The classical and alternative pathways of complement activation. Components with protease activity are shown in green, collectins in blue and anaphylatoxins in red.*

The alternative pathway

C3, factor B, factor D and properdin are the components of the alternative pathway of complement activation. Activation of this pathway does not rely on any specific triggering factors but on a constant, low level of spontaneous activation. A small proportion of circulating C3 becomes hydrolysed and this form of C3 can bind to factor B in the presence of magnesium ions. Bound factor B is cleaved by factor D to give Ba and C3Bb and the latter can activate further C3 to form C3a and C3b. C3b can bind to surfaces and, once attached, bind more factor B. C3b bound to the surface of microorganisms is resistant to the regulatory activity of factor H and factor I so that activation is favoured. In the same way that factor B bound to circulating C3 is cleaved, factor B bound to C3b on surfaces is cleaved by factor D to give C3bBb. This complex is stabilized by properdin and both C3bBb and C3bBbP can cleave further C3 molecules, thus amplifying the process. Another function of the C3bBbP complex is that it can bind to and activate C5 (see below).

The membrane attack complex

The complement components C5, C6, C7, C8 and C9 form the terminal pathway. C5 can be activated by either the classical or the alternative pathway C5 convertases (C4b2a and C3bBbP respectively). Activated C5b binds to C6 and the remaining components, C7, C8 and C9, bind in turn. Six molecules of C9 will bind to this complex and form a pore in the membrane of a cell on which it is present. This can lead to lysis of the cell and is a property used in the haemolytic assays described below.

Biologically active products of complement activation

One of the main functions of the complement system is to deposit C3b on the surface of microorganisms and, as described above, this can occur either by the classical or the alternative pathways. C3b present on the surface of microorganisms increases their uptake by phagocytes, such as neutrophils, via receptors for C3b and also stimulates these cells. Activation of the classical pathway by immune complexes of antibody and antigen increases the solubility of such complexes and aids their removal from the circulation by complement receptors on red blood cells.

As mentioned above, complexes of C5b–9 can cause lysis of microorganisms by the insertion of C9 polymers into the cell membrane. Lysis of bystander cells may occur unless they are protected by the C3 receptor CR1, decay accelerating factor (DAF), membrane cofactor protein (MCP) and CD59 which prevents the polymerization of C9. The activation of C4, C2, C3, factor B and C5 results in relatively small fragments being released. The two that are most important are the anaphylatoxins C3a and C5a, which are vasoactive and release histamine from mast cells. C5a is also a powerful chemotactic agent which activates neutrophils and monocytes.

Control of complement activation

Spontaneous activation of complement needs to be controlled to prevent an inflammatory response occurring unnecessarily. The classical pathway is regulated by the serum proteins C1 inhibitor (C1-inh), C4bp and factor I and by the cell surface molecules membrane cofactor protein (MCP), decay accelerating factor (DAF, CD55) and CR1. The alternative pathway is regulated by factors H and I and MCP, DAF and CR1. All these factors accelerate the decay of one or more of the activated complement proteins or complexes and hence complement activation will only occur if the activating stimulus can generate enough active products to overcome the inhibitory mechanisms.

Assay of Serum Complement Levels

Specimen preparation and storage

Incorrect storage of samples for complement assay can result in decreased levels because some components are extremely labile. For assays of individual components in serum, blood samples should arrive in the laboratory as soon as possible after venepuncture. Blood should be allowed to clot at room temperature for 30 minutes and the sample placed on ice for one hour for clot retraction to occur before separating the serum at 2–4°C. Samples should be aliquotted and stored at –70°C as quickly as practicable. For use, samples should be thawed at 37°C then immediately placed on ice: repeated freezing and thawing will decrease the haemolytic activity of components. Blood collected into EDTA (which prevents further complement activation by chelating calcium and magnesium and hence such samples are suitable for activation product assays) should be kept on ice for as short as time as possible before being spun to produce platelet-poor plasma which is stored as for serum. Samples from tissue culture may benefit from the addition of proteinase inhibitors such as PMSF.

Immunochemical assays

These assays utilize antibodies which are specific for individual complement components

Assay of Serum Complement Levels

Haemolytic complement assays

and are readily available commercially and can be used for nephelometric, ELISA or immuno-diffusion assays (see Chapter 45). The choice of antibody is critical as polyclonal antibodies may recognize breakdown products of the component under investigation and the resulting value obtained may not reflect the level of functional protein present.

The type of assay system used depends on the number of assays being performed, the level of sensitivity required, the level of the analyte and the quality of the antibody available. For instance, nephelometry is used in routine clinical immunology laboratories for measuring C3, C4, C1-inh and C1q in patient samples where levels are 50 μg/ml or above. For cell culture studies however, levels may be as low as 1 ng/ml and ELISA, although more labour-intensive and taking longer to perform, is more practical. Radial immunodiffusion and gel rocket techniques, although time-consuming and not especially sensitive, are relatively simple and can be useful in identifying degradation products and abnormal forms of complement components. An example of the former is the use of double-decker rocket immunoelectrophoresis for the detection of C3d. Ouchterlony testing of normal human serum (NHS) and C8 deficient serum against anti-C8 may reveal lines of partial identity suggesting C8β chain deficiency. The buffers used in these types of assay are those that are optimal for antibody binding, and phosphate buffered saline (PBS) is usually used.

Haemolytic complement assays
CH50 assays
Lysis of red blood cells by complement will occur if the MAC is assembled on the cell membrane and C9 polymers inserted. The assays depend on the presence of all the necessary components and suitable conditions for complement activation. The simplest of these assays is the CH50 which is a quantitative procedure that depends on a sample containing all the classical and terminal complement components, and the components being functionally active. The assay is performed in the presence of calcium and magnesium ions (required for classical pathway activation) and the pathway

is initiated by the presence of IgM on the surface of sheep red blood cells (EA).

A similar assay for the alternative pathway, the APH50, uses rabbit erythrocytes which provide a surface for C3bBb binding. The addition of EGTA, by chelating calcium but not magnesium ions, will prevent any concomitant activation of the classical pathway whilst permitting activation of the alternative pathway.

These assays need to be controlled with samples known to contain all the components e.g. fresh NHS (positive control) and with buffer alone (negative control) to measure spontaneous lysis of the erythrocytes. Quantitation of the assay can be performed by comparing the amount of haemolysis (measured by the optical density of the cell supernatant which is proportional to the amount of haemoglobin released) to a known normal NHS in a one-tube method or by diluting out the test sample to obtain a range of percentage haemolysis. Using the von Krogh equation which describes the curve obtained by plotting the percentage lysis against the sample dilution, the

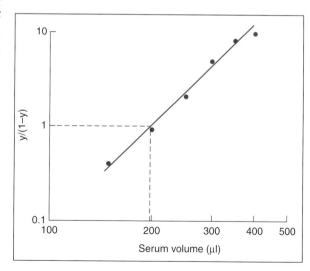

Figure 46.2: *Log-log plot of y/1-y against volume of diluted serum in a CH50 assay: At the point of 50% haemolysis, y/(1-y) = 1 and the volume of diluted serum giving this is shown by the vertical line. y = proportion of cells lysed. (Redrawn from Whaley, K. (ed.) (1985). Methods in complement for clinical immunologists, p 102. Churchill Livingstone, Edinburgh).*

Assay of Serum Complement Levels

Haemolytic complement assays

sample dilution required to obtain 50% haemolysis is calculated and, after taking the initial sample dilution into account, this value is translated into CH50 units/ml. The CH50 unit obtained depends on the amount and nature of the antibody used to sensitize the cells, the erythrocyte concentration and fragility, the ionic strength, divalent cation concentration and pH of the buffer, reaction time and temperature.

CH50 and APH50 assays are used to determine whether or not a patient is genetically deficient in a complement component. A zero value in a CH50 assay but not APH50 indicates a lack of C1, C4 or C2 whilst for a normal CH50 result and zero APH50, a deficiency of properdin, factor B or factor D may be present. Absence of lysis in both assays indicates lack of C3, C5, C6, C7 or C8. Low levels of lysis may occur in C9 deficiency. Low values above zero suggest that the level of one or more complement components is decreased due to consumption in a disease process such as systemic lupus erythematosus or may indicate a heterozygous deficiency state (although complement levels can be variable in these individuals as many components are acute phase proteins).

Haemolytic assays for individual components using complement deficient sera

Assays for the presence and functional activity of individual components can be performed using EA and a serum deficient in the chosen component. Serial dilutions of a test sample are added and lysis of EA will occur only if the component tested for is present and functional. Other components are present in excess so lysis is proportional to the amount of test component. Deficient sera can be obtained commercially but can also be prepared in the laboratory if such assays are performed regularly. Such assays are of lower sensitivity than those described below and are not suitable for regulatory components (C1-inh, factors H and I, properdin).

Haemolytic assays for individual components using pre-sensitized EA

Erythrocytes can be pre-sensitized with early pathway components up to that under test. By adding a sample containing a component under investigation this component can be activated or bound by those already present. Addition of the remaining components will result in lysis if the test component is present and functional. By ensuring that all other components are in excess, the degree of lysis is proportional to the amount of test component. Functionally pure components can be prepared in the laboratory but most are available commercially. The most commonly used pre-sensitized EA are EAC1, EAC4 and EAC14. EAC1 are prepared by adding C1 (e.g. from 5 mM CaCl precipitated guinea pig serum) to EA in a low ionic strength buffer that contains calcium and magnesium. Adding human serum in the presence of EDTA will result in the binding of C4 and C2 and subsequent incubation at 37°C will cause decay of C1 and C2 from the cells, leaving EAC4. EAC14 cells are prepared by adding further C1, again in the presence of calcium and magnesium.

EAC4 cells are used to assay C1 activity by adding dilutions of the test sample followed by guinea pig C2. Haemolysis is achieved by

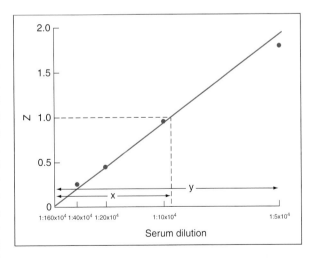

Figure 46.3: *The number of functional molecules per cell (Z) is plotted against the serum dilution in a typical haemolytic titration of an individual complement component. The concentration of the component in this instance is given by y/x × 50,000. (Redrawn from Whaley, K (ed.) (1985). Methods in complement for clinical immunologists, p 107. Churchill Livingstone, Edinburgh).*

Assay of Serum Complement Levels

Haemolytic complement assays

adding the remaining components, usually in the form of rat serum containing EDTA (C^{rat}-EDTA). The concentration of effective molecules of the component under test is measured by plotting the Z value (–ln (1 – %lysis)) against the dilution of the component under test. The straight line plot obtained results from the 'one-hit theory' in that a single effective complement molecule (C1 to C9) results in cell lysis. One unit of complement is taken as that which gives 63% lysis in an assay for that component. If a straight line plot is not obtained then the concentration of one or more components under test is limited.

C4 is assayed using EAC1 by adding dilutions of the test sample, guinea pig C2 and C^{rat}-EDTA as for C1 whilst C2 activity is measured using EAC14. In this case the T_{max} time for the cells (time for maximum C4b2a formation) must be known. The T_{max} varies from batch to batch of EAC14 because it depends upon the amount of C4b present on the cells. In order to assay C3 activity it is necessary to form EAC142. The C4b2a complex on these cells is more unstable than most, hence EAC14^{oxy}2 are prepared, using oxidised C2, to provide increased haemolytic activity of C2.

EAC14 form the starting point of functional assays for alternative pathway components. C2 and C3 are added to form EAC1423 with subsequent removal of C1 and C2 by incubation in EDTA buffer. The resultant EAC43b form an alternative pathway C3 convertase if factor B, factor D and properdin are added. Haemolysis is achieved by adding C^{rat}-EDTA. The activity of factor B, factor D or properdin is measured by omitting the respective pure component and replacing it with dilutions of the test sample, although this method is not suitable for assaying serum factor D, but only pure preparations. Terminal components are assayed by adding C3 and the terminal components up to the one under test to EAC14^{oxy}2. EAC1–8, used for measuring C9 activity, will however undergo spontaneous lysis so must be used as soon as they are prepared.

Functional assays of complement control proteins

C1 inhibitor activity can be assayed by commercial kits which utilize the ability of C1 inhibitor to inhibit a C1s analogue in a colorimetric reaction. C1 inhibitor activity can also be measured by testing the ability of the test sample to inhibit a given level of exogenous C1 added to sensitized EA. If serum is being tested then C1 first has to be removed, for example by precipitating out C1 using phosphate buffer. C1 inhibitor can be allowed to bind to C1 either in the fluid phase before adding to EAC4 with C2, or on EAC14 prior to the addition of C2. For haemolytic inhibitor component assays a 'solo' reaction containing no inhibitor is run in parallel. The inhibitory activity of the test sample is expressed in Z' units and assumes that the inhibition of lysis follows the same 'one-hit' theory as lysis. I is taken as the proportion of C1 lysis which is inhibited and therefore: $I = 1 - e^{-z}$. Hence $Z' = \ln (1 - I)$ or:

$$Z' = \frac{\ln y \text{ in test sample}}{y \text{ in solo}}$$

(where y is the proportion of cells lysed)

When Z in the solo tube is between 0.5 and 1.5, Z' varies linearly with the dilution of C1

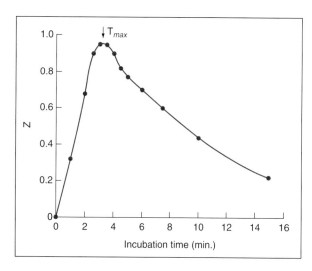

Figure 46.4: *Plot of the number of haemolytic sites (Z) against the incubation time at 30°C in a T_{max} assay. T_{max} is indicated by the arrow. (Redrawn from Whaley, K. (ed.) (1985). Methods in complement for clinical immunologists, p 96. Churchill Livingstone, Edinburgh).*

inhibitor. As for the calculation of Z, Z' is calculated from the graph of serum dilution against Z', taking the initial dilution into account.

Factor H levels can be assayed by measuring the ability of serum to accelerate the decay of the C3 convertase. EAC4b3bBbP are prepared by adding properdin, factor B and factor D to EAC4b3b and the amount of haemolytic activity remaining after decaying the C3 convertase is compared to a solo tube. Factor I activity can be assayed by incubating the test sample with factor H added to EAC43 and then adding factors B and D and testing for residual haemolytic activity.

Detection of complement activation products
Several serum complement proteins are acute phase proteins so during complement consumption, which can occur in conditions such as some types of bacterial infection or immune complex diseases, serum levels may remain normal. Increased complement turnover can be assessed by measuring products of complement activation by using antibodies which distinguish activation products from the native molecule. Commercial kits are available but in-house assays for activation products are easily established if appropriate antibodies are used. ELISAs for C3a, C4a and C5a can be established if standards can be obtained but the clinical usefulness of these assays is limited. Of more help to clinicians are assays for C1s-C1-inh, C3bBbP or C5b-C9, increased levels of which indicate activation of the classical, alternative or terminal pathway respectively.

The latter assays use an antibody against one component such as C1s to bind the complex to an ELISA plate and an antibody against another component of the complex such as C1-inh to detect the complex.

Detection of complement receptors
Antibodies to complement receptors are available commercially and can be used in flow cytometry to detect the presence of receptors on cell suspensions. Some antibodies are also suitable for immunohistochemistry of tissue sections or cytospin preparation if cell morphology is required.

Further Reading

Dodd, Sims (eds) (in press). *Complement. A practical approach*. Oxford University Press. [This is an up-to-date laboratory manual for all aspects of laboratory complement work.]

Phimster G M, Whaley K. Measurement of complement. In *Clinical immunology. A practical approach*. Gooi H G, Chapel H Eds. 1990. Oxford University Press. [This chapter provides guidance as to clinical indications for complement assays as well as methodologies.]

Whaley K (ed) *Methods in complement for clinical immunologists*. 1985: Churchill Livingstone, Edinburgh. [This textbook provides a comprehensive, detailed account of the majority of complement assays, including the preparation of purified components.]

47 CELLULAR IMMUNOLOGY

A Graham Bird

Introduction

Whilst the identification of specific antibodies is relatively straightforward and has resulted in the last three decades in the widespread application of tests to characterize protective, allergic or autoantibody in human disease, the examination of lymphoid populations either in quantitative or qualitative terms still lags far behind. The identification and enumeration of individual lymphoid subpopulations using the combination of specific (usually monoclonal) antibodies and flow cytometry is well established and new techniques employ the identification of intracellular cytokines, cytotoxic granules or markers of activation alongside to give additional information. The assessment of specific lymphocyte function is, however, still poorly standardized, is expensive, labour-intensive and usually requires short- or long-term lymphocyte culture. Such considerations have limited greatly the application of lymphocyte function assays to all but the most specialized immunology diagnostic laboratories.

Lymphocyte Markers and Immunophenotyping

The presence of specific receptors on the surface membranes of individual lymphoid populations allows their reliable identification and quantification. This advance has already found application in two clinical areas: the identification of clonal cells in leukaemias and lymphomas, and in the identification and monitoring of primary or secondary immunodeficiency disease states, particularly HIV infection.

With the increasing understanding of the mechanisms responsible for chronic inflammatory, autoimmune and allergic disease, it is probable that these techniques will find larger application in the monitoring of such diseases and the use of selective immunosuppressive or immunomodulatory therapy in their management.

Early methods for the quantitation of individual lymphocyte subpopulations employed reagents with poor specificity combined with ultraviolet flourescence microscopy to enumerate individual cells, resulting in time-consuming assays with poor performance characteristics.

Monoclonal antibodies

Flow cytometry

<u>Lymphocyte Surface Marker Determination</u>

Qualitative

Monoclonal antibodies

The use of monoclonal antibodies with unique specificity for individual lymphocyte cell-surface antigens has provided reagents which are capable of international standardization of methodology. Individual reagent specificity is classified according to international cluster of differentiation (CD) agreement following regularly updated workshops that assign newly described specificities (for table of the more common specificities, see Table 47.1).

Individual membrane specificities do not always show lineage fidelity and thus may be expressed on other cell populations either uncommonly, at lower density or during malignant transformation of the normal subpopulation cell type. The increasing repertoire of monoclonal antibodies available is permitting the identification and enumeration not only of individual cell populations but also of functional, activation or adhesion molecules which permit the more discriminating analysis of

individual cell types. The binding of one or more monoclonal antibodies is visualized using individual flourochrome dyes which are usually directly chemically conjugated to specific monoclonal antibodies. A fluorochrome dye absorbs light of one wavelength and emits light of a different (longer) wavelength that can be detected by microscopy or directly by photometer. The use of two or three separately labelled monoclonal antibodies allows the simultaneous characterization of individual cell populations with considerable accuracy and speed when combined with flow cytometry.

Flow cytometry

A flow cytometer is an instrument capable of the simultaneous analysis of physical and fluorochrome signals on individual cells sequentially. The instrument comprises a laser source of monochromatic light, fluidics providing a stream of single cells for separate analysis and photodetectors to identify the signals emitted by individual cells. The prodigious amount of data obtained from many thousands of individual cells requires powerful computerization for its subsequent analysis.

Light scatter characteristics reflecting cell granularity together with size allows further identification of individual cells expressing one or more fluorochrome stained monoclonal antibodies. Individual leucocyte populations can be identified by light scatter characteristics, permitting an electronic gate to be placed around individual cell populations which can then be further subdivided and analysed for monoclonal antibody expression.

Table 47.1: Clinically relevant lymphocyte surface marker antigens.	
Antigen	*Characteristics*
CD1	Expressed on cortical thymocytes
CD2	LFA2 sheep erythrocyte T-cell receptor
CD3	T-cell signalling complex found on all mature T cells
CD4	Adhesion molecules on T helper cells recognizing MHC Class I
CD8	Adhesion molecules on T cytotoxic cells recognizing MHC Class I
CD19	Expressed on pre-B and mature B cells
CD20	Expressed on mature B cells
CD25	Low affinity IL2 receptor α chain
CD28	Costimulatory receptor on T cells
CD45RA	Found on native T cells
CD45RO	Found on memory T cells
CD56	Found on NK cells
CD57	Found on 50% NK cells and on some activated CD8$^+$ T cells
CD69	T-cell activation marker
CD71	Transferin receptor present on activated T and B cells

Lymphocyte Surface Marker Determination

The identification of individual lymphoid populations can be either qualitative or quantitative depending on the clinical information required.

Qualitative

This approach is used to examine the presence or absence of individual leucocyte populations, particularly lymphoid populations in suspected immunodeficiency or the identification of an expanded population of cells expressing clonal markers which could represent the presence of a malignant population of lymphoid or other cells. The approach can be applied to cells obtained from blood, bone marrow, tissue aspirates or biopsies. If blood is used, red cell contamination must be removed either by initial separation of leucocytes or by the direct staining of nucleated cells followed by the lysis of red cells.

The identification of benign or malignant lymphoid expansions relies on the principle that individual expressions are largely frozen at an individual differentiation stage that allows an expanded population expressing a combination of antigens, suggesting monoclonality, to be separated from residual normal polyclonal cells during analysis. Still the most valuable clonal marker used is the expression of only kappa or lambda light chains on the surface of an individual B cell monoclonal expression in lymphoma or leukaemia. No equivalent clonal marker for T cells exists and the expression of multiple markers is suggestive rather than conclusive for monoclonality, and receptor gene rearrangement remains the clonal marker of choice for the identification of T cell monoclonality.

The presence or absence of an individual lymphocyte population is very valuable for the diagnosis and classification of individual primary immunodeficiency disease. In severe combined immunodeficiency (SCID) there will be an almost complete absence of lymphocytes bearing T-lymphocyte identification markers, and a relative deficiency of T lymphocytes is characteristic of thymic hypoplasia that accompanies the Di George syndrome. Patients with severe combined immunodeficiency (SCID) can be divided into two groups: a group lacking both T and B lymphocytes (T⁻B⁻SCID); a group with normal or increased B cells but lacking T cells (T⁻B⁺SCID).

The X-linked T⁻B⁺ form of SCID is the most common and results from mutations in the shared γ chain of receptors for the cytokines IL2, IL4, IL7, IL9 and IL15. Autosomal recessive T⁻B⁺ SCID results from mutations of the intracellular Jak3 kinase that binds to the γ receptor chain. The autosomal deficiency of the purine salvage enzymes adenosine deaminase (ADA) and purine nucleoside phosphorylase also gives rise to T-cell deficiency in numbers and function of varying severity, the most severe forms presenting as SCID.

An immunodeficiency of similar severity to SCID is also seen in MHC Class II deficiency in which there is impaired transcription of normal Class II molecules resulting in reduction in CD4+ cell numbers, absence of Class II expression on antigen presenting, dendritic macrophage and B cells and severe defects in T-cell function.

In the X-linked form of antibody deficiency due to mutations in the B lymphocyte tyrosine kinase, the complete absence of serum and secretory antibody is accompanied by a complete lack of peripheral blood and lymph node (but not bone marrow pre-B) B-lymphocyte lineage cells and plasma cells. More subtle immunodeficiencies are now being described in which the lack of stimulation receptors results in a generalized or more specific deficiency, and these deficiencies will increasingly be characterized by flow cytometry. For example, the lack of the co-stimulating molecular CD40 ligand on the surface of activated T lymphocytes results in the complete inability of signalling for B-lymphocyte antibody class switching and affinity (memory) maturation by T lymphocytes. In suspected cases of hyper IgM/CD40 ligand deficiency, T lymphocytes activated by the ionophores DMA and ionomycin should be analysed for the expression of CD40L. The lack of the interferon gamma receptor on macrophages has been identified in kindreds with a specific susceptibility to mycobacterial or salmonella infection.

Quantitative

The precise quantitation of individual lymphocyte populations became necessary with the arrival of HIV infection and the need to monitor asymptomatic infected subjects and initiate clinical decisions before opportunistic infections complicated the management of individual patients.

THE SCIENCE OF LABORATORY DIAGNOSIS

Reports and interpretation
In vitro Assessment of Lymphocyte Function
Introduction
Lymphocyte proliferation

Until recently the quantitation of absolute lymphocyte population numbers has required the integration of three separate laboratory measurements: the total lymphocyte count; the percentage of lymphocytes within the white cell population; the percentage of these lymphocytes that are of the individual subpopulation, e.g. CD4+ cells.

Since each of these analyses was conducted by a different technique and often a different counter with its own measurement error and coefficient of variation, absolute counts were subject to severe inaccuracy. More recently the development of new flow cytometric approaches using either analysis of fixed volumes or comparison against standardized added particle numbers has permitted precise and direct quantitation of absolute cell populations. These techniques allow the development of standardized protocols and the application of internal and external quality control checks that have greatly reduced the amount of intra- and inter-laboratory variation previously encountered in subpopulation enumeration. The whole blood lysis method rather than separation is an essential prerequisite for accurate counting.

Reports and interpretation

In the monitoring of HIV-infected cases, both percentage and absolute values must be reported alongside age-related reference ranges defined from the normal local population.

Single cell counts should be interpreted with caution in view of the considerable measurement and biological variation which is inherent in blood lymphocyte counting. Clinical or therapeutic trial progression should be assessed on the basis of a number of count values taken over three- to six-monthly intervals on occasions when patients are free of acute infections or other problems. In HIV infection, serial results of CD4 cell numbers allow the calculation of slopes of CD4 decline that can be useful in the introduction of specific anti-retroviral therapy or prophylaxis against specific opportunistic infections.

In vitro Assessment of Lymphocyte Function

Introduction

Activation of T lymphocytes *in vitro* results in the expression of new cellular receptors and adhesion molecules, blast transformation and expression of intracellular cytokines and their secretion and eventually cell division and clonal expansion. In the case of B lymphocytes, clonal immunoglobulin synthesis and secretion also occurs.

In clinical practice the assessment of *in vitro* B-lymphocyte function provides little additional information to that obtained from assessment of serum or secretory antibodies and its application is limited to research programmes.

In vitro T-lymphocyte function tests are, however, valuable in the assessment of T-cell competence, particularly in young children with suspected immunodeficiency, where *in vivo* delayed hypersensitivity testing to recall antigens is not available because of lack of prior exposure. In older children or adults, the assessment of T-cell responses to individual antigens assessed either by proliferation or cytokine expression is a valuable assessment either of competence or hyper-responsiveness to individual antigens. Increasingly such techniques are being used to identify more subtle forms of immunodeficiency, particularly those involving defects in intracellular signalling. They can also be used to assess early defects in progressive immunodeficiency such as asymptomatic HIV immunodeficiency, because functional defects are detectable in individual patients before gross qualitative deficiencies such as CD4 lymphocyte depletion become obvious.

Lymphocyte proliferation

Lymphocytes can be activated *in vitro* after short-term tissue culture using four different approaches:

Lectin mitogens

Carbohydrate binding lectins such as phytohaemagglutinin (PHA), concanavalin A (ConA) and pokeweed mitogen (PWM) have been used for many years to activate T lymphocytes polyclonally and, in the case of PWM, secondarily

B lymphocytes. Polyclonal activation is particularly useful in the assessment of suspected severe immunodeficiency in neonates when specific antigen stimulation is of no value because of lack of prior antigen exposure.

Antibodies to T-cell surface activation markers

These also induce polyclonal activation of T lymphocytes directly. Monoclonal antibodies directed against the molecule CD3 of the T-cell signalling protein complex comprising CD3 and the specific T-cell receptor is a particularly valuable approach. Successful standardized approaches have been described using whole blood for short-term lymphocyte cultures. This approach has been useful in the early assessment of patients with asymptomatic HIV infection.

Specific antigens

Antigens derived from natural infections or previous vaccines are valuable in the assessment of lymphocyte function in older neonates, children and adults. Purified protein derivative of mycobacterium, candida, tetanus and streptokinase have all been used and are valuable for looking for more selective immunodeficiency and also in the early assessment of HIV-infected patients. Specific antigen culture takes five to seven days, in contrast to the three days necessary for mitogen or anti-CD3 stimulation.

Allogeneic leucocytes

The use of pooled allogeneic cells that have been inactivated previously by irradiation or mytomycin C treatment as stimulators of T lymphocytes is another useful approach in the polyclonal activation of T lymphocytes. Allogeneic cultures have been employed particularly in the assessment of patients for bone marrow transplantation and offer no particular advantages over mitogen or anti-CD3 stimulation. Allogeneic or mixed lymphocyte cultures take six days to produce satisfactory proliferative readouts.

Quantitation of lymphocyte activation

Until recently, the measurement of proliferation was the only readout of lymphocyte activation frequently employed. Now three approaches are available:

Proliferation responses

The blastogenic response to antigens or mitogens is assessed by the addition of a radioactive precursor such as tritiated thymidine 16 hours before the end of a three-day or six-day culture. At the end of culture, cultured cells are precipitated onto filter paper and the radioactivity measured by liquid scintillation counting. The count is proportional to the level of DNA synthesis occurring within cultures.

Expression of activation markers

A rapid assessment of lymphocyte function can be achieved by the detection of new activation markers on the surface of T lymphocytes in 24–48 hour short-term cultures. Expression of the activation antigens CD69, IL2 receptor α chain (CD25) and transferin receptor (CD71) have all proved useful since they are not expressed or are present on low proportions of resting cells and are expressed on a high percentage of activated T cells. Expression is detected by staining of short-term cultured cells by fluorochrome-labelled monoclonal antibodies followed by flow cytometry quantitation.

Release of cytokines

Activated T lymphocytes and monocytes in culture synthesize and secrete cytokines such as IL2, 4, 5 and 6 and also interferon gamma. Following polyclonal activation by lectins or anti-CD3, individual cytokines can be measured in culture supernate by either ELISA or bioassay. IL2 can be assessed by its capacity to stimulate 3H thymidine uptake by the culture mouse T-cell line CTLL2 which requires exogenous IL2 to maintain its proliferation. This bioassay should be confirmed in the presence of blocking antibodies against IL2 since other cytokines, especially IL15, can also activate this cell line. Methods for the direct identification of cytokines intracellularly using flow cytometry combined with the use of specific monoclonal antibodies against individual cytokines have been described recently. This approach has the additional advantage of being able to identify simultaneously the phenotype of the activated cytokine-secreting cells.

Since it has recently become clear that individual subpopulations of CD4+ T cells produce different sets of cytokines responsible for either cell-mediated or antibody-based and particularly IgE responses against individual antigens, there is now increasing interest in the characterization of cytokine responses in immunodeficiency, autoimmune and infection immune responses. Intracellular pathogens such as *Mycobacterium tuberculosis* and *Borellia burgdorferi* elicit a so-called TH1 response comprising IL2 and interferon gamma whereas HIV and *Toxocara canis* infections elicit predominantly TH2 responses with IL4, 5, 10 being the principal cytokines synthesized and secreted.

At the time of writing, the analysis of cytokine synthesis or secretion has no defined role in the classification or investigation of immunodeficiency, autoimmune or infectious disease and is currently a research technique. Nevertheless, with improved methodologies and standardization, it is likely that these assays will enter the repertoire of investigation in the more specialized immunology laboratories.

Standardization and quality assurance
The recent requirement for a more precise determination of lymphocyte subpopulation results and the need to reduce inter-laboratory variation has driven the development of standardization and quality control for lymphocyte phenotyping.

Guidelines have been produced for the conduct of lymphoid subpopulation quantitation using whole blood lysis methodologies, and a quality control scheme administered as part of the national UKNEQAS quality assurance scheme is organized by Dr J T Reilly, Department of Haematology, Northern General Hospital, Herries Road, Sheffield, S5 7AU, who should be contacted for further details of the scheme.

Lymphocyte function tests are generally not standardized and there is no quality control scheme. It is thus essential that at least one age-matched disease control subject is run in parallel for each assay of lymphocyte function and a range of responses determined for a normal local population before these assays are offered as part of a diagnostic repertoire.

Interpretation of lymphocyte function tests
Patients with severe forms of primary severe combined or T-cell deficiency show absent or minimal proliferation or expression of activation markers after culture with mitogens, antigens or other activators. In the Di George syndrome where peripheral blood T cells can be detected by flow cytometry, usually in reduced numbers, significant reductions in proliferative response are associated with poor prognosis, whereas normal functional tests predict improving T-cell maturation which is often seen in partial Di George cases. In patients with defects in T-cell receptor signalling such as those resulting from the mutation of the T-cell kinase Zap 70, abnormalities in T-cell phenotype, presence of CD4$^+$ blood T cells and absence of the CD8$^+$ T-cell population are associated with absence of CD4$^+$ lymphocyte proliferation to mitogens and anti-CD CD3$^+$, but intact stimulation by phorbol esters.

Further Reading

Arpala E, Shahar M, Dadi H, Cohen A, Roifman C M. Defective T cell receptor signalling and CD8+ thymic selection in humans taking Zap 70 kinase. *Cell* 1994; **76**, 947–958.

Bird A G. Quantification of CD4-positive T lymphocytes. In: *HIV: A Practical Approach*, Vol. 1. J Karn (Ed), 1995: IRL Press, pp. 211–220.

Centers for Disease Control. Guidelines for the performance of CD4+ T-cell determinants in persons with Human Immunodeficiency Virus Infection. *Morbidity and Mortality Weekly Report*. 1992; **41**, 1–19.

CD4$^+$ T Lymphocyte Working Party. Guidelines for the enumeration of CD4+ T lymphocytes in immunosuppressed individuals. *Clin. Lab. Haem.* 1997; **19**, 231–41.

Report of a WHO Scientific Group. Primary immunodeficiency Diseases. *Clin. Exp. Immunol.* 1997; **109** Supl. 1, 1–28.

48   IMMUNE COMPLEX DISEASES AND CRYOGLOBULINS

Siraj A Misbah

Introduction

Immune complexes (IC) are formed whenever antibody encounters antigen. This is a dynamic physiological process which enables potentially harmful exogenous antigens to be cleared by the host's mononuclear phagocytic system (MPS). Failure to clear complexes successfully may lead to immune complex deposition in the capillary basement membranes of glomeruli, skin, synovium and choroid plexus where they trigger an inflammatory response. Inflammation induced by immune complexes is dependent on the ability of complexes to activate complement (determined by immunoglobulin isotype) with the consequent generation of potent proinflammatory mediators (C5a). C5a is a powerful chemoattractant which draws circulating polymorphonuclear leukocytes and monocytes to the site of immune complex deposition, thus serving to amplify tissue damage. The site of immune complex deposition depends partly on the size of the immune complex, as exemplified in the kidney, where small immune complexes are able to pass through the glomerular basement membrane but large complexes are unable to do so and accumulate between the endothelium and the basement membrane.

Several mechanisms ensure that immune complex deposition does not take place in health. These include: (1) Phagocytosis of IC by the MPS. The size of the immune complex is a critical factor in this regard since the MPS is only able to clear small complexes. (2) Integrity of the complement pathway. Proteins of the complement system play a vital role in maintaining IC in solution by coating complexes with C3b (opsonization). This prevents the formation of large immune complex lattices and immune precipitation, in addition IC coated with C3b interact with the C3b receptor (CR1, CD35) on circulating red cells which act as an efficient transporter of immune complexes to the MPS in the liver and spleen (Fig. 48.1). Given the vital role of complement proteins in clearing IC, it is not surprising that patients with primary complement deficiency (especially of early complement components C1, C4, C2) have a high incidence of immune complex disease.

Other factors that influence immune complex deposition include physicochemical properties of antigen and antibody, including

Assays for Circulating Immune Complexes

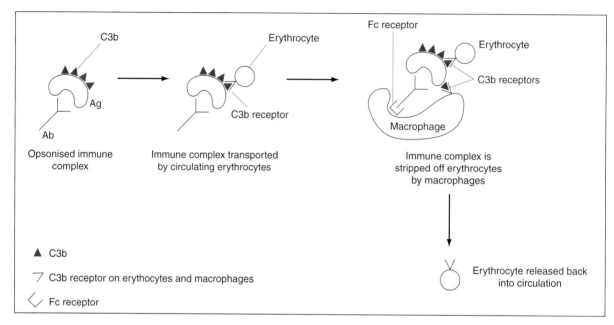

Figure 48.1: *Transport of immune complexes by erythrocytes to mononuclear phagocytes in liver and spleen.*

electrical charge, valency, avidity of antigen–antibody interaction and immunoglobulin isotype, for example IC containing cationic antigens bind tightly to the anionic glomerular basement membrane, causing tissue injury.

Although circulating immune complexes occur in a large number of diseases (Table 48.1), in the majority of cases these complexes are an epiphenomenal or incidental finding. This chapter is confined to those diseases where there is good evidence to support a pathogenetic role for immune complexes: serum sickness, systemic lupus erythematosus (SLE) and mixed cryoglobulinaemia.

Irrespective of the underlying cause, immune complex diseases share several common features which are of clinical significance: (1) Multisystem involvement due to deposition of complexes in the capillaries of the kidney, skin, synovium and choroid plexus. (2) Hypocomplementaemia during periods of active disease. (3) Reduction in circulating immune complex levels by therapy (drugs, plasmapheresis) leads to improvement in disease activity.

Assays for Circulating Immune Complexes

Over 30 assays for the detection of circulating immune complexes were described in the 1970s with the expectation (subsequently unfulfilled) that they would be clinically useful in the diagnosis and management of immune complex disease. These assays were divided broadly into physical methods designed to differentiate between monomeric immunoglobulin and immune complexes and biological methods dependent on the interaction of cell surface receptors or complement with immune complexes (Table 48.2).

The inherent problems with physical methods was exemplified by the polyethylene glycol (PEG) precipitation assay. In addition to precipitating immune complexes, PEG even at low concentrations also precipitates a variety of serum proteins including IgG, thus causing major difficulties in the interpretation of results. Biological methods for the detection of immune complexes based on the recognition of complexes in humoral or cell receptor systems have proved equally unreliable. The Raji cell assay

Table 48.1: Disorders associated with circulating immune complexes.

Immunological	Systemic lupus erythematosus
	Rheumatoid arthritis
	Mixed cryoglobulinaemia
	Felty's syndrome
	Ankylosing spondylitis
	Scleroderma
	Serum sickness
Infections	
Bacterial	*Staphylococcus aureus, Pseudomonas aeruginosa, Streptococcus* sp
Mycobacterial	*M. tuberculosis*
Parasitic	Trypanosomiasis, Onchocerciasis
Malignancy	All forms
Physiological	Normal healthy individuals
	Pregnancy

which used a lymphoblastoid cell line derived from a patient with Burkitt's lymphoma was used widely in the 1970s. Since the assay is based on the ability of lymphoblastoid cells (which possess surface receptors for C1q, C3b, C3d but no surface immunoglobulin) to bind serum immune complexes that have also bound complement, an unacceptably high rate of false-positives was found in patients with anti-lymphocyte antibodies, as in SLE. Although a joint working group of the World Health Organization and the International Union of Immunological Societies (IUIS) in 1981 found four assays analytically acceptable, none of the assays has withstood critical evaluation of its clinical usefulness on account of their highly variable sensitivity, specificity and poor predictive value. In addition the inability of most assays to detect specific antigen within immune complexes was a significant drawback. The joint WHO/IUIS working group concluded that detection of circulating immune complexes is not essential in any human disease and more importantly that the demonstration of circulating immune complexes was not specific for immune complex disease. As a result most clinical immunology laboratories have abandoned immune complex assays and to date there is no evidence to suggest that immune complex assays should be re-introduced into routine clinical practice. In those cases where immune complex disease is suspected, demonstration of immunoglobulin and complement deposits on a biopsy of affected organs (e.g. skin, kidney) is taken as implicit evidence for the presence of immune complex deposits. Assays for circulating immune complexes are a poor substitute for direct immunohistological examination and immune complex disease should under no circumstances be diagnosed primarily on the demonstration of complexes in serum.

Serum Sickness

Serum sickness is a good model to explain immune complex diseases. Von Pirquet in 1908 delineated serum sickness as a distinct entity in children repeatedly immunized with anti-diphtheria serum derived from horses. Serum sickness was clinically manifest as widespread urticaria, fever, lymphadenopathy, arthralgia and proteinuria 8–12 days after the injection of horse serum. The latent period of 8–12 days reflected the time necessary for patients to produce antibodies against horse proteins. Once a sufficient concentration of antibody complexes with circulating antigen, the resultant immune complex load overwhelms the control mechanisms of the body leading to

Table 48.2:   Immune complex assays.

Physical methods – assays dependent on physicochemical properties of complex	Polyethylene glycol precipitation Cryoprecipitation Analytical ultracentrifugation
Biological methods – assays dependent on	
(i) Reaction with antiglobulins (subject to interference by endogenous rheumatoid factors)	Polyclonal rheumatoid factor assay Monoclonal rheumatoid factor assay[*]
(ii) Complement–protein interactions	$^{125}C1q$ binding[*] Conglutinin (a bovine protein that binds immune complexes) dependent assay[*]
(iii) Cell surface receptors	Raji cell radioimmunoassay[*]

[*] Assays found to be analytically acceptable by the WHO/IUIS working group

immune complex deposition and hypocomplementaemia. Clinical improvement is dependent on clearance of circulating complexes which occurs spontaneously after two to three weeks in many patients; a minority may require treatment with steroids to expedite recovery.

More recently serum sickness has been studied extensively in patients with aplastic anaemia receiving horse anti-thymocyte globulin (ATG). The clinical syndrome described in these patients is virtually identical to that described by Von Pirquet, with high levels of circulating immune complexes and hypocomplementaemia coinciding with the occurrence of skin rash and arthralgia. Immunofluorescent studies of biopsied skin revealed abundant deposits of immunoglobulin and C3 in the walls of small blood vessels.

With the decline in use of ATG, drug hypersensitivity reactions are at present the commonest cause of serum sickness. A wide range of drugs may act as haptens and bind to plasma proteins with the ensuing drug-protein complex triggering an immune response, e.g. penicillin, sulphonamides and thiouracils. Drug-induced serum sickness is usually self-limiting providing the offending agent is withdrawn.

Investigation

The diagnosis of serum sickness is usually self-evident by the characteristic clinical presentation in a patient with antecedent drug ingestion. Drug challenges are usually not required and should not be performed routinely. The role of laboratory investigation is limited; while immune complex measurements are likely to show high levels in the circulation, this is seldom performed or required. During the acute stage of the disease, marked hypocomplementaemia (reduced C3, C4) is a feature and provides a useful pointer to systemic immune complex deposition. Tissue biopsies may be required in cases of diagnostic uncertainty and characteristically show immunoglobulin and C3 deposition on direct immunofluorescence of the skin and kidneys.

Systemic Lupus Erythematosus

Systemic lupus erythematosus (SLE) is a common human immune complex disorder

IMMUNE COMPLEX DISEASES AND CRYOGLOBULINS

Systemic Lupus Erythematosus
Investigation of patients with suspected SLE
Autoantibodies as markers of disease

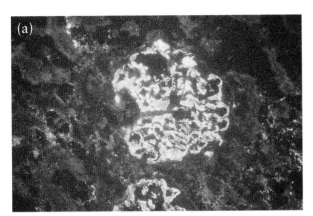

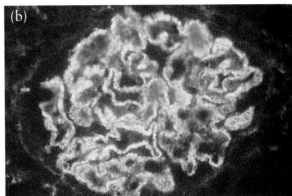

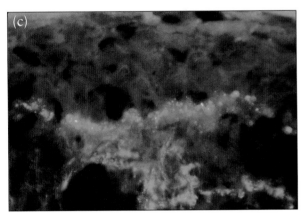

Figure 48.2: *Immunofluorescence of renal and skin biopsies in a patient with SLE. Panel (a) Glomerular IgA deposits in a membranous distribution. (b) Glomerular C1q deposits in a membranous distribution. (c) Granular IgG deposits at the dermo-epidermal junction (lupus band) [courtesy of Dr W. Merchant, Leeds General Infirmary]. [(a) and (b) courtesy of Dr P. Harnden, Leeds General Infirmary].*

with a prevalence of 200 cases per 100 000 population in the UK. In its most florid form, SLE affects the skin, kidneys, joints and central nervous system although many patients may have only single organ involvement at first presentation. Patients presenting with predominant neurological disease pose difficult diagnostic problems which are dealt with later in this chapter. Much of the organ damage in lupus is linked directly to the widespread deposition of immune complexes that occurs in the skin, kidneys and choroid plexus. As in serum sickness, immunofluorescence of skin and kidney biopsies shows deposits of immunoglobulin and complement (Fig. 48.2) while circulating immune complexes are found in a high proportion of patients with active disease. In keeping with the key role of the complement system in processing immune complexes, a range of complement abnormalities are seen in patients with SLE (summarized in Table 48.3).

Investigation of patients with suspected SLE

SLE is associated with a multitude of laboratory abnormalities including polyclonal hypergamma-globulinaemia, leucopenia, hypo-complementaemia and a plethora of autoantibodies in blood. While the polyclonal increase in serum immunoglobulins is a non-specific marker of immune system activation, it results in a raised ESR which acts as a useful diagnostic clue when combined with a normal CRP. Although the inability to mount an acute phase protein response in the face of active disease has long been recognized as a feature of SLE, this is not invariable. Patients with active serositis, chronic synovitis and concomitant bacterial infection are an exception to this dictum.

Autoantibodies as markers of disease

The presence of circulating antibodies to nuclear antigens is the hallmark of active lupus. The ensuing paragraphs will outline the

Systemic Lupus Erythematosus

Autoantibodies as markers of disease

Table 48.3: Abnormalities of the complement system in SLE.

Primary	Total deficiency of early complement components C1q, C1r-1s, C4, C2 associated with high incidence of SLE
	Partial deficiency of C4 with one to two C4 null alleles is seen in approximately 15% of patients with SLE
Secondary	Decreased expression of CR1 is a feature of advanced SLE
	Increased activity of classical and alternative pathway reflected as hypocomplementaemia ($\downarrow$ C3, $\downarrow$ C4)

principles and the clinical utility of the assays used to detect these antibodies.

Antinuclear antibody (ANA)

In clinical practice, the detection of antinuclear antibodies (ANA) as demonstrated by indirect immunofluorescence is the single most useful sign for the diagnosis of SLE. ANA are detected by overlaying rodent tissue or tissue culture cells derived from a human epithelial cell line (HEp-2) with test serum followed by a second antibody, anti-human IgG conjugated to fluorescein. Using rodent tissue, approximately 95% of patients with active untreated disease have high titre ANA (>1 in 80). HEp-2 cells exhibit an even higher degree of sensitivity with approximately 98–99% positivity in patients with untreated disease. Conversely, the likelihood of untreated SLE in a patient with negative ANA on HEp-2 cells is of the order of <1%. A positive ANA result, however, is not specific for SLE since it occurs in a variety of other diseases (Table 48.4).

Several distinctive patterns of ANA are recognized on HEp-2 cells: homogeneous, nucleolar, speckled, peripheral and centromere (Fig. 48.3). With the exception of the centromere antibody, which is a specific marker of the CREST syndrome (calcinosis, Raynaud's phenomenon, oesophageal dysfunction, sclerodactyly, telangiectasia) and scleroderma, none of the other ANA patterns is a reliable indicator of antigenic specificity. In view of this and the occurrence of ANA in many other disease states, it is essential to characterize a positive ANA further in terms of its antigenic specificity. In SLE, a positive ANA by indirect

Table 48.4: Causes of a positive ANA

connective tissue disease.
  SLE
  Sjögren's syndrome
  Polymyositis
  Rheumatoid arthritis
  Vasculitis

Liver disease
  Autoimmune chronic active hepatitis
  Primary biliary cirrhosis
  Alcoholic liver disease

Drugs

Infection

Malignancy

Healthy individuals

immunofluorescence reflects the presence of antibodies to nuclear antigens such as DNA, histones and a group of extractable nuclear antigens (ENA) known individually as Ro, La, Sm and U1-RNP (uridine ribonuclear protein).

Antibodies to extractable nuclear antigens (ENA)

Ro, La and Sm were named after the patients in whom they were first characterized: Robert, Lane and Smith. In conjunction with U1-RNP (uridine ribonuclear protein) these proteins are responsible for splicing and processing mRNA. In contrast to ANA, antibodies to ENA are specific for lupus and related disorders and are therefore helpful in the diagnosis. In addition,

Systemic Lupus Erythematosus
Autoantibodies as markers of disease

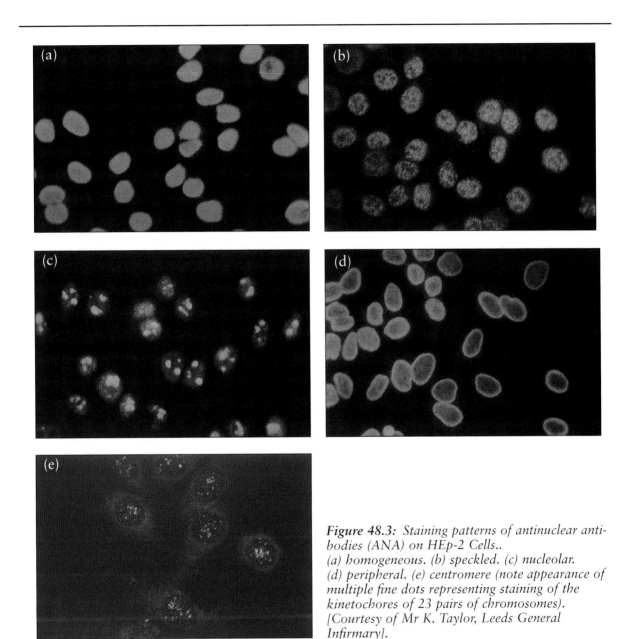

Figure 48.3: *Staining patterns of antinuclear antibodies (ANA) on HEp-2 Cells..*
(a) homogeneous. (b) speckled. (c) nucleolar.
(d) peripheral. (e) centromere (note appearance of multiple fine dots representing staining of the kinetochores of 23 pairs of chromosomes).
[Courtesy of Mr K. Taylor, Leeds General Infirmary].

individual antibodies tend to correlate with certain clinical manifestations; anti-Ro occurs in lupus and Sjögren's syndrome and correlates with cutaneous disease. It is important to recognize that anti-Ro antibodies may occur in the absence of ANA. The ANA negative, Ro positive profile occurs in a minority of patients with lupus (<1% on HEp-2 cells as substrate); on rodent tissue substrate, however, this figure rises to 5% since the Ro antigen is poorly represented in rodent tissue. In 5–25% of pregnant women with lupus, anti-Ro antibodies cross the placenta to cause transient cutaneous lupus in the neonate; more seriously 1–3% of babies born to anti-Ro positive mothers develop permanent congenital heartblock requiring pacemaker insertion. While anti-Ro antibodies occur in isolation in approximately 30% of lupus patients, they are accompanied by anti-La antibodies in 15% of cases. In the latter situation patients are less likely to have renal disease.

Systemic Lupus Erythematosus

Autoantibodies as markers of disease

In addition to the clinical correlates discussed above, the ANA negative anti-Ro positive profile also acts as a marker for underlying primary complement deficiency affecting early complement components. Surveys of patients with homozygous C4 and C2 deficiencies reveal anti-Ro positivity in approximately 50–70% of cases. While the precise mechanism responsible for the association of SLE with primary complement deficiency has not been established, the existence of a hierarchy of disease severity in relation to the missing complement component is well documented; disease severity is greatest in patients with C1q deficiency closely followed by total C4 deficiency. Disease severity in patients with C2 deficiency is comparable to that seen in patients with intact complement pathways.

Anti-Sm antibodies are highly specific for lupus but their prevalence varies with the ethnic background of the patient; 30% of Afro-Caribbean patients are anti-Sm positive in contrast to 10% of Caucasians. In view of the shared peptide sequences between Sm and U1-RNP, antibodies to Sm and U1-RNP tend to occur together.

The presence of anti U1-RNP antibodies in isolation was thought to identify a group of patients with lupus overlap syndromes with additional features of polymyositis and scleroderma. Sharp and colleagues introduced the term 'mixed connective tissue disease' (MCTD) to characterize these patients, who were felt to have a better prognosis in view of the lower risk of renal and neurological disease. Long-term follow-up of the original cohort has questioned the existence of MCTD as a distinct benign entity since many of the patients have subsequently developed renal and neurological disease.

Methods of detection

Immunoprecipitation assays. Antibodies to ENA may be detected by several methods. Initially, many laboraties used countercurrent immuno-electrophoresis (CIE) or the Ouchterlony double diffusion method to demonstrate the presence of antibodies. CIE is performed on agar gels allowing antibody and antigen to migrate in opposite

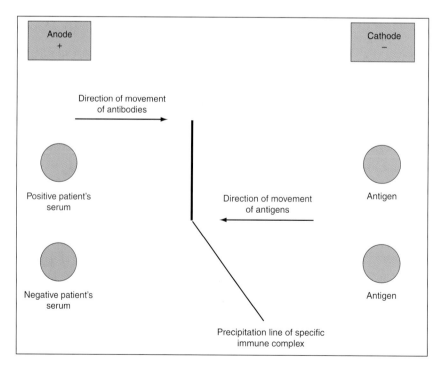

Anode
+

Cathode
–

Direction of movement
of antibodies

Positive patient's
serum

Direction of movement
of antigens

Antigen

Negative patient's
serum

Antigen

Precipitation line of specific
immune complex

Figure 48.4: Countercurrent immunoelectrophoresis [reproduced with kind permission from Chapel H. M., Haeney M. R., Essentials of Clinical Immunology *3rd Ed. 1993 Blackwell Scientific].*

Systemic Lupus Erythematosus

Autoantibodies as markers of disease

directions to meet in the centre of the slide where immunoprecipitation occurs at the appropriate pH (Fig. 48.4). The Ouchterlony double diffusion technique too is based on immunoprecipitation; antigen is placed in the centre well of an agar slide while control and patient's sera are placed in the wells that surround the centre well. After 24–48 hours of incubation precipitin lines are formed denoting the presence of an antigen-antibody reaction. Precipitin identity is established by comparison with precipitin lines produced by previously characterized reference serum. Both CIE and double diffusion are qualitative techniques suitable for detecting high concentrations of specific antibodies (0.1–1.0 μg/ml). Occasionally the results of double diffusion tests may be difficult to interpret. False-negative results may occur if the concentration of antigen is not adjusted to produce a zone of equivalence with the concentration of antibody in patient serum, and multiple precipitin lines of unknown specificity may interfere with identification of clinically significant antibodies. In contrast to double diffusion, CIE exhibits relatively greater sensitivity, speed and the ability to handle more samples. It is, however, technically demanding and the results less clear-cut.

Enzyme immunoassays. More recently, sandwich immunoassays have been developed to detect antibodies to ENA. Briefly, the method involves the addition of patient's serum containing antibody to microtitre plate wells coated with purified or recombinant individual ENA. Antibodies bound to antigen are detected by the addition of a polyclonal or monoclonal anti-human immunoglobulin antibody conjugated with an enzyme or luminescent molecule. The concentration of antibody in patient serum is directly related to the intensity of coloured or fluorescent product. Enzyme immunoassays are more sensitive (analytical sensitivity 1–10 ng/ml) than either CIE or double diffusion. Con-sequently, false-positive results may occur in hypergammaglobulinaemic sera as a result of increased non-specific binding.

Immunoblotting. An additional method for detection of antibodies to ENA is the qualitative technique of immunoblotting (Western blot) (Fig. 48.5). Briefly, antigens from a nuclear extract are separated according to molecular weight by sodium dodecyl sulphate electrophoresis (SDS-PAGE). The separated antigens are then transferred (blotting) to nitrocellulose paper, which is cut into single strips and incubated with patient's serum (commercial strips precoated with individual antigens are also available). Bound antibodies are detected by incubating the strips with an enzyme-labelled anti-human immunoglobulin. In a recent quality control exercise carried out by the Arthritis Foundation and the US Centres for Disease Control, immunoblotting was used to reanalyse anti-ENA specificities in reference sera previously characterized by immuno-fluorescence and double diffusion (Smolen *et al.*). The results of immunoblotting were largely in keeping with double diffusion although differences in individual laboratories were noted in relation to the reporting of additional unspecified bands. This is a recognized phenomenon with immunoblotting due to minor differences in techniques employed by individual laboratories. Immunoblotting is not at present used routinely in clinical immunology laboratories. In view of its specificity, it tends to be reserved for the investigation of patient samples producing discrepant results by standard assays. In those rare patients with compelling clinical evidence of lupus or lupus overlap disorders, in whom conventional assays fail to detect antibodies to DNA and ENA, immunoblotting offers the potential of detecting antibodies to previously uncharacterized antigens.

Antibodies to double-stranded DNA (anti-dsDNA)

Antibodies directed against double-stranded DNA (anti-dsDNA) play an important role in the pathogenesis of organ damage in SLE, particularly in the kidney. Complexes of ds-DNA and IgG anti-DNA antibodies have been demonstrated in eluates of renal biopsies. In keeping with this finding, levels of anti-dsDNA antibodies tend to correlate well with overall disease activity in SLE. In most patients, a rise in anti-dsDNA levels in serum is predictive of a

Systemic Lupus Erythematosus

Autoantibodies as markers of disease

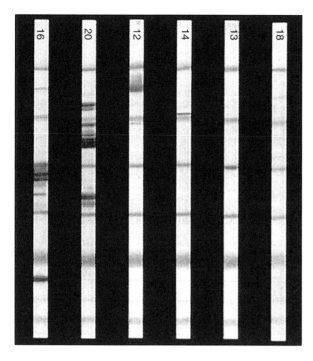

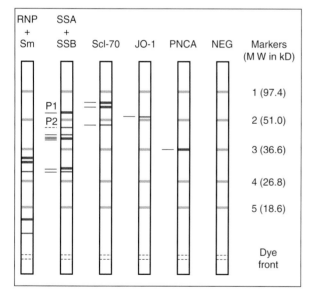

Figure 48.5: *Classic profiles of antibodies to extractable nuclear antigens on immunoblotting (modified with permission from Biodiagnostics Ltd). SS-A and SS-B are alternative terms for ant-Ro, La antibodies respectively. P1 and P2 refer to individual subunits of Ro. Additional antibodies included are anti-Scl 70 (marker for scleroderma), anti-Jo1 (marker of polymyositis with interstitial lung disease), anti-PCNA (proliferating cell nuclear antigen; seen in 2–10% of cases of SLE).*

disease flare. Occasionally a fall in previously elevated anti-dsDNA levels may presage lupus nephritis, presumably a reflection of immune complex deposition in the kidney. While antibodies to double-stranded DNA are highly specific for SLE, occurring in 75–95% of patients with untreated disease, antibodies to single-stranded DNA (ss-DNA) are non-specific, occurring in a variety of other disorders (rheumatoid arthritis, chronic active hepatitis, healthy elderly) in addition to lupus.

Methods of detection
Of the many methods available for detecting anti-dsDNA, most clinical immunology laboratories will use one of the following three assays:

Farr assay The Farr assay employs the use of radiolabelled dsDNA (^{125}I is commonly used as the radioisotope) as antigen. Incubating test serum containing anti-dsDNA with ^{125}I-dsDNA leads to the formation of immune complexes which are precipitated using a saturated solution of ammonium sulphate. The amount of anti-dsDNA is directly proportional to the amount of radioactivity in the precipitate. The concentration of anti-dsDNA in test samples is derived by measuring the amount of ^{125}I labelled DNA in the presence of a reference standard serum containing known amounts of antibody. A WHO standard serum designated Wo/80 is available for assay standardization. Since ammonium sulphate disrupts immune complexes containing antibodies of lower avidity, the Farr assay predominantly detects antibodies of high avidity which correlate well with the presence of severe lupus associated with renal disease. The Farr assay, however, does not detect low avidity anti-dsDNA antibodies which occur in patients with relatively mild lupus.

ELISA. A number of commercial ELISA assays which utilize purified dsDNA (either recombinant or from calf thymus extract) are available for the detection of DNA antibodies. Since dsDNA does not bind directly to plastic wells, most assays utilize DNA complexed to poly-L-lysine or protamine to coat microtitre plates. In contrast to the Farr assay, ELISA assays detect both low and high avidity DNA antibodies. Consequently, the ELISA assay exhibits a higher degree of sensitivity for diagnostic purposes than the Farr assay; however, its relatively lower specificity results in the generation of a significant number of false-positive DNA antibody results in patients without lupus e.g. infections, chronic liver disease.

Indirect immunofluorescence using Crithidia luciliae. Since the large mitochondrion (kinetoplast) of the haemoflagellate *Crithidia luciliae* is composed almost entirely of double-stranded DNA, indirect immunofluorescence studies using *Crithidia* as the antigen exhibit a high degree of sensitivity and specificity for the detection of anti-DNA antibodies in lupus. Commercial slides containing fixed *C. luciliae* are incubated with appropriately diluted test serum followed by the addition of anti-human immunoglobulin antibody conjugated to fluorescein. Samples producing fluorescence confined to the kinetoplast are considered positive (Fig. 48.6). Occasional samples may produce nuclear fluorescence as well but this should be disregarded since the nucleus contains many other antigens in addition to DNA. Although some workers have expressed concern that the kinetoplast may contain histones (basic proteins that bind DNA) leading to false-positive results in anti-histone antibody positive serum, this has not been confirmed. In most cases where contamination with histones is a concern, it is possible to perform immunofluorescence on *Crithidia* slides pretreated with hydrochloric acid, a procedure that removes histones. In view of the difficulties associated with standardization of immuno-fluorescent assays, the *Crithidia* assay is unreliable for serial monitoring of antibody levels.

Which anti-DNA assay to choose?
The ideal assay should be sufficiently sensitive and specific for the diagnosis of lupus, in addition to reflecting disease activity reliably. All three assays described (Table 48.5) fulfil the first criterion with sensitivities >90% in patients with active disease. With regard to specificity, the *Crithidia* and Farr assays

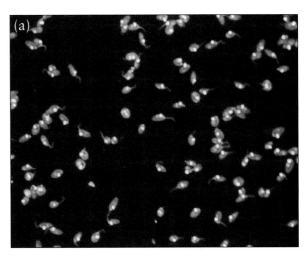

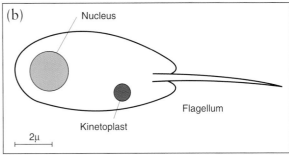

Figure 48.6: (a) depicts fluorescence confined to the kinetoplast of C. luciliae *using serum containing high levels of anti-DNA antibodies from a patient with active SLE. (b) Diagrammatic representation of the anatomy of* C. luciliae *[reproduced with permission from Rose N. R., Macario E. C., Fahey J., Friedman H., Penn G. M. Manual of Clinical Laboratory Immunology 4th Ed 1992, American Society for Microbiology, p. 731].*

(specificity >90%) are superior to ELISA. ELISA assays, by virtue of their propensity to detect low avidity antibodies, are known to produce false-positive DNA antibody results in a significant minority of patients without lupus. Despite this drawback, ELISA assays are used increasingly in clinical practice in view of their high sensitivity, ease of automation, ability to quantify results reliably (useful for serial monitoring) and the lack of radioisotopes in the assay.

The Farr assay is equally suitable for disease monitoring and may indeed be superior to ELISA in predicting the development of disease flares,

Systemic Lupus Erythematosus

Lupus and the anti-phospholipid syndrome

Table 48.5: Comparison of three commonly used anti-dsDNA assays in SLE.

	Farr	Crithidia	ELISA
Sensitivity	High	High	High
Specificity	High	High	Moderate
Detection of high avidity antibodies	+++	++	++
Detection of low avidity antibodies	+	++	+++
Ability to identify individual antibody Isotypes (IgG, IgA, IgM)	No	Yes	Yes
Suitability for monitoring disease activity	Yes	No	Yes

particularly involving the kidney. In a recent randomized Dutch study, patients with a 25% rise in anti-dsDNA levels receiving pre-emptive increases in immunosuppressive treatment had a significant decrease in relapses compared to the control group who were treated conventionally (Bootsma *et al.*). A small proportion of lupus patients may relapse without an accompanying rise in DNA antibodies; similarly a minority of patients may be clinically stable or asymptomatic despite the presence of persistently elevated antibody levels by all three assays.

Lupus and the anti-phospholipid syndrome

Antibodies to phospholipids (APA) act as markers of thrombosis and occur in a third of patients with lupus. The term anti-phospholipid syndrome (APS) was coined to delineate those patients with thrombosis and elevated levels of phospholipid antibodies (Table 48.6). In contrast to other thrombophilic states which result predominantly in venous thrombosis, patients with APS may develop thromboses both of arterial and venous vessels. Clinical manifestations are dependent on which organ is rendered ischaemic (Fig. 48.7). APA may be detected by ELISA or by the prolongation of phospholipid-dependent clotting assays (activated partial thromboplastin time–APTT). APA detected by ELISA using cardiolipin, an acidic phospholipid, as antigen may not always act as a true marker of thrombosis, since many false-positives have been described in patients with infection (bacterial, viral, protozoal), drug therapy and other connective tissue diseases. Indeed the historical false-positive VDRL is due to the presence of APA directed against cardiolipin present in the VDRL reagent. The inability of current ELISA assays to distinguish between thrombosis-associated and non-thrombosis-associated APA has led to difficulties in interpreting the clinical significance of elevated APA levels. The distinction is important since patients with thrombosis-associated APA require intensive long-term anticoagulant therapy, probably for life. Recent

Table 48.6: Criteria for the diagnosis of the anti-phospholipid antibody syndrome[*].

Clinical	Venous and/or arterial thrombosis
	Recurrent fetal loss
	Persistent thrombocytopenia
Laboratory	Persistent elevation of IgG and/or IgM cardiolipin ($ß_2$GPI dependent) antibody[†]
	Lupus anticoagulant

[*] At least one laboratory and one clinical criterion should be present; laboratory tests should be positive on at least two occasions more than three months apart
[†] Measurement of cardiolipin antibody may soon be replaced by direct measurement of antibodies to β_2GPI

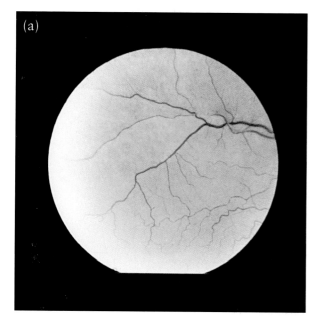

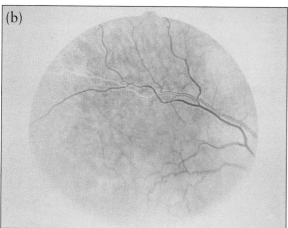

Figure 48.7: *(a) Branch retinal artery occlusion in a patient with SLE and the anti-phospholipid syndrome; the defect is more pronounced in the subtraction angiogram shown in panel (b).*

conventional ELISA assays to differentiate between thrombosis-associated and non-thrombosis-associated APA, there is much interest in assays using purified β_2GPI as antigen. Preliminary evidence suggests that antibodies to β_2GPI are likely to be stronger predictors of thrombosis than conventional cardiolipin antibodies detected by ELISA.

APA which interfere with phospholipid-dependent clotting assays recognize a phospholipid–prothrombin complex and are termed lupus anticoagulants (LAC) in recognition of their occurrence in lupus patients. The term LAC is a misnomer since it is associated with thrombosis *in vivo* rather than haemorrhage. The presence of LAC is suspected from a prolonged APTT which does not correct with the addition of normal plasma, thus suggesting the presence of an inhibitor. Since the demonstration of LAC antibodies indicates functional derangement of clotting, these antibodies correlate more closely with thrombosis than APA demonstrated by ELISA. Most patients with lupus will have LAC as well as cardiolipin antibodies (70%), although a minority of patients will have either cardiolipin antibodies or LAC (15% in each category).

Neuropsychiatric systemic lupus erythematosus (NPSLE)
The role of laboratory investigation
Neurological involvement in SLE is a major problem affecting up to two-thirds of patients at some point in their illness. Whereas approximately 20% of such patients do so on a background of active systemic disease, in the majority of cases systemic disease is quiescent or only mildly active. The physician confronted with a patient with SLE and neurological features has to make the important distinction between neurological disease directly due to lupus (primary), opportunistic infection as a secondary cause and steroid psychosis, since most patients will be on immunosuppressive therapy at the time of presentation. A diverse range of clinical presentations is seen (Table 48.7), reflecting multiple underlying pathogenic mechanisms. At least three hypotheses have been proposed to explain the diverse clinical presentations: anti-neuronal antibodies, throm-

evidence suggests that thrombosis-associated APA is directed largely against beta-2 glycoprotein I (β_2GPI, a serum protein cofactor which binds phospholipids) rather than phospholipids *per se*. Two sources of β_2GPI are found in current assays: human serum test samples and bovine serum used to block ELISA plates. It is thought that the interaction of immobilized cardiolipin with β_2GPI alters its conformation, rendering it immunogenic. In view of the inability of

Systemic Lupus Erythematosus

Assessment of disease activity in SLE

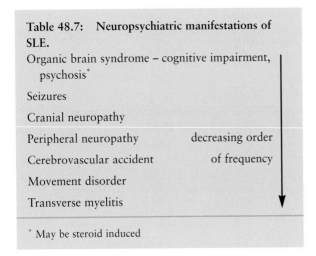

Table 48.7:   Neuropsychiatric manifestations of SLE.

Organic brain syndrome – cognitive impairment, psychosis*

Seizures

Cranial neuropathy

Peripheral neuropathy

Cerebrovascular accident

Movement disorder

Transverse myelitis

decreasing order of frequency

* May be steroid induced

bosis associated with phospholipid antibodies and cytokine-driven disease.

Regrettably, none of the currently available laboratory markers of SLE is sufficiently specific for the diagnosis of primary neurological lupus. Several studies have shown that abnormalities in anti-DNA and complement (C3, C4) levels in either serum or cerebrospinal fluid (CSF) do not discriminate between neurological and non-neurological disease in SLE. Initial enthusiasm for antibodies directed against neurones (lymphocytotoxic antibodies which cross-react with brain tissue and antibodies directly targeted against neuronal antigens) as specific markers for neurological lupus were dampened by studies demonstrating their presence in lupus patients without neurological involvement. Equally, recent claims that antibodies directed against ribosomal P proteins are specific markers of lupus psychosis have been refuted by their demonstration in up to 50% of SLE patients without psychosis.

Examination of CSF is mandatory in all patients with neuropsychiatric SLE to enable cases of infection masquerading as NPSLE to be diagnosed. In a recent prospective study of neurological involvement in SLE, infection (cryptococcal, tuberculosis and pyogenic meningitis) was the underlying cause in approximately 50% of cases. The presence of oligoclonal bands exclusively in CSF favours primary NPSLE but may also occur with infection. In the absence of a specific laboratory marker, the diagnosis of NPSLE remains heavily dependent on traditional clinical acumen.

Assessment of disease activity in SLE

The accurate measurement of disease activity is crucial to the proper management of SLE. Several indices of disease activity have been devised in order to simplify this task and ensure uniformity in clinical studies. Four well-validated systems currently in use are the SLE Disease Activity Index (SLEDAI), Systemic Lupus Activity Measure (SLAM), the British Isles Lupus Activity Group scale (BILAG) and the Lupus Activity Index (LAI). In conjunction with clinical assessment, serological markers of disease activity are a vital aid to the physician in determining the need for immunosuppressive therapy in SLE.

Active disease is accompanied in most patients by a rise in serum anti-DNA levels and a fall in complement (C3, C4) levels. In some patients however, complement measurements do not mirror disease activity. Since C3 acts as an acute phase reactant, a rise in concentration secondary to inflammation or infection would mask consumption due to active SLE. Serum C3 levels are normal in approximately 50% of patients with active disease while C4 measurements are of limited value in patients with C4 null alleles. As a result, several studies have assessed the role of complement breakdown products (C3d, C4d, C5b-9) as markers of disease activity.

In general, complement breakdown products are more sensitive markers of active disease (sensitivity 60–80%) than conventional C3 and C4 measurements. Their relative lack of specificity (specificity 45–80%) has however prevented its widespread adoption in clinical practice. In the absence of the ideal serological marker of disease activity in SLE, the use of serial anti-DNA antibody levels in conjunction with complement (either C3, C4 and/or breakdown products) and CRP represents the most useful laboratory profile for assessing disease activity (Table 48.8).

The place of adhesion molecule assays in the routine assessment of disease activity in lupus is currently under investigation. Preliminary studies suggest that serum levels of VCAM-1 (vascular cell adhesion molecule) are markedly

Table 48.8:   Changes in Anti-DNA antibodies, C3, C4 and CRP in relation to disease activity in SLE.

	anti-DNA	C3	C4	CRP
Active disease	↑	↓	↓	N or sl ↑
Inactive disease	N or sl ↑	N	N	N
Concomitant bacterial infection	N or sl ↑	N, ↑or ↓	N, ↑or ↓	↑

N = Normal   sl = slight

raised in lupus nephritis and appear to correlate with disease activity; E-Selectin and ICAM-1 (intercellular adhesion molecule) levels are unhelpful. Whether measurement of VCAM-1 is superior to existing serological markers of activity will depend on the merits of future prospective studies.

Cryoglobulinaemia

Introduction
The term cryoglobulinaemia is used to denote the presence of cryoglobulins in blood.

Cryoglobulins are immunoglobulins that precipitate reversibly in the cold (4°C), redissolving at higher temperatures (37°C). Three types of cryoglobulins are recognized on the basis of their immunoglobulin composition and associated diseases (Table 48.9). Type I cryoglobulins are composed entirely of monoclonal immunoglobulin (IgG or IgM) and account for approximately 25% of all cryoglobulins. Type II, which are composed of a mixture of monoclonal IgM with rheumatoid factor activity and polyclonal IgG account for a further 25%. Type III cryoglobulins are composed entirely of a mixture of polyclonal IgG and IgM and

Table 48.9:   Classification of cryoglobulins.

	Composition	Disease associations
Type I	Monoclonal immunoglobulin, usually IgM or IgG	Waldenström's macroglobulinaemia Myeloma, lymphoproliferative disease
Type II	Monoclonal IgM rheumatoid factor plus polyclonal IgG	Infections • Viral – hepatitis C, hepatitis B, HIV, Epstein–Barr • Bacterial – endocarditis • Spirochaetal – syphilis, Lyme disease • Parasitic – malaria • Fungal – coccidioidomycosis • 'Idiopathic'-mixed essential cryoglobulinaemia
Type III	Polyclonal IgM rheumatoid factor plus polyclonal IgG[*]	Autoimmune • SLE, rheumatoid arthritis, Sjögren's syndrome 'Idiopathic' • Mixed essential cryoglobulinaemia

[*] Trace amounts of type III cryoglobulins may be found in some normal individuals

Cryoglobulinaemia

Aetiology

Clinical features

Laboratory investigation of suspected cryoglobulinaemia

---

account for the remaining 50%. While the majority of cryoglobulins tend to precipitate at temperatures below 10°C, occasionally a thermolabile cryoglobulin may precipitate in the syringe used for venepuncture if it has not been prewarmed at 37°C. The precise reason(s) for the cryoprecipitation of immunoglobulins is not known.

Aetiology

Cryoglobulinaemia is associated in the majority of cases with an underlying disorder in the form of malignant paraproteinaemia, lymphoma, autoimmune disease or infection. Type I cryoglobulinaemia is associated typically with paraproteinaemia, with only a minority of patients failing to show evidence of underlying lymphoproliferative disease at presentation. In mixed cryoglobulinaemia (types II and III) detailed clinical investigation fails to uncover associated autoimmune disease or infection in up to one-third of patients. These patients were classified originally as having idiopathic or mixed essential cryoglobulinaemia. Since 1992 studies from Italy, US, France and Switzerland have provided convincing evidence that 60–80% of patients with types II and III cryoglobulinaemia have underlying hepatitis C infection. Although some patients with mixed cryoglobulinaemia exhibit features of lymphoproliferative disease, such as monoclonal B-cell populations in bone marrow and clonal immunoglobulin gene rearrangement in peripheral blood lymphocytes, overt lymphoma is uncommon.

The immunopathogenesis of cryoglobulinaemia is poorly understood. A wide range of primary antigen–antibody complexes has been detected in the cryoprecipitates of types II and III cryoglobulins, in addition to the complex of rheumatoid factor and IgG. This has led to the view that the formation of mixed cryoglobulins is the end result of a sequence of events driven by an antibody response either to infective agents or to endogenous antigens, as in SLE.

Clinical features

The clinical manifestations of cryoglobulinaemia are due to a combination of vascular obstruction and immune complex deposition.

Type I cryoglobulins may occur in either sex and mainly cause hyperviscosity and vascular obstruction. In contrast, mixed cryoglobulins (types II and III) affect females in particular and present with diverse clinical features due to deposition of cryoprecipitable immune complexes in blood vessels, causing systemic vasculitis affecting the skin, kidney and joints. Skin biopsies of the characteristic purpuric rash seen in such patients show leucocytoclastic vasculitis with deposition of immunoglobulin and complement. Renal involvement due to membranoproliferative glomerulonephritis with immunoglobulin and complement deposition occurs in up to 50% of all patients with mixed cryoglobulinaemia. Distinctive histological features of cryoglobulinaemic glomerulonephritis include marked glomerular monocytic infiltration, amorphous Congo red negative eosinophilic deposits in capillaries and a double contoured glomerular basement membrane due to an interposition of monocytes. The presence of these features on renal biopsy in a patient with so-called idiopathic glomerulonephritis should prompt a serarch for cryoglobulins. Impaired liver function with a wide spectrum of histological abnormality, ranging from chronic persistent hepatitis to cirrhosis, occurs in up to 70% of patients and is of interest in view of the strong association of hepatitis C infection and mixed cryoglobulinaemia (Fig. 48.8).

Laboratory investigation of suspected cryoglobulinaemia
Processing of samples

The commonest reason for failure to demonstrate circulating cryoglobulins is incorrect sample collection and processing. Meticulous attention in the collection of blood samples is essential. Blood should be collected into a plain tube without anticoagulant and immersed into a flask containing water at 37°C followed by immediate transfer to the laboratory. Failure to collect samples at 37°C enables cryoglobulins to precipitate with the blood clot and hence escape detection. Figure 48.9 illustrates the steps in the detection of cryoglobulins in the laboratory.

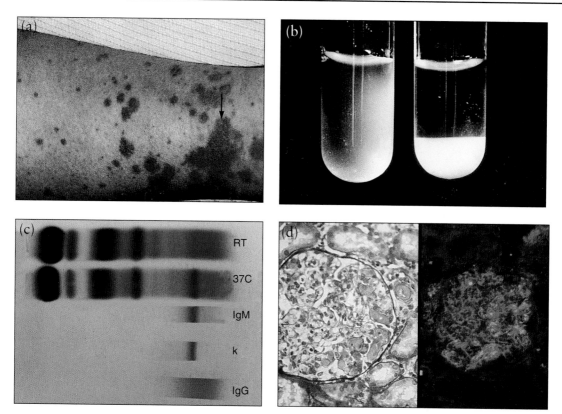

Figure 48.8: *Clinical and laboratory manifestations of mixed cryoglobulinaemia in a patient with hepatitis C. (a) Characteristic purpuric rash on lower limbs; arrow indicates an area of palpable purpura [reproduced with kind permission from Shakil A. O., Bisceglie A. M. New Engl J Med 1994; 331: 1624] (b) Stored serum showing cryoprecipitate after 24 hr incubation at 4°C (right of panel), redissolving on heating to 37°C (left of panel). (c) Zone electrophoresis of serum collected at 37°C shows the redissolved cryoprecipitate as a discrete band in the gamma region which on immunofixation is shown to be composed of monoclonal IgM kappa and polyclonal IgG. Note absence of gamma band on zone electrophoresis of sample collected at room temperature (RT) from the same patient. (d) Renal biopsy showing eosinophilic glomerular deposits of cryoglobulin (pseudothrombi) on routine H and E examination (left of panel) corresponding to coarse deposits (right of panel) of IgG on immunofluorescence [reproduced with kind permission from Graham A. Arthritis and Rheumatism 1992; 35: 1107, Fig. 5].*

Other laboratory features suggesting presence of cryoglobulins

Useful pointers to the presence of mixed cryoglobulins are marked depletion of early serum complement components (C4, C1q) due to activation of the classical pathway by immune complexes. The combination of a low serum C4 and IgM rheumatoid factor is a characteristic feature of mixed cryoglobulinaemia occurring in over 90% of patients. It is a useful rule of thumb that patients with an unexplained low serum C4 and renal or skin disease should be investigated for cryoglobulinaemia.

Cryoglobulins interfere with routine immunochemical measurements of serum immunoglobulins leading to artefactually low levels; they may also interfere with routine full blood count analysis by automated cell counters leading to spurious leukocytosis and thrombocytosis. Collection and analysis of samples at 37°C will prevent these problems.

In addition to characterizing the cryoglobulin, all patients should be investigated for an underlying trigger. In the case of type I cryoglobulinaemia appropriate investigations for lymphoproliferative disease should be

Acknowledgements

Further Reading

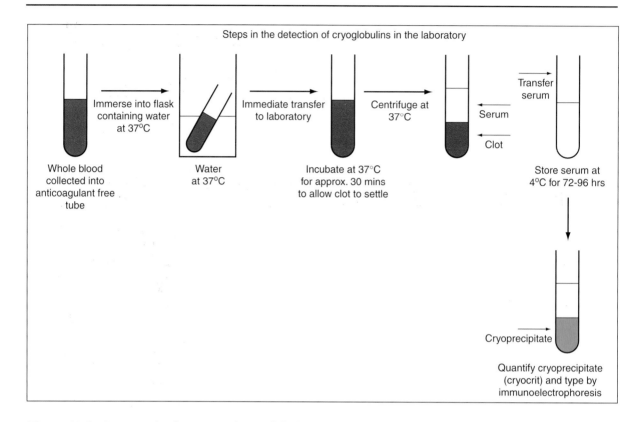

Figure 48.9: *Steps in the detection of cryoglobulins in the laboratory.*

instituted. Patients with mixed cryoglobulinaemia should have hepatitis serology done, including PCR for hepatitis C RNA in order to select those patients who would benefit from alpha interferon therapy. Routine investigation for other infective triggers (endocarditis, syphilis, Lyme disease, malaria, HIV) reportedly associated with mixed cryoglobulinaemia is not warranted in the absence of clues to the contrary.

Acknowledgements

I thank Faye Storey and Tracy Bower for their expert secretarial assistance.

Further Reading

Bootsma H *et al*. Prevention of relapses in systemic lupus erythematosus. *Lancet* 1995; **345**: 1595–1599.

Bruyn G A W. Controversies in lupus: nervous system involvement. *Annals Rheum Dis* 1995; **54**: 159–167.

Buyon J P *et al*. Assessment of disease activity and impending flare in patients with SLE. Comparison of the use of complement split products and conventional measures of complement. *Arthritis and Rheumatism* 1992; **35**: 1028–1037.

Cervera R *et al*. Systemic lupus erythematosus: clinical and immunologic patterns of disease expression in a cohort of 1000 patients. *Medicine (Baltimore)* 1993; **72**: 113–124.

Clinical Immunology. A practical approach Gooi H C, Chapel H (Ed). 1990: Oxford University Press.

<u>Further Reading</u>

Gorevic P. Cryopathies: cryoglobulins and cryofibrinogenaemia. In *Samter's Immunologic Diseases*. 5th Edn. Frank M M, Austen K F, Claman H N, Unaue E R (Ed) 1994: Vol II pp. 951–974.

Lawley T J. Immune complexes. In *Samter's Immunologic Diseases*. 5th Edn. Frank M M, Austen K F, Claman H N, Unaue E R (Ed) 1994: Vol I pp. 321–330.

Lockshin M D. Antiphospholipid antibody – babies, blood clots, biology. Grand rounds at the clinical centre of the National Institutes of Health. *JAMA* 1997; **277**: 1549–1551.

Sharp G C *et al*. Mixed connective tissue disease – an apparently distinct rheumatic disease syndrome associated with a specific antibody to an extractable nuclear antigen. *Am J Med* 1972; **52**: 148–159.

Smolen J S *et al*. Reference sera for antinuclear antibodies II. Further definition of antibody specificities in international antinuclear antibody reference sera by immunofluorescence and western blotting. *Arthritis and Rheumatism* 1997; **40**: 413–418.

ter Borg E J *et al*. Measurement of increases in anti-double-stranded DNA antibody levels as a predictor of disease exacerbation in systemic lupus erythematosus. *Arthritis and Rheumatism* 1990; **33**: 634–643.

Use and abuse of laboratory tests in clinical immunology: critical considerations of eight widely used diagnostic procedures. Report of an IUIS/WHO working group. *Clin Exp Immunol* 1981; **46**: 662–674.

Wong K L *et al*. Neurological manifestations of systemic lupus erythematosus: a prospective study. *Quarterly Journal of Medicine* 1991; **81**: 857–870.

49   HLA TYPING

Mark Hathaway

Introduction

Transplantation is now an accepted medical therapy to replace diseased organs. However, the response of the host's immune system to the transplanted organ remains a major obstacle to a successful outcome. Organ transplants are destroyed by an adaptive immune response by T lymphocytes to 'foreign' or non-self antigens present on the graft. Of the various donor antigens present on allografted tissue that may potentially cause rejection, disparate antigens of the major histocompatibility complex (MHC) are the most important.

When donor and recipient are MHC disparate, an immune response is initiated and directed against a non-self MHC molecule or molecules on the grafted tissue. Although other antigen systems can invoke an allograft-directed immune response, MHC antigens known as human leukocyte antigens or HLA are the most immunogenic. This is because of their ability to bind directly to the T-cell antigen receptor, thus bypassing normal antigen processing which is required to stimulate T-cell responses, and the high frequency of circulating T-cells in peripheral populations with receptor specificity for non-self MHC.

Since differences in MHC antigens provoke such vigorous rejection of allografts, a considerable amount of work has been directed towards donor–recipient MHC matching. Defining the HLA specificity, in an attempt to minimize rejection, through donor–recipient MHC matching is a process known as HLA typing.

HLA Structure and Function

The HLA genes of the human MHC consist of multiple class I, class II and class III loci present on the short arm of chromosome 6. They comprise approximately 4×10^6 base pairs, containing at least 50 genes.

HLA class I proteins consist of an alpha (α) chain that has three subunits, each resembling an immunoglobulin (Ig) domain. When expressed on the cell surface HLA class I molecules are non-covalently bound to the peptide beta-2-microglobulin (β-2M), which is coded for on a separate chromosome. At present there are three well-defined α-chain genes, designated HLA-A, -B, and -C. HLA-A and HLA-B represent the major class I products and serve as targets both for antibody and cell mediated immune responses against transplanted tissue. Their expression is differential, depending on cell type, with cells of the lymphoid lineage having the highest expression and hepatocytes and red blood cells having the lowest. Expression can be altered by inflammatory mediators such as cytokines and this is particularly important in transplantation since upregulation can promote allograft immunogenicity, or increase the susceptibility of allografts to a pre-existing immune response.

HLA class II proteins differ from those of the class I region in terms of structure, function and distribution. They consist of two chains, α and β, and are expressed on the cell surface as $\alpha\beta$ heterodimers HLA class II α and β chain genes are designated HLA-DP, HLA-DQ and HLA-DR, both chains being encoded for in the class II region and having two subunits resembling Ig domains. HLA-DR gene clusters contain an extra β chain gene, whose product can pair with any DR α chain. Therefore, three sets of class II genes can give rise to four types of class II molecules. The distribution of class II proteins is largely restricted to B-lymphocytes and professional antigen presenting cells (APCs), although expression on other cells is inducible following activation. The function of class II molecules has been traditionally considered in terms of their ability to stimulate helper T-cell responses, however, more recent evidence has shown significant cytotoxic antibody and effector T-cell responses directed against class II determinants.

Also encoded for in the MHC are two TAP genes. These are found in the class II region, closely associated with two genes encoding low molecular weight proteins of the proteosome. The genes of the class III region encode the complement components C4 (C4a and C4b), C2 and factor B, together with those for the cytokine tumour necrosis factor (TNFα and β), the steroid synthesizing enzyme 21-hydroxylase, and two heat shock proteins Hsp 70 1H and Hsp 70 2.

Genetics of the MHC

The genes coding for HLA class I α chains and class II α and β chains are linked within the MHC. Although the genes coding for each chain are to be found in separate regions, several genes encoding for each chain have been identified within each region. Because the HLA genes are in close proximity to each other, genetic recombination is rare. Therefore, most offspring inherit an intact set of parental alleles, one from each parent. Such sets of linked genes are known as haplotypes. Certain alleles in particular haplotypes form in greater or lesser frequencies than would be expected if the alleles were at genetic equilibrium. This

phenomenon is known as linkage disequilibrium and may reflect both the recent origin of some alleles and geographical origins and racial breeding patterns.

The products of HLA class I and class II genes are codominantly expressed, therefore heterozygous individuals should express two distinct HLA specificities for each locus (one maternal, one paternal). In addition, because there are three genes for HLA class I and four possible sets for class II, each individual would be expected to express three different MHC class I and four different class II proteins. The number expressed is in fact much higher due to the extreme polymorphic nature of class I and II genes; indeed more than 70 alleles at the same genetic locus have been identified for some class I proteins. For this reason, the probability of HLA genes in two non-identical individuals encoding the same allele is extremely small. Because HLA proteins are extremely immunogenic, the objective, in transplantation, is to get the closest possible match between allograft and recipient, thus minimizing the risk of graft loss to rejection. The technical process of HLA protein identification in a given individual is known as HLA typing.

Mechanics of HLA Typing

Serological typing

Historically, the mixed lymphocyte reaction (MLR) was used to detect HLA variability. In this technique, cells from a potential recipient are co-cultured with 'stimulator' cells of donor origin which have been irradiated so that they cannot respond. T-cells from the recipient are stimulated to proliferate and differentiate in response to disparate HLA antigens usually as a result of CD4+ T-cell recognition of HLA class II antigens and recognition of class I antigens by CD8+ T-cells. Thus 'matched' recipients can be readily identified on the basis of their 'non-responsiveness'. Whilst this technique correlates well with rejection, is extremely sensitive and closely reflects the rejection response itself, its application in the clinical setting is of limited or no value since it takes 5 to 10 days to obtain results and is cumbersome, expensive and technically difficult to perform.

Until recently, the 'traditional' method used to distinguish HLA non-identical individuals employed antibody. HLA-A and -B locus antigens were the first to be defined in this manner, using alloantisera obtained from subjects immunized by blood transfusions, pregnancy or renal allograft rejection. Using this technique, called a microcytotoxicity assay, peripheral blood T lymphocytes (HLA class I antigens) and B lymphocytes (HLA-DR, -DQ) from potential allograft recipients of unknown HLA type are incubated with antiserum of characterized HLA specificity. These cells are then exposed to complement. If antibody reacts with HLA proteins expressed on the cell surface, complement is activated and the cells are killed–complement mediated lysis. In the absence of reaction no lysis occurs. Killing is visualized usually by a two-colour fluorescent dye system, one of which labels all viable cells green. The other can only penetrate killed cells, labelling them red, therefore killing is assessed semi-quantitatively by loss of green cells and is usually expressed as a percentage. Thus, where lysis occurs, the specificity of the antibody identifies which HLA proteins are expressed.

Several types of error are possible with serological typing. A failure to identify a rare or cross-reactive antigen is a frequent problem. This is principally because the relevant antisera either have not been used, or are not available. Linkage disequilibrium, geographical origins and racial breeding patterns are contributing factors, moreover some antigens are expressed at a lower frequency or not at all in certain populations. Such errors are most likely to occur in laboratories using limited numbers of antisera. In addition, a misinterpretation of antiserum reactions can also produce errors. Antiserum may contain more than one antibody, each with differing HLA specificities and even monospecific HLA antibodies frequently cross-react with other HLA antigens. Furthermore HLA typing of DR antigens using serology is particularly susceptible to misinterpretation since B lymphocytes are both more cross-reactive to a wide range of DR antigens and more susceptible to non-specific comple-

ment mediated lysis, giving rise to 'false-positive' results. Technical variations also account for a 15–30% inter-laboratory error in serological typing. Variation in complement activity between batches and quality of antiserum are the main contributory factors.

Serotyping is a rapid method for HLA genotyping, however, the reagents used are not specific enough to determine the precise structural identity of MHC molecules in genetically non-identical individuals. This can only be achieved by direct analysis of the MHC genes themselves.

Molecular typing
Restriction fragment length polymorphism
In recent years, intensive molecular cloning and mapping of the class II region of the MHC has been achieved. Extensive analysis of the organization of specific gene sequences, using a technique known as Southern blotting, has revealed the existence of polymorphisms in the restriction sites that are in the majority of cases allele specific. Therefore, mapping and elucidation of the restriction fragment length polymorphism (RFLP) patterns associated with HLA alleles should facilitate allelic identification in any given individual. The feasibility of HLA typing by detection of RFLPs using DNA probes was first suggested by Wake et al. (1982), who reported HLA-DR region polymorphisms using a full-length DRβ1 cDNA clone. RFLP typing of HLA-DR and -DQ alleles using full-length cDNA probes for DRβ, DQα and DQβ have since been used extensively in an attempt to define accurately the relationship between RFLPs and serological or cellular defined HLA class II specificities.

RFLP analysis is carried out on genomic DNA samples usually obtained from 'buffy coat' leukocytes. Full-length DNA is extracted via sodium dodecyl sulphate (SDS)/proteinase K digestion of the leukocytes and subjected to restriction digestion using the restriction endonuclease Tag-1 or MSP-1. The digest is then electrophoretically separated on a 2% agarose gel and transferred to a nitrocellulose membrane using a Southern blotting technique. Restriction fragment patterns are visualized by hybridization of the blot with complementary

Mechanics of HLA Typing

Molecular typing

radio-labelled cDNA probes, which is then exposed to X-ray film. The hybridization signal patterns generated are then compared with reference tables to enable identification of differing HLA-DR and -DQ specificities.

The merits of this technique are that multiple samples (>30) can be processed simultaneously. In addition, DRβ, DQα and DQβ allelic specificities can be identified from a single sample, since restriction digests can be blotted and probed with one HLA gene specific cDNA (e.g. DRβ) and the blot stripped, washed and reprobed with a cDNA of differing HLA specificity (e.g. DQα or DQβ). Its disadvantages are that RFLP requires extremely careful sample handling and DNA extraction. The DNA must be full length, not partially degraded, since this can radically alter the restriction pattern, giving rise to incorrect banding. In addition, it cannot be used in the clinical transplant setting to HLA type cadaveric donors due to inherent time constraints, since it can take up to three weeks to obtain results. Moreover, the restriction fragment banding patterns are highly complex and inter-locus cross-hybridization of cDNA probes means this technique requires considerable expertise in interpretation. However, the latter problem can be circumvented by the use of short region, or exon specific cDNA probes. In technical terms, RFLP analysis does not directly identify polymorphic DNA sequences in the region coding for HLA antigens, but restriction sites in strong linkage with them. In addition, it relies on the linkage disequilibrium between HLA-DR and HLA-DQ alleles to discriminate between certain HLA-DR alleles that demonstrate similar RFLP patterns; for example DR3 (DQ2) from DR6 (DQ6) and DR7 (DQ2) from DR9 (DQ9). Such an exercise needs great caution when analysing non-Caucasian populations since particular HLA-DR–DQ associations are not always the same. Indeed, later evidence has shown that such associations are not always true in Caucasoid populations as well.

Polymerase chain reaction

At present, the most convenient method of identifying MHC alleles is by a technique known as polymerase chain reaction or PCR. This is a rapid method of selectively replicating particular sequences of genomic DNA. In order to amplify specific DNA regions, such a polymorphic exon of a particular MHC gene, synthetic oligonucleotide primers, complementary to the DNA sequence flanking the region of interest, have to be synthesized. Genomic DNA, extracted in an identical procedure to that for RFLP analysis, is then denatured, at high temperature, in the presence of excess concentrations of the two synthetic oligonucleotides. Cooling then allows the DNA strands to re-anneal so that both primers are bound to their complementary sequence on genomic DNA. The thermostable enzyme DNA polymerase (Taq-polymerase), obtained from the bacterium *Thermus aquaticus*, which is added to the reaction, now elongates the primer, using the genomic DNA between the two primers as its template. The replicated DNA is then denatured into single strands by high temperature and the mixture cooled to facilitate new cycles of annealing and replication. The first extension product is random in length, but all subsequent cycles create products of defined length because the template ends at the first primer. Cycles are then repeated until sufficient DNA is available for sequencing.

Once DNA associated with a particular allele has been defined at the sequence level, oligonucleotide probes can be constructed from regions where differences occur. These sequence specific oligonucleotide (SSO) or allele specific oligonucleotide (ASO) probes can then be hybridized to Southern blotted PCR amplified specific target DNA using a technique called PCR-SSO/PCR-ASO. Such techniques are rapid, cheap and a sensitive way of defining MHC gene structure. However, PCR-SSO/ASO typing techniques require the preparation of multiple blots and labelled probes, at least one probe for each allele at each locus. RFLP typing in contrast requires at most two blots and three probes. Time constraints using PCR-SSO/ASO are similar to DNA-RFLP, only the preparation of target DNA is quicker (5–6 hours compared with 24 hours), blotting and probing taking a similar amount of time. Thus, like RFLP, this technique is only of use in non-urgent clinical applications and therefore cannot be used to HLA type cadaveric donors.

HLA typing by molecular techniques has been revolutionized by the recent introduction of a PCR-based multiple sequence specific primer (PCR-SSP) method. Intensive molecular cloning of HLA class I and class II genes has facilitated the construction of a complete series of SSPs. PCR-SSP maintains the allelic specificity of each primer pair, both by the stringency of the PCR reaction conditions and the design of the oligonucleotide primers, which exploit the ability of Taq polymerase to amplify target DNA sequences that are mismatched to the primer sequence. In reactions where complementarity between DNA and primer is complete, amplification efficiency is 100% and target DNA is replicated. Where there is one or more base pair mismatch between target DNA and the 3′ end of the primer, amplification efficiency is 0% and no products are synthesized. This system for HLA class I and class II typing uses 192 PCR reactions to define HLA-A, -B, -C, DRβ1, DRβ3, DRβ4, DRβ5 and DQβ1 genes. Reaction products are separated electrophoretically using a 1% agarose gel containing ethidium bromide and visualized on an ultraviolet transilluminator.

Complete HLA types can be identified from a single polaroid photograph, hence it has been termed 'phototyping'. This technique has a sensitivity greater than or equal to serology without cross-reaction problems, and can distinguish most heterozygous allelic combinations. It has the advantage both over DNA-RFLP and PCR-SSO/ASO based typing techniques in that it does not require blotting and probing and is therefore cheaper and quicker to perform. Moreover, full HLA typing, from blood to results, can be obtained in three hours, making this technique comparable to serology and thus suitable for HLA typing of cadaveric donors. Indeed PCR-SSP has now superseded serological techniques in many histocompatibility testing laboratories. Another advantage over DNA-RFLP is that PCR-SSP does not rely on full-length DNA to produce results, therefore partially degraded samples can be utilized.

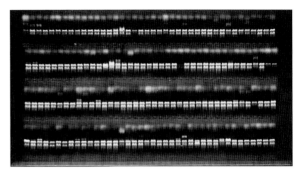

Figure 49.1: *This figure shows typical 'phototyping' results obtained with the 160 reaction set currently in use with the Birmingham liver transplant programme. This gel is overloaded, as indicated by the presence of 'double bands' in the centre of each gel lane resulting from over-amplification of the DR-β positive control. Allelic products appear above the positive control band (except Bw 4/6 and Cw 1). Thus all reactions should amplify the positive control, plus an extra allelic band where specificities are expressed. PCR failure, indicated by 'blank' lanes on the gel, is a frequent problem which may in part be due to sub-optimal DNA or Taq concentrations or poor DNA purity. In the absence of complete allelic specificities such samples require re-typing.*

However, this and other PCR-based techniques are not devoid of problems. Deviation from defined PCR protocols, poor quality DNA (in terms of purity) and unsuitable PCR machines can produce individual PCR failures that result in incorrect or missed antigen assignment. In addition, these high level molecular techniques are no less demanding than serology and require considerable training and expertise if they are to be performed correctly.

Summary

The cell surface glycoproteins of the MHC play a central role in transplant immunology. The MHC was originally determined as the major barrier to transplantation because of the strong rejection response of T lymphocytes to non-self MHC antigens present on the grafted tissue. The HLA proteins of the human MHC are amongst the most polymorphic known, therefore the likelihood of two unrelated individuals expressing the same HLA alleles is very small. Since T-cell antigen recognition is profoundly influenced by MHC polymorphism, the HLA proteins of transplant donors and potential recipients must be identified and the closest possible match sought in order to minimize the risk of graft loss to rejection. The technique of HLA identification, termed 'tissue typing', is indeed used in clinical medicine to match donor to recipient in cadaveric transplant programmes, but can also be used to study the role of the MHC in determining susceptibility to allergic and autoimmune conditions.

MHC genotyping in humans was originally carried out by mixed lymphocyte reaction and then serology. Because of inherent methodological constraints, these methods were supplemented by techniques analysing at the genetic, rather than the expression level. The -DR and -DQ genes of the MHC class II region were the first to be HLA typed by DNA-RFLP. This technique was then replaced by quicker and faster PCR-based methods. Molecular cloning and mapping of the MHC has led to the recent development of a new PCR-based technique that types antigens both of class I and class II regions. Using this technique, HLA genotyping can be carried out on a single sample using multiple PCR and a single gel, with results obtainable from a single polaroid photograph. This system has either replaced, or is replacing, all previous serological/molecular based HLA typing procedures in the majority of histocompatibility testing laboratories.

Further Reading

Bunce M, O'Neill C M, Barnardo M, Krausa P, Browning M J, Morris P J, Welsh K I. Phototyping – Comprehensive DNA typing for HLA-A, HLA-B, HLA-C, HLA-DRβ1, HLA-DRβ3, HLA-DRβ4, HLA-DRβ5 and HLA-DQβ1 by PCR with 144 primer mixes utilising sequence specific primers (SSP). *Tissue Antigens* 1995; **465**: 355.

Janeway C A Jr, Travers P. In *Immunobiology, the system in health and disease* Robertson M, Ward R, Lawrence E (Eds). 1994: Blackwell.

Olerup O, Zetterquist H. HLA-DR typing by PCR amplification with sequence-specific primers (PCR-SSP) in 2 hours: an alternative to serological DR typing in clinical practice including donor: recipient matching in cadaveric transplantation. *Tissue Antigens* 1992; 38: 255.

Wake C, Long E, Mach B. Allelic polymorphism and complexity of the genes for HLA-DRβ-chains: direct analysis by DNA-DNA hybridisation. *Nature* 1982; 300: 372.

SECTION 8
MOLECULAR PATHOLOGY

50 THE POLYMERASE CHAIN REACTION (PCR)

John J O'Leary, Ivan Silva, Volker Uhlmann and Robert J Landers

Historical Background to PCR

DNA was first isolated in 1869 by Miescher, but its double helix structure was not described until 1953 by Watson & Crick.

In 1955, Arthur Kornberg of Stanford University discovered DNA polymerase. This cellular enzyme is involved in DNA replication and repair by catalysing the addition of nucleotides to the 3′ end of an existing DNA chain. The initiation of a new chain requires an existing oligo- or polynucleotide chain, referred to as a primer. The polymerase attaches nucleotides in a new DNA strand, complementary to nucleotides on corresponding positions of the parent DNA strand (template strand). RNA polymerases are involved in the assembly of RNA from a DNA template (transcription).

In the following years, new tools for producing and manipulating DNA were developed. Restriction endonucleases (RE) cut DNA at specific sequences (restriction sites), making it possible to isolate strands of DNA containing specific genes. In 1975, Edwin Southern described a technique for the localization of specific sequences within genomic DNA by electrophoretic transfer techniques. This technique, subsequently known as Southern blotting involves the digestion of genomic DNA by one or more REs and the separation of the resulting fragments by agarose gel electrophoresis. The separated fragments of double-stranded DNA are then separated into single-stranded form and transferred (blotting) from the gel to a solid support (usually a nitrocellulose or nylon filter). The sequence of interest can then be detected using a short fragment of DNA (oligonucleotide probe), which is complementary to the DNA sequence of interest (hybridization) (see Fig. 50.1).

Initially, radioactive labels (i.e. ^{32}P, ^{35}S, ^{3}H) were used for probing, but later non-isotopic labels including biotin, digoxigenin and fluorescein were employed. Three nucleic acid labelling methods are now described, including

Historical Background to PCR

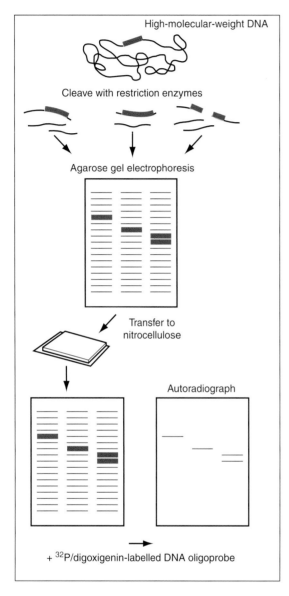

High-molecular-weight DNA

Cleave with restriction enzymes

Agarose gel electrophoresis

Transfer to
nitrocellulose

Autoradiograph

+ ^{32}P/digoxigenin-labelled DNA oligoprobe

*Figure 50.1: Schematic representation of Southern
blot analysis of a genomic DNA fragment.*

enzyme incorporation, chemical derivatization and chemical cross-linking. The enzymatic labelling reactions for DNA include nick translation, random priming and 5′ and 3′ end labelling, utilizing DNA polymerase, Klenow polymerase and DNAase. For RNA detection, riboprobes can be created using SP6, T3 and T7 *in vitro* enzymologies. Alternatively, synthetic oligonucleotides can be conveniently used as probes for DNA and RNA detection

assays. Additionally, PCR probe labelling methods, employing biotin, digoxigenin or fluorescein labelled dNTPs in substituted molar ratios in the PCR reaction mix can also be used for generating probes for any hybridization analysis.

A refinement of Southern blot analysis, of interest to pathologists, was first published in 1969 by two groups working independently in the United Kingdom and the US. The technique called in-situ hybridization allowed for the first time direct correlation between hybridization signals and tissue morphology. The initial reports were followed by application of the methodology to cryostat, paraffin wax, chromosomal and electron microscopic preparations. Since then, numerous DNA and RNA targets have be demonstrated using both isotopic and non-isotopic labels (see Chapter 54).

Analogous techniques for RNA and proteins have been named Northern and Western blotting respectively, as a play on the name Southern. These techniques gained widespread acceptance in the 1970s.

The next significant breakthrough in molecular biology was the development of rapid DNA sequencing techniques. In the chemical method of Maxem & Gilbert the sequence is determined from native DNA itself. DNA is labelled at one end and then exposed to agents that destroy one or two of the nucleotides, resulting in fragments which can be separated and analysed by electrophoresis. The Sanger or dideoxy chain termination method parallels the process of DNA replication. Starting with a primer, a DNA polymerase adds nucleotide triphosphates (dNTPs) producing a complementary DNA strand. Four different reaction mixes, each containing in addition a dideoxynucleotide triphosphate (ddNTP) corresponding to one of the four nucleotides, is added to the new DNA strand and terminates the replication process. This produces DNA fragments of various lengths. The sequence is then determined by separating the resulting DNA fragments of each reaction by gel electrophoresis.

For further progress to be made, techniques allowing the production of large quantities of

THE POLYMERASE CHAIN REACTION (PCR)

A Wonderful New Tool or a Dangerous Weapon?
Basic Methodology

recombinant DNA were necessary. Cloning was the first revolutionary technique described, involving the isolation and production of many copies of a DNA sequence. The DNA fragment of interest is cut using REs and then ligated into other DNA molecules called vectors or cloning vehicles (e.g. plasmids). The vector and the inserted DNA fragment can then be produced in large quantities by transformed bacteria. Subsequently, the cloned sequence can then be extracted and analysed or used directly as a probe for hybridization.

Cloning is however a time consuming process and is not routinely applicable to a busy diagnostic pathology laboratory. This obvious disadvantage was overcome by the development of the polymerase chain reaction (PCR). The technique was first described by Khorana and colleagues in the early 1970s, was developed and named PCR in 1983 by Kary Mullis, who subsequently received the Nobel Prize for chemistry in 1994 for his work on PCR.

A Wonderful New Tool or a Dangerous Weapon?

Since publication of the polymerase chain reaction (PCR) technique in 1985 by Saiki, a plethora of reports and publications on its use in medicine and molecular pathology has been unleashed on the scientific world. Like all new techniques, it suffers from an explosive input from the trained, the wary and the inexperienced.

Occasionally, a technique is developed in an area which improves the ability of the scientist to perform detailed experiments and quickly becomes established as a routine procedure. The polymerase chain reaction represents such a technique in the field of molecular medicine, particularly in the analysis of DNA and RNA.

With this technique, a sequence of DNA can be amplified (from small starting quantities) to an extent that it may be analysed directly for point mutations, polymorphisms, etc. and then sequenced following amplification. The requirement is that the nucleotide sequence of

short regions of DNA flanking the region of interest is known.

DNA polymerase enzymes catalyse copying of DNA in proliferating cells and *in vitro*, if conditions are optimal. What is required is that a template strand and primers (short sequences of complementary DNA) are provided to start the process. By selecting appropriate pairs of primers, millions of copies of a chosen DNA sequence can be amplified in a few hours. This DNA can then be visualized on a size fractionated gel, or analysed further by restriction endonuclease digestion or by hybridization with labelled highly specific probes.

With this technique, it is now possible to study DNA from before birth to even after death. The DNA template can be retrieved from many sources including smears, hair roots, blood spots, paraffin wax-embedded tissues and even single cells, which can then be directly analysed to detect viruses, activated oncogenes, gene defects or to provide forensic or anthropological information.

Basic Methodology

The method was invented by Kary Mullis and originally employed by a group in the Human Genetics Department at Cetus Corporation USA for the amplification of β globin DNA. Two synthetic oligonucleotides that flank the region of interest to be amplified are prepared using the flanking sequences from published data, one complementary to each of the strands (see Fig. 50.2).

DNA is denatured at high temperatures 95°C (denaturation step) to convert double-stranded DNA into two single-strand forms and then reannealled in the presence of a large molar excess of oligonucleotide primers. The primers, orientated with their 3′ ends pointing towards each other, hybridize to opposite strands of the target sequence to be amplified (annealing step) and subsequently prime enzymatic extension by Taq DNA polymerase along the nucleic acid template (extension step) in the presence of four deoxynucleotides (dATP, dCTP, dGTP, dTTP). The end product is then denatured again for another cycle.

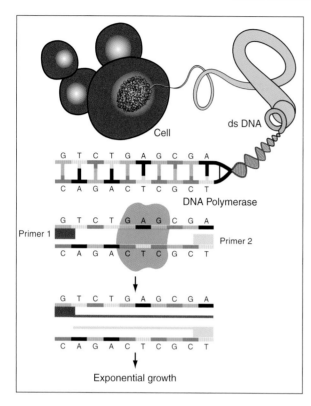

Figure 50.2: *DNA-PCR showing an exponential increase in PCR product.*

This leads ultimately to amplification of the target sequence so that it can be readily detected by gel electrophoresis. After the above three-step cycle, the above procedure is repeated 20 to 50 times depending on the size of the amplified product and the GC content of the amplified template. Amplification of the order of 10^{12} can thus be achieved. As can be seen, the process is highly efficient and allows the use of minute quantities of starting DNA.

The enzyme originally used to catalyse the reaction was the large fragment DNA polymerase derived from *E. coli* known as the Klenow fragment. Today, Taq polymerase, which is stable at high temperatures, allows greater flexibility with the reaction and dispenses with the need to add DNA polymerase with each cycle, as is required with the Klenow fragment. Taq polymerase is obtained from the thermophilic species *Thermus aquaticus* which has been cloned. In addition to greater flexibil-

ity with this enzyme, larger amplified products can now be obtained with Taq XL, which originally were not achievable with thermolabile DNA polymerases. The sensitivity and specificity of the procedure are improved by high annealing and extension temperatures which reduce secondary structure and increase the specificity of the oligonucleotide priming events. The specificity of the reaction can be increased by using the 'nested primer' technique. This uses one or two oligonucleotide primers designed to hybridize to sequences internal to the original set of primers.

Using 1–5% of the original amplification product and fresh deoxynucleotide triphosphates, buffer and enzyme, a further set of amplifications can be performed. This generally results in dramatic increases in the amount of the desired amplified product.

As well as making copies of DNA between two primers, it is also possible to amplify DNA outside of the selected primer pair provided that one of the primers is at the edge of the known DNA sequence. In the normal PCR scenario, primers direct DNA extension towards each other but in 'inverse PCR' primers are selected so that DNA elongation is away from each of the primer pair. The generated DNA template is then cut with a restriction endonuclease and is converted to a circular form by ligation. This circular DNA is subsequently subjected to PCR, in which extension occurs in both directions across the ligation site yielding a linear product consisting of DNA sequences copied from DNA template flanking the primers. Sequencing of the product can then be performed and thus integration sites of viruses, etc, can be determined (see later).

The 'Standard' DNA PCR Assay

Because of the wide variety of applications in which PCR is now being used, it is probably impossible to describe a single set of conditions that will guarantee success in all situations. A standard reaction is typically performed in a 50 or 100 μl volume and in addition to the sample

DNA, contains 50 mM KCl, 10 mM TrisHCl (pH 8.4 at room temperature), 1.5 mM $MgCl_2$, 100 μg/ml gelatin (optional), 0.25 μM of each primer, 200 μM of each deoxynucleotide triphosphate (dATP, dCTP, dGTP and dTTP), and 2.5 units of Taq polymerase.

Amplification can be conveniently performed in a DNA thermal cycler or other automated heating block to denature at 94°C for 20 seconds, anneal at 55°C for 20 seconds, and extend at 72°C for 30 seconds for a total of 30–40 cycles. These general conditions can be used to amplify a wide range of target sequences with excellent specificity.

The 'Standard' RNA PCR Assay

RNA can also conveniently be amplified by the PCR process. The reaction is entitled reverse transcriptase PCR (RT-PCR). In the first round reaction, a cDNA template is made from RNA in the cell. This is achieved using one of several reverse transcriptase enzymes (MMLV, AMV, etc.). To achieve reverse transcription, one of three priming strategies can be employed. The most specific is downstream priming with a target specific primer. The second method employs oligo dTs, which will hybridize any poly A tail RNA species in the sample, giving rise to reverse transcription of many mRNA targets. The final method employs random hexamers, essentially performing a degenerate (non-target specific) reverse transcription reaction. Following reverse transcription, cDNA amplification is then performed with Taq DNA polymerase. Alternatively a one-step RT-PCR assay can be performed using the enzyme rTth polymerase, which possesses both reverse transcriptase and DNA polymerase activity.

Primer Selection ... a Critical Step

Unfortunately, the approach to the selection of efficient and specific primers remains somewhat empirical. It is primer design more than anything else that determines the success or failure of an amplification reaction. Fortunately, the majority of primers can be made to work and the following guidelines are helpful. (1) Primers should be selected with a random base distribution and with GC contents similar to that of the fragment being amplified. It is best to avoid primers with stretches of polypurines, polypyrimidines, or other unusual sequences. (2) Sequences with significant secondary structure, should be avoided particularly at the 3'-end of the primer. (3) Homology of primers and primers with 3' overlaps will increase the incidence of 'primer-dimer' (see below) formation and should be avoided.

Most primers are between 20 and 30 bases in length and the optimal amount to use in an amplification reaction varies. Sequences not complementary to the template can be added to the 5'-end of primers. These exogenous sequences become incorporated into the double-stranded PCR product and provide a means of introducing restriction sites or regulatory elements (e.g. promoters) at the ends of the amplified target sequence. If required, shorter primers or degenerate primers can be used, as long as the thermal profile of the reaction is adapted to reflect the lower stability of the primed template. In general, concentrations ranging from 0.05 to 0.5 μM of each oligonucleotide primer are used.

'Primer-dimer' is an amplification artifact often observed in the PCR product, especially when many cycles of amplification are performed on a sample containing very few initial copies of DNA template. It is a double-stranded fragment, whose length is very close to the sum of the two primers and appears to occur when one primer is extended by the DNA polymerase enzyme over the other primer. In some cases this may overwhelm the reaction.

The exact mechanism by which primer-dimer formation occurs is not clear. The observation that primers with complementary 3'-ends are predisposed to dimer formation suggest that transient interactions that bring the termini of the oligonucleotide primers in close proximity are the initiating event. Several polymerases, including Taq, have been shown to have a weak non-template directed polymerization activity, which can attach additional bases to a blunt-ended duplex.

If such an activity were also to occur on a single-stranded oligonucleotide, there is a good chance that the extension would form a short 3' overlap with the other primer, sufficient to promote dimerization. Formation can be reduced by using minimal concentrations of primers and enzyme.

Changes in PCR Buffer are Critical

Changes in PCR reaction buffer will usually affect the outcome of the amplification procedure. The concentration of $MgCl_2$ seems to have a profound effect on the specificity and yield of an amplification. Concentrations of approximately 1.5 mM are usually optimal (with 200 μM each dNTP), but in some circumstances, different amounts of magnesium may prove to be necessary. Generally, excess magnesium will result in the accumulation of non-specific amplification products and insufficient Mg^{2+} will reduce the yield. More recently, it has been shown that the reduction or elimination of KCl and gelatin may be beneficial. Some protocols include 10% dimethyl sulphoxide (DMSO) to reduce the secondary structure of the target DNA, and Triton X, a detergent used with some Taq enzymes. DMSO can be slightly inhibitory to Taq polymerase and may decrease the overall yield of amplified product.

The deoxynucleotide triphosphates (dATP, dCTP, dGTP and dTTP) are usually present at 50 to 200 μM concentrations. Higher concentrations may tend to promote misincorporations by the polymerase (i.e. 'thermodynamic infidelity') and should be avoided. At 50 to 200 μM, there is sufficient precursor to synthesize approximately 6.5 and 25 μg of DNA, respectively.

Deoxynucleotide triphosphates appear to quantitatively bind magnesium; the amount of dNTPs present in a reaction will determine the amount of free magnesium available. In the standard reaction, all four triphosphates are added to a final concentration of 0.8 mM; this leaves 0.7 mM of the original 1.5 mM $MgCl_2$ not complexed with dNTP. Consequently, if the dNTP concentration is changed significantly, a compensatory change in $MgCl_2$ may be necessary.

The concentration of Taq enzyme typically used in DNA PCR is about 2.5 units per 100 μl reaction. Increasing the amount of enzyme beyound this level can result in greater production of non-specific PCR products and reduced yields of the desired target fragment.

PCR ... Exponential Growth with a Plateau Effect

The amplification reaction in PCR is not infinite. After a certain number of cycles, the desired amplification fragment gradually stops accumulating exponentially and enters a linear or stationary phase. This second stage of the reaction is called the plateau. The point at which a PCR reaction reaches its plateau depends primarily on the number of copies of target originally present in the sample and on the total amount of DNA synthesized. Several possibilities exist to explain the plateau effect, such as exhaustion of primer or dNTP or inactivation of polymerase or dNTP, none of which appear to be significant in a standard reaction in the authors' experience. The most important causes are substrate excess conditions, competition by non-specific products, and product reassociation.

Substrate excess is the result of synthesis of more DNA than the amount of Taq polymerase present in the reaction is capable of replicating in the allotted extension time. For a standard 100 μl DNA PCR assay containing 2.5 units of Taq polymerase, substrate excess conditions begin to occur around 1 μg of DNA. By increasing the extension time and/or increasing the amount of enzyme in the reaction, this problem can be alievated. However from our experience, this is not practical, because in such a case, each succeeding cycle would require the doubling of extension time and/or Taq polymerase to continue exponential growth.

The accumulation of non-specific amplification products is closely related to substrate excess conditions. Here the unwanted DNA fragments compete with the desired fragment for the limited supply of Taq DNA polymerase. This problem can be minimized by increasing the specificity of the reaction so that non-target sequences are not allowed to accumulate.

In the majority of cases, the plateau effect is an integral part of the PCR reaction. Usually, by the time it occurs, sufficient amounts of the desired product have accumulated.

Perfecting the PCR

The concept of differentiating sample preparation from the PCR process needs to be stressed. Contamination is one of the major reasons for misinterpretation of results with the polymerase chain reaction and occurs when exogenous DNA or RNA, proteases, nucleases and various inhibitors of Taq polymerase are introduced into the reaction mix and prematurely terminate the amplification process. The following simple precautions should be adopted from the authors' experience gained from working with the polymerase chain reaction:

Sample preparation
Sample preparation should be carried out in a safety hood (laminar flow cabinet) with the operator(s) using sterile disposable gloves. The UV germicidal lamps present in most good quality safety cabinets quickly damage DNA left on exposed surfaces, making it unsuitable for subsequent amplification. Separate sets of positive displacement pipettes should be set aside for sample preparation and performance of the actual PCR. Aerosolization must be avoided during pipetting, as contamination of the barrel of the pipette will cause spurious results, particularly after repeated experiments.

All tubes, pipette tips and containers must be sterile and disposable.

Master mixes of solutions should be prepared where possible. This reduces greatly the amount of handling time of the individual reagents and

concurrently reduces any inaccuracies that may arise during pipetting procedures. Autoclaving of deionized water and buffer solutions should be performed where possible. It is important to recall that dNTPs, Taq and DNA material to be PCRed must *not* be autoclaved.

Vials containing Taq polymerase, primers and buffers should be opened in a laminar flow hood and opening of these reagents should be reduced to a minimum. Some types of vials supplied commercially have an inherent disadvantage of having caps that are extremely difficult to open. It is profitable to briefly spin down the contents before attempting to open these tubes and thus avoid splashes, which in some laboratories have caused major problems. Solutions that are particularly viscous (e.g. primers with ammonia as the vehicle) also pose problems, and again a spin down step is advised.

Correct concentrations of each of the reaction components must be achieved. Having prepared master mixes, daily working solutions should be aliquoted out. The Ependorf tubes used for the polymerase chain reaction should be sterile, non-siliconized and where possible RNAase free and non-cytotoxic to the sample to be amplified.

Template DNA for amplification, particularly from paraffin wax-embedded material, need not be ultra-pure. However, a report from Higuchi states that in blood samples a product that co-purifies with DNA was seen to inhibit Taq polymerase enzyme. Ideally 10^2 to 10^5 copies of template DNA which equates to 0.1 μg of human genomic DNA should be present in the starting sample. For RNA targets 50–100 ng of tRNA template is required.

Optimization of PCR buffer reagents
The contents of the PCR buffer also need to be critically evaluated. KCl in particular may have deleterious effects on the polymerase chain reaction and if conditions are right may accelerate the synthesis rate of DNA in the solution by 50%. The optimum concentration assessed from calibration experiments (including our own observations) is that no matter what the starting DNA template consists of, 50 mM KCl will suffice for most conditions and a recordable amplified product will be achieved. The addition of low concentrations of urea and

formamide appear to have little effect on the incorporation rate of Taq polymerase. Dimethylsulphoxide (DMSO) has variable effects under certain reaction conditions, where it may inhibit DNA synthesis by almost 50% or conversely accelerate its formation. SDS (sodium dodecyl sulphate) used in some DNA extraction procedures appears to directly inhibit the action of Taq polymerase and therefore care should be taken when using this compound during such procedures. Fortunately, this can be reversed by the addition of detergents such as 0.5% Tween 20 and NP 40.

Magnesium titration experiments should ideally be performed for DNA PCR, and RT-PCR using MMLV and AMV/Taq DNA polymerase assays, to assess the precise concentration required for maximum sensitivity of the PCR. In addition, when using the rTth polymerase system for RT-PCR, the concentration of manganese acetate in the bicine buffering system must be assessed similarly. Taq activity is exquisitely related to the concentration of magnesium ion present in the reaction tube. The 'free' magnesium concentration, itself a function of the deoxynucleotide triphosphate concentration, is the ultimate determinant of Taq polymerase activity and magnesium concentrations should therefore be titrated against dNTP concentration used for the particular reaction. High concentrations of magnesium are directly inhibitory to the extent of 40–50% at 10 mM concentrations of $MgCl_2$.

Primer concentration and construct must be ideal, as primers are the rate-limiting step for the Taq enzyme in PCR. Concentration ranges of 0.1–1.0 μm and AT:GC ratios of 50:50 should be achieved.

Deoxynucleotide phosphates are usually required in concentrations of 200 μm per reaction. Lower concentrations (40–100 μm) have been found to give higher fidelity and specificity with no apparent reduction in the amplified product yield. Higher concentrations (4–6 mM) inhibit Taq polymerase, except for in-cell amplification assays.

Taq polymerase kinetics
Taq polymerase itself has approximately 200 000 units/mg activity and has an extension rate of 150 nucleotides/sec/enzyme molecule with a high temperature system for DNA synthesis (75–80°C). At other temperatures, activity alters with specific activity of 60 nucleotides/sec at 70°C, 24 nucleotides/sec at 55°C, 1.5 nucleotides/sec at 37°C.

Taq DNA itself has no 3' to 5' exonuclease (proofreading activity), but has a 5' to 3' exonuclease activity during polymerization. The half-life of Taq is also temperature dependent, a fact that should be borne in mind when performing PCR processes. Studies show that $T_{1/2}$ is 6 minutes at 97.5°C, 40 minutes at 95°C and 130 minutes at 92.5°C. The problem of incorporation error rates should also be mentioned, and for Taq has been calculated at one error in 75 000 nucleotides polymerized, which is well outside the normal size of amplified fragment generated.

The fidelity (i.e. nucleotide misincorporation frequency) of Taq DNA polymerase (lacking 3'-5' proofreading activity), depends besides other things, on the concentration of free Mg^{2+} and dNTPs, on whether the four dNTPs are balanced, and on heat damage to template DNA and pH. If a DNA polymerase lacks proofreading activity, primers may be elongated in spite of a primer 3' terminus/template mismatch. In the case of Taq, the elongation will strongly depend on the type of mismatch. The following primer 3'-terminus/template mismatches significantly reduce PCR product yield after 30 cycles as indicated: C-C, G-A, A-G to <1%, A-A to <5%. All other mismatches do not decrease product yields.

Temperature profile of the reaction
During PCR itself, problems can arise during the denaturation, annealing and extension steps. Insufficient heating during the denaturation step is a common cause of failure in a PCR reaction. It is very important that the reaction reaches a temperature at which complete strand separation occurs. A temperature of 94°C is adequate in most cases. As soon as the sample reaches 94°C it must be cooled to the annealing temperature. Extensive denaturation is probably unnecessary and limited exposure to elevated temperatures helps maintain maximum polymerase activity throughout the reac-

tion. If the GC content of the template is high, then a higher denaturation temperature is required.

The concept of 'thermal lag' across Ependorf tubes while positioned in the DNA thermal cycler must also be addressed. Care must be taken to ensure that all the samples in the cycler reach the denaturation temperature of 94°C, otherwise incomplete reactions and spurious products will be revealed as well as inadequate amounts of the desired product.

This problem is best overcome, in the authors' opinion, by applying mineral oil or Ampli-wax beads to each of the wells and by the use of a thermocouple and periodic recalibration of temperature ramping curves for temperature changes on the DNA thermal cycler. Most thermal cyclers do not heat the lids of the reaction tubes, except for the 9600 DNA thermal cycler and 7700 DNA sequence detector from Perkin Elmer. Therefore, an overlaying of the amplification mix with light mineral oil is necessary to prevent evaporation. Any evaporation would lead to higher reagent concentration and to a decrease in temperature. In addition, the oil helps to prevent cross-contamination. On the other hand, too much oil slows down the thermal profile. It is necessary to standardize the amount of oil overlay in order to minimize these factors. For most applications, 70 μl oil for 100 μl reactions, 20 μl of oil for 50 μl reactions, and 10 μl oil for 25 μl reactions is probably sufficient. If necessary, oil may be removed with chloroform. In most cases, it is enough to eliminate it from samples prior to electrophoresis, for example, by pushing some air in at the water phase with a pipette. The oil on the outer surface of the tip should be wiped off with a fluff-free paper towel. Positive displacement pipettes should be used for this method of removal in order to prevent cross-contamination.

The temperature at which annealing is performed depends on the length and GC content of the primers. A temperature of 55°C is a good starting point for typical 20-base oligonucleotide primers with about 50% GC content; even higher temperatures may be necessary to increase primer specificity. In general, the longer the primer the higher the annealing tem-

perature must be to ensure adequate annealing conditions. Because of the very large molar excess of primers present in the reaction mix, hybridization occurs almost instantaneously and long incubation at the annealing temperature is not required. If smaller primers are used (15 mer) a lower annealing temperature is required, T_m 45–59°C. If extension is attempted at a higher temperature, 'primer dissociation' follows and the primer will not remain annealed to the DNA template. The problem can be overcome by taking advantage of the partial enzymatic activity of the polymerase at lower temperatures, to extend the primers by several bases and stabilize them. This is accomplished either by an intermediate incubation at 50–60°C or by heating gradually from 40°C to 72°C, i.e. gradual ramping of the temperature.

It is often possible to anneal and extend the primer at the same temperature (two-temperature PCR). In addition to simplifying the procedure to a two-temperature cycle, simultaneously annealing and extending at a temperature greater than 55°C may further improve the specificity of the reaction.

The use of long extension times has in our experience led to excess product formation. When this situation occurs, Taq will begin to extend unusual or misprimed product leading to smearing effects or 'dirty products' on the post-amplification gel.

Avoiding False Positives with PCR

The polymerase chain reaction (PCR) is a powerful, exquisitely sensitive technique. However, some investigators may not be using adequate care in experimental design and execution when using PCR to detect only a few molecules of a target DNA sequence. A false positive or mistyping may occur when the majority of molecules to be detected arise from exogenous sources rather than from the sample itself.

The smaller the starting quantity of DNA, the greater the care that should be taken to avoid spurious amplification. The use of PCR for sensitive detection is complicated by the fact that the product of the amplification serves as the substrate for the generation of more product. A single PCR cycle produces very large numbers of amplifiable molecules that can potentially contaminate subsequent amplifications of the same target sequence. This kind of contamination is called product carryover to differentiate it from contamination by naturally-arising DNA from exogenous sources.

A typical PCR reaction can generate molecules of amplified DNA in a 0.1 mol reaction. To control contamination, prevention of the physical transfer of DNA between amplified samples, and between positive and negative experimental controls, must be eliminated.

To prevent carryover from equipment used in previous experiments, gel apparatus and combs should be soaked in 1 M HCl to depurinate any residual DNA. New razor blades should be used to excise each gel band if this is so desired, and the surface of the UV transilluminator should be covered with a fresh sheet of plastic wrap for each gel. Other potential sources of contamination include purified restriction fragments of target sequence, dot-blot apparatus, microtome blades, centrifuges, centrifugal vacuum devices and dry ice or ethanol baths. Most of these items are also amenable to treatment, if necessary, with 1 M HCl.

The use of the enzyme uracil N-glycosylase (UNG), present in the pre-reaction mix, catalyses the excision of uracil from any potential single- or double-stranded PCR carryover DNA present in the reaction prior to the first cycle of PCR. This effectively destroys DNA or cDNA synthesized from a previous reaction.

The Role of Positive and Negative Controls

The use of highly concentrated solutions of plasmid DNA containing the target sequence as a positive control is generally not a good idea, because it introduces as many amplifiable molecules into the sample preparation area as a typical PCR. When using plasmid DNA con-taining the target sequence as a positive control, the procedure adopted in our laboratory is to dilute the plasmid substantially. Depending upon the detection system, as few as 100 copies of target may suffice as a positive control.

The inclusion of 'anti-contamination primers' has been addressed by Van Den Brule in relation to the amplification of human papilloma virus when using plasmid-inserted viral DNA as positive control material. This problem has apparently arisen in some laboratories, but as yet we have not encountered this problem.

Typically, 'no DNA' reagent controls and negative sample controls with each set of amplifications are included. The reagent controls contain all the necessary components for PCR, except template DNA. Negative sample controls do not contain target sequences, but have gone through all the sample preparation steps.

The amount of PCR product generated is sometimes insufficient, requiring reamplification after enrichment by gel electrophoresis. If the amount of amplified target sequence DNA in a particular gel slice is very low, the problem of cross-contamination from analogous PCR products or plasmid DNA containing the target sequence run in other lanes of the gel must be appreciated.

The Raw Material for the Polymerase Reaction

Direct PCR of tissue DNA

The commonest source of tissue for the histopathologist is paraffin wax-embedded material. 5 μm sections can be subjected to PCR without prior de-waxing. Cytology smears, body fluids such as urine, CSF, pleural aspirates and peritoneal fluids are also an ideal template for the PCR method.

Several tissues including peripheral blood contain enzyme inhibitors and ideally prior extraction of DNA should be performed. Lysis and boiling the tissues for ten minutes is usually adequate to inactivate inhibitors, but usually more satisfactory results are obtained if all the protein is removed by proteinase K incubation and phenol extraction.

Nucleic acid and fixative interactions are varied. Many fixatives have been used for preservation of nucleic acids in tissue specimens, but relatively few with the exception of mercury and chromium salts are known to react with them chemically. In our own department we have examined the interaction of fixative type on DNA extracted from tonsillar material and its suitability for PCR by assessing the ability to amplify β globin gene.

Fixative type and fixation time have long been known to influence the preservation of proteins for immunohistochemistry and it is now clear from our own work and similar observations that they also directly influence the results of PCR. Formal saline, 10% formalin, neutral buffered formaldehyde, Carnoy's and glutaraldehyde fixed tissues usually yield amplifiable DNA.

Formal saline, 10% formalin and neutral buffered formaldehyde and glutaraldehyde induce extensive cross-linking between nucleic acids and proteins. DNA and RNA in their resting native states do not normally react with these fixatives. However, if the fixative solution is heated to 45°C for DNA and 65°C for RNA, uncoiling of the helices occurs. This selective non-reactivity appears to be related to the structure of the nucleic acids, the hydrogen bonded structures of which are only broken at relatively high temperatures when purine and pyrimidine bases become available for reaction with the aldehyde fixative. These reactions may be reversible or irreversible. Depending on the degree of cross-linkage then, it seems conceivable that erratic PCR results may be obtained from tissues fixed with one of the formaldehyde fixatives.

The alcohol fixatives (ethanol and methanol) are known to preserve DNA and histone proteins. From our own observations, Carnoy's fixed tissue yields good results with proteinase K extraction, which is in accordance with similar findings from Greer, Jackson and others. Bouin's (a picric acid fixative) fixed tissue yields variable results. Picric acid derivates are known to react with histone

protein subfractions and basic proteins to form picrates. DNA bound to histone proteins, which are intercalated with picric acid residues, are then unavailable for reaction in the PCR and thus amplification failure could occur.

Disappointing results are also observed with buffered formaldehyde sublimate, Zenker's fluid and Helly's fluid fixed tissues. All these are mercuric chloride-containing fixatives, and mercuric ion in the fixative solution can become deposited and remain bound in the tissues even after vigorous washing. This directly inhibits Taq DNA polymerase activity, if present in high concentrations.

Forty-year-old material has been successfully employed to amplify specific gene sequences, however it has been reported that the size of DNA fragments prepared from samples four to six years old was often much smaller than from comparable samples which were two years old or less.

Tissue RNA as a source of template for PCR

For information on gene expression in a cell or tissue, or the presence of genomic RNA from a retrovirus, RNA is the appropriate template for amplification. Indeed RNA/PCR is much more sensitive than Northern blot or *in situ* hybridization. DNA polymerase will not react directly with RNA templates, therefore use is made of a retroviral enzyme, reverse transcriptase, to catalyse the production of RNA from cDNA (copy DNA), which can then be subjected to PCR under conventional conditions. This technique can yield several million copies of cDNA of the RNA species under investigation, even when starting from minute quantities of material, even from a single cell.

Single cell PCR ... fact or fiction?

From work with *in vitro* fertilized embryos, genetic defects can be detected from single cell preparations at the eight cell stage before implantation has occurred. Embryos can be sexed by the presence or absence of Y chromosome bands using PCR. Gene expression has also been studied from single cell isolates. However, because the starting amounts of DNA and RNA in such an isolate is so small, more amplification cycles are required. The

THE SCIENCE OF LABORATORY DIAGNOSIS

Size and Structure of Amplification Products

The Use of Inosine Substituted Primers ... Does it Benefit the Overall Effects of the PCR Process?

subsequent possibility of 'primer-dimer' formation and errors of fidelity of copying, occurring during the first round of amplification, must be recognized.

Size and Structure of Amplification Products

PCR is very often less efficient with longer products. One possible cause might be the nature of the secondary structure of single-stranded templates. Secondary structures in long products could have up to four deleterious effects.

Firstly, a hairpin or a loop within the fragment, still giving access to a primer at its 3′ terminus, either slows down the polymerase or is degraded through the 5′–3′ exonuclease activity of Taq polymerase. Erlich mentioned the efficient amplification of long fragments with a mutant Taq DNA polymerase lacking 5′–3′ exonuclease activity. The commercially available Stoffel fragment, a truncated Taq, which has the same properties, might be suitable for such purposes.

Secondly, a loop, where the 3′ end of the product anneals somewhere within the product, becomes a primer structure. If such a structure is elongated once, a new primer annealing site is created on the 'wrong' strand. In the next cycles, a product with distinct length (longer than the one wanted originally) may be created and exponentially amplified with only one primer. Similar annealing events may occur at the 3′ end of such generated fragments to a similiar strand of another product (with an identical sequence) and thus leads to identical artifacts. If the created sequences prefer their own intra-strand secondary structure (due to the complementarity of the ends), a shorter product is created. This is the basic feature of a method referred to as 'panhandle PCR'. All this may be checked with Southern blot analysis of gels where many unspecific bands or smears hybridize to a specific probe that contains only internal sequences of the desired product.

One of the major effects of additional components in the PCR is their influence on secondary structure stability. When secondary structures are a problem, the addition of reagents which lower the T_m of dsDNA (e.g. formamide), and an increase in primer concentration to compensate for interference with primer annealing, might improve the yields of long amplification products. Through enzymatic incorporation of the modified nucleotide 7-deaza-dGTP, secondary structures of template DNA may be destabilized, so that it might be amplified more efficiently.

Thirdly, if products are very long, they might preferentially reanneal at particular domains close to one terminus, especially with higher product concentrations. Eventually elongation of a primer on the other end will already have started. Again, the polymerase will be slowed down, or the product will be degraded. If the enzyme 'jumps' to the other strand, a phenomenon similar to that described in the previous paragraph might result, which is exponentially amplifiable with only one primer. But the lengths of such artifacts would be very variable (depending on the jumping location), thus creating a smear, on gel analysis.

Fourthly, with increasing cycle numbers, the PCR products compete with the primers for annealing and create gap- or nick-like sites. These structures are target sites for the polymerase-independent 5′-3′ exonuclease activity of Taq.

The Use of Inosine Substituted Primers ... Does it Benefit the Overall Effects of the PCR Process?

The matching of DNA template and the 3′ position of the primer is critical for the process of PCR. This results from the fact that Taq DNA polymerase lacks a 3′ to 5′ prime exonuclease activity. If a mismatch occurs, then correction is not possible and in the context of diagnostic considerations this may have serious implications.

Inosine is a purine base which is naturally found in the cell as rare nucleotides of tRNA. Its ability to form base pair combinations with A,C,T,G is central to its role in PCR. Knoth *et al.* recently used the inosine approach for internal primer system positioning. Their approach to test the amplification of amino acid sequences with such inosine residues acting as 'wobble bases' to amplify rare cDNA sequences was successful. The one disadvantage with this approach is in the production of the primers themselves. 3′ Inosine primers are difficult to prepare, because inosine-coupled controlled glass columns are difficult to prepare and handle. In the future, this problem of 3′ primer mismatch will be overcome and therefore will become largely irrelevant in PCR amplifications.

Use of Co-solvents and Other Agents to Improve PCR Signals

The amplification process of PCR can be adversely affected by the base composition of the template. GC-rich sequences will initally impede genomic DNA denaturation which is an important step for the critical annealment of the primers to the template, as we have seen. Secondary structures in the chosen DNA template may hinder the extension of primers by Taq polymerase. The use of co-solvents such as dimethylsulphoxide (DMSO) and glycerol can sometimes overcome these difficulties in amplification.

Primer systems and templates in which high GC ratios are problematic include herpes simplex II and cytomegalovirus. Smith *et al.* reported stronger amplification signals of HSV I and II following DMSO and glycerol addition. Glycerol may be inhibitory in some PCR situations and therefore critical evaluation of the use of these types of co-solvents is required for each amplification system.

Another agent used to improve PCR signals, particularly when starting with small quantities of cells, is Chelex. This agent is a polyvalent chelating agent in resin form. Its main use in molecular medicine was to prevent DNA degradation in low ionic strength buffers. By binding heavy metal ions that act as a catalyst in the breakdown of DNA, it acts as a direct inhibitor of DNA breakdown. It is particularly useful in boiled extracts of DNA from small groups of cells. Chelex is best utilized at its natural pH of 10.8 (room temperature) for full enhancement of PCR signal. It appears that heating under alkaline conditions may in addition help disrupt cell membranes and may aid complete denaturation of DNA template. Using this technique and incorporating a cDNA synthesis step, RNA templates may be recovered sporadically.

'Booster PCR' ... for Better Amplification of a Small Number of Target Molecules

Experience has shown that when amplifying very dilute DNA samples (<1000 copies of target), artifacts are marked following the amplification process. This includes primer-dimer formation as well as other low molecular weight products. The formation of such products results in the consumption of primers which are then not available for the desired amplified sequences.

Booster PCR, which should probably be used in cases where artifacts occur, is designed specifically to enhance specificity at the expense of yield. In general, the technique relies on the fact that in the first 15 to 20 cycles, primers are diluted as required to provide a 10-fold molar excess of primers with respect to the expected amount of target sequence. In the remaining cycles, fresh aliquots of the primers are added to the reaction vial, so that the final concentration added is 0.1 μm. In essence, the 'first round' PCR is designed to increase the number of copies of template under dilute primer conditions. In the 'second round', the framed copies of target are amplified preferentially under usual PCR conditions.

The required effect of primer dilution is to reduce the probability of primer to primer collision in a starting environment that has little DNA template. The limitation of the step is the reduction in the yield of amplified DNA, despite allowing a 10-fold excess of primer.

In summary, dividing a standard PCR reaction into two stages, the first designed for specificity, the second for yield, appears to greatly enhance the sensitivity of the amplification process and

Hot Start PCR

Inhibitors of Taq Polymerase Enzyme ... Little is Known!

---

from our experience is of great value in amplification reactions in which artifact formation can be encountered.

Hot Start PCR

A hot start polymerase chain reaction entails the witholding of at least one reagent from the reaction mixture until the reaction tube temperature has reached 60 to 80°C. Currently, hot start amplification with an ampliwax vapour barrier uses a layer of solid wax to separate the retained reagent (s) and the test sample from the bulk of the reagents, until the first heating step of automated thermal cycling melts the wax and convectively mixes the two aqueous layers.

Wax mediated hot start PCR greatly increases the specificity, yield and precision of amplifying low copy numbers of many viral targets. Mispriming events are minimized and in the absence of mispriming, the procedural improvement still suppresses putative primer oligomerization.

Hot start PCR with ampliwax vapour barrier permits routine amplification of a single target molecule with detection by ethidium stained gel electrophoresis. Chou et al. believe that the hot start PCR method which prevents primer annealing to non-target sequences in useful for target copy numbers below approximately 10^3.

The hot start process requires the opening and reclosing of reaction PCR tubes as they sit in the thermal cycler at 60 to 80°C in order to add missing reactants (which are normally enzyme and/or primers). However, with 9600 and 7700 thermocyclers, ampliwax is not required and Taq DNA polymerase can be added directly to the tube at the beginning of PCR.

Theoretically, the hot start PCR is closer to the optimum, in which the DNA polymerase and essential reaction components join after heating. This may be done by mixing the enzyme or other essential reaction components with a pre-heated reaction mixture. But with this procedure, it is difficult to maintain identical conditions for all reaction tubes. Pipettes and tips are not designed for pipetting into hot media, and it becomes difficult to prevent cross-contamination. Generally, those procedures are preferable in which the tubes, once closed and heated, are never opened until thermal cycling is completed.

A good and safe way to perform a hot start PCR is by physically separating the reaction components with various materials that melt at higher temperatures, such as paraffin or agarose. A hot start PCR with agarose may be performed with primers and/or dNTPs pre-cast in agarose. A melted aliquot of the agarose reagent mixture is placed at the bottom of the reaction tube, and the tube is then placed on ice. The gelled agarose/reagent mixture is overlaid with the remaining reaction components and will subsequently melt during the initial heating of the reaction tube.

Inhibitors of Taq Polymerase Enzyme ... Little is Known!

Because PCR is essentially a 'reaction', carefully controlled conditions are required for successful amplification. It is not so surprising to find that the reaction may be susceptible to drugs, metabolites and other biological compounds found in the body fluids of patients.

To date, information on the influence of these inhibitors is sketchy, however the following data have emerged. Modest concentrations of KCl stimulate the synthesis rate of Taq polymerase, the apparent optimum being 50 mM. Higher concentrations inhibit activity and no significant activity is observed at >75 mM KCl. The addition of ammonium chloride, ammonium acetate or sodium chloride to a Taq polymerase activity assay results in mild inhibition. Low urea concentrations and 10% DMSO appear to inhibit Taq activity, the precise mechanism however is not known. It may involve alteration of the T_m (annealing temperature) of the primers used in the reaction, the thermal activity profile of Taq or the degree of product strand separation achieved at a particular denaturation or upper limit temperature.

Sodium dodecyl sulphate used in some DNA/RNA extraction regimes is also known to inhibit Taq activity but this may be reversed by the use of certain non-ionic detergents (Tween 20 and NP 40).

PCR Variants

Reverse transcriptase (RT-PCR) (rtPCR) is used for detection of RNA targets. In this reaction, cDNA (copy DNA) is firstly created using a reverse transcriptase enzyme (e.g. MMVLV RT) and then subsequent amplification of the newly created cDNA follows. Originally the method used a two-step procedure, firstly reverse transcription and secondly DNA amplification. The development of rTth polymerase, which combines reverse transcriptase and DNA polymerase activity, obviates the need for a two-step reaction. This is a major improvement, as it minimizes handling and lowers possible contamination risks.

Asymmetric PCR is a simple and effective method for the production of single-stranded DNA suitable for direct sequencing. It uses unequal molar concentrations of primers in the reaction setup, essentially driving the reaction to single target strand accumulation. This can then be easily sequenced directly, without the need for cloning or the establishment of DNA libraries.

Inverse PCR allows amplification of DNA outside the boundaries of known sequences. This is important in the study of viral tumourigenesis, when attempting to identify possible insertion sites of viruses in host DNA and for the assessment of clonality in lymphoid tumours.

Amplification refractory mutation system (ARMS) is a novel system using primers which are designed so that the 3′ end coincides with a mutated nucleotide base, facilitating allelic discrimination.

Single-strand conformation polymorphism (SSCP) is another method used for the detection of single base changes in DNA and RNA, and relies on the different mobilities of DNA strands containing single base-pair differences, when run on non-denaturing polyacrylamide gels.

Differential display allows the simultaneous genetic analysis of changes in gene expression in cells and tissues. The technique uses a set of primers, one of which will hybridize to a polyadenylated tail present in mRNA (the primer also contains a one- or two-base anchor), the other primer is short and arbitrary in sequence, and anneals in different positions relative to the first primer. A combination of nearly 300 primers is required in order to ensure that each possible mRNA is amplified at least once. The mRNA populations defined by these primers are amplified after reverse transcription and resolved on a DNA sequencing gel. Fragments which display differential expression between the diseased and non-diseased states can easily be excised from the gel. Subsequent cloning of individual mRNAs is then possible. The technique has been specifically useful for the detection of differentially expressed genes in leukaemia, heart disease and diabetes mellitus.

cDNA subtraction PCR can be easily applied to cells enriched by flow cytometry. The subtraction procedure involves three steps leading to the indentification of a collection of full length cDNAs cloned in an expression vector, suitable for direct functional analysis. In the first step, an RT-PCR is performed which amplifies cDNA representing all poly mRNA present in two different samples (X and Y). The PCR produces 3′cDNA stubs of approximately 200–600 bp which can be amplified through multiple rounds of PCR while maintaining the gene expression profile present in the starting mRNAs. The second step involves the reciprocal removal of common sequences from both samples using a biotin/avidin cDNA subtraction protocol. Subtraction product X-Y is enriched for sequences present in X but not in Y and similarly Y-X is enriched for sequences in Y, not found in X. The final step of the reaction involves labelling of the subtraction products X-Y and Y-X, which are then used to screen replica filters from a full length library. cDNA clones are selected that hybridize consistently with one and not the other subtracted probe.

Representational difference analysis (RDA) is a newly developed technique which allows the identification of the differences between two complex genomes. The technique basically involves a genomic subtractive hybridization protocol, which allows the investigator to discriminate sequences present in a tumour specimen from normal control DNA of the same individual.

In situ PCR represents for most histopathologists the marriage of standard old-fashioned histopathology and molecular biology. *In situ* PCR is used to detect single copy target nucleic acid sequences in fixed tissues and cells. It aims to correlate PCR results with morphology. While holding the greatest potential for diagnostic histopathology, it is a technique that needs to gain widespread acceptance.

TaqMan PCR (5′ nuclease assay) (Figs 50.3, 50.4, 50.5 and 50.6) represents a major advance in PCR. It was firstly described by Holland *et al.* in which the 5′-3′ endonucleolytic activity of Taq DNA polymerase was utilized to detect target sequences during amplification by PCR. Included in the PCR mixture is a probe (usually 20–30 mer in length) designed to hybridize within the target sequence and to be non-extendible at the 3′ end. The fluorescent emission activity of a fluorescent reporter molecule attached to the probe at its 5′ end is neutralized by a quencher molecule at the 3′ end. When hybridized to its target sequence, the intact probe shows no signal due to the proximity of the

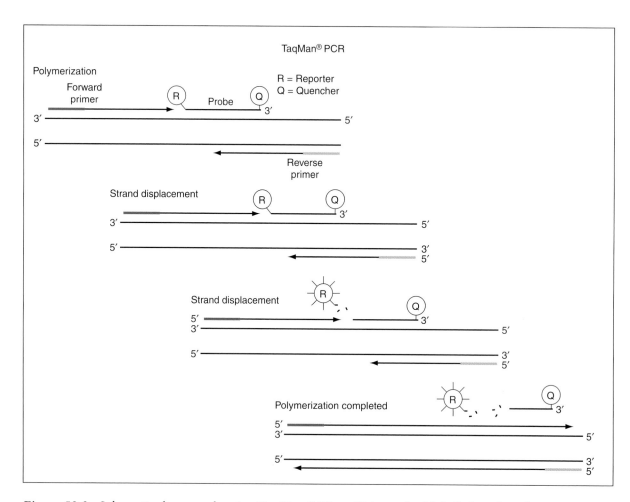

Figure 50.3: Schematic diagram showing TaqMan PCR, utilizing a dual labelled probe. The reporter molecule at the 5′ end of the probe is released due to the exonuclease activity of Taq DNA polymerase.

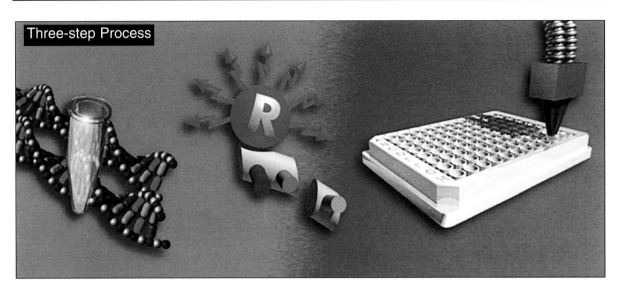

Figure 50.4: Endpoint TaqMan PCR. The specific increase in fluorescence is monitored by a luminescence spectrometer, using a microtitre plate format.

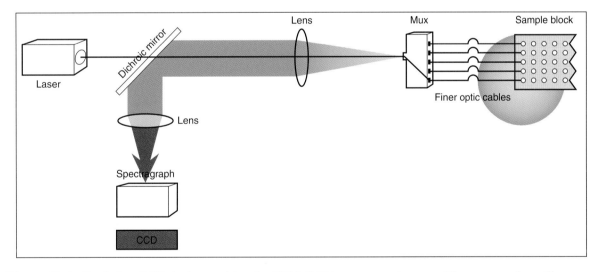

Figure 50.5: Real-time PCR is detected by the 7700 DNA sequence detector. The cartoon here illustrates the operation of this DNA sequence detector. The DNA thermal cycler consists of a 96 well format. The PCR reaction is contained within an optical tube. The top of the tube contains an optical cap, through which a laser beam is shone during the PCR assay. The laser beam is emitted from an Argon laser and transmitted to the reaction tubes via fibre-optic cables. The laser excites the fluorescent reporter and quencher molecules, which emit a fluorescent signal, which is carried back via the fibre-optic cables to a charged couple device (CCD) camera. The signal is then converted into an electronic signal and shown as a graphic interface on a Macintosh computer.

reporter molecule to the quencher molecule. During amplification Taq DNA polymerase, through its 5′-3′ endonucleolytic activity, cleaves the probe into fragments, separating the reporter molecule from the quencher, thus allowing its detection. The level of fluorescence is directly proportional to the amount of specific amplification of the target. The major advantage of

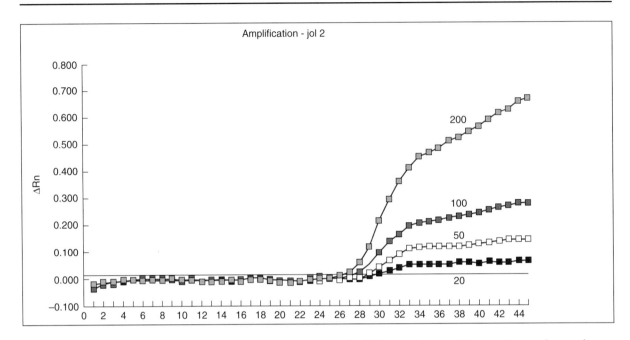

Figure 50.6: Real-time PCR read-out showing an increase in PCR product with increasing cycle number. The DNA template is varied in this assay and has been extracted from the HHV 8 positive BCP-1 cell line.

this technique is its ability to detect specifically amplified DNA or RNA sequences at selected time points in the PCR, thereby allowing direct quantitative real-time DNA and RNA detection. This is achieved using specifically designed equipment (e.g. Perkin Elmer Applied Biosystems 7700 DNA sequence detector). Alternatively, an end-point format can be adopted, in this case using a luminescence spectrometer.

Comparative genome hybridization (CGH) is a new approach in fluorescence *in situ* hybridization, allowing the comprehensive analysis of chromosomal imbalances in entire genomes. Genomic DNA from cell populations to be tested is labelled with modified nucleotides (e.g. dig 11dUTP) and used as a probe to normal metaphase chromosomes of the patient. This can be achieved by rich translation or degenerate PCR. This probe is called the test probe. As an internal control, genomic DNA derived from cells with an normal karyotype is differentially labelled (control DNA probe) and hybridized simultaneously with the test probe. For detection of the hybridized test, and control DNA probes, different fluorochromes are used and each is visualized

with epifluorescence microscopy with selective filters. If the tissue under analysis contains additional chromosomal material, hybridization reveals higher signal intensities at the corresponding target regions of the hybridized chromosome. Conversely, deletions are visible as lower signal intensities. By comparing the hybridization patterns of the test and control probes, changes in signal intensities caused by allelic imbalance can be conveniently identified.

Newer Amplification Techniques

PCR is time consuming, labour intensive and subject to the precautions and constraints of contamination. The newly introduced amplification technique, ligase chain reaction (LCR) (Fig. 50. 7), has a sensitivity of less than 300 molecules. The LCR technique, was first published by Biotechnica International Incorporated and now is developed jointly by Abbott Laboratories and Biotechnica International Incorporated.

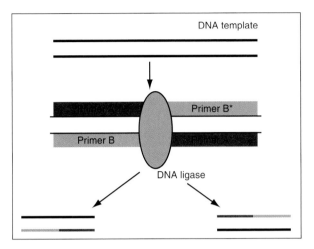

Figure 50.7: Schematic representation of the ligase chain reaction (LCR). See text below for details of the reaction.

The LCR separates in two different steps, firstly the amplification which is performed using a thermal cycler (as in PCR) and secondly detection performed with enzyme immuno-assay (EIA) using the Abbott IIMx analyser with micro particles as solid phase. For the amplification of the target, the region of the genome (usually between 50 to 100 nucleotides in size) is selected and two probes each complementary to one half of the target sequence are synthesized. In addition a second pair complementary to the first set occupy adjacent sites on the other strand of the target. These probes are added in excess to the samples and the double-stranded DNA target is melted by heat denaturation. After lowering the temperature, the probes will hybridize with the complementary sequence of the target. After hybridization, a thermostable DNA ligase from *Thermus thermophilus* will join the two adjacent probes A and B and/or A* and B* respectively. Repeated cycles of heating and cooling will melt the double-stranded structures, allowing them to reanneal with fresh probes that are available in excess. The ligated probe pairs act as new and additional targets for the reaction and thus allow an exponential amplification of the only target.

The detection mechanism utilizes two ligands that are coupled to the probes; the homologous pair A and A* carry a capture ligand at their 5' and 3' termini respectively distal to the ligation site. The other pair B and B* carry signal generating moieties at their corresponding ends. The amplified product is captured on microparticles coated with antibodies to capture ligand. Excess probe is washed away and signal is generated by enzyme immunoassay mediated through the other ligand.

The cloning of the thermostable ligase has enabled this new amplification method (LCR) to both amplify DNA and discriminate a single base mutation.

Allele-specific LCR employs four oligonucleotides, two adjacent oligonucleotides which uniquely hybridize to one strand of the target DNA and a complementary set of adjacent oligonucleotides which hybridize to the opposite strand. Because the reaction uses thermostable DNA ligase, this will covalently link each set provided that there is a complete complementarity at the junction. Because the oligonucleotides from one round serve as substrates during the next round, the signal will therefore be amplified exponentially, which is analogous to PCR amplification as we have seen. A single base mismatch at the oligonucleotide junction will not be amplified and is therefore distinguished. A second set of mutant specific oligonucleotides is used in a separate reaction to detect the mutant allele.

DNA diagnostics employs the tools of molecular biology to detect the presence of bacterial and viral infectious agents, genetic traits and diseases. This demands exquisite specificity to distinguish closely related pathogens or single-allele diseases which may consist of subtle deletions, insertions or single nucleotide substitutions in over three billion base pairs of target DNA. Reliability therefore is required, with faithful amplification of target sequences and with little or no false positives, allowing accurate single base discrimination, low background and either complete automation or the use of simple inexpensive kits. PCR has achieved some of these goals. Small deletions, insertions, or single base mismatches may be detected through the use of allele-specific oligonucleotide hybridization, reverse oligonucleotide, blot dot hybridization, denaturing gradient gel electrophoresis, RNAase or chemical cleavage of mismatched hetroduplexes, fluorescent PCR amplification/detection, allele specific PCR using nested PCR, or polymerase amplification of specific alleles (PASA). Ligase based assays including LCR which accomplish both amplification and single nucleotide discrimination in the same step also achieve many of these goals.

Initially it was apparent that the ligase enzyme could serve as a reporter for the presence of two adjacent strands of DNA hybridized to a complementary target DNA strand. Thermostable ligase discriminated single base mismatches under both LDR (ligase detection reaction using two adjacent probes) and LCR (ligase chain reaction using two pairs of adjacent probes).

LCR amplification aims to discriminate accurately between different alleles while achieving the highest signal to noise ratio possible. LCR did not amplify a T-T, G-T, C-T, or C-A 3′ terminal mismatch as has been reported for some allele specific PCR amplifications. The greatest potential for LCR amplification and detection is its compatibility with a primary amplification of genomic DNA or RNA by either PCR or with the other newly developed technique, 3SR (self-sustained sequence replication).

LCR is compatible with radioactive, fluorescent or enzymatic reporter group incorporation. The combination of PCR and LCR in multiplex PCR/LCR detection assay could rapidly screen large populations for monogenic disease polymorphisms, determine HLA haplotypes for tissue typing and transplantation, or help distinguish single base deletions, or several polymorphisms simultaneously or indeed eliminate ambiguities in DNA identification of individuals for forensic or paternity cases.

3SR relies on RNA transcription which is a process employed by all cellular and viral systems to copy discrete segments of nucleotide sequences into multiple single-stranded RNA molecules. It has been discovered that isothermal replication of a targeted nucleic acid is possible using a concerted three enzyme *in vitro* reaction. This amplification strategy was modelled after the general scheme employed during retroviral replication. In this reaction, activities of avian myeloblastosis virus (AMV) reverse transcriptase (RT), *E. coli* RNAase H and T7 RNA polymerase produced an average ten-fold amplification every 2.5 minutes. Whether these new techniques of *in situ* PCR, LCR or 3SR will attain routine use in clinical medicine still remains to be evaluated.

Uses of PCR in Pathology

PCR is now an established technique and has increased the range and sensitivity of diagnostic procedures. The exquisite sensitivity of PCR is also its major drawback, as contamination and amplification artifacts can give rise to difficulties in the interpretation of results.

Microbiology

In the past the diagnosis of infections was limited by the supply of appropriate material for culture, protein analysis or microscopy. These limitations have been overcome by the introduction of PCR in diagnostic microbiology. It is now possible to detect DNA or RNA of infectious organisms, that are either present in small numbers, slow growing (viruses, mycobacteria, etc.) or in material not suitable for culture. PCR can facilitate the diagnosis of early and latent stages of infection, which cannot be identified by conventional laboratory techniques.

The examination of archival material, allowing retrospective studies, has had great impact and has demonstrated correlations between viral agents and tumourigenesis (e.g. human papilloma virus and cervical carcinoma, Epstein–Barr virus and post-transplant lymphoproliferative disorder (PTLD) and KSHV/HHV-8 and Kaposi's sarcoma). Table 50.1 lists microorganisms which are detectable by PCR in routine clinical samples such as blood, CSF, semen, saliva, faeces, pleural fluid and fixed tissues.

Human genetics

One major use of PCR is in the diagnosis of chromosomal disorders or hereditary diseases, such as Down's syndrome, β-thalassaemia,

Table 50.1: **Microorganisms which can be detected by PCR.**

Viruses	*Bacteria*	*Protozoa*
Adenovirus	Mycobacterium tuberculosis	Toxoplasma gondii
Cytomegalovirus	Mycobacterium paratuberculosis	Plasmodium falciparum
Epstein–Barr virus	Mycobacterium leprae	
Hepatitis A, B, C	Borrelia burgdoferi	
Herpes simplex	Legionella pneumophilia	
HIV 1 and 2	Listeria monocytogenes	
HHV 7, 8	Chlamydia trachomatis	
Human papilloma virus	Helicobacter pyloridis	
HTLV-1		
Lassa virus		
Measles virus		
Rotavirus		

cystic fibrosis and haemophilia. Invasive antenatal procedures, such as chorionic biopsies and amniotic fluid sampling, to obtain fetal cells have an inherent risk to the fetus and can perhaps be replaced by non-invasive techniques. Fetal DNA may be amplified from maternal blood by PCR, and fetal blood cells from the maternal blood can be used for aneuploidy detection and also to determine fetal sex. Fetal cells isolated from maternal cervical mucus have also been used for genetic analysis. Parental testing for genetic disease is made easier by PCR to detect variable numbers of tandem repeats (VNTRs), microsatellite tandem repeats and allele specific sequences in the parental genome. This can be achieved using only a few cells with a fluorescent multiplex PCR approach, analysing 'microsatellite fingerprints' and disease loci in one reaction. Table 50.2 illustrates some of the genetically inherited diseases which can be screened for using PCR.

Tumour biology/oncology

In oncopathology, PCR has led to a better understanding of the pathobiology of malignancy, allowing the analysis of mutations in oncogenes and tumour suppressor genes (e.g. *c-myc*, *p53*, *ras*), the detection of minimal residual disease (MRD), clonality (e.g. B and T cell gene rearrangements in lymphomas) in identifying gene rearrangements (e.g. t(14,18) in follicular lymphomas and the Philadelphia chromosome in chronic myeloid leukaemia) and in the assessment of loss of heterozygosity (allelic imbalance) particularly in colorectal and breast cancer. PCR's greatest versatility is that it allows the examination of formalin-fixed paraffin wax-embedded tissue, in which DNA may be degraded and is therefore not suitable for Southern blotting. Using such archival material, large-scale retrospective genetic analysis of p53, DCC, APC and ras mutations in colorectal cancer, and genome-wide screening for novel tumour suppressor genes/oncogenes

Table 50.2: **Inherited diseases which can be screened for using PCR.**

Beta thalassaemia	Muscular dystrophy
Alpha-1 anti-trypsin deficiency	Osteogenesis imperfecta
Cystic fibrosis	Porphyria
Gaucher's disease	Phenylketonuria
Haemophilia	Sickle cell anaemia
Huntingdon's disease	Tay–Sachs disease
Lesch–Nyhan syndrome	

in any cancer can now be easily undertaken using PCR and fluorescent amplicon detection technologies.

Forensic pathology

PCR has brought significant progress in forensic pathology. It is used in establishing the identity of mutilated corpses or decomposed human remains, in sex determination, in cases of disputed paternity, and in identifying perpetrators of crime. This is based on the amplification of VNTRs or restriction fragment length polymorphisms (RFLPs) and is referred to as DNA fingerprinting. PCR has not only made such evaluations easier, but also possible even with trace amounts or partially degraded biological material (e.g. blood and semen stains, hair), increasing dramatically the range of samples that can be analysed.

Where to from here?

Today, PCR represents a highly specialized research tool with many uses in medical laboratories. PCR methodology is well established, which greatly facilitates genetic, microbiological and virological analysis. The advent of automated thermal cyclers, fluorescent DNA sequencers and real-time PCR sequence detectors (ABI 7700 DNA sequence detector) has also extended the power and repertoire of PCR.

The major advance of PCR is that it can amplify a sequence of DNA from amongst the background of the entire genome (three billion base pairs in the haploid cell), making it exquisitely more sensitive than other molecular biological tools.

In the past number of years many startling advances have been made in PCR technology including *in situ* PCR, direct sequencing of PCR products and quantitative assays using ELISA technology and real-time PCR detectors, which automatically quantitate DNA and RNA loads directly in the starting sample.

New enzymology including the combined reverse transcriptase DNA polymerase enzyme (rTth DNA polymerase), the recently introduced long amplifying Taqs (e.g. TaqXL) and newer sequencing Taqs (e.g. Taq CS) will in the future greatly facilitate the investigation of human disease, making the basic technique of PCR more robust and more easily reproducible.

Microchip-based PCR technologies may have once seemed a dream, but have finally become reality. It is envisaged that these techniques will identify point mutations, subchromosomal regions, viruses, bacteria, etc., in clinical samples, in a high throughput configuration. In cell direct DNA sequencing in time may also be possible if current *in situ* technologies are refined.

Further Reading

Alberts B, Bray D, Lewis J, Raff M, Roberts K, Watson J D, eds. *Molecular biology of the cell.* 3rd edn 1994: Garland, New York. 291–318.

Barany F. Genetic disease detection and DNA amplification using cloned thermostable ligase. *Proc Natl Acad Sci (USA)* 1991; **88:** 189–193.

Brady G, Iscove N N. Amplified representative cDNA libraries from single cells. *Methods in Enzymology* (Chapter 36 'Guide to techniques in mouse development') 1993; **225:** 611–623.

Brule A J C van Den, Class H C J, du Maine M, Melchers W J G, Helmerhorst T, Quint W G V, Meijer C J L M, Walboomers J. Application of anti-contamination primers in the polymerase chain reaction for the detection of human papillomavirus genotypes in cervical scrapes and biopsies. *J Med Virol* 1989; **29:** 20–27.

Chou Q, Russel M, Birch D E, Raymond J, Block W. Prevention of pre-PCR mis-priming and primer dimerization improves low copy number amplification. *Nucl Acid Res* 1992; **7:** 1717–1723.

Further Reading

Erlich H A, Gelfand D, Sninsky J J. Recent advances in the polymerase chain reaction. *Science* 1991; **252**: 1643–1651.

Greer C E, Patterson S L, Kiviat N B, Manos M. PCR amplification from paraffin embedded tissues: effects of fixative and fixation time. *Am J Clin Pathol* 1991; **95**: 117–124.

Holland P M, Abramson R D, Watson R, Gelfand D H. Detection of specific polymerase chain reaction product by utilizing the 5′-3′ exonuclease activity of *Thermus aquaticus* DNA polymerase. *Proc Natl Acad Sci (USA)* 1991; **88**: 7276–7280.

Jackson D P, Lewis F A, Taylor G R, Boylston A W, Quirke P. Tissue extraction of DNA and RNA and analysis by the polymerase chain reaction. *J Clin Pathol* 1990; **43**: 499–504.

Kallioniemi A, Kallioniemi O P, Sudar D, Rutovitz D, Gray J W, Waldman F, Pinkel D. Comparative genome hybridisation for molecular analysis of solid tumours. *Science* 1992; **258**: 818–821.

Knoth K, Roberds S, Potete C, Tamkun M. Highly degenerate inosine containing primers specifically amplify rare cDNA using the polymerase chain reaction. *Nucl Acid Res* 1988; **16**: 10932.

Liang P, Pardee A B. Differential display of eukaryotic RNA by means of the polymerase chain reaction. *Science* 1992; **257**: 967–972.

Lisitsyn N A. Representational difference analysis: finding the differences between genomes. *Trend Genetics* 1995; **11**: 303–307.

Mullis K B, Faloona F A. Specific synthesis of DNA in vitro via a polymerase-catalysed chain reaction. *Methods Enzymol* 1987; **155**: 335–350.

Newton C R, Graham A, Heptinstall LE, Powell S J, Summers C, Kalsheker N, Smith J C, Markham A F. Analysis of any point mutation in DNA. The amplification refractory mutation system. *Nucl Acid Res* 1989; **17**; 2503–2516.

Orita M, Iwahana H, Kanazawa H, Hayashi K, Sekiya T. Detection of polymorphisms of human DNA by gel electrophoresis as single-strand conformation polymorphisms. *Proc Natl Acad Sci (USA)* 1989; **86**: 2766–2770.

Panet A, Khorana H G. Studies on polynucleotides. The linkage of deoxyribopolynucleotide templates to cellulose and its use in their replication. *J Biol Chem* 1974; **249**: 5213–5222.

Saiki R K, Scharf S, Faloona F, Mullis K B, Horn G T, Erlich H A, Arnheim N. Enzymatic amplification of beta-globin genomic sequences and restriction site analysis for diagnosis of sickle cell anemia. *Science* 1985; **230**: 1350–1354.

Sanger F. Determination of nucleotide sequences in DNA. *Science* 1981; **214**: 1205–1210.

Smith K T, Long C M, Bowman B, Manus M M. Using co-solvents to enhance PCR amplification. *Amplifications: A forum for PCR users* 1990; **5**: 18–19.

Southern E M. Detection of specific sequences among DNA fragments separated by gel electrophoresis. *J Mol Biol* 1975; **98**: 503–517.

51 *IN SITU* HYBRIDIZATION

John J O'Leary, Volker Uhlmann, Ivan Silva and Robert J Landers

Introduction

Over the last three or four decades, new techniques employing immunological and molecular biological assays have had a major impact in pathology. The field of molecular biology has expanded dramatically with the development of recombinant DNA techniques which makes sensitive detection of specific DNA and RNA sequences by molecular hybridization now possible.

All nucleic acid hybridization techniques rely on the annealing and re-annealing of complementary sequences of nucleic acid. As one of these nucleic acid assays, *in situ* hybridization (ISH) allows specific identification of genes and, more importantly, gene expression.

ISH differs from other hybridization methods (e.g. Southern, Northern and Western blotting) in that the nucleic acids which are to be identified remain in their cellular environment. Therefore, when one uses a complementary labelled nucleic acid sequence and hybridizes this to the tissue section or smear, the label can subsequently be demonstrated, allowing precise cytological localization of the target sequence. ISH was first described in 1969. Its potential was quickly realized and in the early 1970s it was already being employed for the identification of genomic, viral and messenger RNA sequences in cryostat, paraffin wax, electron microscopic and chromosomal preparations. The general use of ISH was hindered by problems associated with probe preparations. Initially, probes were prepared using crude isolates of nucleic acids. In addition, cumbersome, expensive and dangerous radioactive labels could only be used. These difficulties were overcome by recombinant DNA technology. The development of a biotinylated nucleotide analogue of dTTP, Biotin dUTP, and the development of the DNA labelling method nick translation, greatly facilitated the use of ISH.

Probe Preparation

Several recombinant DNA methods are available for cloning nucleic acid sequences. Double-stranded and single-stranded nucleic acids can be regenerated using recombinant techniques, and single-stranded oligonucleotides can be made using DNA oligo synthesizers.

The cloning principle is similar in all cases and involves the ligation of double-stranded DNA into the genome of a vector followed by amplification of the hybrid (e.g. growth in *E. coli*) in order to produce large quantities of the introduced nucleic acid sequence. For nucleic acids up to 20 kb, plasmid, lambda and

Labelling

Enzyme incorporation of nucleotide analogues

M13 bacteriophage vectors can be used. Cosmid systems are available for larger sequences (see Fig. 51.1).

Labelling

Labels must be attached to or incorporated into nucleic acids so that their annealing with the

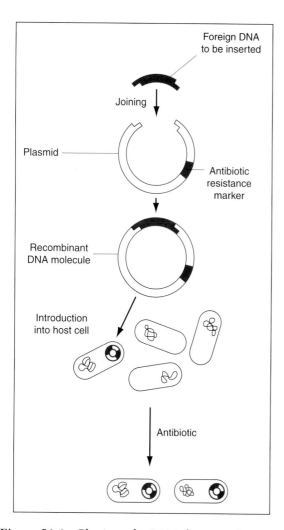

Figure 51.1: *Cloning of a DNA fragment in a plasmid. The gene of interest and the plasmid is cleaved with a restriction enzyme. This generates overhanging ends which hybridize and are then ligated. The new recombinant DNA molecule is then introduced into a colony of bacterial cells, which can be selected by growth in the presence of a specific antibiotic.*

desired target nucleic acid sequence can be visualized. For safety reasons, only non-radioactive labels for ISH are suitable for general use. Three methods of labelling are available: enzyme incorporation of nucleotide analogues, derivatization of nucleic acids and chemical crosslinking with macromolecules. Of the above, enzyme incorporation of nucleotide analogues is the most important. Table 51.1 lists methods for incorporation of labelled nucleotides into probes.

Enzyme incorporation of nucleotide analogues
Among the radioisotopes available, tritium provides the highest autoradiographic resolution. Iodine (^{125}I) provides good resolution and is useful because of the relatively short exposure time. Isotopes of sulphur and phosphorus allow results to be produced within days of hybridization but, frequently, resolution is compromised. Biotin dUTP has largely been responsible for the development of non-radioactive ISH. It is formed by covalent attachment of biotin-*n*-hydroxysuccinimide through an allylamine linker to carbon 5 position of the pyrimidine ring. In addition to being safe, biotinylated probes when stored at −20°C are stable for many months to years. In combination with suitable detection methods, excellent resolution of target sequences can be achieved.

The initial main limitation of bionylated probes lay in the fact that they lacked the sensitivity of radiolabelled probes, but this can be overcome by the use of higher probe concentrations and multiple step (sandwich) detection systems (see Fig. 51.2), giving results equivalent to ^{35}S and ^{3}H labelled probes. For certain probe/target combinations, however, radioactive methods may be of advantage.

Problems do exist when using biotinylated probes. Biotin is present as an endogenous component of several organs and is frequently present in active cells. Reduction of interference by endogenous biotin in tissue sections has been addressed in several publications but none of the techniques described entirely overcome this problem. Because of this, alternative labels with sensitivities equivalent to biotin and not having endogenous tissue distribution have

538

Table 51.1: Methods for incorporation of labelled nucleotides into probes.

Method	Enzyme	Template	Vector	Type and length of sequence
Nick translation	DNAase I DNA polymerase	dsDNA	Plasmid	300–800 dsDNA
Random priming	Klenow polymerase	dsDNA	Plasmid	200–300 dsDNA
Tailing	Terminal transferase	ssDNA	Nil	Depends on length of oligonucleotide
5′ unique primer	Klenow polymerase	ssDNA	M13	Vector labelled as dsDNA, attached to ss unlabelled probe
SP6, T7, T3	RNA	dsDNA	Plasmid	ssRNA

been developed. Among these, digoxigenin dUTP can be substituted for biotin in labelling reactions. The other labels are haptens which can be incorporated into nucleic acids using chemical methods (see Table 51.2).

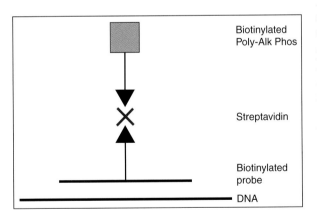

Figure 51.2: Schematic representation of a biotin avidin detection used in in situ *hybridization assays for the detection of biotinylated probes.*

In our laboratory, nick translation is the favoured labelling method. The achievement of correct sequence length when labelling probes is important. When considered along with tissue permeability, the length of the probe determines how easily that particular probe can penetrate and subsequently hybridize with a target sequence. Probes produced by nick translation achieve optimal sequence length (100–300 bp). In addition, newly synthesized labelled nucleic acid sequences have overlapping ends and therefore probe 'meshworks' can readily be formed during hybridization, which by itself amplifies the quantity of label available for detection. Synthesized oligonucleotide probes favour easy penetration, but because they hybridize to only small portions of the target sequence, their sensitivity is compromised. This problem can be overcome by simultaneously hybridizing several oligonucleotides complementary to different sequences within the targeted nucleic acid (cocktail probes). In relation to chemical deriva-

Table 51.2: Hapten molecules and methods for labelling nucleic acids.

Hapten	Group labelled	Mechanism of linkage
Photobiotin	Cytosine	Visible light
Sulphur	Cytosine	Sulphonation with sodium bisulphite stabilized with methylhydroxylamine
Mercury/trinitrophenol	Pyrimidines	Acetoxymercuration
Acetoxy-2-acetyl-aminofluorine	Guanine	Direct interaction

Labelling

Sample preparation and fixation of tissues

---

tization, several chemical techniques can be used to introduce hapten groups into nucleic acids. The major haptens that can be used in such techniques are photobiotin, sulphur, mercury/trinitrophenol and acetoxy-2-acetyl-aminofluorine (see Table 51.2).

Sample preparation and fixation of tissues

The main goal of tissue fixation and preparation is the retention of the maximal level of target cellular DNA and/or RNA, while maintaining cellular architecture and allowing sufficient probe penetration. ISH for the detection of DNA targets has been applied to most histological and cytological preparations. In histopathology, cryostat and paraffin wax-embedded sections as well as cytology smears and cultured cells have been examined. Metaphase chromosome spreads have been examined by light and electron microscopy using ISH. The results of ISH studies can be greatly affected by fixation and processing. The effects of different fixatives on the detection of nucleic acids from paraffin wax-embedded fixed tissues has been examined. Formalin-fixed tissue proved successful for the detection of hybrids using oligonucleotide probes. Bouin's and B5 gave unsatisfactory results. Importantly, large retrospective studies using formalin-fixed paraffin wax-embedded tissue are easily adaptable for use with ISH.

The formaldehyde group of fixatives in particular 'cross-link' DNA to DNA and DNA to histone proteins. In addition, an unwanted effect of formaldehyde fixation is DNA nicking, producing small fragments of double- and single-stranded DNA within the cell. This does not prove to be much of a problem for ISH, but can compromise some PCR reactions (as discussed in Chapter 53).

DNA and RNA nucleases are ubiquitous in the environment. DNA is relatively stable in fixed tissue sections, however mRNA is degraded enzymatically. Consequently, tissue prepared for RNA localization should be fixed or frozen as soon as possible following surgical excision. For the localization of DNA, the type and concentration of fixative does appear to be of major influence. Furthermore, it appears that viral nucleic acid degradation may proceed more slowly, making it possible to use post-mortem tissues for viral *in situ* hybridization studies.

In relation to *unfixed* material, tissue disruption and target sequence loss is commonly encountered and it is therefore essential that all samples are fixed before commencement of the *in situ* hybridization procedure. In *cryostat* fixation regimes, Haase *et al.* concluded that protein precipitating methods based on alcohol and acetic acid mixtures gave the best hybridization signals. Aldehyde fixation has also been used for the demonstration of RNA. Comparative studies have shown the suitability of paraformaldehyde in cell and cryostat preparations for mRNA studies. Routine formalin-fixed paraffin wax-embedded samples are also suitable for demonstration of total and transcript specific mRNA.

Once tissues are cut into sections, the problem of section adhesion to glass slides arises. A definite tendency exists for sections to detach themselves from the glass slides on which they are mounted during hybridization procedures. Many adhesive slide coatings have been suggested but only 3-aminopropyl-triethoxysilane produces consistently reliable results.

Because tissues are routinely fixed in histopathology, proteolytic enzyme digestion is required to expose target nucleic acid sequences. This is particularly important when aldehyde fixation is employed. Such proteolytic enzyme digestion must be carefully controlled; under-digestion yields suboptimal hybridization and over-digestion partial or complete disruption of the tissue. Ideally, a titration assay should be carried out for each tissue in order to obtain optimal results.

However, a recently introduced fixative, Permeafix, utilizing a formaldehyde base and detergent system, can be used directly on cell preparations without the need for proteolytic digestion. Its use with large pieces of tissue is currently being evaluated.

Among successfully used proteolytic enzymes are proteinase K, pepsin and pronase. The addition of 5 mM EDTA to the digestion solution will abolish any nuclease activity that may be present in these products from commercial sources. Some centres (including ourselves) in addition to proteolytic enzyme treatment, use other agents such as HCl and Triton X-100 to aid in unmasking target nucleic acid sequences. In our department, we routinely use acid hydrolysis of membranes combined with Triton X-100 and proteinase K digestion. However, comparative studies fail to demonstrate any advantage in using such 'combination digestion' in the detection of DNA sequences by ISH. Postfixation with paraformaldehyde is useful following unmasking procedures to maintain cellular architecture.

Endogenous biotin may cause problems in some tissues, e.g. liver, kidney, small bowel and ovary. Blocking procedures to suppress biotin detection include sequential application of avidin and biotin, protease type XXIV enzyme digestion and washes with a methanol hydrogen peroxide solution.

Nucleic acid hybridization

Molecular hybridization may be defined as a reaction in which single-stranded target nucleic acid sequences in solution, on filters, or within tissues, and a complementary probe anneal to form double-stranded hybrid molecules. In general, DNA hybridizations involve the use of double-stranded target and probe sequences. It is therefore essential when demonstrating DNA sequences, or when using double-stranded probes, to separate the double-stranded forms into single-stranded configurations. This process is termed denaturation or melting. Typically, this is achieved by using acid, heat or alkali treatment. In relation to nucleotide analogues in which the reporter molecule is biotin, heat denaturation must be used because alkali will remove the reporter molecule by alkaline hydrolysis. The optimal denaturation temperature differs from sequence to sequence and is governed by the percentage of guanine and cytosine residues within that particular sequence. Denaturation of target sequences is in theory not necessary for hybridization, but is advantageous because of secondary structures of DNA and RNA molecules in solution. Denaturation therefore can be seen as creating several fragments which are willing and able for hybridization. If one looks at solution hybridization, the optimum temperature for renaturation of sequences is approximately

25°C lower than the melting temperature (T_m) of the hybrid molecule.

For double-stranded DNA, the T_m is defined as the temperature at which 50% of dsDNA is dissociated, and this is governed by the proportion of guanidine and cytidine residues, the length of the duplex in base pairs (L), the concentration of monovalent cation (C) and the amount of formamide (F) in the hybridization reaction mixture. This set of variables is linked by an equation derived from DNA association in solution.

$$T_m = 81.5 + 16.6 \log M + 0.41 (\% \ G + C) - 0.72 \ F - 650/L$$

Hybridization stringency and post-hybridization washing conditions ultimately determine the degree to which mismatched hybrids are permitted to form. This is particularly important in relation to human papilloma viruses (HPV), where there are many related viral subtypes with significant DNA homology. The T_m of mismatched hybrids is lower than for matched sequences and is governed by the equation

$$T'_m = T_m - x \ (\% \ of \ mismatch): x = 0.5 \ to \ 1.4 \ °C$$

The relationship depends on the nucleotide sequence of the hybrid. Mismatches of the GC-rich segments reduce the T_m by greater amounts than AT mismatches. In relation to human papilloma viruses, the value of 'X' above lies between $0.95 \pm 0.05°C$. If hybridization is carried out at a temperature between T'_m and T_m, theoretically, only matched sequences will hybridize. Conventional stringency conditions (hybridization solutions containing 50% formamide, 2 × sodium chloride, sodium citrate (SSC) at 37°C) represents a T_m of −17°C which allows rapid reannealing, but only distinguishes sequences sharing less than approximately 83% homology. Higher stringencies can be achieved by post-hybridization washes which attain values closer to the T_m as defined above.

The rate of *in situ* hybridization is approximately 10% that of solution reactions, with annealing usually accomplished within three to five hours in the presence of high molecular weight polymers (dextran sulphate). However, longer hybridization times can be used. These polymers establish networks in the hybridization solution and effectively exclude the probe, which as a result is concentrated. The rate of hybridization is increased by increasing probe concentration and consequently this will determine the ultimate amount of hybrid formed. In our own department, overnight hybridizations are employed. Longer hybridization times result in the loss of target sequences.

With some viruses, in particular HPV, the problem of viral types sharing homologous sequences needs to be addressed. Hybridization using high stringency conditions is therefore required to demonstrate individual types, while low stringency conditions reveals closely homologous related sequences.

As we have seen, formamide plays an important role in optimal conditions for hybridization. Its effect on DNA and RNA is different. In DNA hybridization mixtures, hybridization temperatures may be reduced by 0.65°C for each one per cent of formamide added, while with RNA hybridizations the equivalent reduction is 0.38°C. Typically in most laboratories, hybridization is carried out using 50% formamide, which yields incubation hybridization temperatures of approximately 40°C, facilitating the preservation of cellular architecture and target sequences.

Some hybridization protocols include heterologous unlabelled nucleic acid sequences (often derived from salmon sperm DNA). The purpose of such additions is for the formation of electrostatic bonds with positively charged components in the nuclear or cell cytoplasm. Such unlabelled sequences thereby reduce the propensity for similar electrostatic reactions to occur with the labelled probe and thus minimize background staining.

The *in situ* Hybridization Reaction

Hybridization and washing conditions employed in *in situ* hybridization have largely been formulated from solution phase hybridization and using the assumption that nucleic acids within cells and tissues behave in a similar manner to those in solution. The cytoskeleton, because of its structure, impairs diffusion of the applied probe to the target sequence. Fixation and processing, but in particular aldehyde fixation routinely used in histopathology, impede the diffusion of probe further, due to cross-linking of nucleic acids to one another and to nucleoproteins. In relation to archival material, the denaturation of nucleic acid within such material routinely has to be performed at 90–95°C in the presence of 50% formamide and 2 × SSC. This is approximately 37°C above the predicted denaturation temperature as given by the equation above.

The ability of ISH to distinguish between closely related sequences has also been assumed from classical solution phase hybridization kinetics. Herrington *et al.* has examined the problem of HPV type homology (HPV-6 and HPV-11) in relation to ISH. These HPV types exhibit 80% homology of their respective nucleic acid sequences.

Reported incidences of HPV-6 and HPV-11 co-infectivity in cervical biopsy material have been shown to be due to cross-hybridization by HPV-6 and HPV-11 probes with target sequences in paraffin wax-embedded sections. The T_m of matched and mismatched hybrids has been calculated in paraffin wax-embedded sections by increasing the stringency of post-hybridization washes. Post-hybridization stringency is determined primarily by the T_m of hybrids formed. Using such an approach, the linear relationship established between salt, formamide and T_m in solution phase hybridization also holds in relation to archival material. Such analyses have led to the introduction of the term T_m^t which relates to melting temperatures derived by non-ISH analyses using nick translated probes. The endpoint definition of this term can be taken as the midpoint of the temperatures at which signals are absent or just retained under particular washing conditions.

$$T_m^t = 85.7 + 6.4 \log M - 0.42 \,(\% \text{ formamide})$$

It is clear therefore that manipulation of salt and formamide concentrations has a predictable effect on the behaviour of DNA–DNA hybrids which form between closely related sequences. However, non-viral DNA may not behave in an identical manner to HPV sequences.

It is also clear that, following hybridization, firstly low and then high stringency washes should be used for each system examined. Low stringency conditions remove unbound or loosely hybridized probes together with other constituents of the hybridization solution. High stringency may be considered as a 'fine tuning' event for the specificity of probe hybridization, prior to probe detection.

Detection

Detection conditions must not employ temperatures approaching that of the melting point of any hybrids that are formed. Standard autoradiographic and immunohistochemical detection procedures can be employed for detection of radioactive and non-radioactive probes. The detection of radiolabelled probes will not be considered further here.

Detection methods originally described in immunohistochemistry are now used for the detection of non-radioactive labelled hybrids (see Figs 51.2 and 51.3). The strong binding affinity of avidin for biotin has been exploited in many detection protocols. One disadvantage of avidin however is its property of non-specific electrostatic binding to negatively charged groups, among which could be included the phosphate molecules of nucleic acids. Such a propensity to bind electrostatically may be reduced by the use of a high pH buffer as a diluent for the detection reactions and a dried milk blocking step. The closely related streptavidin can be substituted directly for avidin itself. Having an acidic isoelectric point, electrostatic interactions between this compound and tissue sections are minimal.

Other non-specific binding problems arise particularly when using antisera. The use of a bovine serum albumin (BSA) blocking step before the application of the detection reagents will minimize such reactions.

Immunohistochemical 'multistep' detection methods (Figs 51.2 and 51.3) can provide significant amplification of the *in situ* signal compared with single or indirect methods. In particular multistep avidin–biotin complex methods and digoxigenin sandwich techniques yield highly sensitive results. The sensitivity of the detection procedure used and the ultimate localization of the hybrids formed is influenced considerably by the choice of chromogens or chromogenic substrates in the detection method. Fluorescent detection with compounds such as fluorescein isothiocyanate and rhodamine give high sensitivity and precise localization of hybrids. Enzyme conjugate systems provide simultaneous morphological and reaction information and have the added advantage of being permanent preparations. The most commonly used indicator enzymes are horseradish peroxidase and alkaline phosphatase. Following detection, counterstaining of preparations is essential.

Amplified detection using immunohistochemical sandwich techniques are used to enhance signal and therefore sensitivity. The sensitivity of any non-fluorescent or non-isotopic detection system depends on the following: (1) the availability of target sequences for hybridization (dependent on the degree and success of unmasking of nucleic acids in the tissue specimen); (2) the probe type; (3) the reporter molecule used; (4) the affinity of the antibody/avidin for the reporter molecule; (5) the level of amplification by multiple antibody/avidin/enzyme layers and the enzyme chromogen combination.

The affinity of the detection molecule for the reporter used contributes to the sensitivity of the *in situ* protocol. The maximum affinity of

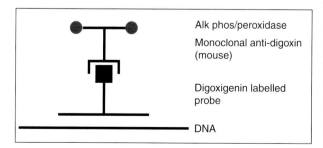

Alk phos/peroxidase

Monoclonal anti-digoxin (mouse)

Digoxigenin labelled probe

DNA

Figure 51.3: Immunocytochemical sandwich technique for the detection of digoxigenin labelled probes in in situ *hybridization.*

Detection

antibodies for antigen (Kd) = 10^{-12} is approximately 1000 times less than that for avidin–biotin. The sensitivity of single-step digoxigenin labelled probe detection (using an antibody conjugate), was examined and found to be less than that for the corresponding system for the detection of biotin.

It has been shown that the use of a three-step amplification system (which employs monoclonal antibodies for both digoxigenin and biotin) with the same second and third steps, achieves equal reporter sensitivity.

Amplification of detection can be achieved by either antibody layering techniques or by enzyme–antibody complexes. The choice of chromogenic enzymes and substrate is also important, but is at the discretion of the user. Alkaline phosphatase-based systems tend to be of greater sensitivity than those employing peroxidase alone. A quantitative assessment of the sensitivity in NISH detection systems is in general difficult to achieve. 'Relative sensitivity' can be assessed by the estimation of the number of positive cells within a given area of comparable tissue sections using different reporter and detection systems. 'Absolute sensitivity' is estimated by analysing the ability of the particular system to detect sequences of known copy numbers in defined cell lines. This can be achieved using CaSki, HeLa and SiHa cell lines that contain multiple copies of HPV. Syrjanen[11] has estimated the sensitivity of biotinylated probes to be 10–50 copies by examining their ability to detect HPV in CaSki and HeLa cells (which contain 50–200 copies of HPV-16 and HPV-18 respectively), but not in SiHa cells which contain one to two copies of HPV-16.

Copy number of virus however probably varies from cell to cell and a more appropriate method perhaps is to analyse the frequency distribution of signals obtained using ISH within the cells screened and to compare the median of the distribution obtained with the average copy number per cell which can be calculated by dot blot hybridization. Amplified detection procedures can increase the sensitivity of an ISH assay ten-fold.

A new technique, tyramide signal amplification (TSA), increases significantly the detection sensitivity of non-isotopic *in situ*

hybridization. Through a direct and indirect cascade system (Figs 51.4 and 51.5), single copy viral genes are easily detected (Fig. 51.6). TSA technology uses horseradish peroxidase (HRP) to catalyse deposition of biotin or fluorescent labelled tyramide in tissue sections, or cell preparations previously blocked with proteins. Using TSA indirect, deposited biotins are detected with a labelled streptavidin. If chromogenic visualization is required, HRP or alkaline phosphatase-labelled streptavidin is followed by the appropriate chromogen. In the direct system, TSA-direct deposits fluorescent labels on the tissue section or cell preparation that can be directly visualized after amplification (see Figs 51.5 and 51.6).

Simultaneous double nucleic acid detection in archival biopsies can also be easily achieved. Histochemical detection techniques for two antigens on the one tissue section or antigen or nucleic acid have been described. The use of non-isotopic reporter molecules allows probe

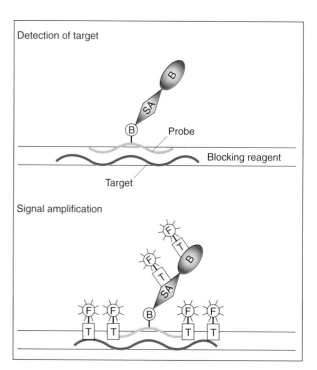

Figure 51.4: *Tyramide signal amplification (TSA) system for detection of low copy viral and mammalian DNA and RNA targets in cells and tissues. Direct system is illustrated here.*

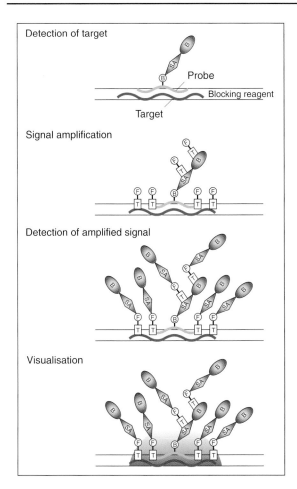

Detection of target

Probe

Blocking reagent

Target

Signal amplification

Detection of amplified signal

Visualisation

Figure 51.5: Indirect tyramide signal amplification system.

detection by fluorescent and non-fluorescent means. Simultaneous detection of two nucleic acids is easily achieved by using one or both of the following schemas: (1) sequential hybridization and detection of probes labelled with the same reporter molecule; or (2) simultaneous hybridization and detection of probes labelled with different reporter molecules.

The Importance of ISH Controls

The specificity of the hybridization reaction must be established. Removal of DNA or RNA prior to hybridization by nucleases allows determination of the particular type of nucleic acid

to which the probe is hybridized. When probes are included in vectors, a labelled vector control to establish the extent to which the vector sequence is contributing to the hybridization reaction must be included with each hybridization reaction. Probe specificity can be examined by competitive inhibition of its reaction with an excess of unlabelled sequence during hybridization. Methodological controls should always be included. Samples or cell lines containing the desired target sequence will establish whether or not the technique is working. Two types of negative control can be included: a sample without any target sequence or a sample that contains target nucleic acid which is hybridized without the addition of labelled probe.

The Chromosomal Assignment of Genes and Interphase Cytogenetics of Solid Tumours ... New Fields for *in situ* Hybridization

Genes and DNA sequences can be mapped to their respective sites and chromosomes by several methods. The most popular are somatic cell hybridization and ISH. ISH techniques involve hybridization of a latent probe to metaphase chromosomal spreads. With the introduction of non-isotopic techniques such as CGH (comparative genome hybridization analysis — see Chapter 50), new frontiers have now been opened. Structural and qualitative changes in the genomic content of premalignant and malignant lesions are in some cases directly correlating with the prognosis of the disease. Such changes may be extremely important in initiation and promotion of neoplasia. The detection of such genomic aberrations has resulted in the growth of flow cytometry and karyotyping. However chromosome analysis of cancer tissue by metaphase cytogenetics is often only possible after tissue culture. *In situ* hybridization procedures using chromosome specific DNA probes have been developed.

545

The Chromosomal Assignment of Genes and Interphase Cytogenetics of Solid Tumours ... New Fields for *in situ* Hybridization

What for the Future?

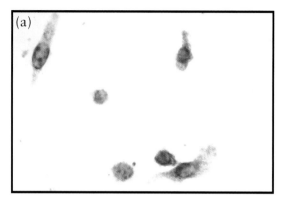

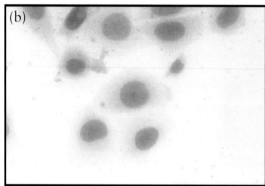

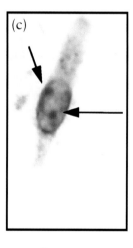

Figure 51.6: SiHa cell HPV-16 NISH using the TSA system, demonstrating the two copies of HPV-16 within the SiHa cell nucleus.

It is clear from these studies that chromosomes occupy discrete areas within interphase nuclei. The ISH method in addition allows the detection of numerical and structural aberations in interphase nuclei. In most instances, probes of the satellite or alphoid family have been used. In rela-

tion to paraffin wax-embedded material, sectioning of nuclei in paraffin wax-embedded sections can result in under-estimation of the real copy number, however.

What for the Future?

ISH for mRNA detection has yet to make a major impact on diagnostic pathology, particularly in areas where problems are encountered with immunohistochemistry. In situations where protein products are rapidly exported from cells, ISH would be of potential use in the identification of mRNA species.

A new probing strategy, peptide nucleic acid (PNA), has recently been introduced. PNA is a new class of molecule, which can hybridize to complementary DNA and RNA sequences with higher affinity than corresponding oligonucleotides, making it an extremely useful tool in Southern and Northern blot analysis, *in situ* hybridization (ISH) and in in-cell amplification techniques (e.g. PCR *in situ* hybridization [PCR-ISH], for localization of DNA targets in the cell; and reverse transcriptase PCR [RT PCR-ISH] for RNA targets). PNA is composed of repeating units of N-(2-aminoethyl)-glycine linked together by peptide bonds. The purine (A and G) and pyrimidine (C and T) bases are attached to the backbone by methylene carbonyl linkages. Unlike DNA, PNA molecules do not contain any pentose sugars or phosphates, making them uncharged.

The enhanced hybridization properties are largely due to the neutral peptide-like backbone of the PNA molecule, which greatly facilitates DNA-PNA and RNA-PNA hybridization. In general, PNA has a high affinity for DNA and RNA, with the stability of DNA/PNA duplexes higher than that of corresponding DNA/DNA duplexes. Because of the neutral backbone of PNA no repulsion between the charged DNA/RNA molecule and the neutral PNA occurs, unlike the repulsion seen with DNA-DNA and cDNA-RNA hybridizations. Importantly, PNA/DNA duplexes are only minimally affected by changes in salt or temperature when performing hybridization analyses, making hybridization easier and allowing greater flexibility with probe melting temperature (T_m). In general, for a 15 base pair PNA/DNA duplex, the increase in T_m over the corresponding DNA/DNA duplex is 15°C at 100 mM NaCl, with approximately similar results reported for RNA/PNA duplexes.

Interestingly, PNAs containing thymidine and cytosine will conveniently form a 2 PNA/DNA triplex. The triplex is composed of a PNA/DNA duplex with a second PNA strand lying outside (Fig. 51.7). These triplexes are extremely stable molecules with strand invasion of the dsDNA molecule, resulting in the formation of a D loop, which may be of potential use to manipulate gene expression, akin to anti-sense oligonucleotides.

PNAs also demonstrate greater specificity than DNA oligonucleotides, with the ability to discriminate single base mutations. A single base mismatch in a PNA/DNA duplex is more destabilizing than the corresponding mismatch in a DNA/DNA duplex. For example, it has been reported that a single mismatch in a PNA/DNA 15-mer lowers the T_m by 10–20°C while the same mismatch in a DNA/DNA duplex lowers the T_m by approximately 4–8°C.

In addition, hybridization times are substantially reduced, again due to the non-charged nature of the PNA molecule. Typical hybridization times are 30 minutes for solution based assays (e.g. Southern, Northern etc.), compared with two to four hours for standard oligonucleotides and overnight for double-stranded probing.

The polyamide backbone in association with purine and pyrimidines makes PNA resistant to nucleases and/or proteases, giving the molecule a longer shelf-life.

The properties of PNAs discussed above make them ideal molecules for use in solution

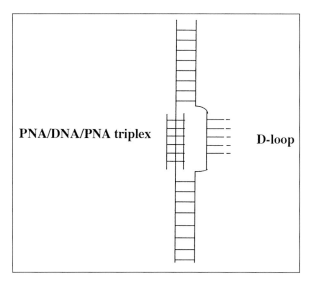

Figure 51.7: *PNA/DNA/PNA triplex and D-loop formation.*

and tissue-based hybridization assays. For NISH, the potential of using short 10–20 mer PNA probes in place of traditional cocktails of oligonucleotides for conventional DNA-DNA *in situ* hybridization and the altered T_m kinetics of PNA/DNA duplexes should make *in situ* hybridizations more reliable, easier to perform and cheaper (Fig. 51.8). The ability to discriminate single point mutations is extremely important in allele specific probing *in situ* and post-PCR amplification. The higher T_m of PNA/DNA duplexes should theoretically allow greater flexibilty in the establishment of T_m (solution) and T_m^t (tissue) for PNA probes.

Finally, automation of some of the detection procedures for *in situ* hybridization will help to bring speed and refinement to the technique, which currently we believe could facilitate greatly its use as a diagnostic tool.

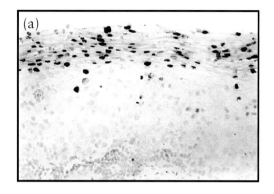

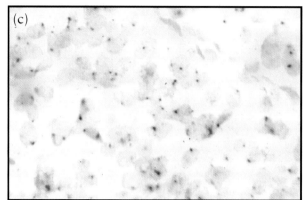

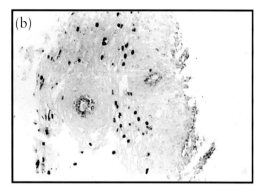

Figure 51.8: (a) HPV-16 NISH in a cervical carcinoma showing dot-like signals within the nucleic of many cells. This illustrates an integrative pattern of HPV-16 in this tumour. (b) HPV-6 NISH in a CIN1 lesion in the cervix, illustrating diffuse signals within superficial epithelial cells. (c) HPV-11 positive condyloma as shown by NISH.

Further Reading

Burns J, Chan T V W, Jonasson J H, Fleming K A, Taylor S, McGee J O'D. Sensitive system for visualizing biotinylated DNA probes hybridized in situ: rapid sex determination of intact cells. *J Clin Pathol* 1985; **38**: 1085–1092.

Burns J, Redfern D R M, Esiri M M, McGee J O'D. Human and viral gene detection in routine paraffin embedded tissue by in-situ hybridization with biotinylated probes: viral localisation in herpes encephalitis. *J Clin Pathol* 1986; **39**: 1066–1073.

Chan V T W, Herrington C S, McGee J O'D. Basic background of molecular biology. In: *In-situ hybridisation: a practical approach.* Polak J, McGee J O'D eds. 1990: Oxford University Press. pp. 1–14.

Egholm M, Buchardt O, Nielsen P E, Berg R H. Peptide nucleic acids (PNA): oligonucleotide analogues with an achiral peptide backbone. *J Am Chem Soc* 1992; **114**: 1895–1897.

Egholm M, Nielsen P E, Buchardt O, Berg R H. Recognition of guanine and adenine in DNA by cytosine and thymine containing peptide nucleic acids. *J Am Chem Soc* 1992; **114**: 9677–9678.

Gall J G, Pardue M L. Formation and detection of RNA–DNA hybrid molecules in cytological preparations. *Proc Natl Acad Sci (USA)* 1969; **63**: 378–383.

Haase A, Brahic M, Stowring L, Blum H. Detection of viral nucleic acids by in-situ hybridisation. *Methods Virol* 1984; **7**: 189–226.

Haase A T, Gantz D, Eble B Walker D, Stowring L, Ventura P, Blum H, Wietgrefe S, Zupancic M, Tourtellotte W, Gibbs C J, Nottley E, Rozenblatt S. Natural history of restricted synthesis and expression of measles virus genes in subacute sclerosing panencephalitis. *Proc Natl Acad Sci (USA)* 1985; **82**: 3020–3024.

Herrington C S, Burns J, Graham A K, Evans M K, McGee J O'D. Interphase cytogenetics using biotin and digoxigenin-labelled probes I: relative sensitivity of both reporter molecules for HPV 16 detection in CaSki cells. *J Clin Pathol* 1989; **41**: 592–600.

Herrington C S, Burns J, Graham A K, Bhatt B, McGee J O'D. Interphase cytogenetics using biotin and digoxigenin labelled probes II: simultaneous differential detection of human papilloma virus nucleic acids in individual nuclei. *J Clin Pathol* 1989; **41**: 601–606.

Herrington C S, Graham A K, Flannery D M J, Burns J, McGee J O'D. Discrimination of closely homologous HPV types by non isotopic in situ hybridisation: definition and derivation of tissue melting temperatures. *Histochem J* 1990: **22**; 545–554.

Herrington C S, O'Leary J J. *PCR in-situ hybridisation*—a practical approach. 1997: IRL Press, Oxford.

Herrington C S, Graham A K, McGee J O'D. Interphase cytogenetics using biotin and digoxigenin labelled probes: III. Increased sensitivity and flexibility for detecting HPV in cervical biopsy specimens and cell lines. *J Clin Pathol* 1991; **44**: 33–38.

Hopwood D. Fixation and nucleic acids. in *PCR in-situ hybridisation*. Herrington C S, O'Leary J J. eds IRL Press, Oxford University Press, in press.

John H A, Birnstiel M L, Jones K W. RNA DNA Hybrids at the cytological level. *Nature* 1969; **223**: 582–587.

Levy E R, Herrington C S. *Non-isotopic methods in molecular biology*. 1995: IRL Press, Oxford.

Matsumoto Y. Simultaneous inhibition of endogenous avidin-binding activity and peroxidase applicable for the avidin–biotin system using monoclonal antibodies. *Histochemistry* 1985; **83**: 325–330.

McDougall J K, Myerson D, Beckmann A M. Detection of viral DNA and RNA by in-situ hybridisation. *J Histochem Cytochem* 1986; **34**: 33–38.

Naoumov N V, Alexander G J M, Eddleston A L W F, Williams R. In-situ hybridisation in formalin fixed, paraffin wax embedded liver specimens: A method for the detection of human and viral DNA using biotinylated probes. *J Clin Pathol* 1988; **41**: 793–798.

Pardue M L, Gall J G. Nucleic acid hybridisation to the DNA of cytological preparations. *Methods Cell Biol* 1975; **10**: 1–16.

Polak J M, McGee J O'D. *In-situ hybridisation: principles and practice*. 1990: Oxford Science Publications.

Syrjanen S, Partanen P, Mantyjarvi R, Syrjanen K. Sensitivity of in-situ hybridisation technique using biotin and ^{35}S-labelled human papillomavirus (HPV) DNA probes. *J Virol Methods* 1988; **19**: 225–238.

Warford A, Lauder I. In situ hybridisation in perspective. *J Clin Pathol* 1991; **44**: 177–181.

52 *IN SITU* AMPLIFICATION

John J O'Leary, Ivan Silva, Volker Uhlmann and Robert J Landers

Introduction

The repertoire of *in situ* amplification has now been extended to include a number of modifications of the initially described technique of *in situ* PCR, to include PRINS (primed *in situ* labelling), cycling PRINS, *in situ* PNA PCR (peptide nucleic acid PCR), IS-TaqMan PCR and allele specific amplification.

The inability to visualize and localize amplified product within cells and tissue specimens has been a major limitation of solution phase PCR, especially for pathologists attempting to correlate genetic events with pathological changes. *In situ* hybridization (ISH) allows localization of specific nucleic acid sequences at the individual cell level, but most conventional non-isotopic *in situ* detection systems do not detect single copy genes, except for those incorporating elaborate sandwich detection techniques as described by Herrington, 1992. Before solution phase PCR amplification can be performed, nucleic acid extraction must be carried out which necessitates cellular destruction.

Recently, a number of studies have described 'hybrid' techniques coupling PCR or other amplification techniques with *in situ* hybridization. The techniques initially were not accepted owing to technological problems. However, extensive optimization of experimental design, dedicated equipment and chemistries have greatly improved the reliability and performance of *in situ* amplification techniques and are rapidly expanding the potential use of these tools in diagnostic pathology.

General Principles

All of the techniques attempt to create double-stranded or single-stranded DNA amplicons within the cell, which can be detected either directly or following an *in situ* hybridization step. For successful application of the techniques, one attempts to achieve a fine balance between adequate digestion of cells (allowing access of amplification reagents) and maintaining localization of amplified product within the cellular compartment and preserving tissue and cell morphology.

The techniques require specific cyclical thermal changes to occur at the individual cell, similar to what occurs in solution phase PCR. These changes initially bring about denaturation of double-stranded DNA (dsDNA) to single-stranded form (ssDNA), if one is amplifying a DNA target. For RNA target specific amplification, the RNA template is already single-stranded and reverse transcription is carried out to create a cDNA template.

Specific short runs of oligonucleotides (primers) are then annealed to the respective ends of the desired target sequence. A thermostable enzyme (Taq DNA polymerase, Klenow fragment or Stoffel fragment) is then used to extend the correctly positioned primers. Subsequent thermocycling increases the copy number of the desired target sequence, in a nucleic acid amplification reaction. However, an exponential increase in amplified product is never achieved, with linear amplification occurring in most situations. This is mainly due to the relative inefficiency of these techniques, owing to problems of accessibility of amplification reagents to the desired nucleic acid sequence, because of the compactness of the nuclear compartment of the cell (containing dsDNA, ssDNA, pre-mRNA and histone proteins).

Once the amplicon is made it must then be detected. If one has used a labelled primer or nucleotide, then the amplicon is labelled and can be demonstrated directly by immunocytochemical techniques. Alternatively, an *in situ* hybridization step (using a single-stranded oligo probe or a double-stranded genomic probe) is carried out post-amplification, adhering to the general rules of standard *in situ* hybridization (see Chapter 51).

Definitions

Several essentially similar techniques are now described including:

DNA in situ PCR (IS-PCR): refers to PCR amplification of cellular DNA sequences in tissue specimens using a labelled nucleotide (e.g. digoxigenin 11dUTP) within the PCR reaction mix. The labelled product is then detected using standard detection techniques as for conventional *in situ* hybridization or immunocytochemistry (Fig. 52.1).

Labelled primer driven in situ amplification (LPDISA): refers to *in situ* amplification of DNA sequences using labelled primers within the PCR reaction mix. The labelled product is then detected as for DNA IS-PCR (Fig. 52.1).

PCR in situ hybridization (PCR-ISH): refers to PCR amplification of cellular DNA sequences in tissue specimens followed by *in situ* hybridization detection of the amplified product using a labelled internal or genomic probe. The labels used can either be isotopic (^{32}P, ^{35}S) or non-isotopic (e.g. biotin, digoxigenin, fluorescein) (Fig. 52.1).

Reverse transcriptase in situ PCR (RT in situ PCR): refers to the amplification of mRNA sequences in cells and tissues specimens by firstly creating a copy DNA template (cDNA) using reverse transcriptase (RT) and then amplifying the newly created DNA template as for DNA IS-PCR.

Reverse transcriptase PCR in situ hybridization (RT PCR-ISH): refers to amplification of RNA sequences in cells and tissues specimens by creating a cDNA template using reverse transcriptase (RT). The newly created cDNA is then amplified, and the amplicon probed with an internal oligonucleotide as in PCR-ISH.

PRINS (primed in situ amplification) and cycling PRINS: amplification of specific genetic sequences in metaphase chromosome spreads or interphase nuclei, using one primer to generate single-stranded PCR product. If many rounds of amplification are utilized then the technique is called cycling PRINS (Fig. 52.2 and 52.3).

In situ PNA PCR (IS-PNA-PCR) and PCR-PNA-ISH: IS-PNA-PCR refers to amplification

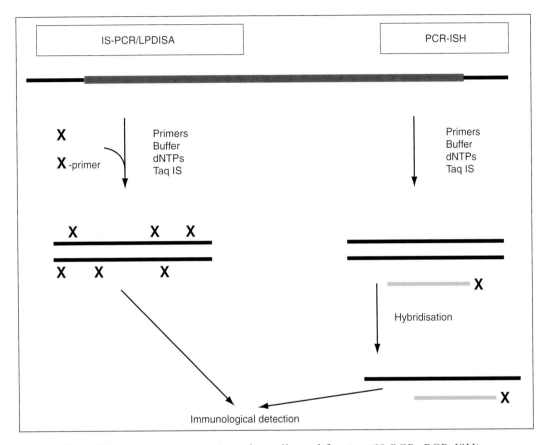

Figure 52.1: *Schematic representation of in-cell amplification (IS-PCR, PCR-ISH).*

of DNA targets using a DNA mimic molecule, peptide nucleic acid (PNA). PNA is a simple molecule, made up of repeating N-(2-aminoethyl)-glycine units linked by amide bonds. Purine (A and G) and pyrimidine bases (C and T) are attached to the backbone by methylene carbonyl linkages. PNA when used as a primer is not elongated by Taq DNA polymerase and therefore can be used in primer exclusion assays, allowing the discrimination of point mutations and direct individual cell haplotyping.

The second reaction which employs PNA is PCR-PNA-ISH; here a 15–20 mer PNA probe is used for the *in situ* hybridization step following amplification. PNAs have higher T_m (melting temperatures) than DNA oligo probes and single point mutations in a PNA-DNA duplex lower the T_m by approximately 15°C as compared to the corresponding DNA-DNA mismatch duplex.

IS-TaqMan PCR: amplification of DNA sequences using a conventional primer pair as in standard PCR. However an internal TaqMan probe is added to the amplification mix. A fluorescent reporter molecule (FAM, HEX, etc.) is placed at the 5′ end of the probe. At the 3′ end, a quencher molecule (again fluorescent, usually TAMRA) is positioned. Once the probe is linearized and intact, the proximity of the quencher to the reporter molecule does not allow any fluorescence from the reporter molecule.

Taq DNA polymerase possess two properties important for the reaction: (1) Y-strand fork displacement (which allows Taq DNA polymerase to lift off a single-strand probe in a Y configuration; and (2) 5′-3′ endonucleolytic activity, which causes cleavage of the linker arm which attaches the reporter molecule to the 5′ end of the TaqMan probe, thereby giving rise to fluorescence if and only if specific amplification has occurred.

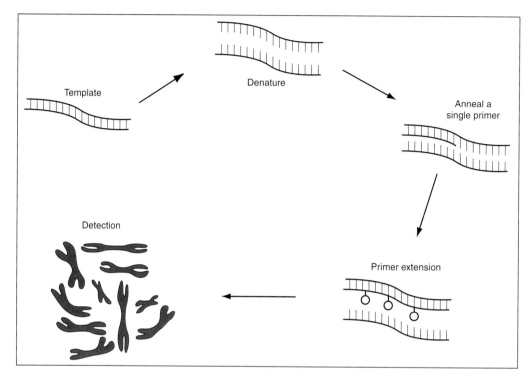

Figure 52.2: *Schematic representation of PRINS.*

In situ allele specific amplification (IS-ASA): this technique utilizes ARMS PCR (amplification refractory mutation system) which has the ability to detect point polymorphisms in human DNA sequences using artificially created base pair mismatches at the 3' end of PCR primers. If the polymorphism matching that of the primer sequence is present, amplification of that sequence will preferentially occur.

Amplification of DNA Targets in Cells and Tissues

Equipment
Several different types of equipment can be used for *in situ* amplification including standard DNA thermal cyclers (using modifications), thermocycling ovens, and specifically dedicated thermocyclers (Perkin Elmer Gene Amp *in situ* PCR system 1000, Hybaid Omnigene/Omnislide and MJB slide thermocycler).

Using a standard thermal cycler, an amplification chamber initially must be created for the slide. This is usually made from aluminium. The aluminium foil boat containing the slide is placed on the thermal cycler, covered with mineral oil and then wrapped completely. However, optimized thermal conduction is never completely achieved. Thermal lag (i.e. differences in temperature between the block face, the glass slide and the PCR reaction mix at each temperature step of the reaction cycle) is commonly encountered. This has been addressed by the newer *in situ* amplification machines, which offer inbuilt slide temperature calibration curves with greater thermodynamic control.

Starting material
Many techniques have been described for performing in cell amplification. In 1990, Haase initially described *in situ* PCR in intact fixed single cells, suspended in PCR reaction buffer. After amplification, cells were cytocentrifuged onto glass slides and the amplified product

Amplification of DNA Targets in Cells and Tissues

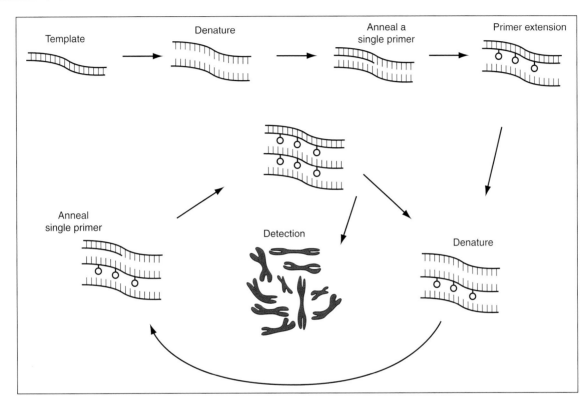

Figure 52.3: *Schematic representation of cycling PRINS.*

detected using *in situ* hybridization. Other early investigators used pieces of glass slides (with cells from cytocentrifuge preparations) in standard ependorf tubes, incubated directly in PCR reaction buffer. More recently techniques using tissues and cells attached to microscope slides have been described with amplification carried out either on heating blocks or in cycling ovens.

For IS-PCR, PCR-ISH, IS-PNA PCR and IS-TaqMan PCR, fixed cells and tissues including archival paraffin wax-embedded material can be used for amplification. Best results are obtained with freshly fixed cells and tissues although successful amplification with old archival material (up to 40 years) has been achieved (personal communication, O. Bagasra).

Fixed metaphase chromosome spreads and interphase nuclei can be used for the detection of specific subchromosomal regions using PRINS and cycling PRINS (Fig. 52.4).

Theoretically, for successful *in situ* amplification to occur, a rigid cellular cytoskeleton must be created which provides a suitable microenvironment allowing access of amplification reagents with minimal leakage of amplified product. Satisfactory results can be obtained with tissues fixed in 1–4% paraformaldehyde, neutral buffered formaldehyde

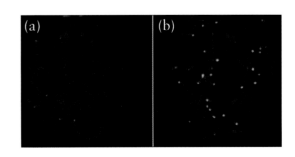

Figure 52.4: *Telomeric specific PRINS and cycling PRINS.*

555

Amplification of DNA Targets in Cells and Tissues

Cell and tissue permeabilization

Amplification

(NBF) and 10% formalin (12–24 hours for biopsy/solid tissue; 10–30 minutes for cytological preparations). Less consistent results are obtained with ethanol and acetic acid fixed tissues. Unfortunately, fixation of cells with formaldehyde fixatives provides a number of drawbacks. Formaldehyde is not easily removed from tissues, even after tissue processing. Aldehyde groups react with DNA and histone proteins to form DNA-DNA and DNA/histone protein cross-links. Formaldehyde fixation also 'nicks' DNA template (random breaks in dsDNA), which may be non-blunt ended (i.e. non-overlapping ends). These nicks may subsequently act as potential priming sites for Taq DNA polymerase leading to incorporation and elongation of labelled and unlabelled nucleotides (e.g. dATP, etc.) analogous to *in situ* end labelling for apoptosis. This process occurs at room temperature leading to spurious results with DNA IS-PCR.

Newer fixatives such as Permeafix (with combined fixative and permeabilization properties) overcome many of the problems associated with the formaldehyde fixatives. In addition, the use of Permeafix obviates the need for proteolytic digestion during the pretreatment of cells for in-cell amplification.

Because repeated cycles of heating and cooling are used during *in situ* amplification, it is imperative that cells and tissues are adequately attached to a solid support (usually glass), so that detachment does not occur. Glass slides are pre-treated with coating agents to ensure maximal section adhesion, the most commonly used being aminopropyltriethoxysilane (APES), Denhardt's solution and Elmer's glue.

Cell and tissue permeabilization

Cells must be adequately digested and permeabilized to facilitate access of reagents. This is can be achieved by protease treatment (e.g. proteinase K, pepsin or trypsin) and/or mild acid hydrolysis (0.01 N–0.1 N HCl). While extended proteolytic digestion is performed for solution phase PCR (often up to 24–48 hours) to overcome DNA/histone protein cross-linking, digestion of cells and tissues for *in situ* amplification is limited by the necessity of maintaining cell morphology, architecture and cell or tissue adhesion. Maximal digestion times and protease concentrations have to be optimized for the particular tissue or cytological preparation employed. Long digestion times compromise cellular morphology but as a result incomplete dissociation of histone protein-DNA cross-links occurs, hindering the progression of Taq DNA polymerase along the native DNA template. Acid hydrolysis probably acts by driving such cross-links to complete dissociation. Alternatively, microwave irradiation of cells and tissue sections can be used to expose nucleic acid templates. Short pulses of microwave irradiation (with or without proteolysis) using a citrate buffer, analogous to antigen retrieval for immunocytochemistry, effectively allow access of amplification reagents to the desired target sequence and in addition, favours the performance of post-amplification immunocytochemistry.

Following this (if a non-isotopic labelling method is used), a blocking step must be employed depending on the method used for post-amplification detection of product (e.g. peroxidase or alkaline phosphatase detection systems). For peroxidase detection systems, endogenous peroxidase is quenched by incubation in a 3% H_2O_2 solution with sodium azide, while 20% ice-cold acetic acid blocks intestinal type alkaline phosphatase.

Amplification

Successful amplification is governed by; (a) careful optimization of cycling parameters; (b) appropriate design of primer pairs (taking into account their T_m i.e. specific melting temperature, their ability to form primer-dimers and uniqueness); and (c) optimization of Mg^{2+} concentrations, needed to drive the amplification reaction.

Due to reagent sequestration (see below), higher concentrations of amplification reagents are required during *in situ* amplification than for conventional solution phase techniques, including primers, dNTPs and Mg^{2+}. Mg concentrations in particular have to be carefully optimized, with satisfactory amplification occurring for most applications at 2.5–5.5 mM (Fig. 52.5).

Amplification of DNA Targets in Cells and Tissues
Post-amplification washing and fixation
Detection of amplified product

Amplification reagent volumes vary depending on the surface area of the cell preparation or tissue section used. This is important as patchy amplification may occur over the surface of the slide due to volume variations consequently leading to localized amplification failure. When using the Perkin Elmer Gene Amp *in situ* PCR 1000 system, 50 μl are used.

Initial denaturation of DNA can be achieved before amplification either during permeabilization or following the fixation process. Alternatively, it may be performed at the beginning of the amplification protocol itself. Denaturation can be achieved using heat, heat with formamide, or alkaline denaturation. In addition, most investigators advocate the use of 'hot start' PCR to reduce mispriming and primer oligomerization, and Nuovo has suggested the addition of single-strand binding protein (SSB) derived from *E. coli*. The precise mode of action of this protein is unknown but it functions in DNA replication and repair by preventing primer mispriming and oligomerization.

Optimization of cycling parameters has to be performed for each particular assay. As preservation of cellular morphology is important, one aims to use the lowest number of cycles and to minimize product diffusion. Most protocols employ 25–30 rounds of amplification, exceptionally 50 cycles. Some investigators have performed two successive 30-cycle rounds with the addition of new reagents, including primers and DNA polymerase between each round; a modification of this is 'nested' PCR, where internal primers 'nested' within the amplicon produced during the first round are added.

Primer selection has evolved around two strategies: single primer pairs or multiple primer pairs with or without complementary tails. Multiple primer pairs have been designed to generate longer or overlapping product with the obvious advantage of localization of amplicons and minimal product diffusion. However, if hot-start PCR is employed, single primer pairs usually suffice.

Post-amplification washing and fixation

Post-fixation with 4% paraformaldehyde and/ or ethanol can be employed to maintain localization of amplified product. When performing PCR-ISH, an oligonucleotide or genomic probe is applied at this stage. To achieve maximum specificity, the probe should hybridize to sequences internal to the amplified product only. However, genomic probes not restricted to these sequences appear to provide comparable results.

Following *in situ* amplification, most protocols include a post-amplification washing step (using sodium chloride, sodium citrate [SSC], formamide and varying washing temperatures) to remove diffused extracellular product which may result in non-specific staining and generation of false-positive results. The stringency of the wash is defined by the set of conditions employed (i.e. SSC concentration, percentage formamide used and the washing temperature). The investigator attempts to achieve a washing 'window' where the signal to background noise ratio is maximal.

Detection of amplified product

Non-isotopic labels (e.g. biotin, digoxigenin, fluorescein) are more widely used and when used

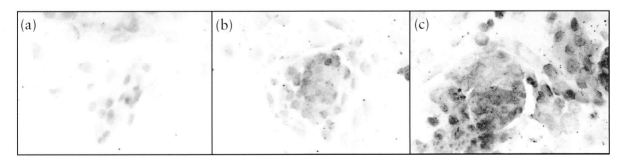

Figure 52.5: *Magnesium chloride effect in in-cell DNA amplification. (a) 3.0 mM. (b) 3.5 mM. (c) 4.5 mM.*

THE SCIENCE OF LABORATORY DIAGNOSIS

Amplification of DNA Targets in Cells and Tissues

Detection of amplified product

Reaction, tissue and detection controls

Amplification of RNA Targets in Cells and Tissues

Cell and tissue preparation

in conjunction with a 'sandwich' immunohisto-chemical detection technique appear to provide similar degrees of detection sensitivity to isotopic labels. These may vary from one-step to five-step detection systems as for conventional immuno-cytochemistry. The product is finally visualized by either a colour reaction (e.g. NBT/BCIP or AEC chromagens) or fluorescence.

Nuovo has described the performance of post-amplification immunocytochemistry, the obvious advantage being co-localization of product with the cell of interest e.g. endothelial cell or macrophage. However, attempts to reproduce this by various groups, including our own, have been disappointing and it is likely that most epitopes do not withstand repetitive thermal cycling.

Reaction, tissue and detection controls
An extended panel of controls must be per-formed for each individual assay. These include parallel solution phase PCR, omission of primers and/or Taq DNA polymerase, irrel-evant primers and/or probes, known negative controls and reference control genes.

The following controls are required in PCR-ISH:

(1) reference control gene e.g. β-globin or pyruvate dehydrogenase (PDH); (2) DNase digestion; (3) RNase digestion; (4) target primers with irrelevant probe; (5) irrelevant primers with target probe; (6) irrelevant primers with irrelevant probe; (7) reference control gene primers with the target probe; (8) target primer one only; (9) target primer two only; (10) no Taq; (11) no primers; (12) omit the reverse transcriptase step in RT IS-PCR or RT PCR-ISH; (13) *in situ* hybridization con-trols for PCR-ISH and RT PCR-ISH; (14) detection controls for immunocytochemical detection systems.

For DNA *in situ* PCR, controls (1), (2), (3), (8) to (11) together with a setup including one target primer and one irrelevant primer pair are used.

Reference control genes, including the use of a single copy mammalian gene such as PDH, are important to assess the degree of amplification in the tissues section or cell preparation. When amplifying DNA targets, the addition of DNase should abolish the signal. If this does not occur,

the signal may have resulted from spurious amplification or alternatively may represent either RNA or cDNA. RNase pre-treatment is mandatory in the assessment of RNA targets (*in situ* reverse transcriptase[RT] PCR) and should be included in the amplification of DNA templates to minimize false positive signals originating from cellular RNA.

The use of a reference control gene primer pair in conjunction with target specific probe assesses the degree of 'stickiness' of the target probe sequence. The addition of only one primer in the amplification mix generates a single-stranded PCR with a quantitative and qualitative reduction in the amount of product synthesized. Irrelevant primers with irrelevant probe should not generate a signal. The specificity of the *in situ* hybridization compo-nent of PCR-ISH is assessed by employing an irrelevant probe with target-specific primers.

The role of primer–primer dimerization and primer oligomerization in the generation of false positive signals is assessed by excluding Taq DNA polymerase, whereas the contribu-tion of non-specific elongation of nicked DNA in tissue sections is examined by the exclusion of primers. The latter is an extremely important control for IS-PCR when using labelled nucleotides. In the assessment of RT-IS PCR, omission of the reverse transcriptase step is important to ensure adequate DNase digestion.

As in routine *in situ* hybridization, hybridiza-tion controls and detection controls are essen-tial to exclude false positive or negative results due to failure of the ISH step or aberrant stain-ing of tissues by the detection system.

Amplification of RNA Targets in Cells and Tissues

Cell and tissue preparation
The same basic principles apply for RNA in-cell amplification as for DNA in-cell amplification. The techniques specifically designed for ampli-fication of RNA targets are RT IS-PCR and RT PCR-ISH. In general, RNA targets are easier to amplify than DNA targets, because of the increased number of starting copies of target.

IN SITU AMPLIFICATION

Amplification methodology and chemistries
Controls for RNA *in situ* amplification
Problems Associated with the Techniques

Once cells or tissues are removed form the body, RNA degradation begins almost instantaneously. In addition, the environment including fingers, gloves and bench tops is rich in RNases. Fixative solutions contain specific RNases that degrade RNA, and tissue processing again contaminated by RNases minimizes the amount of target RNA that can be amplified.

Ideally for RNA *in situ* amplification, an RNase-free working environment should be created. For optimal preservation of RNA in tissue sections, immediate fixation in RNase-free solutions should be carried out. Alcohol, acetic acid with alcohol, Permeafix and neutral buffered formaldehyde fixatives made up in autoclaved DEPC (diethylpyrocarbonate) treated water should be used. All protocols for unmasking of nucleic acid again should employ where possible RNase-free conditions.

Amplification methodology and chemistries

The amplification of RNA targets in cells and tissue is simple to perform, using currently available chemistries. Firstly a cDNA template is created using a reverse transcriptase enzyme, usually Moloney mouse leukaemia virus (MMLV) RT or AMV RT followed by amplification of the newly synthesized cDNA template. A labelled nucleotide (e.g. biotin 11 dUTP) or a labelled primer can be used (RT IS-PCR). Alternatively, a post-amplification *in situ* hybridization step may be employed (RT PCR-ISH).

The above techniques employ a two-step approach, i.e. reverse transcription and then amplification. We have now described a single-step methodology using the rTth DNA polymerase enzyme that obviates the need for splitting the reaction. rTth polymerase possesses both reverse transcriptase and DNA polymerase activity, and is obviously suited for *in situ* amplification applications.

Controls for RNA *in situ* amplification

Similar controls as for DNA *in situ* amplification are required. Omission of the reverse transcriptase step will obviously yield a faint or negative result depending on whether RT IS-PCR or RT PCR-ISH is used. Of importance for RNA

assays is the optimal digestion of DNA in cells and tissue sections, which in many cases can be difficult to remove.

Problems Associated with the Techniques

Many groups have encountered problems with the performance of *in situ* PCR and as yet no universally applicable technique is available. Success is influenced by a number of factors including the type of starting material, fixation conditions and target to be amplified.

DNA IS-PCR is particularly fraught with difficulties, especially when using paraffin wax-embedded material. Here, non-specific incorporation of labelled nucleotide sequences may occur in the presence of Taq DNA polymerase occurs (Fig. 52.6).

PCR-ISH is more specific, especially if a hot-start modification is employed or alternatively if multiple primer pairs are used. PCR-ISH protocols, in general, are more sensitive but, in contrast to solution phase PCR, are less efficient with apparent linear amplification only. The degree of amplification is difficult to assess and contradictory estimates have been documented in the literature. Nuovo has reported a 200 to 300-fold increase in product, in contrast to Embretson and colleagues who estimate an increase of 10 to 30-fold only. Our experience would tend to support the latter figure.

The major limitation with DNA IS-PCR, as previously mentioned, is the non-specific incorporation of nucleotides into damaged DNA by Taq DNA polymerase. This is cycle and DNA polymerase dependent and may occur in the absence of primers and/or with a hot-start modification. Therefore, the routine use of DNA *in situ* PCR with labelled nucleotides is as yet not feasible due to the risk of generating false signals.

However, Gosden has reported the use of strand break joining in chromosomal work to eliminate spurious incorporation during *in situ* PCR. Pre-treatment with di-deoxy blockage has also been documented to eliminate non-specific incorporation, but this is not always successful.

Problems Associated with the Techniques
Sequestration of reagents

Diffusion of amplicons and back diffusion

Patchy amplification

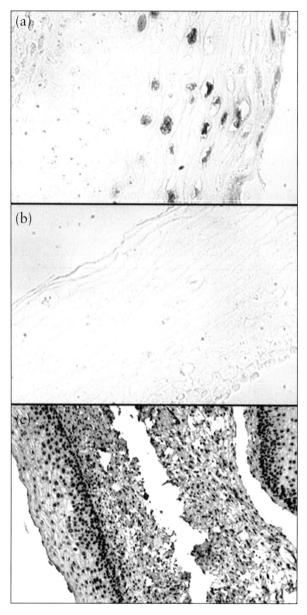

Figure 52.6: (a) PCR-ISH of a cervical biopsy showing intranuclear amplicons. (b) Parallel NISH control, which is negative. (c) Non-specific incorporation phenomenon seen with DNA IS-PCR using labelled nucleotides.

Another approach has been strand 'super-denaturation' i.e. where dsDNA is denatured at high temperatures. The DNA is then maintained in a denatured state for an extended period of time (5–10 minutes) but again, this has produced inconsistent results.

Sequestration of reagents
In contrast to solution phase PCR, increased concentrations of reagents are required for successful *in situ* amplification (usually of the order of two to five times). This is due to reagent sequestration as a result of reagents adhering to slides or to the coating materials used. An additional possibility is that the reagents may intercalate with fixative residues left in tissues. However, it has been documented that pre-treating slides with 0.1%–1% bovine serum albumin (BSA) allows a reduction in reagent concentration, which may function by blocking this sequestration.

Diffusion of amplicons and back diffusion
An inevitable consequence of *in situ* amplification is product diffusion from the site of synthesis, which may occur as a result of permeabilization and/or cell truncation (see below). One can reduce the number of cycles. Another frequently employed strategy is to post-fix the slides in ethanol or paraformaldehyde which helps to maintain localization of product. Alternative approaches include overlaying the tissue section with agarose and/or incorporation of biotin-substituted nucleotides (analogous to *in situ* PCR). This latter modification promotes the generation of bulkier products which are less likely to diffuse. Heterologous sourcing of single-stranded PCR product also decreases the back diffusion phenomenon (O'Leary *et al.*, submitted).

Patchy amplification
In any in-cell amplification assay, 30–80% of cells containing the target sequence of interest stain at any one time. There are many reasons for this including non-uniform digestion of cells, failure to completely dissociate DNA-histone protein cross-linkages which interfere with DNA polymerase progression along the template, and cell truncation. This latter factor is an inevitable consequence of microtome sectioning where cell 'semi-spheres' are created. As a result, the nuclear contents are truncated giving rise to two possibilities: either the desired target sequence may not be present or the target sequence may be present but the product may have diffused out.

Table 52.1: Targets amplified by investigators using *in-situ* amplification.
Viruses (DNA and RNA)

- HIV-1 (mononuclear cells, sperm, fixed brain tissue, macrophages, oral mucosal epithelial cells)
- HPV-6,11, 16,18 etc (cervical biopsies, cell lines)
- HBV, HCV (liver biopsies)
- CMV (archival paraffin embedded tissues)
- HHV-6, HHV-8/KSHV (Kaposi's sarcoma, lymphomas, etc.)
- HSV-DNA/RNA (trigeminal ganglia, disseminated encephalitis)
- LGV (lympho granuloma venerum)

Oncogene/tumour suppressor genes

- p53 mutations (paraffin wax-embedded tissue)
- gene rearrangements (t11;22 in PNET, t14;18 in follicular lymphoma)
- ras mutations (H, Ki, N-ras, codon 12, 13 and 61)
- chromosome mapping (PRINS and cycling PRINS)
- T cell receptor gene rearrangements and immunoglobulin heavy and light V chains

Growth factors, markers of malignancy and other biological markers

- Metalloproteinases and their inhibitors
- EGF receptor mRNA expression
- Endothelial receptor mRNA
- Nitric oxide synthase in multiple sclerosis

Current Applications

In situ amplification techniques and protocols are, as yet, largely being developed. Several groups have documented their success with the identification of single copy sequences in cells and low copy number DNA sequences in tissue sections, including viral DNA sequences (e.g. HIV, HPV, MMTV provirus, CMV, HBV, KSHV) especially in latent infection (see Table 52.1).

Endogenous human DNA sequences have also been examined, including single copy human genes, chromosomal rearrangements and translocations (see Table 52.1).

Table 52.2: Potential uses of *in situ* amplification techniques in pathology.

- Detection of viral genes in tissues e.g. HPV, EBV, CMV, KSHV, HIV-1 and 2
- Detection of bacterial species e.g. *Mycobacterium tuberculosis*, leprae, bovis, etc.
- Detection of mammalian structural genes in embryogenesis and dysmorphogenesis
- Detection of point mutations in oncogenes and tumour suppressor genes
- Single cell allelic discrimination and individual cell haplotyping e.g. cystic fibrosis, thalassaemias, etc.
- Detection of chromosomal translocations e.g. T(11;22), T(14;18), etc.
- Quantitative *in situ* amplification for viral load and oncogene expression (IS-TaqMan PCR)
- Assessment of loss of heterozygosity (LOH) and allelic imbalance
- Forensic identification of tissues, e.g. HLA-DQ, etc.

This has exciting potential, particularly with regard to the amplification of tumour-specific sequences including translocations, e.g. t(11;22) in PNET, T-cell receptor gene rearrangements and point mutations.

As general expertise with these techniques improves, the potential in terms of research and clinical applications is enormous (see Table 52.2).

Further Reading

Bagasra O, Hauptman S P, Lischner H W, Sachs M, Pomerantz R J. Detection of human immunodeficiency virus type 1 provirus in mononuclear cells by in situ polymerase chain reaction. *N Engl J Med* 1992; **326**: 1385–1391.

Bagasra O, Seshamma T, Pomerantz R J. Polymerase chain reaction in situ: intracellular amplification and detection of HIV-1 proviral DNA and other gene sequences. *J Immunol Methods* 1993; **158**: 131–145.

Bagasra O, Seshamma T, Hanson J, Bobroski L, Saikumari P, Pestaner J P, Pomerantz R J. Applications of in-situ PCR methods in molecular biology: I. Details of methodology for general use. *Cell Vision* 1994; **1**: 324–335.

Boshoff C, Schultz T F, Kennedy M M, Graham A K, Fisher C, Thomas A, McGee J O'D, Weiss R A, O' Leary J J. Kaposi's sarcoma associated herpes virus (KSHV) infects endothelial and spindle cells. *Nature Medicine* 1995; **1**: 1274–1278.

De-Mesmaeker A, Altmann K H, Waldner A, Wendeborn S. Backbone modifications in oligonucleotides and peptide nucleic acid systems. *Curr Opin Struct Biol* 1995; **5**(3): 343–355.

Embretson J, Zupancic M, Beneke J, Till M, Wolinsky S, Ribas J L, Burke A, Haase A T. Analysis of human immunodeficiency virus-infected tissues by amplification and in situ hybridisation reveals latent and permissive infection at single cell resolution. *Proc Natl Acad Sci (USA)* 1993; **90**: 357–361.

Gosden J R. *PRINS and in-situ PCR protocols*. 1997: Humana Press, New Jersey, USA.

Gosden J, Hanratty D, Starling J, Fnates J, Mitchell A, Porteous D. Oligonucleotide primed in situ DNA synthesis (PRINS): A method for chromosome mapping, banding and investigation of sequence organisation. *Cytogenet Cell Genet* 1991; **57**: 100–104.

Haase A T, Retzel E F, Staskus K A. Amplification and detection of lentiviral DNA inside cells. *Proc Natl Acad Sci (USA)* 1990; **87**: 4971–4975.

Herrington C S, de Angelis M, Evans M F, Troncone G, McGee, J. O'D. Detection of high risk human papilloma virus in routine cervical smears: strategy for screening, *J Clin Pathol* 1992; **45**: 385–390.

Herrington C S, O'Leary J J eds. *PCR in situ amplification – a practical approach*. 1997: IRL Press, Oxford.

Holland P M, Abramson R D, Watson R, Gelfand D H. Detection of specific polymerase chain reaction product by utilizing the 5' to 3' exonuclease activity of *Thermus aquaticus* DNA polymerase. *Proc Natl Acad Sci (USA)* 1991; **88**: 7276–7280.

Lewis F A. *An approach to in-situ PCR*. 1996: PE Applied Biosystems.

Nuovo G J, Gallery F, MacConnell P, Becker P, Bloch, W. An improved technique for the detection of DNA by in-situ hybridisation after PCR amplification. *Am J Pathol* 1991; **139**: 1239–1244.

Nuovo G J, MacConnell P, Forde A, Delvenne, P. Detection of human papilloma virus DNA in formalin fixed tissues by in-situ hybridisation after amplification by PCR. *Am J Pathol* 1991; **139**: 847–850.

Nuovo G J. *PCR in-situ hybridisation. Protocols and Applications*. 1992: Raven Press, New York.

Nuovo G J. In situ detection of PCR amplified DNA and cDNA; a review. *J Histotechnol* 1994; **17**: 235–246.

Nuovo G J, Gallery F, Horn R, MacConnell, Bloch W. Importance of different variables for enhancing in situ detection of PCR amplified DNA. *PCR Methods and Applic* 1993; **2**: 305–312.

Nuovo G J, MacConnell P B, Simsir A, Valea F, French D L. Correlation of the in situ detection of polymerase chain reaction-amplified metalloproteinase complementary DNAs and their inhibitors with prognosis in cervical carcinoma. *Cancer Res* 1995: 55: 267–275.

O'Leary J J, Browne G, Landers R J, Crowley M, Healy I B, Street J T, Pollock A M, Murphy J, Johnson M I, Lewis FA, Mohamdee O, Cullinane C, Doyle C T. The importance of fixation procedures on DNA template and its suitability for solution phase polymerase chain reaction and PCR in-situ hybridisation. *Histochemical J* 1994; 26: 337–346.

O'Leary J J, Browne G, Johnson M I, Landers R J, Crowley M, Healy I B, Street J T, Pollock A M, Lewis F A, Andrew A, Cullinae C, Mohamdee O, Kealy W F, Hogan J, Doyle C T. PCR in-situ hybridisation detection of HPV 16 in fixed CaSki and fixed SiHa cells – An experimental model system. *J Clin Pathol* 1994; **47**: 933–938.

O'Leary J J, Chetty R, Graham A K, McGee J O'D. In situ PCR: pathologists dream or nightmare? *J Pathol* 1996; **178**: 11–20.

Patterson B K, Till M, Otto P, Goolsby C, Furtado M R, McBride L J, Wolinsky S M. Detection of HIV-1 DNA and messenger RNA in individual cells by PCR driven in situ hybridisation and flow cytometry. *Science* 1993; **260**: 976–979.

53 RESTRICTION ENDONUCLEASES, SOUTHERN, NORTHERN AND WESTERN ANALYSIS, MICROSATELLITE PCR AND DNA FINGERPRINTING TECHNIQUES

John J O'Leary, Ivan Silva, Volker Uhlmann and Robert J Landers

Restriction Endonucleases

Restriction enzymes (REs) are bacterial proteins that cut long, linear DNA molecules into smaller fragments. Restriction endonucleases are a major tool in recombinant DNA technology. A restriction enzyme recognizes a specific sequence in DNA such as AGCT and cuts DNA wherever this combination of bases occurs in the genome. The enzymes are isolated from bacteria and are named with a three or four letter sequence, usually followed by a roman numeral (e.g. *Eco*RI). The prime function of REs is to destroy bacteriophages or other viruses that invade bacteria. Bacteria have developed these enzyme systems to cut the invading DNA sequences of viruses, etc., thereby rendering the virus harmless. Importantly, the nucleotides of the bacteria's own DNA are methylated to protect them from autodigestion by the bacteria's own REs.

Table 53.1 lists some examples of commonly used REs in molecular biology. The number of cut sites in lambda bacteriophage DNA is given. The hundreds of restriction enzymes now available provide a very powerful tool in the molecular analysis of DNA molecules.

Southern Blot Analysis

Southern blot analysis was first described by Edwin Southern in 1975 (see Chapter 53). The technique allows the analysis of DNA frag-ments from a wide variety of samples. The technique proceeds as follows.

Southern Blot Analysis

Table 53.1: Examples of commonly used restriction endonucleases.

Enzyme	Recognition sequence	Number of sites in bacteriophage lambda
BamHI	G/GATCC	5
BglII	A/GATCT	6
DdeI	C/TNAG	>50
EcoRI	G/AATTC	5
HindIII	A/AGCTT	6
PstI	CTGCA/G	18

DNA is extracted from a clinical sample. The extracted DNA is then incubated with a restriction enzyme (e.g. BglII). This enzyme cuts the entire human genome into tens of thousands of fragments ranging from 100 to 20 000 bases in size. These fragments are then run on an electrophoretic gel and size sorted. The smallest fragments move most rapidly through the gel. For demonstration of the fragments, the gel is stained with an intercalating DNA dye such as ethidium bromide. The second step involves transfer of the resolved DNA to a solid support, such as nitrocellulose or nylon. Nitrocellulose or nylon binds DNA. To do this, the nitrocellulose paper is placed on top of the gel slab, which is then covered with absorbent paper. DNA is wicked out of the gel by using a transfer solution such as 20 × SSC (sodium chloride, sodium citrate). Overnight transfer is usually achieved. For laboratories performing many blots, vacuum blotting is commonly used.

After blotting the gel, the membrane is now hybridized with a labelled (isotopic or non-isotopic) probe, to the region of interest, using a suitable solution called a hybridization buffer. Hybridization is usually carried out in a plastic bag (hybridization bag). The probe is a cloned fragment of DNA that has a complementary sequence to the DNA fragment of interest. During the hybridization period, the probe seeks out its complementary sequence. The specificity of the binding of the probe to its complementary sequence is called the stringency (see Chapter 54). The stringency of the probing technique can be varied by adjusting the temperature of hybridization, salt concentration of the hybridization mix, and adding additional agents such as formamide. After hybridization, the blot is washed and detected. Figure 53.1 shows a Southern blot analysis of lambda DNA, a normal patient DNA and DNA from the HL 60 cell line (a leukaemic cell line) for the myeloperoxidase gene (a reference 'housekeeping gene'), with different enzyme patterns illustrated.

Southern blot analysis has been successfully applied to the analysis of many diseases including sickle cell anaemia and cystic fibrosis and for the detection of the Philadelphia chromosome (Ph) in chronic myeloid leukaemia.

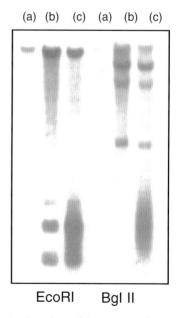

Figure 53.1: Southern blot autoradiograph. (a) Lambda DNA, (b) normal human DNA and (c) HL-60 (leukaemic) DNA was examined using the myeloperoxidase gene. No obvious differences are seen between DNAs.

Northern and Western Blots

The Southern blot analysis can be used to detect alterations in DNA sequences, by looking for differences in DNA fragments after digestion with a restriction endonuclease. Northern blot is analogous to Southern blotting except that it analyses RNA molecules. Western blot analyses protein.

mRNA is an unstable molecule, making Northern blot technically difficult to perform, even in experienced hands. Northern analysis begins with the extraction of RNA from the cell. Cells are initially lysed in the presence of strong RNase inhibitors, in order to prevent destruction of endogenous RNA within the cell by ubiquitous RNases present in the environment. Isolation of RNA from crude cell extracts is usually performed by chromatographic separation. mRNA is then electrophoresed in an agarose gel. Restriction digestion is not required, because RNA molecules are already small as compared to their larger DNA counterparts. After electrophoresis, blotting is carried out analogous to Southern transfer (as described above). Hybridization is then carried out using a labelled probe specific to the mRNA molecule of interest.

Western blotting is an analogous technique for the analysis of proteins within the cell. Proteins are electrophoresed through a gel so as to separate the molecules according to size, and are then transferred to a membrane and hybridized with an antibody against the specific protein of interest.

Alternative techniques have now developed to short-cut classical transfer techniques describe above. Included among these are dot and slot blots (where one dots DNA or RNA samples directly onto a membrane).

Microsatellite PCR Analysis

Microsatellites (also called simple repeat sequence length polymorphisms or short tandem repeat polymorphisms), are defined as arrays of short stretches of nucleotide sequences scattered throughout human DNA, repeated between 15 and 30 times. Several authors however distinguish between microsatellites (two base pair repeats) and short tandem repeats (STR); three to five base pair repeats. Microsatellites belong to the family of repetitive non-coding DNA sequences which are classified as follows:

Satellite sequences: arrays with repeat sizes ranging from 5 to 100 bp, usually arranged in clusters up to 100 megabases (Mb). These are usually located in the heterochromatin near chromosomal centromeres and telomeres and are not variable in size within populations, as compared with other members of this family.

Minisatellite sequences: arrays with repeat sizes of 15–70 bp which range in size from 0.5 to 30 kilobases (kb). Minisatellites are found in euchromatic regions of the genome and are highly variable in repeat size within the population.

Microsatellite sequences: arrays with a repeat of two to six bases pairs, highly variable in size, but ranging around a mean size of 100 bp. Microsatellites are found in euchromatin and allele sizes in populations characteristically exhibit multiple size classes distributed about a population mean.

Microsatellites were originally described in eukaryotic genomes as stretches of dT-dG alternating sequences with varying lengths. Subsequently it was shown that these microsatellites could easily be amplified using PCR, particularly dT-dG and dC-dA dinucleotide repeat microsatellites. Importantly, these repeat sequences showed the Mendelian codominant inheritance of the size polymorphisms.

In order of decreasing abundance, dA, dA-dC, dA-dA-dA-dN, dA-dA-dN and dA-dG repeats were identified as the most frequent sequence motifs in human microsatellites.

(dC-dA)n microsatellites are estimated to number between 35 000 and 100 000 copies in the human genome, giving a marker density of one microsatellite every 100 000 bp. Although widely distributed, microsatellites are not evenly distributed along chromosomes, being particularly underrepresented in subtelomeric regions of the genome.

567

Microsatellite PCR Analysis
Microsatellite PCR

The informativeness (polymorphic informa-tion content PIC) of dinucleotide microsatel-lites increases with increasing average number of repeats. The human genome contains approximately 12 000 (dC-dA)n microsatellites with PIC >0.5 (700 of which have PIC ≥0.7). Tri- and tetranucleotide microsatellites have been identified at a frequency of one every 300–500 kb on chromosome X. About half of these microsatellites appear to be informative.

The precise function of repeat sequences in the human genome is not known. The initial occurrence of short repeat sequences could be due to chance alone, or they may have arisen as mutations from poly(dA)n sequences at the 3′ end of adjacent *Alu* repeat sequences. The selective prevalence of (dC-dA)n repeats can be explained by the methylation of dC residues at the 5′ dG-dC 3′ sequences normally present in the human genome. Methylated dC residues can be deaminated, producing a transition of dC to dT. This process leads to an abundance of 5′ dC-dA 3′ motifs in the genome. Subsequent expansion of the repeat sequence may be due to slippage synthesis during DNA replication. This will then create polymor-phisms differing by a few repeats each time. Additional sequence motifs may subsequently arise because of mutations of the expanded dC-dA repeats.

It was initially thought that repeat sequences possessed a functional role in the genome, either directly via gene regulation or indirectly as hot spots for recombination. CAG trinu-cleotide repeats are transcribed to polygluta-mine tracts. In addition, DNA binding proteins specific to di- and tri-nucleotide repeats have been identified and it has recently been sug-gested that some repeats may act as a site for nucleosome assembly *in vitro*.

Microsatellite PCR
PCR amplification of microsatellite DNA sequences follows the basic broad principles of a normal solution phase PCR (see Chapter 53). Like a standard PCR, the reaction mixture con-sists of the sample DNA, two primers, four deoxynucleotides, a buffer containing magne-sium chloride and Taq DNA polymerase, com-bined in a single tube assay.

When performing microsatellite PCR the following should be borne in mind.

DNA template: starting DNA template can be extracted from a wide variety of sources, including formalin-fixed tissues, paraffin wax-embedded blocks, cytological smears and cell aspirates. The extraction protocol used depends largely on the individual investigator, but can include proteinase K digestion followed by phenol-chloroform purification and ethanol precipitation, simple boiling or chelex treat-ment of cells and tissues. DNA degradation (due to fixation, etc.) must be considered when one is performing microsatellite PCR. This requires that each assay is optimized for each primer pair under investigation.

Primers: 20 mers are best used for microsatel-lite PCR with a GC content of 35–55%. The matched GC content of the primers should be within 5%. Additional precautions need to be taken to ensure non-complementarity, no sec-ondary structure and non-homology with *alu* repeat sequence, which are often located near microsatellites. Primers should ideally be sited as close to the microsatellite as possible, ensur-ing optimal amplification. Optimal annealing temperature range is 3–12°C above the theor-etical T_m values and require empirical opti-mization. The concentration of primer used varies between 0.1 and 0.3 μM.

dNTPs: deoxynucleotide concentrations between 20 and 100 μM are suitable. These concentra-tions are lower than standard solution phase PCR, and reflect the specificity and fidelity required for microsatellite PCR.

PCR buffers: the buffer for each assay should ideally be optimized for each assay. Initially it is advisable to prepare six buffers (100 mM Tris-HCl, 500 mM KCl and 1% Triton-X 100) at two magnesium concentrations (15 and 30 mM) and three pH values (pH 8.0, 8.5 and 9.0). Simultaneous amplification under the same cycling conditions with these six buffers is a useful aid to optimization. The addition of bovine serum albumin (BSA), glycerol, for-mamide and ammonium sulphate have been reported to increase specificity, and should be used if initial optimization is unsuccessful.

Thermocycling: the accurate scoring of allelic fragments can be severely affected by spurious amplification bands, which are due to mispriming events. High annealing temperatures and short extension times (given that the nucleotide incorporation rate of Taq DNA polymerase is 35–150 nucleotides per second at 70–80°C, and the size range of allelic fragments is small) is advised. Hot start PCR and heat soaked PCR (involving incubation of the DNA template at 94°C for 30 minutes before adding Taq DNA polymerase) are recommended to increase specificity. Touchdown PCR (using high initial annealing temperatures, and reducing by 1–2°C in each successive cycle) has been suggested as a way of bypassing the need to optimize individual PCR thermal cycling conditions.

Detection and scoring of microsatellites: polyacrylamide gel electrophoresis (PAGE) is the usual means to resolve microsatellite PCR amplicons. Specific oligoprobing can also be performed using a specific probe that will only recognize the desired repeat sequence. 'Stutter bands' are often encountered on PAGE gels, making interpretation very difficult in some assays. Stutter bands are additional bands differing by 1 to 2 bp in size. They arise probably due to slippage synthesis by Taq DNA polymerase (akin to the mechanism that may be involved in the formation of microsatellites in the first place). It is also possible that Taq DNA polymerase fails to read through the repeat sequence, or due to the 3' terminal addition of nucleotides by Taq DNA polymerase, or due to differences in the migration of (dC-dA)n and (dG-dT)n strands (when both strands are labelled).

There are several methods which can be used for the detection of microsatellite amplicons.

Radioactive methods have traditionally been used for the detection and quantitation of microsatellite PCR, using either a labelled nucleotide triphosphate in the PCR reaction mix (α^{32}P-dCTP) P-dCTP or a single labelled (gamma 32) γ^{32}dATP labelled primer (Fig. 53.2). The primer end labelled approach mini-

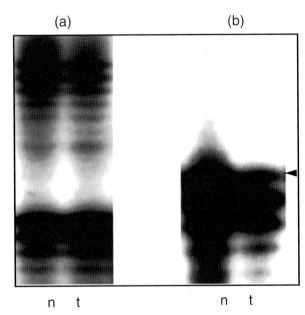

(a)   (b)

n   t   n   t

Figure 53.2: Autoradiograph showing an allelic imbalance (AI) assay in normal (n) and tumour DNA (t) from the same patient. (a) No loss of heterozygosity. (b) Loss of heterozygosity in the tumour sample.

mizes additional bands on the gel and facilitates analysis. Products are resolved on sequencing gels, fixed, dried and autoradiographed, with or without intensifying screens. Pre-flashing of the X-ray film is important to ensure linearity. Optical densitometry is then used for quantitation of PCR products.

Non-radioactive method include ethidium bromide staining (which offers low detection sensitivity: only >10 ng of dsDNA can be detected), silver staining (with attendant problems of background and non-linear deposition of silver).

Fluorescence analysis offers the most sensitive and reliable method for the detection of microsatellite PCR amplicons (Figs 53.3, 53.4 and 53.5). The advantage of analysing multiple polymorphic markers using an automated DNA sequencer was first described by Skolnick & Wallace in 1988. In 1992, Ziegele *et al.* reported the use of an automated DNA sizing technology, for genotyping microsatellite loci, using a four-colour fluorescence technique.

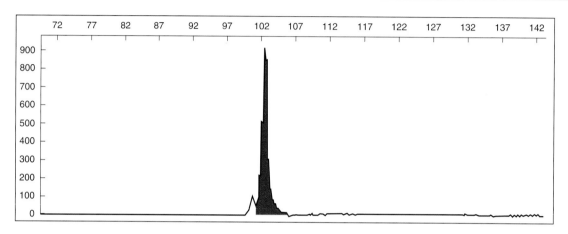

Figure 53.3: *Electrophoretogram of a chromosome 11 microsatellite analysis showing an uninformative homozygous case (one allelic peak).*

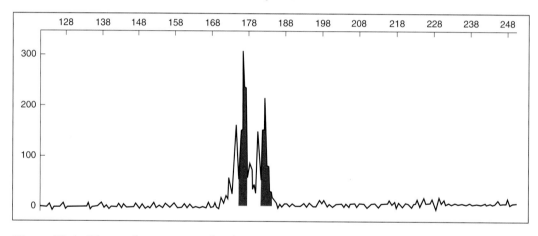

Figure 53.4: *Electrophoretogram of a chromosome 11 microsatellite analysis showing an informative heterozygous case, with two allelic peaks.*

In this method, fluorescent phosphor-amidites are linked to the 5′ end of one of the primers in a PCR assay. The labels used include FAM (blue), TAMRA (yellow), JOE (green), and ROX (red). In addition, newly introduced fluorescently labelled dNTPs (R110, blue; R6G green; TAMRA, yellow) can be used to internally label the PCR product.

Use of Microsatellites in Pathology

Genome analysis

The Human Genome Project (HGP) is attempting to construct a physical map of the entire human genome, to consist of unique genomic landmarks at an average spacing of 100 kB. When completed in 1998/99, the map will consist of 30 000 marker loci, distributed evenly throughout the genome. The National Insti-tutes of Health (NIH) interim goal of a 2–5 centimorgan (cM) map by 1995/96 has been achieved.

Initially, restriction fragment length polymorphisms (RFLPs) were proposed as the DNA markers of choice permitting the reliable detection of genes for dominant diseases. RFLPs suffer from one major disadvantage, in that they exhibit low heterozygosity. The analysis of RFLPs is also tedious and laborious.

The most informative members of this class, VNTRs (variable number of tandem repeats) or

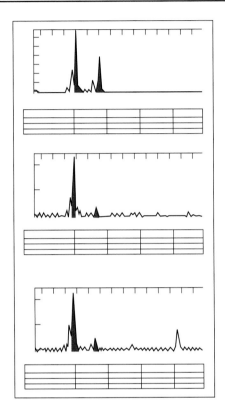

Figure 53.5: Electrophoretogram of a chromosome 11 microsatellite analysis in normal glandular intra-epithelial neoplasia (GIN) and invasive adenocarcinoma of the cervix. Note the decrease in the size of the allelic peak in the middle and bottom panels, indicating that AI is present both in GIN and the invasive adenocarcinoma.

regions of chromosomes, where microsatellites tend to be sparsely distributed. Currently, the number of Genoma Database (GDB) marker loci, scorable by PCR with heterozygosities greater than 69%, is in excess of 3000 (see Table 53.2). The current microsatellite map of the human genome gives a 0.7 cM resolution.

Microsatellites can be used easily for linkage analysis studies. Owing to the enhanced density of microsatellite markers, linkage analysis is now no longer limited to monogenic markers, and has been successfully applied in the study of early onset Alzheimer's disease and in mapping BRCA1 in breast cancer.

In addition to linkage analysis, allele sharing and association studies can easily be performed using microsatellite PCR, to identify novel disease loci. In allele sharing, one attempts to prove that the inheritance pattern of a chromosomal region is not consistent with random Mendelian inheritance, with association studies testing whether a disease and an allele show correlated occurrences in a defined population. Allele sharing has been successfully applied by Davis *et al.* in their genome-wide study of type I diabetes mellitus, in which they identified 18 chromosomal regions with evidence for linkage, identifying three new genes involved in diabetes mellitus, IDDM3, IDDM5 and a locus on chromosome 18. Other genes have similarly been identified including apolioprotein E in Alzheimer's disease and angiotensin converting enzyme in myocardial infarction.

Allelic imbalance/loss of heterozygosity (LOH) studies

Allelotyping of the entire 23 pairs of chromosomes has been performed by Vogelstein *et al.*

minisatellites, tend to cluster at the ends of chromosomes, where telomeric shortening occurs independent of tumourigenesis, as part of the normal ageing process. Minisatellites however give good coverage of centromeric

Table 53.2:	Human genome maps.			
Year	Group	Marker	Loci No.	Resolution (cM)
1981	Keats	Classical	53	16
1987	CRI	RFLP	403	10
1992	Genethon	CA	814	4.4
1992	NIH/CEPH	Mixed	1416	3.0
1994	Genethon	CA	2066	2.9
1994	CHLC	Mixed	5840	0.7

Use of Microsatellites in Pathology

Microsatellite markers in human disease

in colorectal cancer. Allelic imbalance assays use the Knudson hypothesis of deleted anti-oncogenes. Loss of heterozygosity (LOH), the loss of an allelic band in a tumour versus constitutional DNA from the same individual is now universally recognized as indicative of putative tumour suppressor genes. Cawkwell *et al.* have applied microsatellite PCR technology for the analysis of microdissected tissues from archival paraffin wax-embedded material. With small starting amounts of DNA, allelic amplification is difficult to distinguish from allelic loss, and therefore the term allelic imbalance (AI) is used.

Individuals are either heterozygous or homozygous at microsatellite loci (see Figs 53.3 and 53.4). Allelic imbalance is calculated as a ratio; the numerator and denominator being the ratios of the intensities of the two allelic peaks in the tumour and constitutional DNA (Fig. 53.5). At least 30% tumour load is required for AI/LOH assays, although recent reports using flow cytometry suggests a figure as low as 10% tumour cells. Using such AI/LOH assays, the search is now on to identify novel tumour suppressor genes in many solid and non-solid tumours (see Table 53.3).

Microsatellite markers in human disease
Microsatellite expansion in disease
Mutations in repeat sequences may be a common cause of human disease. In myotonic dystrophy (MD) and the fragile X syndrome, expansion of microsatellite repeats has been identified. The expansion is linked to parental copy number and it is known that such repeats predispose to mutations. In the fragile X syndrome, expansion of the CCG trinucleotide repeat in the 5′ untranslated region of the FMR1 gene on chromosome X, causes methy-lation at the CpG residues, both in the repeat region and also in the adjacent FMR1 promoter, effectively stopping transcription of the gene. In myotonic dystrophy, the degree of expansion of the non-coding 3′ trinucleotide repeat is associated with disease severity and the age of onset. Table 53.4 lists common microsatellite markers which are associated with disease.

Microsatellite instability (MSI) in human disease
Microsatellite instability was first discovered in the search for causal mutations in hereditary non-polyposis colorectal cancer (HNPCC), an autosomal dominant syndrome, in which there is a predilection to colorectal and endometrial tumours. In HNPCC kindreds, there is linkage to the marker D2S123 on chromosome 2p. In addition, microsatellite instability was present throughout the genome. This was represented by microsatellites of varying size. These groups of patients became known as RER+ (replication error positive). It is estimated that the total number of mutations at microsatellite loci in replication error positive (RER+) tumour cells could be up to 100-fold that in RER– cells, suggesting a mutation affecting DNA replication, or repair, thereby predisposing to replication errors. Studies in mutator mutants of *Saccharomyces cerevisiae* and *Escherichia coli* showed that mutations in the mismatch repair genes, PMS1, MLH1 or MSH2 and Mut S produced an RER+ phenotype. The mechanism of error is explained by slippage DNA synthesis, whereby DNA polymerases slip on the repeat motif during normal cellular replication, with subsequent correction of the frame shifts by the mismatch repair complex, thereby predisposing to the RER+

Table 53.3:	Tumours associated with allelic imbalance/loss.		
Breast	1p, 1q, 3p, 6q, 11p, 11q, 13q, 16q, 17p, 17q	Hepatocellular	8p, 13q, 16q, 17p
Lung	3p, 5q, 8p, 11p, 13q, 17p	Cervical	3p, 11q, 17p
Renal	3p, 5q, 17p	Ovarian	3p, 6q, 11p, 13q, 17p
Colorectal	1p, 2p, 5q, 8p, 11q, 13q, 14q, 17p	Testicular	3p, 11p, 17p
Gastric	13q, 18q	Prostate	8p, 10q, 16q
Pancreas	1p, 3p, 6q, 8p, 11p,q, 17p	Melanoma	6q, 9p, 11p

RESTRICTION ENDONUCLEASES, SOUTHERN, NORTHERN AND WESTERN ANALYSIS

Use of Microsatellites in Pathology
Forensic and population study applications of microsatellites
DNA Fingerprinting

Table 53.4: Microsatellites associated with disease.

Repeat sequence	Association
Mononucleotide Dinucleotide Trinucleotide	HPNCC
Dinucleotide Trinucleotide Tetranucleotides	Various human cancers
CCG	Fragile X syndrome FRAXA FRAXE FRAXF
CAG	Spinal and bulbar muscular atrophy Myotonic dystrophy Huntington's disease Spinocerebellar ataxia (type 1) RED-1 Machado–Joseph disease Haw–River syndrome

phenotype. Thus was discovered hMSH2, homologous to the yeast MSH2 gene, whose protein product has been shown to be a DNA mismatch binding protein. Other mismatch repair genes involved in the pathogenesis of HNPCC include hMLH1, hPMS1 and hPMS2. Indeed, analysis of sporadic tumours belonging to the HNPCC spectrum also reveal a significant proportion of cases with multiple replication errors. Some small cell lung tumours (with multiple primary sites) are also now shown to demonstrate the RER+ phenotype.

Forensic and population study applications of microsatellites

Population studies reveal that microsatellite alleles segregate in a Mendelian fashion in families. The *de novo* mutation rate for tri- and tetranucleotide repeats (STRs) ranges from 2.3 to 15.9×10. Therefore new mutations are not a significant problem in identity determination. STRs are therefore ideally suited for use in medical and forensic identification and are admissible in court. Using fluorescent techno-

logy as little as 100 pg of DNA target can be used for the direct identification of an individual.

In addition, a number of markers of genetic diversity have been utilized to construct a phylogenetic tree of human populations, in order to understand fully population mobility traits and evolutionary trends. Genetic similarity can be interpreted as evidence of shared ancestry, though most genetic variation in humans exists between individuals within races.

DNA Fingerprinting

The establishment of identity in forensic medicine and in paternity cases is of utmost importance. Fingerprinting has long been the only method of identification of human subjects. Recombinant DNA testing now has the potential to replace conventional hand fingerprinting. Just like the fingerprint, the human genome is different for every individual (except for genetically identical twins). Of the six billion base pairs making up the diploid content of a

DNA Fingerprinting

human cell, one person differs from another by about three million base pairs, or at least 0.5% of the genome. Some of these differences between individuals are due to mutations, thereby affecting the phenotype of the individual, although most mutations are silent with no constitutive effect. Most changes do not occur within coding regions of the genome, and therefore do not affect the phenotype of the individual. These alterations are called *polymorphisms* (incidental variations in the genome, with no effect on gene expression). Many of the polymorphisms that constitute differences in individuals occur in areas called 'spacer DNA'. These are short segments of DNA that repeat a variable number of times (see microsatellites, above).

When a sperm or an egg is formed by the process of meiosis, the number of spacer segments in the germ cell changes in a random fashion. A fertilized zygote is formed at the moment of conception by the combination of two haploid genomes (from haploid germ cells) to give a diploid cell. The diploid zygote has different numbers of spacer elements than

either of its parents. This forms the basis of DNA fingerprinting.

The human genome is present in every cell of the body, and all cells serve as sources of material for DNA fingerprinting. DNA is very stable: indeed a dried blood sample can be tested many years after a crime.

Several recombinant DNA technqiues are useful for DNA fingerprinting, employing both PCR and Southern blot techniques. One technique utilizes variable numbers of tandem repeats (VNTRs), typically six to eight bases in length, repeating 6 to 20 times. The randomness of VNTRs throughout the genome of an individual gives that individual a unique serial number, akin to a 'bar-code' on the side of a carton of corn flakes. Figure 53.6 illustrates schematically how the mapping pattern of VNTRs from two different individuals can be used in DNA fingerprinting. In this illustration, three different regions with VNTRs are used (A, B and C). A restriction enzyme digestion site (indicated by the vertical arrows) on either side of the VNTR releases the DNA fragments containing that VNTR. More copies of the

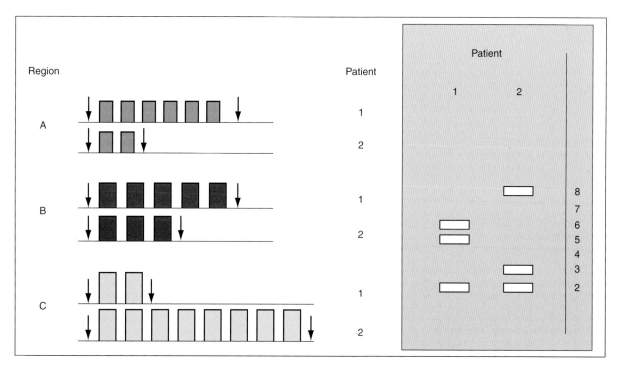

Figure 53.6: Schematic diagram illustrating a typical DNA fingerprinting assay using the VNTR method.

tandem repeat results in larger DNA fragments being cut. In region A, patient 1 has six repeats, patient 2 has two repeats. In region B, patient 1 has five repeats and patient 2, three. In region C, patient 1 has two repeats and patient 2 has eight. Southern blot analysis of the restriction digest electrophoresis, probed for the VNTR sequences, establishes the banding pattern and size of each band for a particular patient. Figure 53.6 only shows a three region analysis, but in practice, many regions (up to 1000 or more) can be probed for using such a methodology. This increases the specificity of the DNA fingerprint, effectively giving a 'barcode' result as mentioned previously.

PCR can be used to detect specific site differences in DNA, which also form a unique DNA signature for that individual. PCR methods are now commonly employed to examine variations in regions of the HLA-DQ locus of the human histocompatibility system (HLA). Employing PCR means that minute quantities can be used (as little as 100 pg), as compared to Southern analysis which requires 10 μg, a 10^6-fold difference in starting DNA template concentrations. More importantly, however, PCR can be used with degraded DNA samples, which are often the only means of forensic identification.

DNA fingerprinting is offered by several companies and hospital laboratories worldwide, particularly in the investigation of rape, paternity suits, and forensic identification of human remains.

There are however problems associated with DNA fingerprinting techniques. False DNA left at a crime scene can totally confound a DNA fingerprinting result. In addition, some cosmetics contain human DNA (e.g. shampoos), which if one was using hair samples for DNA fingerprinting analysis, again may make interpretation of the result extremely diffficult. In routine histopathology, DNA fingerprinting is sometimes resorted to, to sort out mis-labelled tissue specimens from different individuals, where the diagnosis carries serious implications for one individual.

Further Reading

Braaten D C, Thomas J R, Little R D et al. Locations and contexts of sequences that hybridize to poly (dG-dT).(dC-dA) in mammalian ribosomal DNAs and two linked X genes. Nucl Acids Res 1988; 16: 865–881.

Brook J D, McCurrach M E, Harley H G et al. Molecular basis of myotonic dystrophy: expansion of a trinucleotide (CTG) repeat at the 3′ end of a transcript encoding a protein kinase family member. Cell 1992; 68: 799–808.

Cawkwell L, Bell S M, Lewis F A, Dixon M F, Taylor G R, Quirke P. Rapid detection of allele loss in colorectal tumours using microsatellites and fluorescent DNA technology. Br J Cancer 1993; 67: 1262–1267.

Davies J L, Kawaguchi Y, Bennett S T et al. A genome wide search for human type I diabetes susceptibility genes. Nature 1994; 371: 130–136.

Edwards A, Hammond H A, Jin L, Casket, C T, Chakraborty R. Genetic variation in five trimeric and tetrameric tandem repeat loci in four human population groups. Genomics 1992; 12: 241–253.

Goate A, Chartier–Harlin M C, Mullan M et al. Segregation of a missense mutation in the amyloid precursor protein gene with familial Alzheimer's disease. Nature 1991; 349: 704–706.

Hall J M, Lee M K, Newman B et al. Linkage of early onset familial breast cancer to chromosome 17q21. Science 1990; 250: 1684–1689.

Koreth J, O'Leary J J, McGee J O'D. Microsatellites and PCR genomic analysis. J Pathol 1996; 178: 239–248.

Litt M. PCR amplification of TG microsatellites. In: McPherson M J, Quirke P, Taylor G R eds. PCR – a practical approach. 19??: IRL Press; Oxford. pp. 85–89.

Further Reading

Lynch H T, Lanspa S, Smyrk T, Boman B, Watson P, Lynch P. Hereditary non-polyposis colorectal cancer (Lynch syndromes I & II). Genetics, pathology, natural history and cancer control, Part 1. *Cancer Genet Cytogenet* 1991; **53**: 143–160.

Richards R I, Holman K, Yu S, Sutherland G R. Fragile X syndrome unstable element, p(CCG)n, and other simple tandem repeat sequences are binding sites for specific nuclear proteins. *Hum Mol Genet* 1993; **2**: 1429–1435.

Ross D W. *Introduction to molecular medicine*. 1996: Springer Verlag, Berlin.

Shriver M D, Jin L, Chakraborty R, Boerwinkle E. VNTR allele frequency distributions under the step-wise mutational model: a computer simulation approach. *Genetics* 1993; **134**: 983–993.

Skolnick M H, Wallace R B. Simultaneous analysis of multiple polymorphic loci using amplified sequences polymorphisms (ASPs). *Genomics* 1988; **2**: 273–279.

Tautz D, Renz M. Simple sequences are ubiquitous repetitive components of eukaryotic genome. *Nucl Acid Res* 1984; **12**: 4127–4138.

Tomfohrde J, Silverman A, Barnes R *et al*. Gene for familial psoriasis susceptibility mapped to the distal end of human chromosome 17q. *Science* 1994; **264**: 1141–1145.

Tyler Smith C, Willard H F. Mammalian chromosome structure. *Curr Opin Genet Dev* 1993; **3**: 390–397.

Vogelstein B, Fearon E R, Kern S E *et al*. Allelotype of colorectal carcinomas. *Science* 1989; **244**: 207–211.

Weber J L. Informativeness of human (dC-dA)*n*.(dG-dT)*n* polymorphisms. *Genomics* 1990; **7**: 524–530.

Ziegele J S, Su Y, Corcoran K P *et al*. Application of automated DNA sizing technology for genotyping microsatellite loci. *Genomics* 1992; **14**: 1026–1031.

54   DNA SEQUENCING

Steven J Picton

The Beginnings of DNA Sequencing

Publication of the methods for routine determination of the base sequence of isolated DNA did not emerge until some 20 years after the report of the three-dimensional structure of the DNA double helix in 1953. Some early chromatographic sequencing methods used tRNA templates since these were both very short and the nucleic acid template was available in substantial amounts. The first intact molecule whose sequence was determined was a simple 80-base yeast tRNA published as early as 1965. Around the start of the 1970s routine DNA sequencing became reality with the discovery and isolation of DNA restriction enzymes, essentially molecular scissors to cut up the complex genome templates, and DNA polymerases that enabled the template fragments to be copied *in vitro*. These enzymes enabled small DNA fragments to be isolated from much larger sequences and then used as templates for *in vitro* synthesis of new labelled or tagged DNA. This provided one route for base sequence determination.

Utilizing the techniques of primed DNA synthesis and subsequent separation of the DNA products by polyacrylamide gel electrophoresis, the 5.4 kb genome of the bacteriophage ØX was determined in 1976 and published in 1977. With almost a quarter century having now passed from Crick & Watson's paper, 1977 was marked by not one new sequencing methodology but publication of two ways of determining the base sequence of DNA. These published methods, now synonymous with the DNA sequencing process, provided the final breakthrough in both the rate of sequencing possible and size of fragments for which base composition could be determined in a single reaction. The dideoxy chain termination technique was used to sequence the 16.5 kb human mitochondrial genome, and chemical degradation methodology[2] allowed analysis of the 40 kb T7 bacteriophage genome.

These two techniques, and modifications to them, remain as the backbone of almost all present-day sequencing strategies, the dideoxy chain termination method being used for most genome projects and the basis of the current commercially available automated fluorescent sequencing instruments.

The ability to determine DNA sequences rapidly has now revolutionized the science of molecular genetics. DNA sequences from diverse sources have been obtained and vast repositories, such as the EMBL database, DDBJ and GenBank exist as international stocks of nucleic acid sequences. These data banks serve as a nucleic acid library to which scientists have electronic access in order to study evolution, mutations and phylogeny, and ultimately to apply the sequence information to the characterization of complete biological systems.

Entire genome sequencing projects are currently under way, the aim being to obtain the nucleic acid sequence of entire organisms to shed light on the biological significance of individual sequences and study the evolution of individual genes and mutations within genes that may lead to specific diseases or susceptibility to the onset of certain types of cancer. Ten years after routine sequencing of nucleic acids became possible, the GenBank database contained approximately 15 million nucleotides. The rate of deposition of sequence data practically doubled in each of the subsequent five years, reaching 120 million bases in 1992. Increasing levels of sequencing automation have allowed continuing expansion in the rate of data submission.

Until this decade the establishment of genome projects was largely dismissed as too expensive, too time consuming and of little short-term benefit. The sequencing process itself remained for the scientist, until automation, a thankless and repetitive pursuit. Automation of the process, both the chemistry and data analysis along with increasing understanding of the potentials of the sequence data obtained for reverse genetics has led to the flurry of sequencing activity in the past five years in which the nucleic acid sequence itself now serves as the raw material to stimulate future research.

Of all of the genome projects there can be few scientists in any field who are unaware of the efforts collectively called the Human Genome Project (HGP). This undertaking is a truly international project of a planned 15 year duration. The HGP project was initiated in 1990 with the aim of discovering and sequencing all of the projected 50 000 to 100 000 human genes. The ultimate objective of the HGP is to sequence, database and make available the entire three billion bases that make up the human genome. As submitted to the worldwide web in 1996 by the HGP, details of 6289 individual genes have been identified. The physical mapping of the human genome is currently two years ahead of schedule and over four million bases have been sequenced generating a largest contiguous sequence of some 885 000 bases.

The following sections will describe the methodology of DNA sequencing, automation of the sequencing process and modifications to the process as the result of the discovery of new polymerases.

DNA Sequencing: Back to Basics

Genes, the individual units of biological inheritance, carry the detailed instructions for the activities of all cells in the organism, with individual genes encoding a specific biologically active product. These complex genetic instructions, or arrays of multiple genes, are coded in long strands of DNA, the chromosomes. Information in the DNA sequences encode such determinants as eye colour, height, and susceptibility to certain genetic diseases. The sequence of the DNA strands determine how the instructions are read and interpreted into the production of polypeptides. If mutations occur through changes to DNA structure, affecting the base sequence of the gene, it is possible that the protein produced will be inactive or will function in an aberrant way. The study of specific mutations in an individual's genetic makeup forms the basis of such applied areas as genetic counselling and prenatal genetic testing.

Chemical Sequencing of DNA, the Maxam-Gilbert Approach

One of the earliest methods of determining the nucleotide sequence of a section of isolated DNA was the chemical sequencing of the DNA strand, more usually referred to as the Maxam–Gilbert technique and published in 1977. In this method isolated single-stranded DNA is labelled, generally with a radioisotope marker, at its terminus and is then partially degraded by subjecting the labelled template to a series of base-specific cleavage reactions. Conditions are designed so that only a limited number of each of the cleavage reactions occurs within a given DNA strand. Four different chemical modifications occur in separate reaction tubes, with G residues being methylated using dimethylsulfate in one tube, G and A residues being methylated by formic acid, C and T being removed by hydrazine and C alone being removed by hydrazine in the presence of sodium chloride. Following each of the specific chemical reactions the template in the tube is treated with piperidine, which then cleaves the DNA where there is a chemically modified or missing base.

Since the starting DNA template is end-labelled and the components of the reaction and its kinetics can be closely controlled so that the lengths of the labelled fragments can identify the position of the individual bases, the combination of reactions yields a 'ladder' of fragments that vary in size from one another by a single base. This array of cleaved products generated can then be subjected to polyacrylamide gel electrophoresis to resolve fragments of different lengths and the ladder of radio-labelled products can be then visualized and analysed by autoradiography, the process of exposing the radiolabelled fragments in the gel to X-ray film to produce an image of the fragments. In the early days it was possible to read only some 100 bases from the point of labelling, making the sequencing of long fragments of DNA time-consuming and tedious. Since the publication of this method many modifications have been made both to optimize the sequencing chemistry and to improve the spatial separation of the labelled fragments, in some cases the use of one metre long gel separation systems has enabled the number of bases that can be resolved from a single reaction to approach 600 or more. Other modifications have included rapid labelling protocols for the DNA fragment and the substitution of chemicals required for the chemical degradation to render the reaction process less hazardous to the scientist. Although the Maxam–Gilbert method of sequencing DNA is still utilized in some laboratories, it has many disadvantages and its popularity, judged by publication of new sequence information, is decreasing.

Sequencing by Chain Termination, the Sanger Methodology

The Sanger or chain termination method of sequencing DNA is now the main workhorse of the major genome initiatives. The principle of this method is simple: an isolated fragment of DNA or entire plasmid, cosmid or PCR product is denatured to its single-stranded form by heat or alkali treatment. A short synthetic oligonucleotide primer is annealed to its complementary sequence encoded on one of the single-stranded templates. The 3′ end of the primer/template duplex is then used as the initiation site for polymerase action and a complementary DNA strand is synthesized using dNTPs as precursors (Fig. 54.1 and 54.2).

Chain termination chemistry has been used in conjunction with either labelled oligonucleotide primers (Fig. 54.1) or by incorporation of labelled nucleotides during the extension reaction (Fig. 54.2). Early chemistry employed polymerases such the Klenow fragment of DNA polymerase I or used the bacteriophage-derived T7 DNA polymerase or its variants. In more recent times thermostable polymerases such as AmpliTaq DNA polymerase and its variants have been exploited to carry out the chain termination chemistry by the marriage of chain termination and the PCR process. Such an approach is termed cycle sequencing (Fig. 54.3).

In a standard chain termination sequencing approach, four separate synthesis reactions are required. Each of the individual reactions contains a small amount of one of the four dideoxynucleotide triphosphates (ddNTPs). When the growing strand of DNA being synthesized incorporates a specific ddNTP the reaction elongation reaction is terminated since the ddNTP lacks the 3′-hydroxyl group required for further chain elongation. By careful control of the ratio of ddNTP to dNTP in each of the four reactions one achieves a random but low level incorporation of each of the ddNTPs into the growing strands of DNA and creates an array of fragments with a common 5′ end, defined by the primer, but terminating at each possible position where the specific ddNTP could have been incorporated. The average length of such chains can be manipulated by altering the ddNTP to dNTP ratios to ensure that all of the products can be easily resolved by polyacrylamide gel electrophoresis.

By carrying out four reactions, with each of the four ddNTPs present, and then resolving

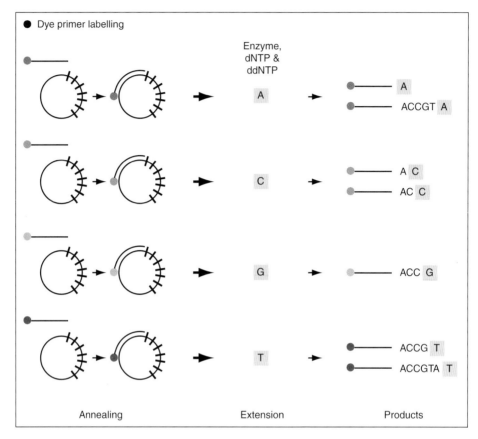

Figure 54.1: *Sanger or chain termination sequencing chemistry employing fluorescent dye labelled primers. Four different dye labelled primers (A, C, G and T termination) are used in four separate extension and termination reactions. At completion of the reactions the contents of the four tubes are pooled and loaded onto a single lane of a polyacrylamide gel. The ladder of dye labelled products are separated by electrophoresis and detected in real time.*

the four reactions, A, C, G and T terminated, side by side on a resolving gel we again produce the characteristic ladder of fragments that enables the sequence to be read. Common labelling strategies include incorporation of radiolabelled dNTPs followed by autoradiography or chemiluminescent detection of the terminated products.

The Need and Quest for Automation

As the requirement for ever more DNA sequence data increased, the highly complex manual strategies became severely limiting for generation of data from large numbers of templates, and the search began for methods that would automate and speed the process of both the sequencing chemistry and the acquisition of data from the gels on which the data was to be resolved.

At the outset of the sequencing of nucleic acids radioisotopic markers were the only method of detection of the fragments and such labelled fragments were separated by acrylamide gels and the isotopic bands visualized following autoradiography. Four reactions, A, C, G and T were required for each template and the reactions were then loaded into adjacent lanes on the gel. Following separation and autoradiography the sequence was determined by 'reading' the band pattern from the bottom

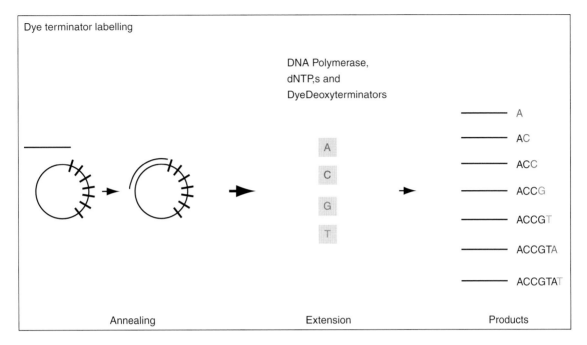

Figure 54.2: *Sanger or chain termination sequencing chemistry employing dye labelled dideoxy terminators. Dideoxy terminators, with each of the four possible ddNTPs being labelled with a different fluorescent dye, are incorporated by a polymerase during the extension phase of the sequencing reaction. The ladder of dye labelled products are separated by electrophoresis and detected in real time.*

to the top of the autoradiograph, representing fragments of ever increasing length until the resolving power of the gel became limiting. The requirement to use four lanes for each template reaction was a major limitation on the number of samples that could be processed simultaneously on one gel and further required high levels of template. The manual reading of the autoradiographs was a lengthy and tedious job. Manual reading is also highly prone to human error in both interpretation of the data on the X-ray film and errors in transcription from the sequence on the autoradiograph to the sequence on a piece of paper or typed directly onto a computer. In many cases the resulting X-ray films were read by two people for verification and DNA sequence was required and compared from reactions carried out on both of the DNA strands, giving both the forward and reverse sequence for comparison.

The increase in the speed with which DNA sequence data can be obtained has come from stepwise improvements to the basic sequencing chemistries, including the use of thermostable polymerases, template preparation methods, increased resolution of acrylamide gels and electrophoresis apparatus. The major gains in speed have come from the automation of the process of running, reading and processing the ladders of DNA fragments that are the sequence information and from the software that enables sequences to be quickly aligned, compared and edited electronically.

As sequencing chemistry, particularly the Sanger chain termination methodology, has become more robust the DNA template requirements for the reactions have fallen. A wealth of mini-column purification cartridges is now available that can prepare small amounts of clean DNA templates for sequencing in a matter of minutes rather than the days that were required to perform plasmid preparation by banding on caesium gradients in ultracentrifuges. Longer and thinner acrylamide gels and variants on the cross-linking reagents used to prepare the matrix have allowed better resolution of longer fragments. Wedge or gradient gels can give a more even spacing of the

The Need and Quest for Automation

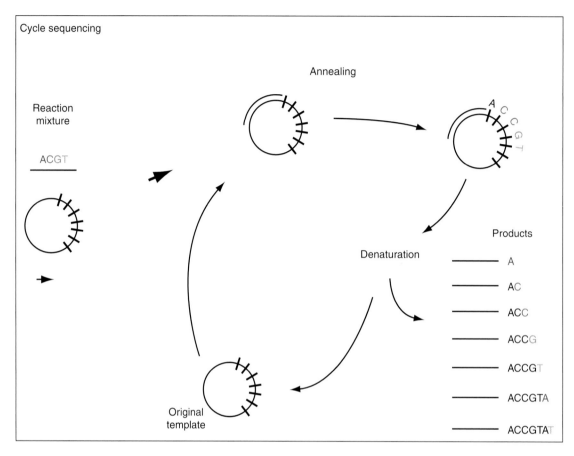

Cycle sequencing

Annealing

Reaction mixture

ACGT

Products

A

AC

ACC

ACCG

ACCGT

ACCGTA

ACCGTAT

Denaturation

Original template

Figure 54.3: Chain termination cycle sequencing. In a combination of the Sanger chain termination method and the PCR process the original DNA serves as a template for a linear PCR reaction. In each of 25 rounds of PCR cycling a ladder of dye labelled terminated fragments are produced from the templates. Following the extension step the subsequent denaturation then allows the same DNA molecules to serve again as a template for production of more dye-labelled products.

resolved fragments over an increased size range and aid interpretation.

The quantum leap in terms of automation of the sequencing process arose from the use of fluorescent reporter dyes as the molecule for the detection of the sequencing ladder. In conjunction with laser excitation of the dyes as they migrate through the gel and direct optical detection of the fluorescent fragments in real time (Fig. 54.4 and 54.5), full automation of data acquisition was possible.

Essentially two methods of using this approach, coupled with gel based electrophoretic separation, have to date been commercialized, the single dye four-lane loading systems (Pharmacia ALF and LI-COR) and the four-dye

single lane loading systems (PE Applied Biosystems, Fig. 54.6). The latter single lane approach has been the method of choice for both large-scale and large sample number application groups. The four-dye single lane instrumentation allows for higher sample throughput and consistent results among the large numbers of samples processed on a single run. Further advantages are seen since electophoretic mobility artefacts do not cause mis-calling between adjacent lanes. This can occur with the single dye four-lane approach since this requires comparatively uniform migration across four individual lanes, A, C, G and T, to produce the sequence data.

In the most recent chemistry utilized on PE Applied Biosystems PRISM Automated

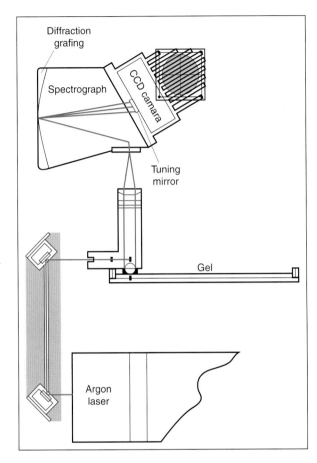

Figure 54.4: *Real time scanning fluorescent detection system as used on the ABI PRISM 377. As the fluorescently labelled DNA fragments migrate down through the gel they pass a region where a laser beam is scanned across the glass plates that sandwich the gel. The laser energy excites the fluorescent dyes and emissions from the fragments are captured by the detection system and fed to a computer for analysis. The laser light is scanned at a constant speed across the full width of the gel enabling multiple lanes of data to be collected on each pass.*

Sequencing Systems, four different fluorescent dyes, each with a characteristic emission frequency, are utilized as the reporting label for the dideoxy terminator sequencing reaction, each specific dye being associated with a specific dideoxy chain termination at one of the bases A, C, G or T. This approach allows the simultaneous inclusion of all four dyes in a single chain termination reaction and allows for the loading of the entire completed reaction into a single lane on the gel (Fig. 54.4). The latest ABI PRISM 377XL system has the capability to run, detect, analyse and base call 64 different sequenced templates simultaneously with individual read lengths of in excess of 700 base pairs being reported. Such capacity can enable the production of nearly 50 000 bases of sequence data in a single electophoretic run. Such machines and their predecessors are now the mainstay of the genome laboratories worldwide.

As mentioned previously, a marriage of the technologies of the Sanger chain termination methodology and PCR cycle sequencing involves a linear PCR amplification of the target DNA. The method lends itself ideally to templates of low yields (such as PCR products) or those of very large size such as the direct sequence determination of cosmids or inserts cloned in lambda vectors. The cycling reaction repeats rounds of primer annealing, extension and chain termination (Fig. 54.3), allowing a 25-fold increase in the level of product generated from the target material. When coupled with the single tube fluorescent chain termination methodology (Fig. 54.4) this approach enables 96-well format production of 96 cycle sequencing reactions carried out simultaneously in under three hours, and further allows rapid automation of both the pipetting and cycling reactions, so that a robot platform such as the ABI PRISM 877 can produce hundreds of sequencing reactions unattended in a working day.

In another modification of the basic Sanger methodology, direct chain termination sequencing of PCR products completely removes the need for the preparation of plasmid templates. One simply amplifies the inserted sequence of interest, using the conserved sequences present in most cloning vectors, purifies the PCR product by any one of a number of column or membrane separation products and then uses an aliquot of the template for a subsequent cycle sequencing reaction. It is becoming increasingly common to directly sequence specific short PCR products. Such a process has many advantages for rapid gap closure required by the genome groups, verification of recombinant plasmids and obtaining short

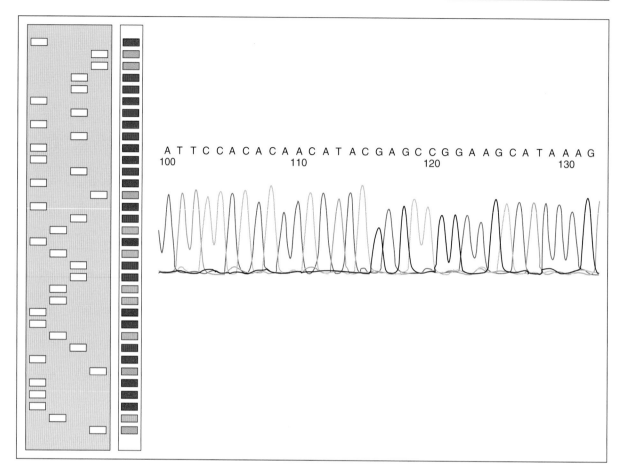

Figure 54.5: Simultaneous multi-colour detection as used on the ABI PRISM 377. The fluorescent emissions from the dye-labelled DNA fragments are split into their individual spectral components by the spectrograph and focused onto the surface of a CCD camera. The camera is calibrated such that each of the four different fluorescent dyes is recognized individually and assigned to an specific base. This enables the software to call the nucleotide sequence after the entire collection of data has been completed.

segments of sequence from unknown cDNAs prior to screening against databases of known sequences. Direct sequencing of products removes the need to carry out the tedious subcloning of the PCR product into a vector and removes the need to purify plasmids, thereby removing any manipulations.

The Future of Nucleic Acid Sequencing

It would appear that the majority of genome laboratories, both in the public sector and within the pharmaceutical industry, now accept that at present any further increases in the speed of sequence acquisitions will come from small, multiple stepwise improvements to currently available automated sequencing platforms and chemistries rather than from a revolutionary new technology. Limitations of length dictate that we have focused on the current commercially available systems for automated sequencing.

Other developments are never far away but often their complexity means that they remain unique research tools and never reach the commercial marketplace. For readers interested in novel and emerging, potentially commercial,

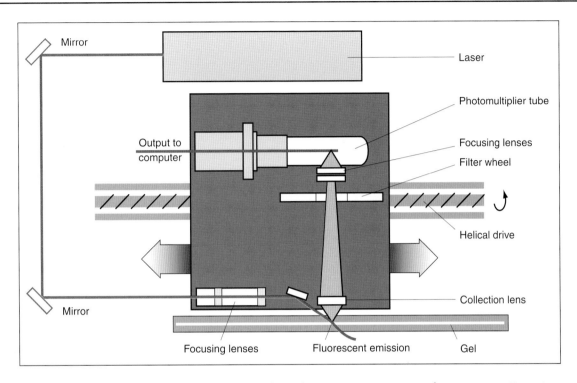

Figure 54.6: *Four dye single lane analysis as used on the ABI PRISM series of instruments. By using four spectrally distinct reporter dyes it is possible to load the entire sequencing reaction into a single lane of the acrylamide gel. Such an approach allows increased numbers of samples per gel and removes error associated with non-uniform fragment migration across the gel. The fluorescent bands are processed to produce the characteristic sequencing chromatogram and call the nucleotide sequence.*

approaches to DNA sequence generation it is suggested that areas of sequencing by hybridization to oligonucleotides, atomic probe microscopy, mass spectrometry and multiple chip arrays are those to be watched with interest.

In terms of speeding the current electophoretic acquisition of DNA sequence data, PE Applied Biosystems have now released an automated single capillary-based platform, the ABI PRISM 310. Capillary-based systems can offer a substantial increase in separation speed with runs completing in minutes rather than hours. Potentially such platforms could lend themselves to multiple arrays although simultaneous sequence detection across multiple capillaries presents a considerable technical challenge. At a recent European meeting a new 96-capillary array system under development

was presented by Molecular Dynamics. Whether such multiple capillary technology proves to be robust, reproducible and cost-effective in the long term remains to be seen, but at present much effort continues in the search to improve speed, throughput and accuracy and to drive down reagent costs with current technology so that the genome projects come to completion within the time and budget constraints.

Acknowledgements

I am grateful to Iain Comely and Angela Bardon from the UK Perkin Elmer Applied Biosystems Training group for allowing the reproduction of their figures in this chapter.

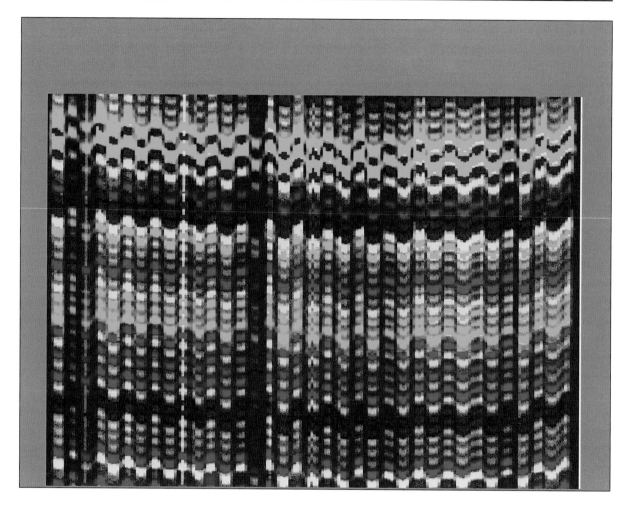

Figure 54.7: *Gel image of a sequencing gel. This electronic image represents the fluorescent sequencing ladders from multiple templates that were loaded and separated simultaneously on a four dye single lane instrument.*

Further Reading

Adams M D, Fields C, Venter J C (eds). *Automated DNA Sequencing and Analysis*. 1994: Academic Press, London.

Ansorge W, Sproat B, Stegemann J, Schwager C, Zenke M. Automated DNA sequencing: ultrasensitive detection of fluorescent bands during electrophoresis. *Nucl Acids Res* 1987; **15**: 4593–4602.

Howe C J, Ward E S (eds). *Nucleic Acids Sequencing*. 1992: IRL Press, Oxford.

Hunkapillar T, Kaiser R J, Koop B F, Hood L. Large-scale and automated DNA sequencing determination. *Science* 1991; **254**: 59–67.

Innis M A, Myambo K B, Gelfand D H, Brow M A. DNA sequencing with Thermus aquaticus DNA polymerase and direct sequencing of polymerase chain reaction-amplified DNA. *Proc Natl Acad Sci (USA)* 1988; **85**: 9436–9440.

Maxam A M, Gilbert W. A new method for sequencing DNA. *Proc Natl Acad Sci (USA)* 1977; **74**: 560–564.

Prober J M, Trainor G I, Dam R J, Hobbs F W, Robertson C W, Zagursky R J, Cocuzza A J, Jensen M A, Baumeister K. A system for rapid DNA sequencing with fluorescent chain-terminating dideoxynucleotides. *Science* 1987; **238**: 336–341.

Sanger F, Nicklen S, Coulson A R. DNA sequencing with chain-terminator for inhibitors. *Proc Natl Acad Sci (USA)* 1977; **74**: 5463–5467.

Smith L M, Sanders J Z, Kaiser R J, Hughes P, Dodd C, Connell C R, Heiner C, Kent S B, Hood L E. Fluorescence detection in auto-mated DNA sequence analysis. *Nature (London)* 1986; **321**: 674–679.

Tabor S, Richardson C C. DNA sequence analysis with a modified bacteriophage T7 DNA polymerase. *Proc Natl Acad Sci (USA)* 1987; **84**: 4767–4771.

INDEX

prothrombin fragment assays, 365
prothrombin time, 358–60
  correction studies, 359
  oral anticoagulant control, 359–60
protozoan parasites, 255, 256–7
Prussian blue, 270, 276, 340
psammoma bodies, 118
Pseudomonas, 149, 154, 155
pure red cell aplasia, 271
puruvate kinase deficiency, 351
pus microscopy, 136–7

Q
quinacrine banding (Q-banding), 370–1

R
radial immunodiffusion (Mancini technique), 462, 466
radioimmunoassay (RIA), 216, 220
  ferritin levels, 341
  platelet release investigations, 317
radioimmunometric methods, 175
radioisotope platelet release investigation, 317
radiotherapy-associated cytological changes, 112, 113
Raji cell assay, 486–7
reagent strips *see* dry reagent chemistry
red blood cell inclusion bodies, 300
red cell abnormalities, 266–7
red cell count, 287
red cell distribution width (RDW), 287–8
red cell flow cytometry, 327
red cell indices, 287–8
red cell morphology, 265, 274
red cell zinc protoporphyrin, 341, 343
Reed–Sternberg cell, 116, 283
reference intervals, 391–3
regressive staining, 19
renal pathology, 51
replication banding, 373–5
representational difference analysis (RDA), 238, 239, 527–8
reptilase time, 362–3
resorcin fuchsin, 20
respiratory syncytial virus (RSV), 189, 192, 220
respiratory tract bacteria, 166
restriction endonucleases, 311, 565
restriction fragment length polymorphism (RFLP), 232, 234
  haemoglobinopathies, 302
  HLA typing, 507–8
reticulin staining, 20
reticulocyte counting, 293, 330–1
retinoblastoma protein (pRb), 94
reverse banding (R-banding), 371–2
reverse phase high performance liquid chromatography (HPLC), 451, 452, 453
reverse transcriptase *in situ* PCR (RT *in situ* PCR), 552, 558
reverse transcriptase PCR *in situ* hybridization (RT PCR-ISH), 552, 558
reverse transcription polymerase chain reaction (RT-PCR), 165, 527
rhesus system, 320
  incompatibility, 353
rhinovirus, 193
rhodamine, 37

riboprobes, 514
ribotyping, 166
Rickettsia, 156
rifampicin, 168, 179
rimantadine resistance, 247
ristocetin platelet aggregation test, 308–9, 317
rocket immunoelectrophoresis, 466–7, 474
Romanowsky stains, 18, 24, 109, 256, 265
rotary microtome, 12
rotavirus, 200, 201–2, 207
rubella, 216, 217, 219, 221, 223

S
Salmonella, 149, 154
satellite sequences, 567
scanning electron microscopy (SEM), 46, 56–8, 126, 198–9
scanning electron microscopy (SEM) — image analysis-microanalysis systems, 63
scanning transmission electron microscopy (STEM), 55–6
Schilling (cobalamin absorption) test, 340
scrapie, 241
scrapings, 104, 107
screening tests, 394, 395
selection in fluid media, 141–2
sensitivity (true positive rate), 120, 394, 395
separation techniques, 449–57
sequestration crisis, 347
serological tests, 215–22
  agglutination, 172–3
  blood products screening, 221–2
  complement fixation tests, 173
  donor tissue/organ screening, 221–2
  enzyme-linked immunosorbent assay (ELISA), 174
  fluorescent antibody tests, 174
  fungal pathogens, 253–4
  HLA typing, 506–7
  immunity verification, 221
  microbiology, 171–5, 220–1
  parasitology, 259–60
  precipitation tests, 173
  principles, 215–16
  radioimmunometric methods, 175
  techniques, 216–20
serotonin assay, 452
serum protein electrophoresis, 455, 456, 462–3
serum sickness, 486, 487–8
severe combined immunodeficiency (SCID), 481
sexually transmitted diseases, 124, 125, 137
shell vial immunofluorescence (DEAFF test), 192, 193, 212
Shiff's reagent, 18
Shigella, 149, 154
sickle cell disease, 275, 296, 346, 347, 349, 566
sickle solubility test, 297
sickle/thal disease, 349
sideroblastic anaemia, 276, 282
silver impregnation, 20, 23, 24
simultaneous coupling, 28
single-beam photometer (colorimeter), 420
single-strand conformation polymorphism (SSCP), 527
skeletal muscle enzyme histochemistry, 29–30, 31
skin disorders, 51, 64, 136, 200, 205
sledge microtome, 12
slide writers, 4–5
small round structured viruses (SRSV), 201, 202–3